HANDBOOK OF DIABETES MEDICAL NUTRITION THERAPY

Edited by
Margaret A. Powers, MS, RD, CDE
Consultant
Health Promotion and
Nutrition Communications
Powers and Associates
St. Paul, Minnesota

AN ASPEN PUBLICATION®
Aspen Publishers, Inc.
Gaithersburg, Maryland
1996

Library of Congress Cataloging-in-Publication Data

Handbook of diabetes medical nutrition therapy/
edited by Margaret A. Powers.—2nd ed.
p. cm.
Includes bibliographical references and index.
ISBN 0-8342-0631-5
1. Diabetes—Diet therapy. 2. Diabetes—Nutritional aspects.
I. Powers, Margaret A., RD.
[DNLM: 1. Diabetic Diet. WK 818 H236 1996]
RC662.H36   1996   616.4'620654—dc20
DNLM/DLC
for Library of Congress
95-36825
CIP

Aspen Publishers, Inc., grants permission for photocopying for limited personal or internal use.
This consent does not extend to other kinds of copying, such as copying for general
distribution, for advertising or promotional purposes, for creating new collective works,
or for resale. For information, address Aspen Publishers, Inc.,
Permissions Department, 200 Orchard Ridge Drive, Gaithersburg, Maryland 20878.

Aspen Publishers, Inc., is not affiliated with
the American Society of Parenteral and Enteral Nutrition.

The authors have made every effort to ensure the accuracy of the information herein, particularly with regard to drug selection and dose. However, appropriate information sources should be consulted, especially for new or unfamiliar procedures. It is the responsibility of every practitioner to evaluate the appropriateness of a particular opinion in the context of actual clinical situations and with due consideration to new developments. Authors,editors,and the publisher cannot be held responsible for any typographical or other errors found in this book.

Editorial Resources: Ruth Bloom

Library of Congress Catalog Card Number: 95-36825
ISBN: 0-8342-0631-5

Printed in the United States of America

1 2 3 4 5

To Michael, Jessica,
Colin, and Martin

Table of Contents

Contributors

Betty Brackenridge, MS, RD, CDE
President
Learning Prescriptions
Phoenix, Arizona

Sydne K. Carlson, MS, RD, CDE
Dietitian Nutrition Specialist
Diabetes Education
University of Iowa Hospitals and Clinics
Iowa City, Iowa

Anne Daly, MS, RD, CDE
Director
Nutrition and Diabetes Education
Springfield Diabetes and Endocrine Center
Springfield, Illinois

Linda M. Delahanty, MS, RD
Clinical and Research Dietitian
Department of Dietetics
Massachusetts General Hospital
Boston, Massachusetts

Samuel S. Engel, MD
Clinical Assistant Professor of Medicine
Diabetes Center
Albert Einstein College of Medicine
  of Yeshiva University
Bronx, New York

Cade Fields-Gardner, MS, RD
Director of Services
The Cutting Edge
Cary, Illinois

Marion J. Franz, MS, RD
Director
Nutrition and Publications
International Diabetes Center
Minneapolis, Minnesota

Judith M. Gaare-Porcari, MS, MBA, RD
Assistant Director
Clinical Nutrition
North Shore University Hospital
Manhasset, New York

Patti Bazel Geil, MS, RD/LD, CDE
Diabetes Nutrition Educator
Department of Dietetics and Nutrition
University of Kentucky Medical Center
Lexington, Kentucky

Sandy Gillespie, MMSc, RD, LD, CDE
Nutrition Specialist
Atlanta Diabetes Associates
Atlanta, Georgia

Beverly Holt Halford, MPH, RD, CDE
Control Diabetes Services
Braintree, Massachusetts

Harold J. Holler, RD, CDE
Governance Team
Association Management Group
The American Dietetic Association
Chicago, Illinois

Lea Ann Holzmeister, RD, CDE
Clinical Nutritionist
Phoenix Children's Hospital
Phoenix, Arizona

Monica Joyce, RD, CDE
Program Director
Diabetes Program
Gerald W. Sobel, MD and Robert J. Sobel,
    MD, Private Practice
Chicago, Illinois

Pamela Goyan Kittler, MS
Food and Nutrition Consultant
Sunnyvale, California

Karmeen D. Kulkarni, MS, RD, CDE
Director
Nutrition Services
Diabetes Health Center
Salt Lake City, Utah

Carolyn Leontos, MS, RD, CDE
Nutrition Specialist
University of Nevada Cooperative Extension
Las Vegas, Nevada

**Melinda Downie Maryniuk, MEd, RD,
    FADA, CDE**
Program Manager
Affiliated Centers Program
Joslin Diabetes Center
Boston, Massachusetts

Sue McLaughlin, RD, LD, CDE
Nutrition Consultant/Diabetes Specialist
St. Joseph Villa Homecare
Omaha VA Medical Center
Omaha, Nebraska

Kristen McNutt, PhD, JD
President
Consumer Choices, Inc.
Winfield, Illinois

Boyd E. Metzger, MD
Professor of Medicine
Center for Endocrinology, Metabolism,
    and Molecular Medicine
Northwestern University Medical School
Chicago, Illinois

Mark E. Molitch, MD
Professor of Medicine
Center for Endocrinology, Metabolism, and
    Molecular Medicine
Northwestern University Medical School
Chicago, Illinois

Julie O'Sullivan-Maillet, PhD, RD
Associate Dean
Academic Affairs and Research
Chairman
Department of Primary Care
University of Medicine and Dentistry of New
    Jersey
Newark, New Jersey

Carol Rees Parrish, RD, CDE, CNSD
Nutrition Support Specialist
Division of Gastroenterology/Department of
    Nutrition Services
University of Virginia Health Sciences Center
Charlottesville, Virginia

Joyce Green Pastors, MS, RD, CDE
Assistant Professor of Education in Internal
    Medicine
University of Virginia Diabetes Outreach
    Program
Charlottesville, Virginia

William H. Polonsky, PhD, CDE
Assistant Clinical Professor
Department of Psychiatry
University of California, San Diego
Head
Health Psychology Division
Balboa Medical Center
San Diego, California

Michael J. Powers, MA
Education Consultant
Powers and Associates
St. Paul, Minnesota

Margaret A. Powers, MS, RD, CDE
Health Promotion and Nutrition
    Communications Consultant
Powers and Associates
St. Paul, Minnesota

Maryanne Grinvalsky Richardson, RD, CDE
Diabetes Nutrition Specialist
Education Program for Young People with Diabetes
Mount Sinai School of Medicine
New York, New York

David A. Sirois, DMD, PhD
Assistant Professor and Director
Division of Oral Medicine
Department of Oral Pathology, Biology, and Diagnostic Sciences
University of Medicine and Dentistry of New Jersey
New Jersey Dental School
Newark, New Jersey

Linda G. Snetselaar, PhD, RD
Director of Nutrition Research Projects
Adjunct Assistant Professor
Department of Internal and Preventive Medicine
University of Iowa
Iowa City, Iowa

Max E. Stachura, MD
Professor
Department of Medicine
Medical College of Georgia
Chief
Endocrine Service
VA Medical Center
Augusta, Georgia

Kathryn P. Sucher, ScD, RD
Professor
Department of Nutrition and Food Science
San Jose State University
San Jose, California

Susan L. Thom, RD, LD, CDE
Partner and Clinical Specialist
Diabetes Associates
Cleveland, Ohio

Lesley Fels Tinker, PhD, RD
Nutrition Scientist
Women's Health Initiative
Fred Hutchinson Cancer Research Center
Seattle, Washington

Riva Touger-Decker, PhD, RD
Assistant Professor and Director
Master of Science in Clinical Nutrition Program
Department of Primary Care
School of Health Related Professions
University of Medicine and Dentistry of New Jersey
Clinical Assistant Professor
Department of Oral Pathology, Biology, and Diagnostic Sciences
New Jersey Dental School
Newark, New Jersey

Linda V. Van Horn, PhD, RD
Professor of Preventive Medicine
Northwestern University School of Medicine
Chicago, Illinois

Elizabeth A. Walker, DNSc, RN, CDE
Assistant Professor
Department of Epidemiology and Social Medicine
Diabetes Research and Training Center
Albert Einstein College of Medicine of Yeshiva University
Bronx, New York

Hope S. Warshaw, MMSc, RD, CDE
Nutrition Consultant
Freelance Writer
Hope Warshaw Associates
Alexandria, Virginia

Sylvia Wassertheil-Smoller, PhD
Professor
Department of Epidemiology and Social Medicine
Head
Department of Epidemiology and Biostatistics
Albert Einstein College of Medicine of Yeshiva University
Bronx, New York

Madelyn L. Wheeler, MS, RD, CDE
Coordinator
Dietetics Research
Diabetes Research Training Center
Indiana University School of Medicine
Indianapolis, Indiana

Judith Wylie-Rosett, EdD, RD
Professor of Epidemiology
Albert Einstein College of Medicine of Yeshiva
    University
Bronx, New York

Forewords

THE CHALLENGE OF MOVING FORWARD

The next decade promises to be an exciting and challenging time for dietitians in general and, specifically, for dietitians specializing in nutrition related to diabetes management. It is exciting because we have more and more studies documenting the effectiveness of medical nutrition therapy for many acute and chronic diseases as well as for wellness and disease prevention. This is also true in the field of diabetes. The Diabetes Control and Complication Trial (DCCT) completed in 1993 reaffirmed that education, nutrition, and blood glucose monitoring are essential to achieve the treatment outcomes of intensive diabetes management. The DCCT began as a study intending to use only insulin adjustments to achieve optimal control, but as the study progressed it became clear that there was more to managing diabetes than just adjusting insulin. Following a meal plan, treating hypoglycemia appropriately, responding to hyperglycemia, and consistently eating snacks were all nutrition-related factors associated with improved glycated hemoglobin levels. Traditionally, dietitians have educated people with diabetes about nutrition and diabetes, but the DCCT required that they become more than educators—they also become involved in patient medical care. Blood glucose monitoring results were used to integrate insulin regimens with usual eating and exercise patterns of the person with diabetes. They were also used to adjust insulin regimens to achieve desired outcomes, to tailor nutrition instruction, determine appropriate hypoglycemic treatments, and to determine snack and insulin changes for exercise. *Dietitians became educators and clinicians integrally involved in decisions relating to overall diabetes management.* It became essential for dietitians to develop skills in diabetes management if nutrition and dietitians were to be truly integrated into the team management of diabetes. Because the person with diabetes is the key decision maker, helping individuals make life-style changes and correct decisions were major factors in the success of the study.

For individuals with non–insulin-dependent diabetes mellitus (NIDDM), the Diabetes Nutrition Guidelines study documented the important role of dietitians and nutrition in the management of NIDDM. In a controlled clinical trial, patients were randomized into basic or practice guideline nutrition care and compared to a similar group of patients with no nutrition intervention. The first two groups who received nutrition care from dietitians had significantly improved glucose control by three months. However, after the intervention ended, there was a gradual increase in glucose levels, suggesting the need for ongoing nutrition interventions. This was in contrast to the group with no intervention from a dietitian who had no improvement in glycemia during the same time period. Furthermore, when dietitians acted on the outcomes of the nutrition interventions by making recommendations to the physicians for changes in medical therapy, the extra time the dietitians spent became cost effective.

The documentation of the role that nutrition plays in diabetes management, however, brings with it challenges. Integrating nutrition into the overall management of diabetes requires skills above and beyond what is provided in traditional training programs. We must keep current not only with what is new and important in the field of nutrition, but also in overall diabetes management.

We are also challenged to measure our effectiveness by evaluating and documenting the outcomes that result from our clinical care. It is not enough to just give advice—follow-up is essential. We must know if the recommendations given have lead to the desired outcomes and treatment goals. If not, we need to take action. Other team members need to know that nutrition therapy has accomplished what can be done or what the patient is willing and able to do. This information with recommended changes for medical therapy to other team members is an important role for dietitians to take. Furthermore, we must also document outcomes. One or two studies are not enough. We need continued statistics documenting the effectiveness of medical nutrition therapy.

Becoming better clinicians and documenting effectiveness is essential, but in this time of change in how medical care is provided, this also is not enough. Every dietitian needs to become more politically and administratively active. Reimbursement either by third-party payors, by managed care, or by health maintenance organizations (HMOs) will be essential to survival. It was all too comfortable to have the cost of nutrition services included in the cost of the hospital stay. In the future, every hospital or clinical service will need to be covered, either by the patient or by reimbursement. If we are not active in seeking reimbursement we will be left with skills that patients will not have access to. What a loss for patients and for our profession.

This wonderful text can help update our nutrition knowledge and skills for the management of diabetes. Applying the knowledge and skills and measuring effectiveness will be our responsibility. But don't forget the bigger picture—we must also get involved in the "business" of our profession as well!

Marion J. Franz, MS, RD, CDE
Director, Nutrition and Publications
International Diabetes Center
Minneapolis, Minnesota

****

THE TIME HAS COME

As we move toward the end of the 20th century, it is a time to reflect upon the tremendous accomplishments and advances in diabetes care, management, and education. The 75th anniversary of the discovery of insulin will be recognized in 1996. The 100th anniversary of Dr. Elliot P. Joslin's world renowned diabetes practice will be celebrated in 1998 and the Diabetes Care and Education Practice Group of The American Dietetic Association will mark its 20th birthday also in 1998.

One of the areas that has advanced the most is the role and scope of practice of the dietitian involved in the care and management of the person with diabetes. During the nearly 20 years I have worked in diabetes care, some of the changes I have noticed include:

- The Exchange List approach to meal planning has gone from the only recognized teaching option to one of at least four main approaches to meal planning.
- *Diabetic diets* have become *meal plans* and *nutrition care* has become *medical nutrition therapy.*
- A meal plan is no longer defined simply as one where the individual may not eat sugar. There is no scientific evidence to justify the restriction of sucrose.
- The Diabetes Care and Education Practice Group's mailing list, a special interest group of the American Dietetic Association, has grown from 150 to over 4,000 individuals.
- Nurses, who had been the primary educators for all diabetes education including nutrition, now share that responsibility with other team members including dietitians, exercise physiologists, and mental health counselors.
- The dietitian's role has moved from just planning the meals and conducting the nu

trition education to playing an integral role on the team, teaching all aspects of diabetes care and education, working closely with other disciplines and using results of self-monitoring of blood glucose to fine tune blood glucose by balancing food, medication, and exercise.

Although only nine years have passed since the first edition of *Handbook of Diabetes Nutritional Management* was published, much has happened in the field of diabetes to warrant a revision. Key advances in diabetes management addressed in this book include the refinement of technology which has further enhanced self-monitoring of blood glucose and insulin pump therapy, the benefits of intensive insulin therapy as demonstrated by the Diabetes Control and Complications Trial, the science behind the behavior change process and individual goal setting, the release of the 1994 American Diabetes Association Nutritional Guidelines, and the publication of a whole new series of diabetes nutrition education materials.

The time has come to celebrate our successes. Maggie Powers is to be commended for her role in expanding the role of nutrition in diabetes care and advancing the knowledge of dietitians through the publication of this book. She has been a very strong advocate of expanding the dietitian's role to include more than just teaching food-related topics. The *Handbook of Diabetes Medical Nutrition Therapy* is an essential reference book for every diabetes dietitian educator's shelf.

Yet at the same time, we cannot sit back for much still remains to be done. The *Handbook of Diabetes Medical Nutrition Therapy* is the most comprehensive resource for dietitians to use in practicing state-of-the-art care. On the other hand, it does not provide all the answers because there are many research questions that remain to be solved. Dietitians need to continuously improve their communication and counseling skills to best reach their clients. We need to evaluate the outcomes of our practice by assessing whether or not the nutrition counseling made any measurable improvements in care. And, we need to work to have medical nutrition therapy and diabetes self-management training covered by third-party payers.

One thing that has not changed is the importance of teamwork and empowering the client with diabetes to take control. It is the person with diabetes who is in the driver's seat—and not the physician or diabetes educator. As Dr. Elliot P. Joslin wrote in 1935:

> I look upon the diabetic as a charioteer and his chariot as drawn by three steeds named Diet, Insulin, and Exercise. It takes will to drive one horse, intelligence to manage a team of two, but a man must be a very good teamster who can get all three to pull together.

Melinda Downie Maryniuk,
MEd, RD, FADA, CDE
Program Manager
Affiliated Centers Program
Joslin Diabetes Center
Boston, Massachusetts

Preface

Knowledgeable diabetes health care team members can have a tremendous impact on their client's health and well-being. This book, the second edition of the *Handbook of Diabetes Nutritional Management,* provides you, dietitians and other health care professionals, the information you need to provide comprehensive diabetes care and self-management training.

The contributors to this edition are experts. They have written outstanding chapters that will guide you in providing excellent care. This book reviews background information and research to support practice-based interventions. I encourage you to use this book as a reference guide to therapy as well as an authoritative text that provides detailed support and research background for interventions.

Medical nutrition therapy is more than handing out a diet. It encompasses the many elements that influence a person's food choices from hypoglycemic reactions to psychosocial and developmental issues to reimbursement practices. This book serves as a rich resource for anyone who needs to understand and provide nutrition therapy.

Margaret A. Powers
March 1996

Acknowledgments

There are many people who make a book like this possible. First are the authors who are dedicated to providing quality care to persons with diabetes. Their knowledge of the issues that influence our interventions will ultimately benefit our clients/patients.

Second is Aspen Publishers, Inc. for their strong interest in publishing nutrition textbooks that are practical and research based. Ruth Bloom was especially helpful in bringing the book to publication.

The third group of people to acknowledge for their support during this project is my family—Michael, Jessica, Colin, and Martin, who lent support in many ways.

Part I

Understanding Diabetes

Chapter 1

Pathophysiology

Max E. Stachura

Diabetes mellitus is a chronic disorder characterized by hyperglycemia and metabolic abnormalities involving carbohydrates, proteins, and lipids. Long-term complications arise from damage to blood vessels, nerves, kidneys, and eyes. As the most common endocrine disorder, it is estimated to affect 15 million people in the United States alone. However, the affected population is not homogeneous. There are several distinguishable diabetic syndromes, and ethnicity plays an important role.

Ongoing investigations of diabetes have significantly enhanced our understanding of its etiologies, the mechanisms through which tissue damage occurs, and the benefits that can be derived from tight metabolic control. Protocols for insulin and oral hypoglycemic agent delivery have become more sophisticated. Measurement of capillary blood glucose and hemoglobin glycosylation have enhanced evaluation of metabolic control by both the diabetic individual and the health professional team.

Successful management, however, remains the primary responsibility of the affected individual who must use this monitoring information to modulate therapeutic protocols in real-life settings beyond the direct influence of health professionals. In many ways, health care personnel are simply coaches. Our client-patients are successful when during daily living they themselves apply self-management principles that we have taught. Therefore, one critical measurement of our effectiveness is how well the diabetic individual functions without us.

HISTORICAL BACKGROUND

In approximately 500 BC, the Egyptian Ebers Papyrus described an illness associated with excessive urination and thirst. About 600 BC, a semimythological Indian physician, Susruta, described an illness characterized by extreme thirst and copious passage of a sweet urine. Because of its predilection for the rich, Susruta ascribed it to gluttonous overindulgence. In 1st century Greece, Aretaeus used the term diabetes from a root meaning "to run through a siphon." His was the first known complete clinical description of this condition in which flesh and limbs melted down into urine. The Latin word for honey, mellitus, was not added until 1674 when in England Thomas Willis made a distinction between this condition and other causes of excessive urination.

Two French physicians, Bouchardat and Lancereaux, anticipated more modern understanding of the disease by proposing in the mid-1800s that the diabetic population could be divided into two types: "diabetes gras" or fat and "diabetes maigre" or thin. Their concept was not widely accepted at the time, and most physicians continued to think in terms of a single disease that varied only in severity.

Langerhans described the pancreatic islets in 1869. Von Merring and Minkowski produced diabetes in dogs by pancreatectomy in 1889, and by 1900 pancreatic islet ß-cells had been noted to be damaged in people dying of diabetes. On this background, Banting and Best demonstrated in 1921 that measurable manifestations of diabetes could be reversed by injecting an extract of islet tissue called insulin. It seemed logical to conclude that diabetes was basically an insulin-deficiency syndrome.

"Juvenile-onset" type I diabetes was demonstrably an insulin-deficiency state. However, bioaassays for circulating insulin suggested in the 1950s that some diabetic individuals were not insulin-deficient. In fact, they possessed as much or more insulin-like material as did nondiabetic individuals. Yalow and Berson's[1] development of a specific insulin radioimmunoassay allowed them to confirm oversecretion of insulin in some diabetic individuals and to suggest either inappropriate insulin release or cellular resistance to insulin action as the cause.[2] Karam et al[3] ascribed the observed insulin resistance to obesity in 1963. In 1977, Bar and Roth[4] suggested that the insulin resistance of obese type II diabetic individuals resulted from reduced cellular insulin receptors and that obesity reduced receptor number similarly in diabetic and nondiabetic individuals. Two years later, Bar et al[5] demonstrated reduced receptors in nonobese type II diabetic patients, documenting intrinsic as well as obesity-related receptor reduction in type II diabetes. Also in 1979, Larner et al[6] suggested that a malfunctioning intracellular messenger, normally generated by insulin-receptor interaction, played a role in the pathogenesis of type II diabetes.

Other investigators demonstrated that normal insulin secretion in response to glucose was biphasic and that the first or acute phase of insulin response to intravenous glucose in type II individuals with fasting glucose in excess of 140 mg/dL is essentially absent[7,8] despite its presence in response to nonglucose stimuli.[9,10] By contrast, the second phase of insulin secretion in response to intravenous glucose is reduced to a degree that correlates with the severity of the diabetes.[7,11] Also, one component of the general concept of "glucose toxicity"[12] is the observation that hyperglycemia can itself impair insulin secretion.

The liver came to be understood as an additional active participant in the development of hyperglycemia. Hepatic glucose uptake is normal in type II diabetes,[13] but hepatic glucose output is abnormally increased with or without simultaneous obesity.[14,15] By contrast, hepatic glucose output is normal in impaired glucose tolerance.[16]

Thus, the term diabetes mellitus has come to be understood to describe a group of disorders with a common manifestation, hyperglycemia. Relative or absolute insulin deficiency, impaired insulin action or insulin resistance due to decreased cellular receptors and/or postreceptor defects, and excessive hepatic glucose output are contributing factors. They, in turn, interact differently in diabetic individuals depending on their genetic and environmental background, as well as on other concurrent pathology (see Table 1-1).

NORMAL PANCREAS

The pancreatic head is framed medially by the duodenal C loop into which the pancreatic duct empties through the sphincter of Oddi after joining the common bile duct. The pancreatic tail extends toward the spleen, passing below and behind the stomach. The organ's two major functions are to produce many of the enzymes needed for digestion (exocrine) and to produce hormones critical to the body's regulation of fuel use (endocrine).

Islets of Langerhans

Embedded in the enzyme-producing acinar tissue that forms the bulk of the pancreas are clusters of endocrine cells, the islets of Langerhans. They secrete hormones that are important components of the body's mechanisms for regulating the diverse, asynchronous, and varying fuel distribution needs of tissues.[17] These integrated cell clusters have all the functional requirements of a fuel distribution regulatory system including the ability to (1) sense the need for or availability of key fuels, (2) promote storage of overabundant fuel supplies or the recovery from storage of scarce fuel, and (3) vary the flux

Table 1-1 Classification of Diabetes and Other Categories of Glucose Intolerance

Classification	Former Terms	Characteristics
A. Diabetes		
I. Insulin-dependent diabetes mellitus (IDDM), Type I	Juvenile-onset diabetes Ketosis-prone diabetes Brittle diabetes	Low or absent endogenous insulin Onset generally in youth Dependent on exogenous insulin for life Ketosis prone

II. Non–insulin-dependent diabetes mellitus (NIDDM),
  Type II
  Obese
  Nonobese
	Adult-onset diabetes
	Maturity onset diabetes
	Ketosis resistant diabetes
	Stable diabetes
		Insulin levels normal, elevated, or depressed
		Not ketosis prone
		Onset generally after age 40
		Majority obese
		Insulin resistant
		May require OHA or insulin for control of symptoms

III. Diabetes associated with certain conditions or syndromes	Secondary diabetes	Hyperglycemia present at a level diagnostic of diabetes Cause of diabetes may be result of drugs, pancreatic disease, hormonal disease, or unknown
B. Gestational Diabetes (GDM)	Gestational diabetes	Elevated glucose with onset in pregnancy Associated with increased risk of congenital malformations Increased risk for later developing DM
C. Impaired Glucose Tolerance (IGT)	Borderline diabetes Chemical diabetes	Defined by plasma glucose criteria and OGTT Plasma glucose levels greater than normal, but less than diabetic
D. Previous Abnormality of Glucose Tolerance (Prev AGT)	Subclinical diabetes Prediabetes Latent diabetes	Previous hyperglycemia or IGT, but currently has normal glucose tolerance May develop DM
E. Potential Abnormality of Glucose Tolerance (Pot AGT)	Prediabetes Potential diabetes	Never had IGT or DM, but is at greater risk Strong family history of DM or obesity

Source: Adapted with permission from the American Diabetes Association Inc. National Diabetes Data Group, "Classification and Diagnosis of Diabetes and Other Categories of Glucose Intolerance," *Diabetes* (1979;28:1042–1043), Copyright © 1979.

of a specific fuel through circulation while maintaining its concentration within narrow limits.

The normal human pancreas contains about 1 million islets, most in the pancreatic tail. Each islet is populated by several cell types (Table 1-2). ß-Cells are dominant, representing 60 to 80% of islet cells,[18] but the cellular composition of islets is heterogeneous. In particular, glucagon and pancreatic polypeptide distribution is anatomically uneven, possibly explaining enhanced insulin secretion in response to glucose by the dorsal portions of the pancreas compared

Table 1-2 Pancreatic Islet: Cell Types and Hormones

Cell Type	Primary Hormonal Content [a]
α	Glucagon
ß	Insulin
δ	Somatostatin
PP	Pancreatic polypeptide
δ₁ [b]	Vasoactive intestinal polypeptide
EC [b]	Serotonin, Substance P
G [b]	Gastrin

[a] Many additional hormones have been identified in these cells (eg, adrenocorticotrophic hormone-related peptides, calcitonin gene-related peptide, cholecystokinin, endorphin, glicentin, glucagonlike polypeptide, met-encephalin, pancreastatin peptide YY, prolactin, and thyrotropin-releasing hormone), some only at particular stages of growth and development.

[b] Each of these cell types represents less than 1% of total islet cells.

with the ventral.[19] There is even heterogeneity of ß-cells within an individual islet in that cells exhibit different sensitivities for glucose-induced insulin secretion,[20] so that as glucose concentrations rise, more ß-cells participate in the insulin secretory response.[21]

There is also evidence for cell-to-cell interaction within the islet to modulate hormone secretion. Direct communication can occur through gap junctions between adjacent cells.[22] Distinct islet architecture, both of cells and vascular blood flow, allows upstream cells to influence downstream cells within the islet.[23] Diffusion of cell secretions also creates a paracrine tonic bath, modulating the environment in which the cells function.[24] Thus, metabolic activity results from a net hormonal balance rather than from the isolated action or fluctuation of any one hormone. Defined anatomic relationships must exist among islet cells for normal fuel metabolism to occur.[25] Pancreatic islets and their individual cells act both as units and as integrated components of a whole tissue.

Insulin

The ß-cell manufactures a long single-chain molecule (preproinsulin), trims and folds it (proinsulin), and then removes a specific connecting (C) peptide to produce the 51-amino-acid double-chain polypeptide known as insulin.[26] The 21-amino-acid A chain is connected to a 30-amino-acid B chain by two disulfide bridges.

Insulin secretion in the fasted state is minimal, basal circulating levels ranging from 8 to 15 µU/mL. The primary stimulus that increases insulin secretion rates is a rise in the glucose concentration of blood perfusing the pancreas[27]; a change as small as 0.5 mg/dL glucose is detected by the normal ß-cell. Most amino acids, especially anginine and leucine, are potent stimulators of insulin secretion in humans. Although dietary fat does influence insulin secretion per se, it also stimulates release of gastric inhibitory peptide, which in turn enhances insulin secretion in response to glucose. Insulin secretion is also under direct neural control, and a "cephalic" phase of insulin secretion in anticipation of food has been demonstrated.

After food ingestion, circulating insulin concentrations rise within minutes, peak at about 100 µU/mL in about 30 minutes, and then gradually return to baseline over the next 3 hours. Lean normoglycemic adults secrete a total of 20 to 30 units of insulin per day. Meal- or glucose-induced insulin secretion is actually biphasic.[8] Within 1 or 2 minutes after food ingestion, a rapid burst of insulin release occurs and is complete within 10 minutes (even if a contrived maintenance of high glucose is produced by infusion[27]). A second secretory phase begins 5 to 10 minutes after the initial increase and continues as long as the ß-cells are stimulated.

Initial-phase insulin secretion derives from pre-formed storage granules. Late or second-phase secretion derives from both storage and new insulin synthesis. Because of how the hormone is manufactured, insulin and C-peptide are released in equimolar amounts. A small amount of unprocessed proinsulin is also released. C-peptide has no known biologic activity in humans.[27] The effects of proinsulin (present in increased amounts in the plasma of non–insulin-dependent diabetes mellitus [NIDDM] patients[28]) are under active investigation but appear to be trivial.

Glucagon

Glucose is normally the sole source of energy for the human brain, which consumes approximately 6 g/h. To maintain the fuel needs of the central nervous system, a staunch defense against hypoglycemia has evolved. Glucagon is the most important hormone in this defense mechanism. Glucagon is a single-chain, 29-amino-acid polypeptide secreted into the hepatic portal circulation by islet α-cells. The liver removes about 25%. Glucagon stimulates hepatic cells to produce cyclic adenosine monophosphate, the principal intracellular signal for glucagon-mediated hepatic glucose production through glycogenolysis (breakdown of stored glycogen) and gluconeogenesis (formation of new glucose). Increasing the glucagon concentration without changing the insulin concentration will double glucose production within 15 minutes.[29]

Whereas insulin secretion is stimulated by a rise of plasma glucose, glucagon secretion is triggered by a falling plasma glucose concentration. Thus, glucagon secretion normally varies inversely with the plasma glucose concentration,[30] counterbalancing the effects of insulin and protecting against extreme fluctuations of the plasma glucose level in response to sudden changes in body fuel supply and demand.

Amino acids (especially adenine and arginine, but not branched-chain amino acids) or protein meals,[31] stress hormones such as epinephrine, cortisol, growth hormone, and ß-endorphin,[30,32] and exercise[33] enhance glucagon secretion.

Somatostatin

α-Cells that produce somatostatin comprise about 5% of the islet population. An inhibitory hormone that can act on α- and ß-cells, somatostatin is widely distributed in the body's neural and endocrine tissues. Depending on its location, it can function as a neurohormone, a neurotransmitter, a local regulatory agent, or a classic hormone. Because it inhibits the release of both insulin and glucagon, its discovery suggested possible major roles in fuel homeostasis.

Two species of the molecule were defined, somatostatin-28 and -14. Somatostatin-14 is secreted by islet α-cells, and somatostatin-28 originates in the gut in response to the absorption of fatty meals.[34] Somatostatin-28 is preferentially bound by ß-cells and is a more powerful inhibitor of ß-cell secretion.[35] Somatostatin's role in the integration of gut absorption of fuels, their distribution to body cells, and the interplay of insulin and glucagon in fuel homeostasis remains unclear. In the insulin-deficient state, in which glucagon's effects on hepatic glycogenolysis, gluconeogenesis, and ketogenesis are unopposed, endogenous hyperglycemia and ketoacidosis are lessened by suppressing glucagon secretion using somatostatin.[36] However, simultaneous suppression of preserved ß-cell function worsens metabolic control.[37] Two recent publications are worthwhile reviews of this problem of intraislet interactions and the integration of insulin, glucagon, and somatostatin action.[38,39]

Pancreatic Polypeptide

Originally regarded a contaminant during insulin purification, pancreatic polypeptide is secreted by the islet PP cell. The cell makes up 10% of islet cells and is predominantly found in the periphery of islets located in the pancreatic head. Pancreatic polypeptide is secreted in response to hypoglycemia,[40] and a reduction of this response is seen in some diabetic patients,[41] especially those with a reduced epinephrine response to hypoglycemia.[40,42] As with somatostatin, its role in intraislet communication and the integration of hormonal regulation of fuel homeostasis is unclear at this time.

METABOLIC HOMEOSTASIS IN THE NORMAL HUMAN

During fuel homeostasis, the normal human being maintains (1) plasma glucose concentrations within narrow limits independent of glucose flux through the plasma compartment, (2) an adequate supply of emergency carbohydrate in the form of liver and muscle glycogen, diverting excess consumption to adipose tissue, (3) an adequate supply of protein for body structure and enzyme functions, and (4) body stores of protein in preference to fat during fasting.

Fuel Deposits

Carbohydrate: a normal 70-kg human has access to about 300 g of mobilizable carbohydrate in the form of plasma glucose and hepatic glycogen. An additional 400 to 500 g carbohydrate is in muscle glycogen; this carbohydrate is almost entirely used by the exercising muscle, and it is not readily available to support circulating plasma glucose levels.

Protein: normal 70-kg humans contain about 6 kg protein, virtually all of it in the form of vital body structures such as muscles and enzymes. Loss of more than one-third of this protein is not well tolerated, producing marked muscle weakness, including impairment of basic tasks such as breathing and coughing.

Fat: the average 70-kg human carries about 15 kg adipose tissue, which contains only 10% water by weight. By contrast, 2 to 3 g of water per gram of glycogen and 3 to 4 g of water per gram of protein are obligated. Thus, adipose tissue stores are of the highest energy density. Oxidation of adipose tissue yields 6 to 8 calories/g, close to the theoretical 9 calories/g from pure triglyceride. Adipose tissue is the body's most efficient way to store mobilizable energy.

Hormone–Fuel Interrelationships

Pancreatic insulin and glucagon work with several nonpancreatic hormones (including steroids, growth hormones, and catecholamines) to coordinate fuel mobilization and storage with body need. Insulin and glucagon are the primary hormonal determinants of the adaptive changes that occur during metabolism of ingested nutrients. Their metabolic effects can best be presented in terms of the fed (characterized by higher circulating insulin concentrations) and fasted (characterized by higher circulating glucagon concentrations) states.

Fed State

Food ingestion immediately stimulates ß-cell insulin secretion while α-cells decrease glucagon secretion almost simultaneously.[36] Increasing insulin concentrations result in a generally anabolic state through paired stimulatory and inhibitory effects on carbohydrate, protein, and fat metabolism (Table 1-3).

The liver has a central role in the metabolic response to food ingestion. Increased insulin and decreased glucagon shift the liver to glycogen synthesis and curtail hepatic glucose release. In the normal fed state, about 60% of ingested glucose is taken up by the liver, the magnitude of this effect being determined by the portal vein insulin concentration.[43]

Muscle cell sensitivity to insulin is related to how recently it has been exercised and the quantity of glycogen already stored; sensitivity to insulin is markedly increased after exercise.[44] Muscle cell storage of amino acids as protein is also stimulated by insulin.

Table 1-3 Insulin's Actions

Promotes
• Entry of glucose into cells
• Storage of glycogen
• Storage of fat
• Storage of protein

Inhibits
• Synthesis of glucose
• Breakdown of glycogen
• Breakdown of fat
• Breakdown of protein

In adipose tissue, glucose is primarily converted to glycerol, the backbone of stored triglyceride. Only a small fraction is converted to adipose tissue glycogen. Insulin stimulates adipose tissue uptake of circulating triglyceride by enhancing lipoprotein lipase activity while simultaneously exerting an antilipolytic effect through inhibition of hormone-sensitive lipases.

Fasted State

In fasting, a catabolic state occurs in which the processes discussed above are reversed and glucose is diverted from most other tissues to maintain its supply to the central nervous system. The brain's constant glucose supply in fasting depends on a decline of circulating insulin concentrations to basal levels of 10 to 15 µU/mL and the ability of glucagon to maintain hepatic glucose production at a rate that will prevent hypoglycemia. This shift in hormone balance induces endogenous glucose production through glycogenolysis and gluconeogenesis.

For the first 8 to 12 hours of fasting, plasma glucose concentrations are maintained by the steady release of hepatic glucose at 2 to 3 mg/kg per minute, about 75% of which derives from glycogenolysis and the remainder from gluconeogenesis. Most of this glucose supplies the central nervous system. Even though skeletal muscle constitutes 40 to 45% of total body mass, it uses less than 20% of fasting hepatic glucose production because the fasting plasma insulin concentration is too low to enhance muscle glucose uptake. As fasting continues, hepatic glycogen stores are depleted, being essentially gone by 24 hours. Thus, the role of gluconeogenesis in maintaining hepatic glucose output becomes increasingly important. For the first 3 to 7 days of continued fasting, protein catabolism is the principal supplier of substrate for hepatic glucose production. Beyond 7 days, loss of amino acids from skeletal muscle protein is minimized by ketone production resulting from lipolysis. Ketones then take the place of glucose as the major fuel source for the central nervous system.

As plasma insulin declines in the fasting state, adipose tissue escapes from insulin's antilipolytic effect and hormone-sensitive lypase activity increases. Lipolysis releases glycerol, which is used by the liver as a substrate for gluconeogenesis, and free fatty acids, of which some are used by the liver but most are consumed by skeletal muscle.

Protein is catabolized during fasting with release of skeletal muscle amino acids at the rate of from 0.5 to 1.0 g/kg per day. Alanine and glutamine make up two-thirds or more of total α-amino-nitrogen loss. Alanine is used as a substrate for gluconeogenesis by the liver. Glutamine is distributed primarily to the kidney and gut.

In summary, plasma insulin and glucagon are biologic antagonists whose concentrations are primary regulators of normal fuel homeostasis in normal humans. Skeletal muscle and adipose tissue use of glucose is insulin-dependent. Insulin stimulates the storage of glucose as glycogen in the liver. It is the chief modulator of protein synthesis in muscle tissue and triglyceride synthesis in adipose tissue. It also inhibits endogenous glucose production. Glucagon is secreted in response to low glucose in a fashion similar to other counterregulatory hormones (epinephrine, cortisol, and growth hormone). It stimulates hepatic glucose production through glycogenolysis and gluconeogenesis and also inhibits glucose storage.

In the nondiabetic state, the balanced metabolic effects of insulin and glucagon, together with the other counterregulatory hormones, prevent fluctuations in the plasma glucose level despite changes in body fuel source and flux.

METABOLIC HOMEOSTASIS IN DIABETES

In general terms, metabolism in diabetes can be described as a runaway fasting state. Both fasting and diabetes are characterized by reduced insulin activity. In diabetes, this results from an absolute or relative (resistance) decrease in insulin concentration. Plasma glucagon concentrations are increased in both fasting and diabetes. As a result, both fasting and diabetes are associated with increased glycogenolysis, gluconeogenesis, and lipolysis.

Because an effective amount of insulin is not available, the balance between insulin and glucagon is lost. There is no longer coordination and equality between the amount of glucose leaving and entering the circulation, and hyperglycemia results. Adequate tissue supply is maintained but only in the presence of an elevated plasma glucose level. The degree to which the insulin effect is lost is a determinant of the clinical presentation of the disorder. Teleologically, it may not be surprising that tissue damage occurs with hyperglycemia, since the renal threshold for glucose establishes a plasma level above which glucose is discarded from the body. In the broadest of terms, to permit or delay the development of diabetes-related complications, glucose control at levels below that renal threshold is necessary. The process of fuel homeostasis is short-circuited in diabetes, and the body attempts to rid itself of a troublesome by-product of that dysregulation.

Target blood glucose levels should be individualized for each person with diabetes. Starting guidelines are provided in Table 1-4.

PATHOGENESIS OF INSULIN-DEPENDENT DIABETES MELLITUS (TYPE I DIABETES)

Genetic Factors

Genetic factors are important in the development of insulin-dependent diabetes mellitus (IDDM), and there is evidence in humans that more than one gene contributes. In 1974, geneticists discovered that certain histocompatibility locus (HLA) antigens were commonly found in children who developed IDDM. HLA antigens are glycoproteins present on all human cell membranes. The genes determining them are located on the short arm of chromosome 6. Specific areas of the gene complex, termed loci, are identified by letters and numbers (eg, B8, D3). These antigens are believed to be involved in the detection and destruction of foreign substances in the body, such as viruses and bacteria.

In 1974, evidence was presented that certain HLAs are found more frequently among IDDM patients than among normal individuals.[45,46] For example, a B8 or B15 antigen confers a two- or threefold increased risk, and both together increase the risk tenfold. CW3 is present in twice as many IDDM patients as in normal individuals. About 70% of identical twins who carry two gene alleles (DR3, DR4) known to be at high risk for developing IDDM will be concordant for the disease.[47]

If IDDM were caused solely by genetic factors, the concordance rate in identical twins would be expected to approach 100%. However, other factors, such as whether one parent or both have IDDM and which is the affected parent when there is only one, also influence likelihood.[48] Just possessing an HLA antigen commonly associated with IDDM does not guarantee the individual will develop IDDM. However, it does mean an increased chance of developing

Table 1-4 Glycemic Control for People with Diabetes

Biochemical Index	Nondiabetic	Goal	Action Suggested
Preprandial glucose (mg/dL)	< 115	80–120	< 80, >140
Bedtime glucose (mg/dL)	< 120	100–140	< 100, >160
Hemoglobin A_{1c} (%)	< 6	< 7	> 8

Values are for nonpregnant individuals. "Action suggested" depends on individual patient circumstances.

Hemoglobin A_{1c} is referenced to a nondiabetic range of 4.0–6.0% (mean 5.0%, standard deviation 0.5%).

Source: Reprinted with permission from American Diabetes Association, Standards of Medical Care for Patients with Diabetes (position statement). *Diabetes Care.* 1995;18[1]:8–15. Copyright © 1995, American Diabetes Association.

IDDM. In general, within the white population, for example, first-degree relatives of an IDDM individual are 10 to 12 times more likely to have IDDM than are individuals without such a first-degree relative. It follows that more people carry genes associated with IDDM than actually develop the condition.

Autoimmunity

It appears that many individuals genetically predisposed to IDDM actually develop the disease when an environmental event or stress factor that would not so influence a normal individual triggers a series of events that result in damage to, or destruction of, pancreatic ß-cells. Viruses are one example. Onset of IDDM has been reported to coincide with or follow infections with mumps, rubella, cytomegalic, measles, encephalitis, polio, Epstein-Barr, and coxsackie B4 viruses.

If because of an HLA-associated defect, the body fails to identify a particular foreign invader, pancreatic ß-cells could undergo attack. ß-Cell destruction could be either immediate or through gradual inactivation. Alternatively, ß-cell characteristics could be altered in such a way that some of their components are identified as foreign substances, triggering the production of antibodies. Antibodies directed at the virus also could cross-react with ß-cell components.

Evidence linking the presence of circulating antibodies with the development of other specific endocrinopathies has been present for decades (primary hypothyroidism, Graves' disease, idiopathic adrenal insufficiency). MacCaren et al[49] used human insulinoma cells to demonstrate circulating autoantibodies in IDDM. They found sera to be positive for islet cell surface antibodies in 85 to 90% of patients within 1 week of the diagnosis of IDDM. Antibody detectability decreased with time, so that only 10 to 20% were positive after 1 year. Cytoplasmic islet cell antibodies have been demonstrated.[50] These also diminish with time; they are detectable in only 20% of IDDM patients 3 years after diagnosis.

However, conversion to antibody positivity in an identical twin of an IDDM patient, for example, does not necessarily mean immediate development of the disease. Progressive deterioration of insulin secretion can occur over several years.[51] Loss of first-phase insulin release can precede hyperglycemia by years, and oral glucose tolerance can be normal when intravenous glucose tolerance testing reveals inadequate insulin secretion.[52] Even when this insulin response to glucose is essentially lost before the onset of overt diabetes, stimulation with tolbutamide, glucagon, and/or arginine may induce insulin release.[52] However, by the time overt IDDM presents itself, most ß-cells have been destroyed.[53]

PATHOGENESIS OF NON–INSULIN-DEPENDENT DIABETES MELLITUS (TYPE II DIABETES)

Genetic Factors

Type II diabetes is not a single disease process. There are many etiologies and a heterogeneity of disease processes that converge on a common denominator, hyperglycemia. It is, therefore, not surprising that the details of inheritance are equally heterogeneous and undefined. Nevertheless, inheritance of NIDDM is clearly more common than is IDDM. When an identical twin has NIDDM, the chances are 90 to 100% that NIDDM will appear in the other twin as well.[54]

Environment also plays such an important role in the pathogenesis of NIDDM that it has been called a disease of civilization. Its prevalence clearly increases as urbanization, working patterns, and dietary habits evolve from primitive to industrial modes, perhaps associated with a more abundant food supply. The latter is especially an issue to the extent that it leads to increased obesity, insulin resistance, and impaired insulin secretion.

Insulin Secretion

Normal subjects exhibit biphasic insulin release. Early-phase insulin release is rapid (minutes) and derives from pre-formed insulin pools. Late-phase insulin release is protracted and derives from both stored and newly synthesized sources. In NIDDM, early-phase insulin secretion is markedly diminished or lost and late-phase insulin secretion is prolonged. There is thus a failure of insulin levels to decrease appropriately in response to hypoglycemia.[55] There is a delay of insulin decline after meals.[56] The plasma glucose eventually returns to normal but only at the expense of insulin overproduction during the late secretory phase. In fact, the overall insulin response is elevated even though the early insulin response is lost. The reactive hypoglycemia frequently found in mild NIDDM or impaired glucose tolerance may also result from this delayed decline of postprandial insulin levels.[56] Further, the importance of deficient early-phase insulin secretions in NIDDM was demonstrated in human studies in which it was replaced with appropriately timed insulin infusions[57]: a marked improvement in the postprandial excessive glucose rise resulted.

Insulin Resistance

Basal and meal-stimulated plasma insulin levels in NIDDM may be normal, reduced, or even increased.[58] At issue is the fact that resistance to insulin action at the cellular level is present in most NIDDM patients, even in the absence of the increased insulin resistance associated with obesity. Their level of fasting hyperglycemia appears to be directly proportional to the degree of insulin resistance. The resistance is manifest in both hepatic and muscle tissue.

Hepatic resistance results in an inappropriately high level of glucose production in the fasted state, as well as an inappropriately low level of glucose uptake in the fed state. Muscle resistance impairs glucose uptake. Resistance may be attributed to defects in the insulin receptor, to reduced concentrations of receptors on the cell surface, and/or to postreceptor defects within the cell.

Insulin must first bind to the cell membrane receptor before glucose can be transported across the cell membrane. Insulin resistance, secondary to impaired insulin binding, is present in most individuals with impaired glucose tolerance and in essentially all type II diabetic individuals whose fasting plasma glucose level exceeds 140 mg/dL. This reduced insulin binding appears to result from a decreased number of available receptors rather than from decreased receptor affinity. Cell receptor level is also influenced inversely by the basal insulin level: the higher the basal insulin level, the lower the receptor concentration. Thus, any manipulation that will lower basal insulin secretion, such as diet and weight loss, will increase receptor concentration and decrease insulin resistance.

Most investigators agree, however, that decreased insulin receptor binding does not explain all the insulin resistance of NIDDM even when obesity is excluded. Involvement of a more distal step, one or more postreceptor defects, is likely and contributes to the etiologic heterogeneity of NIDDM.

As our knowledge of the intricacies of this condition continues to expand, it becomes increasingly apparent that each affected individual has his or her own unique case of diabetes mellitus. A team approach to management is necessary, but actions of the affected individual are the principal determinants of success.

REFERENCES

1. Yalow RS, Berson SA. Immunoassay of plasma insulin in man. *Diabetes*. 1961;10:339.

2. Yalow RS, Berson SA. Plasma insulin concentrations in non-diabetic and early diabetic subjects. *Diabetes*. 1960;9:254.

3. Karam JH, Grodsky GM, Forsham PH. Excessive insulin response to glucose in obese subjects as measured by immunochemical assay. *Diabetes*. 1963;12:197.

4. Bar RS, Roth J. Insulin receptor status in disease states of man. *Arch Intern Med*. 1977;137:474.

5. Bar RS, Harrison LC, Muggo M, et al. Regulation of insulin receptors in normal and abnormal physiology in humans. *Adv Intern Med*. 1979;24:23.

6. Larner J, Galasko G, Cheng K, et al. Generation by insulin of a chemical mediator that controls protein phosphorylation and dephosphorylation. *Science*. 1979;206:1408.

7. Brunzell JD, Robertson RP, Lerner RL, et al. Relationships between fasting plasma glucose levels and insulin secretion during intravenous glucose tolerance tests. *Clin Endocrinol Metab.* 1976;42:222.

8. Pfeifer MA, Halter JB, Porte D Jr. Insulin secretion in diabetes mellitus. *Am J Med.* 1981;70:579.

9. Palmer JP, Benson JW, Walter RM, Enamck JW. Arginine stimulated acute phase of insulin and glucagon secretions in diabetic subjects. *J Clin Invest.* 1976;58:565.

10. Robertson RP, Porte D. The glucose receptor: a defective mechanism in diabetes mellitus distinct from the beta-adrenergic receptor. *J Clin Invest.* 1976;52:870.

11. Ward WK, Beard JC, Halter JB, et al. Pathophysiology of insulin secretion in non–insulin-dependent diabetes mellitus. *Diabetes Care.* 1984;7:491.

12. Rossetti L, Giaccari A, DeFronzo RA. Glucose toxicity. *Diabetes Care.* 1990;13:610.

13. Ferrannini E, Reichard G, Bevilacqua S, et al. Oral glucose disposal in non-insulin dependent diabetics. *Am Diabetic Assoc.* 1984;33:66A. Abstract.

14. Garvey WT, Olefsky JM, Griffin J, et al. The effects of insulin treatment on insulin secretion and action in type II diabetes mellitus. *Diabetes.* 1985;34:222.

15. Bowen HF, Moorehouse JA. Glucose turnover and disposal in maturity-onset diabetes. *J Clin Invest.* 1973;52:3033.

16. Olefsky JM. Pathogenesis of non–insulin-dependent (type II) diabetes. In: Degroot LJ, Besser M, Burger HG, Jameson JL, eds. *Endocrinology.* 2nd Ed. Philadelphia, Pa: WB Sanders Co; 1989.

17. Unger RH, Orci L. Role of glucagon in diabetes. *Arch Intern Med.* 1977;137:482.

18. Orci L, Baetens D, Rufener C. Hypertrophy and hyperplasia of somatostatin-containing ß cells in diabetes. *Proc Natl Acad Sci USA.* 1976;73:1338.

19. Trimble ER, Halban PA, Wolheim CB, Renold AE. Functional differences between rat islets of ventral and dorsal pancreatic origin. *J Clin Invest.* 1982;69:405.

20. Grodsky GM. A threshold distribution hypothesis for packet storage of insulin. II. Effect of calcium. *Diabetes.* 1972;21(suppl 2):584.

21. Salmon D, Meda P. Heterogenicity and contact-dependent regulation of hormone secretion by individual B cells. *Exp Cell Res.* 1986;162:507.

22. Meda P, Perrelet A, Orci L. Gap junctions and cell-to-cell coupling in endocrine glands. *Mol Cell Biol.* 1984;3:131.

23. Stagner JI, Samols E, Bonner-Weir S. Beta to alpha to delta pancreatic cell islet perfusion in dogs. *Diabetes.* 1988;37:1715.

24. Stefan Y, Meda P, Neufeld M, Orci L. Stimulation of insulin secretion reveals heterogenicity of pancreatic B cells in vivo. *J Clin Invest.* 1987;80:175.

25. Hopcroft DW, Mason DR, Scott RS. Structure–function relationships in pancreatic islets: support for intraislet modulation of insulin secretion. *Endocrinology.* 1985;117:2083.

26. Chan SJ, Kwok SCM, Steiner DF. The biosynthesis of insulin: some genetic and evolutionary aspects. *Diabetes Care.* 1981;4:4.

27. Porte D Jr, Bagdade JD. Human insulin secretion: An integrated approach. *Ann Rev Med.* 1970;21:219.

28. Rubenstein AH, Kuzuya H, Horwitz DL. Clinical significance of circulating C-peptide in diabetes mellitus and hypoglycemia disorders. *Arch Intern Med.* 1977;137:625.

29. Felig P, Wahren J, Hendler R. Influence of physiologic hyperglucagonemia on basal and insulin-inhibited splanchnic glucose output in normal man. *J Clin Invest.* 1976;58:761.

30. Unger RH, Dobbs RE, Orci L. Insulin, glucagon, and somatostatin secretion in the regulation of metabolism. *Am Rev Physiol.* 1978;40:307.

31. Unger RH, Orci L. Glucagon and the A cell. *N Engl J Med.* 1981;304:1518.

32. Gorich JE, Charles MA, Grodsky GM. Regulation of pancreatic insulin and glucagon secretion. *Am Rev Physiol.* 1976;38:353.

33. Wahren J, Felig P, Hagenfeldt L. Physical exercise and fuel homeostasis in diabetes mellitus. *Diabetologia.* 1978;14:213.

34. D'Alessio DA, Sieber C, Beglinger C, Ensink DW. A physiologic role for somatostatin-28 as a regulator of insulin secretion. *J Clin Invest.* 1989;84:857.

35. Mandarino L, Stenner D, Blanchard W, et al. Selective effects of somatostatin-14, -25, and -28 on in vitro insulin and glucagon secretion. *Nature.* 1981;291:76.

36. Unger RH, Aguilar-Parada E, Muller WA, et al. Studies of pancreatic alpha cell function in normal and diabetic subjects. *J Clin Invest.* 1970;49:837.

37. Christensen J, Hansen A, Lundbalk K. Somatostatin in maturity onset diabetes. *Diabetes.* 1978;27:1213.

38. Weir GC, Bonner-Weir S. Islets of Langerhans: the puzzle of intra islet interactions and their relevance to diabetes. *J Clin Invest.* 1990;85:983.

39. Marks V, Samols E, Stagner J. Intra-islet interactions. In: Flatt PR, ed. *Nutrient Regulation of Insulin Secretion.* London: Portland Press; 1992:41.

40. White NH, Gingerich RI, Levandoski LA, et al. Plasma pancreatic polypeptide response to insulin-induced hypoglycemia as a marker for defective glucose

counter-regulation in insulin-dependent diabetes mellitus. *Diabetes.* 1985;34:870.

41. McGrath BP, Stern AI, Esler M, Hansby J. Impaired pancreatic polypeptide release to insulin hypoglycemia in chronic autonomic failure with postural hypotension; evidence for parasympathetic dysfunction. *Clin Sci.* 1982;63:321.

42. Kennedy FP, Bolli GB, Go VLW, et al. The significance of impaired pancreatic polypeptide and epinephrine response to hypoglycemia in patients with insulin dependent diabetes mellitus. *J Clin Endocrinol Metab.* 1987;64:602.

43. Felig P, Wahren J. Influence of endogenous insulin secretion on splanchnic glucose and amino acid metabolism in man. *J Clin Invest.* 1971;50:1702.

44. Garreto LD, Richter EA, Ruderman NB. Increased insulin sensitivity of skeletal muscle following exercise. *Diabetes.* 1981;30:63A.

45. Nerup J, Platz P, Anderson OO, et al. HL-A antigens and diabetes mellitus. *Lancet.* 1974;2:864.

46. Cudworth AG, Woodrow JC. Evidence for HL-A linked genes in "juvenile" diabetes mellitus. *BMJ.* 1975;3:133.

47. Stefan Y, Orci L, Malaisse-Lagae F, et al. Quantitation of endocrine cell content in the pancreas of non-diabetic and diabetic humans. *Diabetes.* 1982;31:694.

48. Kloppel G, Drenck CR, Oberholzer M, Heitz PU: Morphometric evidence for a striking B-cell reduction at the clinical onset of type I diabetes. *Virchow Arch.* 1984;403:441.

49. MacCaren NK, Huang SW, Foyk J. Antibody to cultured human insulinoma cells in insulin dependent diabetes mellitus. *Lancet.* 1975;1:997.

50. Bottazzo GF, Landrum R. Separate autoantibodies to human pancreatic glucagon and somatostatin cells. *Lancet.* 1976;2:873.

51. Srikanta S, Ganda OP, Jackson RA, et al. Pre-type I diabetes: common endocrinologic course despite immunologic and immunogenetic heterogenicity. *Diabetologia.* 1984;27:146.

52. Ganda OP, Srikanta S, Brink SJ, et al. Differential sensitivity to beta cell secretagogues in "early" type I diabetes mellitus. *Diabetes.* 1984;33:516.

53. Gepts W. Islet cell morphology in type I and type II diabetes. In: Irvine WJ, ed. *Immunology in Diabetes.* Edinborough: Teviot Scientific Publications; 1982:255–266.

54. Tattersal RB, Pyke DA. Diabetes in identical twins. *Lancet.* 1970;2:1120.

55. Hosker JP, Burnett MA, Matthews DR, Turner RC. Suppression of insulin secretion by falling plasma glucose levels is impaired in type 2 diabetes. *Diabetic Med.* 1988;5:856.

56. Liu G, Coulston A, Chen Y-D, Reaven GM. Does day-long absolute hypoinsulinemia characterize the patient with non-insulin dependent diabetes mellitus? *Metabolism.* 1983;32:754.

57. Bruce DG, Chisholm DJ, Storlien LH, Kraegen EW. Physiologic importance of deficiency in early prandial insulin secretion in non–insulin-dependent diabetes. *Diabetes.* 1988;37:736.

58. National Diabetes Data Group. Classification and diagnosis of diabetes mellitus and other categories of glucose intolerance. *Diabetes.* 1979;28:1039.

Chapter 2

Complications of Diabetes Mellitus and Implications for Nutrition Therapy

Mark E. Molitch

The complications of diabetes mellitus may be divided into two major categories: acute and chronic (Exhibit 2-1). The acute complications are directly related to rapid changes in metabolism and include diabetic ketoacidosis (DKA), hyperosmolar hyperglycemic nonketotic "coma" (HHNK), and hypoglycemia. These complications are, in part, preventable and require immediate therapeutic intervention. The chronic complications, such as vascular disease, nephropathy, neuropathy, and retinopathy, are less directly related to the altered metabolic milieu of diabetes. However, the Diabetes Control and Complications Trial[1] has now shown definitively that the rates of initial development and subsequent progression of such complications can be markedly reduced by therapy directed at regulating blood glucose levels close to the normal range. The dietitian plays a critical role in helping the person with diabetes achieve the control necessary to avoid short-term complications and postpone or prevent long-term complications.

ACUTE COMPLICATIONS

Diabetic Ketoacidosis

Currently, 5 to 8% of all diabetes-related deaths are due to DKA, and 5 to 8% of episodes of DKA result in death.[2,3] In most cases, the deaths are associated with conditions that may have triggered the DKA and that undoubtedly contributed to the mortality, such as infection and arterial thrombosis.[3,4] DKA has a significant individual and public health impact; it results in about 75,000 hospital admissions in the United States annually, at an estimated cost in 1983 dollars of $225 million.[2] DKA occurs far more often in individuals with insulin-dependent diabetes mellitus (IDDM) than with non–insulin-dependent diabetes mellitus (NIDDM) and thus is found mostly in younger individuals, accounting for about 30% of diabetes-related hospital admissions in the 0 to 14-year age group and about 6% of such admissions in the 45- to 64-year age group.[2]

Pathophysiology

The metabolic derangements of DKA occur because of a deficiency of insulin relative to the levels of the various counterregulatory hormones: glucagon, epinephrine, cortisol, and growth hormone.[4–6] This imbalance may occur because of failure to take insulin or because of an excess of these counterregulatory hormones that occurs with stress. Such stress is usually physical, such as from infection, tissue injury (myocardial infarction, fractured femur, etc), or surgery, but it may also rarely be psychological. The degrees of insulin deficiency and insulin/counterregulatory hormone imbalance needed to cause DKA are usually found only in individuals with IDDM. Rarely, very major stress, such as myocardial infarction, raises the counterregulatory hormone levels to such a degree that DKA occurs in an individual with NIDDM.

As a result of this insulin/counterregulatory hormone imbalance, substrates (amino acids and

Exhibit 2-1 Complications of Diabetes Mellitus

Acute Complications
Ketoacidosis
Hyperosmolar hyperglycemic nonketotic coma
Hypogylycemia

Chronic Complications
Ophthalmologic
—Retinopathy—background, proliferative
—Glaucoma
—Cataract
Macrovascular
—Coronary
—Cerebral
—Peripheral
—Hypertension
Nephropathy
Neuropathy
—Polyneuropathy
—Radiculopathy
—Mixed nerve mononeuropathy
—Amyotrophy
—Autonomic neuropathy
Infections
Osteopenia

free fatty acids) are mobilized in peripheral tissues and are delivered to the liver for gluconeogenesis and lipid metabolism (Table 2-1). This altered balance also results in increased hepatic glucose output caused by both glucose overproduction and increased glycogen breakdown.[4-6] This increased hepatic glucose output, coupled with decreased metabolism of glucose by insulin-deficient tissues, results in progressive hyperglycemia. The resultant glycosuria and osmotic load cause obligate urinary sodium and water losses that lead to dehydration and further rises in blood glucose levels. Nausea and vomiting commonly occur, perhaps due to the concomitant ketosis, and further worsen the state of dehydration and hyperglycemia.[4,6] As can be seen from the above discussion, prior dietary indiscretion has little to do with the hyperglycemia of DKA.

The altered insulin/counterregulatory hormone balance causes an increased lipolysis in peripheral tissues, with an increased delivery of free fatty acids (FFA) to the liver.[4-6] Further-

more, this imbalance results in the alteration of hepatic metabolic pathways from those favoring re-esterification of FFA to triglyceride to those favoring oxidation of FFA to form ketoacids (acetoacetic acid and ß-hydroxybutyric acid).[4-6] This buildup of ketoacids causes a metabolic acidosis with lowered blood pH, a using up of bicarbonate buffers with lowered serum bicarbonate levels, and partial respiratory compensation that results in a lowered pCO_2 in arterial blood.[3-6]

Laboratory Findings

Other biochemical abnormalities accompany the hyperglycemia and ketoacidosis and will be found on the initial laboratory evaluation (Exhibit 2-2). Serum potassium levels are usually elevated because of an attempt at cellular buffering of the excess acid in which intracellular potassium is exchanged for intravascular and extracellular hydrogen ions.[4,6] Nonetheless, total body potassium stores are markedly depleted (3 to 5 mEq/kg body weight) because of the prior diuresis.[4,6] During therapy, potassium rapidly enters cells, leading to hypokalemia. Once insulin administration and fluid therapy have begun, urine flow is established, and potassium levels have fallen to normal, potassium replacement is

Table 2-1 Effects of Insulin/Counterregulatory Hormone Imbalance

	Insulin/Counterregulatory Hormone Imbalance
Blood Insulin	↓
Blood counterregulatory hormone	↑
Peripheral substrate mobilization	
Lipolysis	↑
Proteolysis	↑
Glycogenolysis	↑
Hepatic glycogenolysis	↑
Hepatic gluconeogenesis	↑
Tissue glucose uptake	↓
Hepatic FFA re-esterification	↓
Hepatic ketogenesis	↑

Exhibit 2-2 Laboratory Findings in Diabetic Ketoacidosis

Glucose	↑	
Acetoacetate	↑	
ß-Hydroxybutyrate	↑	
pH	↓	
Bicarbonate	↓	
pCO$_2$	↓	
Sodium	↓	
Potassium	↑	↓
Phosphate	↑	↓
Amylase	↑	
Creatinine	↑	

begun. When serum potassium levels are low on admission, total body depletion is very severe, and potassium replacement should begin immediately.

Serum sodium levels are usually low on admission for three reasons: (1) the osmotically active glucose draws water from the cells into the intravascular space, "diluting" the sodium level (about 1.6 to 1.8 mEq Na$^+$ lowering for every 100 mg/dL glucose elevation above 100 mg/dL)[4]; (2) severe hypertriglyceridemia accompanying the metabolic decompensation may displace some of the aqueous component of the blood, and sodium is present only in the aqueous component[3]; and (3) the dehydration stimulates volume receptors in the right atrium so that vasopressin is secreted, which causes retention of water by the kidney distal tubules. When the serum sodium is elevated, then free water deficits are usually very great.

Hyperphosphatemia (>4 mg/dL) is present initially in 95% of patients and seems to be due to a transcellular shift that is related to the acidosis and hyperglycemia.[4] As with potassium, hyperphosphatemia may mask total body depletion of phosphorus from prior diuresis-induced urinary losses. Again as with potassium, therapy with insulin causes a shift of phosphorus back into cells, and hypophosphatemia is common.[4] Rarely, marked hypophosphatemia may be associated with severe muscle weakness. However, in most cases it is asymptomatic, and a prospective randomized study has shown that routine intravenous (IV) phosphate replacement is of no

benefit and may even be harmful, causing symptomatic hypocalcemia.[3–6] Generally, phosphate is not replaced until levels fall below 1.0 mEq/L.[5]

In some patients presenting with ketoacidosis, serum amylase levels are elevated. Salivary, not pancreatic, amylase levels are increased,[7] and in general, pancreatitis is not a worry with respect to restarting oral intake. Serum creatinine may also be elevated initially, but this is an artifact due to the cross-reaction of acetoacetate in the automated creatinine assay.[8] Blood urea nitrogen elevations may reflect the patient's degree of dehydration.

Clinical Presentation

Patients with DKA are usually thirsty from their dehydration and hyperosmolar state, polyuric, weak, and short of breath, with deep sighing respirations (Kussmaul breathing) indicating respiratory compensation. They may also complain of nausea, vomiting, and abnormal discomfort. Altered consciousness may be present, depending on the degree of hyperosmolality of the blood. Patients with DKA may also have symptoms related to an underlying precipitating illness. Examination usually reveals an ill-appearing person who is tachycardic, possibly hypotensive, and tachypneic. Observations should be made regarding the underlying illness.[3–6]

Treatment

Insulin is the mainstay of treatment. When given in adequate amounts, regardless of the rate, it will correct the insulin/counterregulatory hormone imbalance by halting lipolysis, ketoacid formation, and glucose output by the liver and permitting glucose uptake by the tissues.[3–6,9] Currently, the usual approach is to give regular insulin as an initial 0.1 U/kg loading dose followed by a constant IV infusion at the rate of 0.1 U/kg per hour. A rate of fall of glucose of 100 to 150 mg/dL per hour may be expected. When glucose levels of 150 to 250 mg/dL are reached, the insulin infusion rate is decreased to 1.5 U/h to 2.0 U/h, and 5% dextrose is begun at a rate of about 100 mL/h. Alternatively, regular insulin can be given subcutaneously every 4 to 6 hours based on blood glucose measurements. Insulin should never be omitted in this acute period because DKA will likely recur; the dose of insulin should be reduced when glucose levels are low.[3–6,9]

Most patients have a 3- to 5-L fluid deficit on admission.[3–6] Normal saline is administered initially at a rate of 500 to 1000 mL/h for the first few hours, and when the blood pressure is stable, 0.45N saline may be substituted to provide needed free water. As mentioned above, potassium replacement is given when normal potassium levels in the blood are achieved at a rate of about 20 mEq/h. Phosphorus therapy is needed only in symptomatic patients who have severe hypophosphatemia (<1.0 mg/dL).[5] Bicarbonate is needed only when the acidosis is very severe (pH <7.1) or if the pH is maintained above 7.1 only by intense respiratory effort and the bicarbonate buffering capacity is severely compromised (serum bicarbonate <4 mEq/L). In these circumstances, bicarbonate is given only to raise the pH to >7.2.[3,4,6]

Patients usually feel much better within 12 to 14 hours after beginning treatment. Depending on any underlying, precipitating illness and their appetite, patients can usually begin eating their usual diet after this initial 12 to 24 hours. At that point, they can also begin their usual insulin regimen. If they are not well enough then, a combination of parenteral 5 or 10% glucose and hypocaloric liquid feeding is usually given. Regular insulin is then given subcutaneously on an every-6-hour regimen based on blood glucose levels, again never omitting a dose but just reducing the dose in the event of hypoglycemia. Ketoacidosis itself seems to impair nerve function so that autonomic neuropathy with gastroparesis may be made transiently worse. Metoclopramide may be helpful in improving gastric emptying, but merely delaying the time of insulin administration with respect to gastric emptying may suffice. The 1- to 2-day recovery period is a good time to reinforce nutritional guidelines and other aspects of treatment.

Hyperosmolar Hyperglycemic Nonketotic Coma

In HHNK, patients develop severe hyperglycemia and associated hyperosmolality without ketosis. As a cause of diabetic coma, HHNK is one-sixth as frequent as DKA but is more common in older individuals, usually older than the age of 65.[2] Most individuals with HHNK have NIDDM, and in many, it is the first presenting sign of diabetes.[5,10] Symptoms of polyuria, polydipsia, fatigue, and lethargy usually develop over 3 to 7 days in HHNK, as opposed to a 1- to 2-day period in DKA.[3,5,10] Neurologic manifestations, including coma, are often the presenting finding. Mortality is high, occurring in about 20 to 40% of patients, and is often due to interaction of the HHNK with the underlying precipitating illness.[3,5,10]

The mechanisms leading to the hyperglycemia are similar to those in DKA. The retention of some endogenous insulin secretion is the likely reason that lipolysis and ketogenesis are limited.[10] Fluid deficits are similar, however. Patients must be admitted to the hospital, where management with insulin and fluids is similar to that for DKA.[3,5,10] In older individuals, care must be taken to avoid overhydration and precipitation of congestive heart failure.[3] Although potassium replacement is needed, bicarbonate and phosphate treatment are not needed. After resolution of the acute illness and any underlying precipitating disorder, the diabetes may often be managed with diet alone or oral agents plus diet. Reinstitution of standard dietary measures depends on the speed of recovery of the patient and his or her appetite and can usually be done in 1 to 2 days.

Hypoglycemia

Hypoglycemia is the most common acute complication of diabetes and results from an imbalance of glucose entry into and exit from the blood. In patients managed by diet alone, hypoglycemia is very rare. In some patients with mild impairment of glucose tolerance, a delay in insulin secretion results in relative hyper-insulinemia at a time when postprandial glucose absorption has already decreased, thereby causing mild hypoglycemia about 3 to 4 hours after eating.[11] Some individuals have very rapid gastric emptying, resulting in a similar situation of still elevated insulin levels when glucose levels have decreased to baseline postprandially, a condition referred to as alimentary hypoglycemia.[12]

The oral sulfonylurea drugs uncommonly cause hypoglycemia. It is very rarely seen with acetohexamide (Dymelor) and tolazamide (Tolinase), occurs somewhat more commonly with tolbutamide (Orinase) and glipizide (Glucotrol), but is most common with chlorpropamide (Diabinese) and glyburide (Micronase, Diabeta).[13] When hypoglycemia does occur with these agents, it may be prolonged and severe; patients experiencing severe reactions usually need to be hospitalized and treated with IV dextrose for up to 24 to 48 hours. With glyburide, mild reactions also may occur and may be corrected by reducing the dose. Hypoglycemia does not occur with metformin.

In patients under insulin management, hypoglycemia usually occurs either because of (1) inadequate nutrient intake around the time of the peak action of the insulin or (2) increased exercise, which may increase the rate of glucose usage and the rate of absorption of insulin from the exercising limb into which it has been injected. Careful matching of food intake to the peak times of insulin action, with a judicious use of snacks, is necessary to avoid hypoglycemia. Self-monitoring blood glucose (SMBG) before and after exercise allows the patient to eat additional snacks if necessary. Reduced insulin dosage is often needed on days when the patient is exercising (see Chapter 6).

The normal hormonal response of the body to hypoglycemia is a release of the counterregulatory hormones: glucagon, epinephrine, cortisol, and growth hormone. Careful studies by several groups have shown that glucagon and epinephrine are by far the most important hormones in causing the blood glucose to increase after an episode of hypoglycemia.[14–17] Rebound hyperglycemia may occur as the release of these counterregulatory hormones and their effects on hepatic glucose production combine with the cessation of maximum insulin effect and extra eating because of symptoms. Whether the release of counterregulatory hormones alone can cause rebound hyperglycemia is controversial. By performing SMBG several times a day, patients can now discern daily patterns of glycemia that allow the detection of this phenomenon. Unexplained fasting hyperglycemia requires the patient to set an alarm clock to wake up at 3:00 A.M. to detect asymptomatic nocturnal hypoglycemia. On close questioning, however, most patients experiencing such episodes remember having had nightmares or waking up with a headache or with bedclothes wet from perspiration during the episode.

Some individuals with long-standing IDDM seem to lose their ability to release, first, glucagon and, later, epinephrine in response to hypoglycemia.[14–17] Some studies have suggested that intensive insulin therapy with the frequent development of hypoglycemia may itself cause this loss.[14–17] Such individuals often lose the premonitory warning signs of hypoglycemia that are predominantly due to epinephrine release, a condition referred to as "hypoglycemia unawareness." Such individuals may proceed rapidly into an altered mental state and sometimes develop coma or seizures. When this occurs, new, higher blood glucose goals must be set with the patient. Avoiding severe hypoglycemic reactions under these circumstances outweighs the potential benefit of maintaining very "tight" metabolic control. Prevention of hypoglycemia centers around alteration of diet, insulin, and exercise to meet these higher glucose targets. Prevention of repetitive hypoglycemia also restores the epinephrine response to hypoglycemia, and so after a period of time, the patient can again try for better glycemic control.[17]

Treatment

The acute reaction must be treated promptly, when symptoms are minor, to prevent the development of more severe symptoms, such as altered consciousness and seizures. Ten to 20 g of rapidly absorbable simple sugars is effective in raising blood glucose levels from hypoglycemic to normoglycemic and not hyperglycemic levels.[18] Symptoms usually abate within 15 minutes with this dose. To avoid hyperglycemia, a second dose of glucose should usually not be ingested until these 15 minutes have elapsed. Patients must carry a readily absorbable amount of simple carbohydrate with them at all times. Glucose tablets, rather than candy, are often preferred for treatment of hypoglycemic reactions because patients are less likely to nibble on these tablets when they are not hypoglycemic. When reactions are severe with loss of consciousness, oral glucose intake is contraindicated because of the risk of aspiration. Under these circumstances, glucagon can be given subcutaneously by a relative or friend or by emergency medical help, or intravenous 50% glucose may be required.

CHRONIC COMPLICATIONS

Morbidity and Mortality

Although people with diabetes comprise only 4.5% of the population in the United States, health care expenditures for diabetes totaled $105.2 billion, 14.6% of the total of $720.5 billion for U.S. health care expenditures in 1992.[19] These are direct costs for health care expenditures and do not include indirect costs such as lost wages and earnings resulting from disability and premature death, which are also considerable.[20] The chronic complications of diabetes account for far more morbidity and mortality than the acute complications. About 50% of hospital admissions for diabetes involve chronic complications,[21] and people with diabetes have a two- to threefold increased number of days lost from work compared with those without diabetes.[22] Deaths related to these chronic complications make diabetes the seventh leading cause of death.[23] In patients with IDDM, renal and car-

diovascular deaths occur 56 and 13 times higher than would be expected in the general population.[24] The long-term complications of diabetes obviously have an enormous impact on society, as well as on the individual with diabetes. To the extent that these complications are related to the level of blood glucose and lipid control, the dietitian has a significant role in their prevention. Also, modifications of diets in patients with renal failure, hypertension, and heart failure are essential once these complications occur.

Pathogenesis of Complications

The exact relationships between the abnormal metabolic milieu of diabetes and the morphologic changes that result in the long-term complications of diabetes remain to be clarified. Hypotheses abound, however.

Polyol Pathway

In tissues where insulin is not necessary for glucose transport—the lens, retina, nerves, kidneys, blood vessels, and islets of Langerhans—glucose enters in direct proportion to the ambient blood glucose level. Some of these tissues, such as lens and retina of the eye and the nerves, display many of the complications of diabetes. In these tissues, glucose is converted to the sugar alcohol sorbitol via the enzyme aldose reductase, and sorbitol, in turn, is converted to fructose via the enzyme sorbitol dehydrogenase (Figure 2-1). Sorbitol and fructose are only slowly metabolizable and diffuse poorly out of the cell. They therefore accumulate in these tissues, especially the lens and, being osmotically active particles, cause water to enter the cell with subsequent swelling, electrolyte imbalance, and cellular dysfunction.[25–27]

In peripheral nerves, and possibly retinal capillary endothelial cells, it is possible that the activity of this pathway is related to complications in a more indirect way by reducing the intracellular levels of another sugar alcohol, myoinositol. Lowered levels of myoinositol cause a reduction in intracellular sodium-potassium ATPase activity and phosphoinositide metabo-

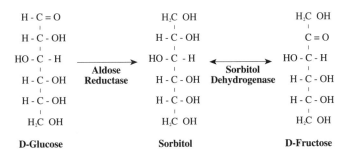

Figure 2-1 Sorbitol Pathway

lism, resulting in altered function.[26] Correction of the lowered nerve myoinositol content by dietary myoinositol supplementation[26,28] or inhibition of the aldose reductase enzyme with an inhibitor such as sorbinil[26,28] results in a moderate improvement in nerve conduction velocity and modest clinical improvement in some patients with neuropathy, but neither approach has been approved by the U.S. Food and Drug Administration.

Protein Glycosylation

The nonenzymatic glycosylation of hemoglobin is well known as hemoglobin A1c and measurement of this moiety has served as a useful indicator of diabetes control. Other proteins in the body may be similarly glycosylated in direct proportion to ambient glucose levels. In proteins that turn over more slowly than hemoglobin, such as albumin, crystallins, collagen, elastin, fibrinogen, low-density lipoprotein (LDL), high-density lipoprotein (HDL), and myelin, further reactions, rearrangement, and dehydration may occur, resulting in end-products that are brown ("browning") and participate in protein-protein cross-linking.[29,30] In proteins that turn over very slowly or not at all, these advanced glycation end-products (AGE) accumulate over the lifetime of the person.[29,30] These products may then alter many physiologic processes by changing (1) enzymatic activity, (2) binding of regulatory molecules, (3) cross-linking of proteins, (4) protein susceptibility to pro-

teolysis, (5) DNA template function, (6) macromolecular (eg, LDL) recognition and endocytosis, and (7) protein immunogenicity.[29,30] Recent studies have shown that aminoguanidine, an inhibitor of AGE formation, is able to prevent AGE-induced cross-linking in collagen and structural alterations in laminin.[29,30] In studies in rats, aminoguanidine treatment resulted in decreases in microaneurysm formation, the development of acellular capillaries, the deposition of protein in intercapillary spaces in the retina, urinary albumin excretion, basement membrane thickening and mesangial expansion in the kidney glomeruli, and axonal atrophy while increasing motor and sensory nerve conduction velocity.[29] Phase II and III studies in humans with diabetes are just now beginning.

Basement Membrane Abnormalities

One of the pathologic hallmarks of diabetes is thickening of capillary basement membranes in such tissues as the retina, renal glomerulus, and nerve Schwann cells. Biochemical abnormalities of the glomerular basement membrane in diabetes have been found, including an increased attachment of disaccharides to hydroxylysine and complex heteropolysaccharides to asparagine in the collagen.[31] It is not known whether these changes also occur in other tissues. The relationships of these biochemical abnormalities to the visible thickening of the basement membranes and the final endpoint of clinical disease are not known.

Atherosclerosis

The process of atherosclerosis is accelerated and more extensive in people with diabetes for several reasons.[32,33] In diabetes, the vascular endothelium is abnormal, in part due to abnormalities of prostacyclin metabolism, decreased plasminogen activator activity, impaired plasmin degradation of glycosylated fibrin, AGE-mediated increased procoagulant activity, and decreased lipoprotein lipase activity. This abnormal endothelium permits increased platelet adhesion and aggregation to occur.[33] Glycosylation of collagen in the vessel wall causes an increased rigidity of the wall and an enhanced ability to bind LDL.[33] In people with diabetes, circulating levels of LDL, very low-density lipoprotein, and triglycerides tend to be elevated and HDL levels are decreased, resulting in cholesterol deposition and atherosclerotic plaque formation at these damaged endothelial sites.[33] Altered platelet function permits thrombosis to occur more readily in these diseased vessels.[33]

In patients with NIDDM, there appears to be an association of insulin resistance, hyperinsulinemia, obesity, elevated LDL cholesterol levels, hypertension, and atherosclerotic vascular disease in cross-sectional studies, a clustering sometimes referred to as syndrome "X" (Figure 2-2). Although these risk factors and manifestations cluster together, the exact cause and effect are not known. However, it is thought that the insulin resistance and resultant hyperinsulinemia may be central to the pathogenesis of some of or all the manifestations (for reviews of this area, see references 32,34,35).

Patients with NIDDM or IDDM have much greater risks for atherosclerotic cardiovascular disease if they have renal disease. This risk is manifest even at the earliest stage of nephropathy when there is an abnormal leak of albumin into the urine, a phenomenon referred to as microalbuminuria (20 to 200 µg/min).[36,37] Researchers at the Steno Hospital in Copenhagen have postulated that there may be common pathogenetic mechanisms for microalbuminuria and accelerated atherosclerosis, including alter-

Syndrome "X"

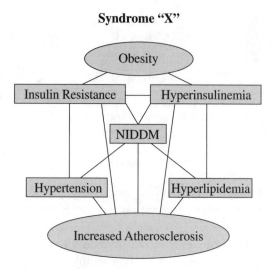

Figure 2-2 Interrelationships between Insulin Resistance, Hyperinsulinemia, Diabetes Mellitus, Hypertension, Hyperlipidemia, and Obesity in Patients with NIDDM

ations of the extracellular matrix such as decreased density and/or sulfation of heparan sulfate-proteoglycan.[36]

Relationship of Diabetic Control to Long-Term Complications

The Diabetes Control and Complications Trial (DCCT) has now definitively demonstrated that glycemic control is of paramount importance in the development of the microvascular and neuropathic complications of IDDM. However, it is clear that many patients suffer few or even no complications, despite having more than 25 to 30 years of poorly controlled diabetes. Yet in other patients with diabetes of much shorter duration, complications abound. Obviously, some genetic substrate influences the rate of progression and type of complications in any single individual. Family longevity, exercise, stress, diet, underlying lipid abnormalities, smoking, hypertension, and possibly other risk factors also are important.

Early studies that attempted to show that blood glucose control influenced complications were marred by several problems. The populations studied were often quite heterogeneous, including patients with IDDM and NIDDM and various age groups. Often the risk factors mentioned above were not considered. It is only in the past few years that the techniques of SMBG, insulin pump therapy, and multiple daily injections of insulin have allowed people with diabetes to achieve glucose levels even approaching normoglycemia. Hemoglobin A1c measurements now also allow objective evaluations of long-term control. Using these measures of achieving control and prospective randomization of subjects with IDDM between "usual" versus intensive insulin management, some short-term studies with relatively small numbers of patients showed modest benefit with regard to retinopathy and nephropathy, but others did not.[38-43]

The DCCT was a multicenter, randomized prospective trial in which 1441 carefully selected subjects with IDDM (726 with no retinopathy at baseline, the primary prevention cohort; 615 with mild retinopathy at baseline,

the secondary cohort) were randomized into conventional and intensively treated groups.[1] These subjects were followed for a mean of 6.5 years, with the minimum time of follow-up being 4.5 years and the maximum being 9 years. The mean quarterly glycohemoglobins and seven-point glucose profiles were 9.1% and 231 ± 55 mg/dL in the conventional group and 7.2% and 155 ± 30 mg/dL in the intensive group, respectively.

Intensive therapy reduced the mean risk for the development of retinopathy by 76% in the primary prevention cohort and by 54% in the secondary intervention cohort compared with conventional therapy (Table 2-2). Furthermore, progression to proliferative or severe nonproliferative retinopathy was reduced by 47% and the need for laser photocoagulation by 56%. The development of microalbuminuria (urinary albumin excretion rate ≥40 mg per 24 hours) was reduced by 39% and clinical albuminuria (urinary albumin excretion rate ≥300 mg per 24 hours) by 54% in the combined cohorts. Clinical neuropathy was reduced by 60% by intensive

Table 2-2 Development and Progression of Long-Term Complications of Diabetes in the Study Cohorts and Reduction in Risk with Intensive as Compared with Conventional Therapy

Complications	Primary Prevention			Secondary Intervention			Both Cohorts
	Conventional Rx	Intensive Rx	Risk Reduction (%)	Conventional Rx	Intensive Rx	Risk Reduction (%)	Risk Reduction (%)
	(rate/100 pt-yr)			(rate/100 pt-yr)			
>3-step sustained retinopathy	4.7	1.2	76	7.8	3.7	54	63
Severe nonproliferative or proliferative retinopathy	—	—	—	2.4	1.1	47	47
Laser treatment	—	—	—	2.3	0.9	56	51
Urinary albumin excretion							
≥40 mg/24 hr	3.4	2.2	34	5.7	3.6	43	39
≥300 mg/24 hr	0.3	0.2	44	1.4	0.6	56	54
Clinical neuropathy	9.8	3.1	69	16.1	1.0	57	60

Source: Adapted with permission from The Diabetes Control and Complications Trial Research Group, The Effect of Intensive Treatment of Diabetes on the Development and Progression of Long-Term Complications in Insulin–Dependent Diabetes Mellitus, *New England Journal of Medicine* (1993;329:977-986), Copyright © 1993, Massachusetts Medical Society.

therapy in the combined cohorts. Although there was a 41% reduction in the number of macrovascular events (myocardial infarction, stroke, amputation, etc), because of the small number of events occurring in each group, this was not statistically significant. LDL cholesterol levels were reduced significantly by intensive therapy, however. Hypoglycemic reactions were the most significant adverse event of intensive therapy, occurring at a two- to threefold increased rate. Over the course of the study, patients in the intensive group also gained, on average, 4.6 kg more than did patients in the conventional group.

Thus, the DCCT has now proved that intensive therapy, with the goal of achieving near-normoglycemia, is able to cause a marked reduction in the development and progression of retinopathy, nephropathy, neuropathy, and possibly macrovascular disease. However, this occurs at the expense of a two- to threefold increased risk of severe hypoglycemia and modest weight gain.[1] Challenges remain in how to implement intensive therapy safely and economically in the larger diabetes community. Although it is likely that improved glycemic control will result in a similar improvement in the long-term complications occurring in patients with NIDDM, this remains to be proved.[44] It is hoped that the Prospective Diabetes Study being carried out in the United Kingdom in patients with NIDDM will give a similar answer when it concludes.[45]

Eye Disease

Diabetes is the leading cause of new blindness between the ages of 20 and 74 in adults in the United States.[46] Vision-threatening proliferative diabetic retinopathy (PDR) may develop in as many as 50% of patients with IDDM and 13% of patients with NIDDM after 20 years of disease,[47] assuming conventional therapy for diabetic control has been used. About 63,000 new cases of PDR occur each year in the United States.[48] Ninety-five percent of this disability can be prevented by timely, proper ophthalmologic evalu-

ation and treatment.[46] Patients with IDDM should be seen by an ophthalmologist initially within 5 years of diagnosis and those with NIDDM within 1 year of diagnosis.[49] All patients should be seen at least yearly thereafter or more frequently if symptoms or other problems develop. Because some women experience a worsening of retinopathy during pregnancy, they should be screened before pregnancy and then during each trimester to assess for progression.[49]

Retinopathy

By 20 years after the initial diagnosis of diabetes, more than 95% of people with IDDM will have developed background diabetic retinopathy (BDR).[47] For people with NIDDM, this figure is about 80% for those who take insulin and 50% for those who do not take insulin.[47] However, as mentioned above, only about 50% of patients with IDDM and 13% of those with NIDDM progress to PDR, with pre-DCCT-type management of diabetes.[47] In BDR, leakage or blockage of small retinal vessels causes microaneurysms, hemorrhages, exudates, and edema that are visible with the ophthalmoscope. Vision is not usually impaired with background retinopathy. However, in 5 to 10% of people with background retinopathy, the edema at some time involves the macula, which is the area of high central visual acuity, and may cause impaired vision.[47] Laser photocoagulation may delay or prevent reduction in visual acuity when this occurs.[47] In proliferative retinopathy, it is thought that the retina becomes hypoxic because of the diseased vessels. This hypoxia results in the production of new blood vessels (neovascularization) on the surface of the retina. These fragile new vessels may hemorrhage more severely than the old vessels, often directly into the vitreous. Hemorrhage into the vitreous or over the macula results in loss of vision. New vessels may also regress, leaving a fibrous band that may contract and cause retinal detachment.[47]

As discussed above, the DCCT has demonstrated that improved metabolic control can significantly delay the initial development of the first microaneurysm and even more markedly retard the progression from less severe to more severe forms of retinopathy.[1] Laser photocoagulation has proved to be remarkably successful in retarding or preventing the progression from preproliferative to proliferative retinopathy.[47] Surgery can also be performed to remove vitreous material that contains hemorrhage and scarring (vitrectomy).[47]

Glaucoma

Glaucoma is a condition of increased intraocular pressure that has several causes and may damage the retinal nerve fiber layer. The risk of glaucoma is increased from 1.8% in the general population to 2.4% in individuals with NIDDM and by age 65, 7.5% of individuals with NIDDM have glaucoma.[50]

Cataracts

Cataracts are opacities developing in the lens of the eye that occur commonly as people age. However, the risk in people with diabetes is increased almost twofold and cataract formation is the most frequent cause of severe visual loss in individuals with NIDDM.[50] Cataracts seem to be one of the few complications of diabetes in which the accumulation of sorbitol can be directly implicated.[50] This sorbitol is not dietary sorbitol but rather glucose converted to sorbitol in the presence of aldose reductase, which is found in the lens. Cataract extraction is successful in restoring vision in more than 90% of patients.

Vascular Disease

Vascular complications are sometimes divided into macro- and microvascular disease. The former conditions are discussed in this section. Microvascular disease refers to retinal disease, renal glomerular disease, and certain neuropathies.

Coronary Artery Disease

Atherosclerotic coronary artery disease is the single most common cause of death in adults with diabetes in the United States.[32] The prevalence of ischemic heart disease is increased two- to threefold in diabetic men and three- to fourfold in diabetic women in comparison to matched nondiabetic controls.[32] Although the presence of coronary artery disease does not correlate well with the duration or severity of diabetes[32] at any age, someone with diabetes has more extensive coronary artery disease than a matched control.[51] Although myocardial infarctions are more commonly asymptomatic or "silent" in people with diabetes, perhaps due to coexisting cardiac sensory neuropathy, people with diabetes who have an acute myocardial infarction are three times more likely to have a fatal outcome.[32] This may be related to the overall tendency to more extensive coronary artery disease in diabetes. Long-term survival after a myocardial infarction similarly is markedly reduced in people with diabetes.[32] Manifestations of coronary artery disease other than myocardial infarctions, such as angina pectoris and congestive heart failure, are also increased two- to fourfold in people with diabetes.[32] The question of whether there exists a cardiomyopathy separate from macro- or microvascular disease remains controversial.[52]

Cerebrovascular Disease

The risk of stroke is increased two- to fourfold in people with diabetes and is generally of the ischemic occlusive type rather than hemorrhagic.[53] Strokes are more likely to result in death in people with diabetes compared with those without it.[53] Carotid artery occlusive disease not resulting in stroke is increased more than tenfold.[53] Risk factors for this occlusive disease include age, hypertension, and increased blood cholesterol.[53] Those with carotid artery narrowing also frequently have other complications of diabetes, such as retinopathy, proteinuria, and neuropathy.[53]

Peripheral Vascular Disease

Diabetes accounts for about 50% of all nontraumatic amputations in the United States.[54] Such amputations result from a combination of trauma to a foot that has impaired sensation from neuropathy and impaired circulation, with resultant poor healing and infection. Reduced peripheral circulation may result in pain in the legs during exertion (intermittent claudication), ulceration, and gangrene (extensive necrosis of the skin and underlying tissue). Intermittent claudication occurs at a fivefold increased rate compared with nondiabetic individuals.[54] These complications are increased by increasing age, duration of diabetes, elevation of blood glucose levels, hypercholesterolemia, hypertension, male sex, and smoking.[54] Nonetheless, it is not uncommon for gangrene of a toe to be the finding that initially causes the patient to seek medical attention. The duration of prior asymptomatic disease in such cases is unknown but could be many years.

Hypertension

Hypertension is two to three times more common in people with diabetes.[55] In both types of diabetes, essential hypertension may occur. However, when IDDM and hypertension are present, most patients have developing nephropathy, which may at the time of initial detection of hypertension be only at the microalbuminuric stage.[55] In such patients, treatment of the hypertension will slow the rate of progression of nephropathy.[56] Nonpharmacologic interventions such as weight loss, lowered dietary sodium, exercise, and restriction of alcohol intake are usually used initially and always concomitantly with pharmacologic agents.[55] Specific treatment with angiotensin-converting enzyme (ACE) inhibitors appears to have a selective additional benefit in slowing this rate of progression so that this class of antihypertensive medications has become the initial treatment of choice.[56] Many patients will have been started on ACE inhibitors because of the development of microalbuminuria even in the absence of hypertension, so that with the development of subsequent hypertension, the above nonpharmacologic maneuvers may be added.[56] In some individuals, the expanded intravascular fluid volume may exacerbate hypertension, and if dietary sodium restriction and ACE inhibitors are not fully effective, diuretics may be added. In general, diuretics are avoided because of their tendency to worsen glucose tolerance and raise LDL cholesterol levels.[56]

Patients with NIDDM may also have hypertension associated with nephropathy, but it much more commonly is associated with obesity, insulin resistance, hyperinsulinemia, and lipid abnormalities (see above). In patients with nephropathy, ACE inhibitors are again used early in treatment along with nonpharmacologic measures.[56] In those without nephropathy, great emphasis is placed on these nonpharmacologic measures, as they will overall reduce insulin resistance, blood pressure, and dyslipidemias.[55]

Because some patients with diabetes and hypertension and mild nephropathy have hyporeninemic hypoaldosteronism, ACE inhibitors may often bring out significant hyperkalemia. Because of the substantial special benefits of ACE inhibitors, they are often continued even under these circumstances. Dietary restriction of potassium is often necessary, and sometimes potassium-binding resins, such as Kayexalate, may be needed.

Neuropathy

By 20 years known duration of diabetes of either type, almost 50% of people will have neuropathy.[28] There are many different types of neuropathy (Table 2-3), with distal symmetric polyneuropathy being the most common and best known. It is this type of neuropathy that causes loss of sensation in the feet and hands, leading to foot injury and amputation. Distal polyneuropathy may be due to disordered sorbitol/myoinositol metabolism, and its onset can be delayed by improved glucose control.[1] As mentioned earlier, myoinositol feeding and aldose reductase inhibitors may cause some improvement.[26,28] Symptomatic relief of pain, usually a burning sensation in the feet, can also be achieved in some patients with tricyclic antidepressants, neuroleptic drugs, and topical capsaicin.[28] Radiculopathy occurs when a spinal nerve

Table 2-3 Diabetic Neuropathies

Neuropathy Type	Manifestations	Nerve Structure Involved
Polyneuropathy	Sensory loss and sometimes pain in feet and hands	Nerve terminals
Radiculopathy	Sensory loss and pain in dermatome distribution	Nerve root
Mononeuropathy	Sensory loss, pain, weakness in mixed nerve distribution	Mixed cranial or spinal nerve
Amyotrophy	Weakness, muscle atrophy, pain	Nerve terminal on muscle
Autonomic	Visceral disease	Autonomic nerves

root is affected, causing loss of sensation and pain along the affected dermatome. Occasionally, it may present as abdominal pain.[28] A mixed spinal or cranial nerve may also be affected, causing pain, loss of sensation, and weakness in its distribution. Cranial third nerve palsies (ptosis of the lid of one eye) fall in this category. These two types of neuropathy are probably due to occlusion of the small blood vessels supplying the affected nerve, and return of function over several months without any intervention is the rule.[28]

Amyotrophy is of uncertain etiology and causes weakness and wasting of muscles in the pelvic girdle in association with pain in these muscles and weight loss. There are no sensory changes.[28] Men with this syndrome may also experience impotence. When weight loss is particularly severe, this has been termed diabetic neuropathic cachexia.[57] Spontaneous recovery is the rule after about 1 year, although antidepressant therapy may speed this improvement. It is not clear whether this is truly a unique syndrome or whether depression is the root cause, brought on by the diagnosis and painful neuropathy and resulting in the impotence and weight loss. However, dietitians should be alert for unexplained weight loss in older men with diabetes who also have these associated symptoms.

Autonomic neuropathy involves nerves to the viscera and is perhaps the most disabling form of neuropathy. Patients with evidence of cardiac autonomic neuropathy have a significantly lower survival rate.[28] Of concern to dietitians are the abnormalities of the gastrointestinal tract that interfere with food absorption. Esophageal motility may be affected, especially in individuals with peripheral neuropathy.[28] When severe, it may cause dysphagia. Gastroparesis diabeticorum is a condition in which vagal neuropathy causes delayed gastric emptying.[28] This delay in gastric emptying often results in a mismatch between the therapeutic timing of insulin's peak action and absorption of food when the insulin is conventionally given before meals. The time of insulin administration should be delayed as long as necessary to correct this mismatch. Patients with this disorder usually complain of nausea, early satiety, and frequent vomiting. Often, the vomitus contains undigested food. Small meal sizes may be helpful. Such patients may benefit from treatment with metoclopramide (Reglan) and cisapride (Propulsid), drugs that work on smooth muscle to coordinate gastric, pyloric, and duodenal motor activity, thereby improving gastric emptying.[28] When given before meals and at bedtime, these drugs have been found to be very helpful in reducing symptoms and improving gastric emptying in controlled trials.[28]

Uncontrollable diarrhea, especially nocturnal, is another manifestation of autonomic neuropathy affecting intestinal peristalsis. Steatorrhea is present in 30 to 50% of patients with diarrhea.[28] Bacterial overgrowth is occasionally present, and some improvement may be seen in some patients with rotating antibiotic therapy.[28]

When bile salt retention contributes, bile salt chelation with cholestyramine may be beneficial.[28] If steatorrhea is present, some patients benefit from pancreatic enzyme supplements.[28] Also, some patients respond to clonidine, an α-adrenergic agonist that is thought to stimulate the cells of the gut mucosa to resorb fluid and electrolytes.[28] Octreotide, a somatostatin analog, and lithium have also been tried.[28] The usual dietary changes recommended in the presence of diarrhea may be of some help as well. Autonomic neuropathy may also affect the bladder, causing urinary retention; sexual organs, causing impotence; and heart and blood vessels, causing tachycardia and orthostatic hypotension.[28]

Nephropathy

Diabetic nephropathy develops in about one-third of people with IDDM and 5 to 10% of people with NIDDM by 20 to 25 years' duration of diabetes.[50,58,59] The nature of diabetic nephropathy and the specific concerns for the dietitian are discussed in detail in Chapter 23.

Other Complications

Infections

The presence of an infection often causes a worsening of diabetes control. Conversely, diabetes itself may predispose to certain specific infections, such as a severe external otitis due to *Pseudomonas*, a severe sinus infection due to the fungus mucormycosis, urinary tract infections, vulvovaginal candidiasis, tuberculosis, pneumonia due to gram-negative organisms and *Staphylococcus*, gallbladder infections, and skin and soft tissue staphylococcal and necrotizing mixed aerobic and anaerobic infections.[60] Often candidiasis may be the presenting complaint leading to the diagnosis of diabetes. Periodontal and gum infections may also be more common.[61] This propensity to infections may be related to the known deleterious effects of hyperglycemia on leukocyte chemotaxis, phagocytosis, and bactericidal activity.[62,63]

Osteopenia

Osteopenia has been found in many patients with both IDDM and NIDDM in excess of what would be expected for age and sex.[64] No specific abnormalities of calcium, vitamin D, parathyroid, or bone metabolism have yet been found as the cause of this problem.[65]

Pancreatic Exocrine Insufficiency

Mild-to-moderate impairment of the secretion of amylase, trypsin, chymotrypsin, lipase, and bicarbonate has been found in many subjects with both IDDM and NIDDM.[66-68] In one study, the degree of deficiency was related to the duration of diabetes,[68] but in another it was not.[66] Improvement of diabetic control resulted in some improvement in enzyme secretion.[68] Clinically, there are no signs of exocrine insufficiency in these patients. However, Harano et al.[68] demonstrated that 50 g of carbohydrate as starch resulted in significantly lower blood glucose levels than 50 g of carbohydrate as maltose in subjects with diabetes.[68] In nondiabetic subjects, the attained glucose levels were the same with both forms of carbohydrate. These data suggest that the decrease in amylase may actually be of some clinical significance.

REFERENCES

1. Diabetes Control and Complications Trial Research Group. The effect of intensive treatment of diabetes on the development and progression of long-term complications in insulin-dependent diabetes mellitus. *N Engl J Med*. 1993;329:977–986.

2. Fishbein HA. Diabetic ketoacidosis, hyperosmolar nonketotic coma, lactic acidosis, and hypoglycemia. In: Harris MI, Hamman RF, eds. *Diabetes in America*. 1985;XII,1–22. NIH Publication no. 85-1468.

3. Berger W, Keller U. Treatment of diabetic ketoacidosis and non-ketotic hyperosmolar diabetic coma. *Bailliere's Clin Endocrinol Metab*. 1992;6:1–22.

4. Fleckman AM. Diabetic ketoacidosis. *Endocrinol Metab Clin North Am*. 1993;22:181–207.

5. Siperstein MD. Diabetic ketoacidosis and hyperosmolar coma. *Endocrinol Metab Clin North Am*. 1992;21:415–432.

6. DeFronzo RA, Matsuda M, Barrett EJ. Diabetic ketoacidosis. A combined metabolic-nephrologic approach to therapy. *Diabetes Rev.* 1994;2:209–238.

7. Warshaw AL, Feller ER, Lee KH. On the cause of raised serum-amylase in diabetic ketoacidosis. *Lancet.* 1977;1:929–931.

8. Molitch ME, Rodman E, Hirsch CA, et al. Spurious serum creatinine elevations in ketoacidosis. *Ann Intern Med.* 1980;93:280–281.

9. Heber D, Molitch ME, Sperling MA. Low-dose continuous insulin therapy for diabetic ketoacidosis. *Arch Intern Med.* 1977;137:1377–1380.

10. Ennis ED, Stahl EJVB, Kreisberg RA. The hyperosmolar hyperglycemic syndrome. *Diabetes Rev.* 1994;2:115–126.

11. Hofeldt FD, Dippe S, Forsham PH. Diagnosis and classification of reactive hypoglycemia based on hormonal changes in response to oral and intravenous glucose administration. *Am J Clin Nutr.* 1972;25:1193–1201.

12. Permutt MA. Postprandial hypoglycemia. *Diabetes.* 1976;25:719–736.

13. Groop LC. Sulfonylureas in NIDDM. *Diabetes Care.* 1992;15:737–754.

14. Tamborlane WV, Amiel SA. Hypoglycemia in the treated diabetic patient. *Endocrinol Metab Clin North Am.* 1992;21:313–327.

15. Cryer PE. Iatrogenic hypoglycemia as a cause of hypoglycemia-associated autonomic failure in IDDM. A vicious cycle. *Diabetes.* 1992;41:255.

16. Gerich J, Mokan M, Veneman T, Korytkowski M, Mitrakou A. Hypoglycemic unawareness. *Endocrinol Rev.* 1991;12:356–371.

17. Cryer PE, Fisher JN, Shamoon H. Hypoglycemia. *Diabetes Care.* 1994;17:734–755.

18. Brodows RG, Williams C, Amatruda JM. Treatment of insulin reactions in diabetics. *JAMA.* 1984;252:3378–3381.

19. Rubin RJ, Altman WM, Mendelson DN. Health care expenditures for people with diabetes mellitus, 1992. *J Clin Endocrinol Metab.* 1994;78:809A–809F.

20. Entmacher PS, Sinnock P, Bostic E, et al. Economic impact of diabetes. In: Harris MI, Hamman RF, eds. *Diabetes in America.* 1985;XXX,1–13. NIH Publication no. 185-1468.

21. Sinnock P. Hospital utilization for diabetes. In: Harris MI, Hamman RF, eds. *Diabetes in America.* 1985; XXVI,1–11. NIH Publication no. 85-1468.

22. Drury TF. Disability among adult diabetics. In: Harris MI, Hamman RF, eds. *Diabetes in America.* 1985; XXVIII,1–22. NIH Publication no. 85-1468.

23. Harris MI, Entmacher P. Mortality from diabetes. In: Harris MI, Hamman RF, eds. *Diabetes in America.* 1985; XXIX,1–48. NIH Publication no. 85-1468.

24. Dorman JS, LaPorte RE. Mortality in insulin-dependent diabetes. In: Harris MI, Hamman RF, eds. *Diabetes in America.* 1985;XXX,1–9. NIH Publication no. 85-1468.

25. Winegrad AI. Banting lecture 1986: does a common mechanism induce the diverse complications of diabetes? *Diabetes.* 1987;36:396–406.

26. Greene DA, Sima AAF, Stevens MJ, Feldman EL, Lattimer SA. Complications: neuropathy, pathogenetic considerations. *Diabetes Care.* 1992;15:1902–1925.

27. Mandarino LJ. Current hypotheses for the biochemical basis of diabetic retinopathy. *Diabetes Care.* 1992;15:1892–1901.

28. Vinik AI, Liuzzi FJ, Holland MT, Stansberry KB, LeBeau J, Colen LB. Diabetic neuropathies. *Diabetes Care.* 1992;15:1926–1975.

29. Brownlee M. Glycation products and the pathogenesis of diabetic complications. *Diabetes Care.* 1992;15:1835–1843.

30. Vlassara H. Recent progress on the biologic and clinical significance of advanced glycosylation end products. *J Lab Clin Med.* 1994;124:19–30.

31. Reddi AS. Diabetic microangiopathy. 1. Current status of the chemistry and metabolism of the glomerular basement membrane. *Metabolism.* 1978;27:107–124.

32. Donohue RP, Orchard TJ. Diabetes mellitus and macrovascular complications. *Diabetes Care.* 1992; 15:1141–1155.

33. Schwartz CJ, Kelley JL, Valente AJ, Cayatte AJ, Sprague EA, Rozek MM. Pathogenesis of the atherosclerotic lesion. Implications for diabetes mellitus. *Diabetes Care.* 1992;15:1156–1167.

34. Reaven GM. Insulin resistance and compensatory hyperinsulinemia: role in hypertension, dyslipidemia, and coronary heart disease. *Am Heart J.* 1991;121:1283.

35. Karam JH. Type II diabetes and syndrome X: pathogenesis and glycemic management. *Endocrinol Metab Clin North Am.* 1992;21:329–351.

36. Deckert T, Kofoed-Enevoldsen A, Nørgaard K, Borch-Johnsen K, Feldt-Rasmussen B, Jensen T. Microalbuminuria. Implications for micro- and macrovascular disease. *Diabetes Care.* 1992;15:1181–1191.

37. Viberti G-C, Yip-Messent J, Morocutti A. Diabetic nephropathy. Future avenue. *Diabetes Care.* 1992;15:1216–1225.

38. The Kroc Collaborative Study Group. Blood glucose control and the evolution of diabetic retinopathy and albuminuria. A preliminary multicenter trial. *N Engl J Med* . 1984;311:365-372.

39. Beck-Nielsen H, Richelsen B, Mogensen CE, et al. Effect of insulin pump treatment for one year on renal function and retinal morphology in patients with IDDM. *Diabetes Care.* 1985;8:585-589.

40. Lauritzen T, Frost-Larsen K, Larsen HW, Deckert T for the Steno Study Group. Two years' experience with continuous subcutaneous insulin infusion in relation to retinopathy and neuropathy. *Diabetes.* 1985;34(suppl 3):74–79.

41. Feldt-Rasmussen B, Mathiesen ER, Deckert T. Effect of two years of strict metabolic control on progression of incipient nephropathy in insulin-dependent diabetes. *Lancet.* 1986;2:1300–1304.

42. Dahl-Jørgensen K, Hanssen KF, Kierulf P, Bjøro T, Sandvik L, Aagenæs Ø. Reduction of urinary albumin excretion after 4 years of continuous subcutaneous insulin infusion in insulin-dependent diabetes mellitus. The Oslo Study. *Acta Endocrinol (Copenh).* 1988;117:19–25.

43. Reichard P, Nilsson B-Y, Rosenqvist U. The effect of long-term intensified insulin treatment on the development of microvascular complications of diabetes mellitus. *N Engl J Med.* 1993;329:304–309.

44. Eastman RC, Sievert CW, Harris M, Gorden P. Implications of the Diabetes Control and Complications Trial. *J Clin Endocrinol Metab.* 1993;77:1105–1107.

45. UK Prospective Diabetes Study Group. UK Prospective Diabetes Study (UKPDS). VII. Study design, progress and performance. *Diabetologia.* 1991;34:877–890.

46. Klein R. Eye-care delivery for people with diabetes. An unmet need. *Diabetes Care.* 1994;17:614–615.

47. Davis MD. Diabetic retinopathy. A clinical overview. *Diabetes Care.* 1992;15:1844–1874.

48. Klein R, Klein BEK, Moss SE. Epidemiology of proliferative diabetic retinopathy. *Diabetes Care.* 1992;15:1875–1891.

49. Screening guidelines for diabetic retinopathy. *Ann Intern Med.* 1992;116:683–685.

50. Herman WH. Eye disease and nephropathy in NIDDM. *Diabetes Care.* 1990;13(suppl 2):24–29.

51. Vigorita VJ, Moore GW, Nutchins GM. Absence of correlation between coronary arterial atherosclerosis and severity or duration of diabetes mellitus of adult onset. *Am J Cardiol.* 1980;46:535–542.

52. Sunni S, Bishop SP, Kent SP, et al. Diabetic cardiomyopathy. *Arch Pathol Lab Med.* 1986;110:375–381.

53. Biller J, Love BB. Diabetes and stroke. *Med Clin North Am.* 1993;77(3):1–16.

54. Bild DE, Selby JV, Sinnock P, Browner WS, Braveman P, Showstack JA. Lower extremity amputation in people with diabetes. Epidemiology and prevention. *Diabetes Care.* 1989;12:24–31.

55. Arauz-Pacheco C, Raskin P. Management of hypertension in diabetes. *Endocrinol Metab Clin North Am.* 1992;21:371–394.

56. Molitch ME. ACE inhibitors and diabetic nephropathy. *Diabetes Care.* 1994;17:756–760.

57. Ellenberg M. Diabetic neuropathic cachexia. *Diabetes.* 1974;23:418–422.

58. Breyer JA. Diabetic nephropathy in insulin-dependent patients. *Am J Kidney Dis.* 1992;20:533–547.

59. Humphrey LL, Ballard DJ. Renal complications in non-insulin-dependent diabetes mellitus. *Clin Geriatr Med.* 1990;6:807–825.

60. Wheat LJ. Infection and diabetes mellitus. *Diabetes Care.* 1980;3:187–197.

61. Williams RC Jr, Mahan CJ. Periodontal disease and diabetes in young adults. *JAMA.* 1960;172:776–778.

62. Rayfield EJ, Ault MJ, Keusch GT, et al. Infection and diabetes: the case for glucose control. *Am J Med.* 1982;72:439–450.

63. Marhoffer W, Stein M, Maeser E, Federlin K. Impairment of polymorphonuclear leukocyte function and metabolic control of diabetes. *Diabetes Care.* 1992;15:256–260.

64. Hui SL, Epstein S, Johnston CC Jr. A prospective study of bone mass in patients with type I diabetes. *J Clin Endocrinol Metab.* 1985;60:74–80.

65. Heath H III, Lambert PW, Service FJ, et al. Calcium homeostasis in diabetes mellitus. *J Clin Endocrinol Metab.* 1979;49:462–466.

66. Domschke W, Tympner F, Domschke S, et al. Exocrine pancreatic function in juvenile diabetics. *Dig Dis.* 1975;20:309–311.

67. Frier M, Saunders JHB, Wormsley KG, et al. Exocrine pancreatic function in juvenile-onset diabetes mellitus. *Gut.* 1976;17:685–691.

68. Harano Y, Kim IC, Kang M, et al. External pancreatic dysfunction associated with diabetes mellitus. *J Lab Clin Med.* 1978;91:780–790.

Part II

Setting and Achieving Management Goals

Chapter 3

Medical Nutrition Therapy for Diabetes

Margaret A. Powers

Medical nutrition therapy (MNT) for diabetes requires the application of nutritional, medical, and behavioral sciences. The combination of these three disciplines provides the dietitian with an exciting opportunity to affect positively the health and well-being of people with diabetes.

This impact is because MNT is integral to diabetes care. Food selection, preparation, and portion size, and timing of consumption affects the diabetes medication prescription, activity adjustments, and achievement of diabetes goals. Food also is a focus of much of what diabetes educators teach including exercise, hypoglycemia, insulin adjustment/algorithms, timing and frequency of blood glucose monitoring, evaluating blood glucose monitoring records, and prevention/treatment of complications such as hypertension, nephropathy, and gastroparesis.

Prior to teaching clients about exercise, hypoglycemia, insulin adjustment, etc., the health care team needs to know what food choices the client is making and what changes they might be willing and able to make, if necessary. Too frequently this information is not obtained and integrated into diabetes care due to the lack of an experienced dietitian on the diabetes care team and/or inadequate intervention time with the dietitian for the client to learn self-management skills and behaviors. Health care teams need to accommodate their practices to offer clients this needed therapy and should seek reimbursement for it.

MNT includes:

- assessing nutritional, medical, and social behaviors that influence food choices and medical conditions
- developing a nutrition prescription based on usual eating behaviors and medical needs
- recommending medication/therapy changes to the primary care provider
- providing self-management training
- evaluating therapy outcomes

This chapter reviews past interest in nutrition in diabetes care and summarizes current nutrition therapy recommendations. The reader is encouraged to refer to individual chapters that explore these nutritional recommendations, intervention strategies, and reimbursement practices in further detail.

PAST FOCUS ON NUTRITION THERAPY

Before Insulin

Nutrition therapy was the focus of diabetes management before the discovery of insulin. Many theories and approaches have been recommended and have re-emerged over the years (see also Appendix 3-A). In 1550 BC, even before it was known that glucose was involved in diabetes, high-carbohydrate diets were prescribed.

Later, in the 6th century, it was thought that consuming starchy foods was the cause of diabetes, and a low-carbohydrate diet was advocated. In the 17th century, high-carbohydrate diets returned as a means to replace sugar lost in the urine. In the 18th century, high-protein and high-fat diets were typical. Concern was raised about the palatability of the diet in both the 18th and 19th centuries. It was recognized that, if the diet was not tolerated, it would not be followed. Yet, the primary nutrition theme continued to be one of high fat, low carbohydrate, and low calorie. At the same time, a few individuals were still convinced that the diet needed to replace lost sugar and recommended diets high in carbohydrate (milk, rice, potatoes, or oats).

1921 to 1950

The focus on nutrition changed after the discovery of insulin in 1921. Insulin was viewed as a miracle[1] as it saved lives through its anabolic and anticatabolic roles (promotes the storage of carbohydrate, protein, and fat and prevents the degradation of their storage components). Food intake could be increased and nutritional status improved. As insulin use increased, became more purified, and had fairly standard actions, it was clear that a consistent food intake was needed.

In 1935, E.P. Joslin wrote, "In teaching diabetic patients their diet, I lay emphasis on carbohydrate values, and teach to a few only the values for protein and fat.... If a patient will grasp the carbohydrate values of seven types of food and use his common sense, he will seldom make egregious errors." He goes on to note, "Diabetic patients have too much to do in their daily work to be encumbered with unnecessary details of arithmetic. An attempt to force accuracy to the extent of a gram may result in loss of accuracy to the extent of an ounce by the patient giving up weighing entirely."[2] This thoughtful perspective remains important today.

1950s to 1960s

Many exciting events have occurred since 1950 and are reviewed in detail elsewhere.[3] The exchange system, in 1950, was developed through a collaborative effort of the American Dietetic Association, American Diabetes Association (ADA), and the diabetes branch of the U.S. Public Health Service to develop consensus on food values and design a simplified method of meal planning.[4] This committee was not en-

tirely comfortable with the term "exchange," but there was agreement on an alternative term.[5] The preplanned diets that resulted were not originally intended for widespread distribution to patients. They were to serve as the basis of management in "average" cases of diabetes.[6] Their use expanded because (1) they saved the dietitian calculation time when education time was limited, and (2) other health professionals distributed them independent of the dietitian.[3] This resulted in a diminished focus on individualizing nutrition care, which was not the intent of the group designing the system for meal planning.

1970s to 1980s

With the emergence of the self-help movement in the mid-late 1970s, the need to listen to the client's concerns helped focus attention on education and behavioral change. Self-monitoring of blood glucose (SMBG) became available at this time and increased in accessibility throughout the 1980s. Several nutrition issues in the 1980s helped focus attention on nutrition, including the approval of several low-calorie sweeteners, increased choices of lower-calorie foods, and research on glycemic index, fiber, starch blockers, and fish oils. There appeared to be an interest in finding the "miracle" that would make nutrition therapy easier. However, what often was needed was individualized nutrition therapy. Lack of reimbursement for nutrition therapy hindered referrals to a dietitian. The distribution of preprinted exchange diets, which many clients thought were too restrictive and not conducive to their eating preferences, diminished clients' interest in nutrition education.

The emphasis on the exchange system for all persons with diabetes was shifting by the early 1980s. Despite the need to individualize nutrition intervention and provide ongoing nutrition education, lack of reimbursement continued to hinder proper nutrition therapy for many persons with diabetes. One or two short sessions for nutrition intervention were not conducive to individualizing the meal plan and to providing adequate self-management training, which contributed to the perceived inadequacy of nutrition therapy.

1990s

Health care reform challenges in the mid-1990s struggled to include nutrition therapy as a reimbursable service.[7] In the early 1990s the Diabetes Care and Education Practice Group of the American Dietetic Association, published four papers summarizing nutrition therapy for non–insulin-dependent diabetes mellitus (NIDDM, type II diabetes), adults with insulin-dependent diabetes (IDDM, type I diabetes), children and adolescents with IDDM, and pregnancy and diabetes.[8–11] In 1994, the American Diabetes Association revised its nutrition recommendations.[12] Many were startled because it did not specify the percentage of calories from carbohydrate and fat and it stated that sucrose and other simple sugars could be included in a diabetic meal plan (see Table 3-1). The position paper stresses the need for a nutrition assessment before developing a nutrition prescription and management plan as well as the importance of

an experienced dietitian as part of the diabetes care team.

The Diabetes Control and Complications Trial (DCCT) results announced in 1993 set an agenda for diabetes care that focuses on achieving euglycemia. The DCCT results demonstrate that any improvement in blood glucose control makes a difference in delaying the onset and progression of diabetes complications.[13] From the DCCT model we learned that

1. nutrition can now be considered the most critical and pivotal component of diabetes care in achieving target blood glucose goals for persons with IDDM or NIDDM
2. dietitians are true partners in diabetes care and research and should make management recommendations beyond diet.[14]

Dietitians were influential in screening patients for the study protocols and determining their ability to make and maintain behavioral changes, as well as providing intensive nutrition therapy, and self-management training and recommending changes to improve overall care.[15] This type of nutrition-focused care has become the model for diabetes medical nutrition therapy.

Table 3-1 Overview of Calorie Distributions in Diabetic Diets

Date	Distribution of Calories (%)		
	Carbohydrate	Protein	Fat
1921[a]	20	10	70
1950[b]	40	20	40
1971[c]	45	20	35
1979[c]	50–60	12–20	<35
1986[c]	up to 55–60	0.8 g/kg[d]	<30
1994[c]	Varies[e]	10–20	Varies[f]

[a] Distribution of diet offered first person on insulin.

[b] Distribution of first exchange diets.

[c] Recommendations by the American Diabetes Association.

[d] Usually 12 to 20% of total calories.

[e] Based on nutrition assessment.

[f] Less than 10% saturated fat.

CURRENT AND FUTURE NUTRITION PRACTICE

We now see increased emphasis on individualized nutrition therapy and the DCCT approach to diabetes care.[12–15] The current role of the dietitian in diabetes care is defined in the 1995 Scope of Practice Paper[16] (see Exhibit 3-1). It outlines responsibilities of dietetic practitioners with varying levels of credentialing. The dietitian is a crucial member of the diabetes health team whose expertise helps shape the diabetes treatment plan.

Nutrition Practice Guidelines

Nutrition practice guidelines for type I and II diabetes provide further guidance and expecta-

Exhibit 3-1 Scope of Practice for Qualified Dietetics Professionals in Diabetes Care and Education

Dietetic Practitioner	Responsibilities
Dietetic Technician, Registered (DTR)	• Completes a nutrition assessment • Provides basic diabetes nutrition information • Explains restaurant dining and alcohol use guidelines • Provides label-reading guidelines • Recommends use of modified foods, as appropriate • Collaborates and communicates with health care providers (MD, RN, RD, etc)
Registered Dietitian (RD)	All the above, plus the following • Negotiates nutrition goals with the client • Provides individualized eating plan (not just an exchange list; may use any other meal-planning approach) • Recommends and implements modifications to eating plan to address complications of diabetes • Recommends behavior modification, as appropriate • Evaluates and adjusts patient's meal plan and goals based on blood glucose levels • Explains management of hypoglycemia and hyperglycemia • Provides sick day guidelines for food intake • Develops/maintains educational resources appropriate to practice needs • Monitors outcomes of medical nutrition therapy and revises therapy as needed • Monitors and collects data on referral patterns and reimbursement practices • Advocates for legislation to improve diabetes care • Participates as a member of the multidisciplinary diabetes care team • Uses a variety of nutrition intervention and behavioral management approaches • Coordinates exercise and nutrition management strategies
Registered Dietitian, Certified Diabetes Educator (RD/CDE)	All the above, plus the following • Provides in-depth information on the pathophysiology of diabetes and overview of diabetes management • Provides sick day management guidelines, beyond food intake • Teaches the use of blood glucose meters, in some cases • Interprets blood glucose results and discusses adjustments in food, insulin, or medication • Interprets appropriate laboratory results and recommends changes in therapy • Reviews the impact of insulin preparation and injection skills/techniques, in some cases • Guides clients to establish problem-solving skills • Assists with client selection as candidates for intensive insulin therapy • Recommends protocols to ensure quality diabetes care • Refers clients to other team members, as appropriate

Source: Reprinted with permission from Diabetes Care and Education Practice Group. Scope of Practice for Qualified Dietetics Professionals in Diabetes Care and Education. *Journal of the American Dietetic Association* (1995;95:607–608), Copyright © 1995, American Dietetic Association.

tions as to the role of the dietitian in diabetes care and provide guidelines for nutrition intervention.[17,18] They take the current nutrition recommendations and outline timeframes for intervention and expected outcomes (see Appendixes 3-B and 3-C). Evaluating the appropriateness of the nutrition prescription and intervention plan requires more than a periodic weight check. The dietitian needs to be involved in monitoring blood glucose records, glycated hemoglobin values, lipid profiles, albuminuria, blood pressure, and other pertinent laboratory values and physical signs and symptoms.

Education Materials/Meal-Planning Approaches

New education materials developed in 1995 by many dietitian volunteers of the American Dietetic Association and the American Diabetes Association strengthen the commitment of both organizations to individualize the educational approach to meal planning used to fulfill the nutrition prescription.[19]

The Future

As we look at the future of diabetes care, it is clear that scientific advances will provide improved technology to detect and monitor diabetes, as well as new medications and improved delivery methods. These changes must not detract from the importance of MNT. Advances in nutrition therapy need to center around methods to improve behavioral change, as that is the major challenge that faces most persons with diabetes. Also, access to nutrition therapy and self-management training for all persons with diabetes is a critical advance that needs to be made in the health care delivery system to improve diabetes care outcomes.

CLINICAL GOALS AND NUTRITION RECOMMENDATIONS

The current clinical goals of medical nutrition therapy for diabetes are listed in Exhibit 3-2. These goals provide overall direction to nutrition therapy. It may be most practical to focus on one goal at a time, which will usually have a positive impact on another goal. The challenge in nutrition therapy is to develop a nutrition prescription and intervention plan that will be followed and optimizes the individual's ability to achieve these goals.

Specific nutrition intake recommendations are given in Exhibit 3-3. Percentage of calories

Exhibit 3-2 Clinical Goals of Medical Nutrition Therapy

1. ***Achieve and maintain as near-normal blood glucose levels as possible*** by balancing food intake with insulin (either endogenous or exogenous) or oral glucose-lowering medications and activity levels

2. ***Achieve optimal blood lipid levels***

3. ***Provide adequate calories*** for maintaining or attaining reasonable weights for adults, normal growth and development rates in children and adolescents, increased metabolic needs during pregnancy and lactation, or recovery from catabolic illnesses

4. ***Prevent, delay, or treat nutrition-related risk factors or complications*** such as hypoglycemia, short-term illness, exercise-related problems, renal disease, autonomic neuropathy, hypertension, and cardiovascular disease

5. ***Improve or maintain overall health through optimal nutrition***

Source: Adapted with permission from American Diabetes Association. Nutrition recommendations and principles for people with diabetes mellitus (position statement). *Diabetes Care.* 1995;18 (suppl 1):16–19, Copyright © 1995, Amercian Diabetes Association.

or distribution of food is not specified so that individualization of each is emphasized. Although the American Diabetes Association in each of its past nutrition recommendations has stressed individualization, when percentages are provided for the macronutrients, they have been too quickly defined as the prescription for all persons with diabetes. Therefore, the 1994 recommendations do not give a total percentage for carbohydrate or fat, whereas protein intake is based on the recommended dietary allowance (RDA).[11]

Setting Goals

Specific clinical and behavioral goals should be discussed, negotiated, and established with each individual client. Short-term goals should

Exhibit 3-3 Nutrition Recommendations for Persons with Diabetes

	Nutrition Recommendations and Principles
Calories	• Sufficient to attain and/or maintain a reasonable body weight for adults, normal growth and development for children and adolescents, and increased to meet needs during pregnancy and lactation or for recovery from catabolic illness • Reasonable body weight is defined as the weight an individual and health care provider acknowledge as achievable and maintainable, both short term and long term
Protein	• 10–20% of daily calories—no less than adult RDA (0.8 g/kg per day) with evidence of macroalbuminuria; adjust for very young children, pregnant and lactating women, and some elderly

Fat	• Individualized, based on the nutrition assessment and treatment goals
	For those older than 2 years old:
	  –Saturated fat <10% of daily calories, <7% with elevated low-density
	    lipoproteins
	  –Polyunsaturated fat up to 10% of total calories
	  –Predominately monounsaturated fat
	• Total fat varies with treatment goals
	  – ~30%—normal weight and normal lipids
	  – <30%—obese, elevated low-density lipoproteins
	  – ~<40%—elevated triglycerides unresponsive to fat restriction and weight loss

Cholesterol	<300 mg/d
Carbohydrate	• Individualized based on the patient's eating habits • Difference after protein and fat goals have been met • Total amount more important than the source • Percentage and distribution vary with insulin regimens and treatment goals
Sweeteners	• Sucrose need not be restricted, must be substituted as carbohydrate • Nutritive sweeteners (fructose, sugar alcohols) have no advantage over sucrose • Nonnutritive sweeteners approved by the Food and Drug Administration (acesulfame-K, aspartame, saccharin) are safe to consume
Fiber	• 20–35 g/d, same as general population • Generally not beneficial to glycemic control at these amounts
Sodium	• <3000 mg/d, same as general population • <2400 mg/d in mild-to-moderate hypertension • <2000 mg/d with nephropathy, hypertension, and edema
Alcohol	• Moderate usage (ie, <2 alcoholic beverages daily for adults unless otherwise indicated) (eg, alcohol abuse, hypertriglyceridemia)
Vitamins/Minerals	• Same as general population • Magnesium replacement possibly needed if at high risk—glycosuria, ketoacidosis • If at high risk, determine if replacement is necessary with laboratory test

Source: Adapted with permission from American Diabetes Association. Nutrition recommendations and principles for people with diabetes mellitus (position statement). *Diabetes Care.* 1995;18(suppl 1):16–19, Copyright © 1995, American Diabetes Association.

Exhibit 3-4 Examples of Short-Term Goals

Type of Short-Term Goal	More Challenging Goal	More Achievable Goal
Behavioral	Keep food record for 1 month	Keep food record for 4 days
Behavioral	Eat breakfast at 7:00 everyday	Eat breakfast at 7:00 on work days and at 8:00 on nonwork days
Behavioral	Test blood glucose levels before all meals, 1.5 hours postprandially, and at bedtime for next 2 weeks	Test with noted frequency for 3 days, then call dietitian
Clinical	Keep all premeal blood glucose levels at less than 115	Keep 75% of premeal blood glucose levels at less than 120

be achievable in a short period of time; if they are not, perhaps they are not the right goals for that individual. Examples are found in Exhibit 3-4.

Long-term goals take more time to achieve and build on the achievement of short-term goals. Each individual should be set up for success when establishing goals. Communicating with the team facilitates selecting the best goals for an individual while remembering that the person with diabetes is most important in establishing goals. The dietitian may wish to use the change framework presented in Exhibit 3-5 when discussing goals with the client and team.

NUTRITION PRESCRIPTION

One step in nutrition therapy that has frustrated many dietitians is receiving a nutrition prescription (diet order) that has been based only on a person's height and weight rather than their eating habits, life style, ability to change, support systems, and cultural, ethnic, and financial considerations. The 1994 ADA Nutrition Recommendations and the Nutrition Practice Guidelines state that a nutrition assessment is necessary before writing a nutrition prescription. This can be compared with the need to complete a physical and medical assessment before writing a medication prescription.

Some physicians will request that the dietitian write the prescription; in other cases, the physician must legally be the one to write the pre-

---

Exhibit 3-5 Framework for Implementing Health Behavior Changes

Step 1. Immediate Plan—This plan is developed based on a minimal assessment and is initiated quickly. It is necessary when there is inadequate time for a full assessment (eg, a meal tray is needed on admission to the hospital).

Step 2. Goal-Directed Plan—This plan is based on achievable short-term goals agreed on by the client and diabetes educator.

Step 3. Realistic Plan—This plan includes the maximum changes that the client is capable of making.

Step 4. Optimal Plan—This is the ideal meal plan that would coincide perfectly with the client's eating habits, life style, and medical needs. It would result in the achievement of optimum clinical goals.

Source: Adapted from MA Powers and PD Cook. The process of diabetic meal planning, in A Van Son, ed. *Diabetes and Patient Education: A Daily Nursing Challenge* (p 54) with permission of Appleton & Lange, © 1982.

Table 3-2 Strategies for Diabetes Medical Nutrition Therapy

Strategy	IDDM	NIDDM[a] Obese	NIDDM[a] Nonobese	Gestational Diabetes	Impaired Glucose Tolerance
Regular timing of meals	H	M	M	H	L
Consistency of day-to-day intake	H	M	M	H	L
Meal spacing	M	H	M	M	L
Fat modification[b]	M	H	H	M	H
Sucrose limitation	M	M	M	M	M
Exercise	M	H	H	M	H
Exercise snack	H	L	L	M	L
Caloric restriction	L	M	L	L[c]	M[d]
Other nutritional variables[e]	M	M	M	M	M
Blood glucose monitoring	H	H	H	H	L

Note: H, high priority; M, moderate priority; L, low priority.

[a] Persons taking insulin may need to follow more closely IDDM strategies of timing and consistency.

[b] Partially dependent on blood lipid levels.

[c] Weight gain should follow weight grid for pregnancy.

[d] If overweight, weight reduction is encouraged.

[e] Dependent on other medical conditions (eg, hypertension, renal disease, food allergies).

scription. It is the dietitian's responsibility to review the nutrition prescription once the nutrition assessment is complete. The prescription should reflect the individual's therapy goals as well as the nutrition assessment.

When obtaining a nutrition consult or making a referral for nutrition therapy, the physician may write a general nutrition prescription such as (1) diabetic meal plan to achieve clinical goals of diabetes nutrition therapy, (2) nutrition therapy to achieve as near-normal blood glucose as possible, (3) a meal plan to improve diabetes control and blood lipids, (4) a diet for improved glycemia, or (5) a diet for diabetes and hypertension. A physician's presciption may facilitate reimbursement for medical nutrition therapy.

The dietitian can further define the nutrition prescription by summarizing the meal plan/nutrition therapy intervention:

- weight reduction meal plan based on general eating guidelines, 1200 to 1500 calories, three meals and one snack; client will be seen three times over the next 2 months

- 2400-mg-sodium meal plan, weight maintenance

- carbohydrate-counting meal plan, adjusting carbohydrate and meal timing to achieve target blood glucose goals

NUTRITION THERAPY STRATEGIES

Nutrition therapy strategies differ for the various types of diabetes and are summarized in Table 3-2. Persons with type I diabetes need to be more consistent with their food intake than those with type II diabetes, making portion sizes and macronutrient (especially carbohydrate) content of their diet key educational concepts. Those with type II diabetes are often overweight, making weight management a frequent priority. Because only a 10- to 20-lb weight loss is needed to obtain an improvement in metabolic control, less emphasis is being placed on weight loss for ongoing therapy.[12,20] A continuous emphasis on weight loss often burdens the client with behavioral goals that may be unobtainable or not maintainable. Refocusing nutrition therapy on metabolic control for those with type II diabetes may result in a secondary benefit—weight loss.

The pregnant woman who has previously diagnosed diabetes (either IDDM or NIDDM) generally follows strategies for the person with IDDM. Persons with impaired glucose intolerance should follow guidelines for a healthy diet and life style. These guidelines include emphasizing the nutritional recommendations in Exhibit 3-3, increasing activity, and reducing stress. It is not mandatory to be extremely rigid about these approaches but rather sound, practical advice should be provided that may prevent or delay the development of NIDDM.

MEDICAL NUTRITION THERAPY FOR INSULIN-DEPENDENT DIABETES MELLITUS (TYPE I DIABETES)

The person with IDDM has usually experienced significant weight loss, polyuria, and polydipsia before diagnosis. The initial nutrition prescription must consider the nutrient needs to replenish fluid, muscle mass, glycogen stores, and fat stores. The nutrition assessment should probe usual eating habits before the above-noted symptoms occurred. Many clients are interested in nutrition at this time but may be overwhelmed with the total amount of information being presented. Initial level education is outlined in Appendix 3-B. Since many are young at the time of diagnosis, the "client" will often include the person with diabetes, and their parent(s) or other care providers. These additional "clients" will have separate educational and support needs to be addressed.

There is no "easy" age or time to change eating habits, as there will always be obstacles to confront. Diabetes often forces the issue of making healthy food choices and learning about food preparation, which can result in healthier food choices for the entire family. The health care team plays an important role in maximizing the importance of nutrition therapy at the time of the initial diagnosis. The challenge to the dietitian is

to capture the clients' interest in nutrition therapy as a critical component of diabetes therapy and one that can be adjusted throughout their life to meet their life style, food preferences, and metabolic needs. The dietitian needs to continually work with the client to maintain a "base" meal plan as nutritional, medical, and behavioral needs/desires change and recommend insulin adjustments to the physician. Medication changes should be made in lieu of creating abnormal eating patterns that may be difficult to maintain.

Consistency versus Flexibility

The nutritional emphasis for the person with IDDM is less flexible than for the person with NIDDM. The insulin-dependent person must be more precise in balancing food intake with exogenous insulin and activity. Once insulin has been injected, it will continue to work regardless of what is eaten or what activity is performed. The injected insulin will not alter its action if more or less food is eaten.

The initial meal plan should provide specific guidelines that promote consistency in food intake while the insulin regimen is being established or adjusted. Nutrition therapy should include discussions of the triad of diabetes management (food, insulin, and activity). The dietitian should work closely with these clients in reviewing blood glucose monitoring records, healthy food choices, eating behaviors, and exercise habits. Often, initial education based on the exchange system or its equivalent in structure provides a solid foundation for flexibility once control has been established.

Most persons with IDDM will take at least two injections of insulin in a split, mixed regimen. This allows for some flexibility in the amount of short-acting insulin taken, which can be adjusted based on a premeal blood glucose level, amount of food to be eaten, or activity changes. At the same time, a base pattern of management should be established and easily reverted to if the flexibility makes it difficult to obtain good control. Some persons need several meal plans based on their activity and schedule changes. The person with IDDM should not exercise without making a management adjustment (unless it is a consistent part of their therapy) and monitoring his or her blood glucose.

The DCCT examined the influence nutrition behaviors had on improved glucose control in the intensively treated clients.[21] This study found that consistency was a positive contributor despite the many tools provided to the clients to enable them to increase their flexibility. The four behaviors associated with improved glucose control were (1) adherence to a meal plan, (2) appropriate treatment of hypoglycemia, (3) prompt response to hyperglycemia (more insulin and/or less food), and (4) consistent consumption of prescribed evening snack.

Insulin Regimens and Algorithms

The insulin prescription has often been implemented when the dietitian first consults with a newly diagnosed individual with IDDM. However, the dietitian should review the insulin prescription based on the nutrition assessment and make recommendations with this additional knowledge to the physician if necessary. At the time of diagnosis and periodically throughout the course of the diabetes, the dietitian should assess life-style patterns that may influence timing of insulin injections and dosage requirements (eg, eating smaller, more frequent meals; switching to a vegetarian diet; having irregular sleep patterns that influence meal times; having gym classes at different times). Monitoring blood glucose records for 3 or more days will indicate when a change needs to be made in the insulin regimen. The medication prescription must be written by the physician unless documented consent has been given by the physician to the diabetes educator (dietitian, nurse, or other).

With previously diagnosed individuals, the dietitian should complete a review of medications as a usual part of the nutrition assessment. Often it is the dietitian, with the detailed nutri-

tion and life-style information, who can best recommend adjustments in the insulin regimen to improve glycemic values. One study showed that the dietitians' involvement in recommending medication adjustment resulted in improved diabetes control as well as cost savings.[22] The chapters on medication and monitoring will help new diabetes educators to be more comfortable with this aspect of nutrition therapy.

Three or more injections of insulin a day or an insulin pump allow clients to adjust a premeal short-acting insulin based on their current blood glucose value and what they plan to eat. For instance, if the morning short-acting insulin dose is 5 U and the client plans to eat more, he or she can easily take additional insulin before breakfast so that the prelunch blood glucose value falls within the target goal. Anticipating a change in the base pattern and making a management adjustment is often better than "playing catch-up." If an increase was not made, in this example, at breakfast and extra food was eaten, the prelunch blood glucose would be elevated.

Dietitians need to be involved in developing such insulin algorithms (insulin adjustment guides). Specific algorithms guide clients in making insulin adjustments at different times of the day based on blood glucose monitoring results. The adjustments often differ at different times of the day and provide guidance for

1. *The current blood glucose level*: Example: if the blood glucose is between 120 and 150 before lunch, take an additional 1 U of short-acting insulin; if blood glucose level is between 150 and 180 before lunch, take an additional 2 U of short-acting insulin. Adjustments and ranges of blood glucose values will vary for different individuals.

2. *Future needs:* Planning ahead for anticipated food intake and activity. Example: if an extra 10 to 15 g of carbohydrate is to be eaten at breakfast, client might take an additional 1 U of short-acting insulin; if an extra 10 to 15 g of carbohydrate is to be eaten at lunch, client might take an additional 2 U of short-acting insulin. Blood

glucose monitoring must be performed to determine the best algorithm for each individual.

Another type of algorithm gaining interest and use involves adjusting the time interval between taking an insulin dose and eating a meal. The time interval is based on the current blood glucose level and the action of insulin. Appendix 3-D provides an example of how an individualized time algorithm might be developed. It should be used in conjunction with the insulin algorithm as appropriate. The use of insulin analogs will also affect the timing of insulin injection. The analogs initiate their action much quicker than human or animal insulins. Their quick absorption from the injection site results in higher serum insulin levels earlier with a shorter duration. This may result in lower glucose excursions during and immediately after meals. This reduces the chance for late hypoglycemia which may occur with insulins that have a longer action time. A regimen including a rapid-acting analog will be especially useful by those who have irregular eating schedules and are not always able to take their insulin the usual 1/2 hour before eating.

Medical nutrition therapy puts the client's interests first (life style, food preferences) and uses insulin regimens and insulin and time algorithms to promote gylcemic control.

Fat and Sucrose

A low fat intake as outlined in Exhibit 3-3 is recommended. People with type I diabetes have plasma cholesterol, very low-density lipoprotein-cholesterol (VLDL-C), low-density lipoprotein-cholesterol (LDL-C), and triglyceride concentrations similar to those of the general population but have higher-than-normal high-density lipoprotein-cholesterol (HDL-C) levels.[20] Elevated plasma lipids occur in uncontrolled diabetes due to the breakdown of body fat (triglycerides) for energy and should revert to normal once glycemic control is achieved.

Sucrose can be part of a healthy eating plan but is not actively encouraged. "Scientific evidence has shown that the use of sucrose as part of the meal plan does not impair blood glucose control in individuals with diabetes."[12] Working "sweets" into the diet may actually facilitate adherence to the meal plan. When consumed, they should be counted as carbohydrates and other carbohydrates should be appropriately reduced at the meal or snack. Blood glucose monitoring will show the effects of the meal plan changes.

Weight Management

Weight management was typically not a concern in the person with type I diabetes until the use of the insulin pump and multiple daily injections (three or more injections per day). Persons who adjust their insulin or use an insulin pump have a tendency to gain weight. This is usually due to the flexible insulin coverage for increased food intake. Also, improved control can result in weight gain because the body becomes more efficient in food metabolism and glucose loss through the urine (glycosuria) is diminished. The health care team frequently views weight gain as an obstacle to overcome and focuses their attention on it. Whether much is said or not said, the client knows it has become an issue and may become overly focused or obsessed with it rather than focusing on glycemic control. In addition to the basic health questions that an increasing body weight raise, many people, especially women, desire to be "thinner." It has been reported that one-third of women with type I diabetes omit insulin at some time intentionally to promote weight loss[23] (see Chapter 30).

Individuals in the DCCT intensive control group gained an average of 4.6 kg after 5 years in the study.[24] Glycemic control in this group led to reduced risk of microvascular complications. The World Health Organization Multinational Study of Vascular Disease in Diabetes (WHO-MSVDD) examined the mortality risks of obesity in persons with IDDM.[25] It concluded that "except in very lean people with IDDM, body weight is not significantly associated with mortality. Thus, efforts to improve glycemic control should not be restricted by concerns about the effects of weight gain on mortality."

MEDICAL NUTRITION THERAPY FOR NON–INSULIN-DEPENDENT DIABETES MELLITUS (TYPE II DIABETES)

Obese Type II

Because strict day-to-day consistency of food intake is not usually necessary, many people with NIDDM can learn about the basic meal plan through basic eating guidelines, sample menus, or a counting approach (calories, carbohydrate, or fat). The dietitian should help the client select a meal plan that provides the correct amount of structure to guide the client in meal planning. A client deficient in basic food composition knowledge may benefit from a brief (1 to 2 months) use of an exchange system meal plan approach.

Weight Management

Most people with NIDDM are obese and are often encouraged to lose weight. This therapy focus is shifting. The 1994 ADA nutrition recommendations state that the emphasis for medical nutrition therapy in type II diabetes should be placed on achieving glucose, lipid, and blood pressure goals. A decreased focus on weight reduction is recommended due to the poor success rate in long-term maintenance of weight loss. If initiated, mild-to-moderate weight reduction of 10 to 20 lb is recommended.

Lending additional support to a decreased emphasis on weight loss is the WHO-MSVDD.[26] The WHO-MSVDD found no strong relationship between body mass index (BMI) and mortality in NIDDM. BMI was positively associated with age, blood pressure, and cholesterol and negatively associated with duration of diabetes, retinopathy, and use of insulin. In addition to this study's own data, it cites studies that showed

- obese persons with diabetes had a better survival experience than did nonobese subjects[27,28]
- in male and female Pima Indians with diabetes, the lowest mortality risk was found in those with a BMI between 35 and 40[29]

- nondiabetic persons whose weight cycles have particularly high mortality rates[30]

The study group concluded that there is little evidence of a relationship between BMI and mortality in people with NIDDM except in the most obese subjects.

The WHO-MSVDD did show that Europeans with an initial BMI of less than 29 who lost weight during the follow-up period had a significantly increased mortality risk compared with those whose weight remained the same. Only those in the most obese group, BMI greater than 29 kg/m, showed a mild reduction in mortality risk with weight loss. Unfortunately, waist-to-hip ratio was not obtained during this study to add any data to the association of central obesity with insulin resistance and increased risk of mortality.[31,32]

Central (android) obesity can be documented by measuring the waist at the widest girth using the umbilicus as a reference point and the hips at the widest girth observed with the client standing. The waist measurement is divided by the hip measurement; a ration of greater than 0.85 is considered upper body or central obesity.

Nutrition strategies that are recommended for obese individuals with type II diabetes are lowering fat intake, spacing meals, and exercise. These approaches to improved glucose and lipid control may serve as the priorities unless the clients feel strongly about weight reduction. If they do, mild-to-moderate weight loss of 10 to 20 lb achieved through a combination of calorie reduction and exercise may be attempted, for it is the clients' commitment that will determine long-term success. Monitoring laboratory values will determine if the weight loss has an effect on clinical goals, including blood glucose and lipid levels, and blood pressure. Based on the WHO-MSVDD, clients with a BMI greater than 29 may be the best candidates for weight reduction. It is known that caloric restriction has an important effect on glucose metabolism in obese persons with NIDDM that is independent of weight loss.[33–35] Just 7 days of caloric restriction can produce dramatic improvements in glycemic control and decrease diabetes medication needs. This short intervention may help break the cycle of chronic hyperglycemia and increasing medications and offers the dietitian an additional therapy strategy to achieve glycemic control.

Meal Spacing

Research shows that persons with diabetes can improve glycemic control with weight reduction. Perhaps the success of this improvement is in improved spacing of food intake. Rather than consuming daily nutrients in two to three meals, spacing out the distribution throughout the day has been shown to be beneficial.[36–38] Clients with NIDDM usually are able to produce adequate insulin, although it may take longer for the insulin to lower blood glucose because the acute or first-phase insulin release is delayed. If meals are spaced 4 to 5 hours apart, the premeal blood glucose values may be at acceptable levels to maximize endogenous insulin secretion. Others may find smaller, more frequent meals more compatible with their endogenous insulin production. SMBG will help determine the ideal spacing and meal size.

Fat and Sucrose

Fat modification is a high priority due to the cardiovascular complications associated with diabetes. Persons with type II diabetes have a two- to threefold increase in the prevalence of dyslipidemia than persons without diabetes.[39] The most frequent lipid abnormalities in persons with type II diabetes are hypertriglyceridemia, increased VLDL-C, and reduced HDL-C.[20]

Sugars can be part of the meal plan. However, consideration should be given to the total nutrient consumption of the food. Frequently, sugar is combined with fat that may affect blood lipid and weight goals. Also, hypertriglyceridemia would warrant a reduction in sugar and possible total carbohydrate.

Exercise

Insulin resistance is associated with persons with type II diabetes. Studies show that exercise improves insulin's action, yet the effects of physical training disappear within days when discontinued.[40] Continued regular exercise is recommended as an adjunct therapy to nutrition therapy to promote weight reduction/maintenance and improved insulin sensitivity.[41]

Nonobese Type II

In nutrition therapy for nonobese individuals with type II diabetes, the priority is to determine a meal pattern that is acceptable to the individual, aids glycemic control, and promotes control of blood lipids and weight stability. Dietary modifications, such as adjusting the amount of carbohydrate calories eaten at one time (ie, converting a large carbohydrate breakfast to a smaller breakfast and morning snack, if desired), may reduce postprandial blood glucose levels. Day-to-day consistency is not as mandatory as for persons with type I diabetes, even when nonobese persons with NIDDM require insulin because they produce some endogenous insulin. Small frequent feedings may help them to use endogenous insulin more efficiently. The evaluative tool most beneficial to determine the effects of a meal plan is blood glucose monitoring.

Clients with Type II Diabetes Requiring an Oral Hypoglycemic Agent

If blood glucose levels are elevated and nutritional intervention alone does not lower glucose levels, an oral hypoglycemic agent (OHA) may be prescribed (see guidelines in Chapter 5). Normalizing glycemic and lipid values are still the priorities if the person is overweight, as the use of an OHA does not eliminate the importance of "diet." More regular meal times are usually recommended when an OHA is taken than with dietary intervention alone. Hypoglycemia is a concern for persons taking a sulfonylurea OHA (but not a biguanide) as well as those taking insulin. The dietitian should provide education and treatment guidelines.

Clients with Type II Diabetes Requiring Insulin

Some persons with type II diabetes require insulin to control blood glucose levels. These clients need to be more careful about the timing of their meals and day-to-day consistency due to the continuous action of the injected insulin. They may require an exercise snack or insulin adjustment to prevent hypoglycemia when they exercise. Usually a reduction of insulin is recommended, if that is possible, to enhance the benefit of the exercise without replacing the expended calories.

An evening dose of an intermediate-acting insulin has been gaining interest.[42] This therapy may not require the attention to timing of meals and day-to-day consistency as compared with when insulin is taken in the morning. It is a therapy that dietitians may want to suggest if fasting blood glucose levels continue to be elevated with nutrition therapy alone or already supported with an OHA. Excessive manipulation of food intake may be unnecessary with this adjunct therapy.

GESTATIONAL DIABETES MELLITUS

The woman with gestational diabetes mellitus (GDM) is typically at the end of her second trimester or into her third trimester when diagnosed. Usually, the morning sickness and nausea related to the first trimester have ended. Toward the end of pregnancy, the woman may not tolerate large meals due to the growing fetus and may require frequent small meals/snacks. The diabetic meal plan guidelines should emphasize timing of meals, consistency of intake, inclusion of an evening snack, and healthy food choices. The evening snack is often as late as possible to prevent starvation ketosis. Some women have two evening snacks [eg, one at 7:30 P.M. and one at 10:00 P.M. or may need to eat the second snack in the middle of the night]. Blood glucose monitoring is important in determining meal spacing and portion sizes. The initiation of insulin may be necessary and should not be viewed as "diet failure," but as a natural progression of the individual's current pregnancy.

MNT during a pregnancy can lead to improved eating behaviors and health habits after pregnancy. For the woman with GDM this may

prevent the development of NIDDM. It is recommended that the dietitian schedule routine postpartum visits that coincide with obstetric and pediatric appointments, and stress the importance of the mother staying healthy as she begins to focus attention on her newborn.

IMPAIRED GLUCOSE TOLERANCE

The prevalence of impaired glucose tolerance (IGT) in the United States is estimated to be about 11% in the 20- to 74-year-old population.[43] Rates of progression to NIDDM vary between 20% and 50% over a 2- to 12-year period with the remainder reverting to normal or remaining with IGT.[44] These figures may increase with recent evidence indicating an increased prevalence of IGT in children of diabetic mothers.[45] It seems prudent to be aggressive in providing medical care, including MNT, that will prevent or slow the development of diabetes. Several studies address this.

First, the development of IGT in children of diabetic mothers has been found to be potentially preventable by minimizing fetal hyperinsulinism by optimal metabolic control throughout gestation.[45] MNT plays a strong role in achieving this. Second, a 2-year study by Bourn et al[44] suggests that a diet and exercise program can significantly improve a range of clinical and metabolic variables. They found that a weight loss of at least 5 kg resulted in clinically significant improvements in glucose tolerance. Weight loss has been reported by others to reduce the progression from IGT to NIDDM.[45,46]

Providing MNT for those at risk for developing IGT and those who have IGT could potentially preserve one's quality of life and reduce health care needs and costs by preventing or slowing the onset of NIDDM.

CONCLUSION

Nutrition intervention by a skilled dietitian results in health-care cost savings and improved glycemia.[22] Each setting that provides diabetes care must overcome obstacles that prevent clients from receiving adequate MNT. This requires the health care team to become strong advocates of MNT and support interventions to achieve the clinical goals of MNT. MNT is more than designing a meal plan and providing one or two education sessions. It is integral to diabetes care as it provides the client knowledge, skills, and behaviors to self-manage their day-to-day variations with ease and finesse.

REFERENCES

1. Bliss M. *The Discovery of Insulin*. Chicago, Ill: The University of Chicago Press; 1982.
2. Joslin EP. *The Treatment of Diabetes Mellitus*. Philadelphia, Pa: Lea and Febiger; 1935.
3. Powers MA. A review of recent events in the history of diabetes nutritional care. *Diabetes Educ*. 1992;18:393–400.
4. Caso EK. Calculation of diabetic diets. *J Am Diet Assoc*. 1950;26:575–583.
5. Cassell JA. *Carry the Flame: A History of the American Dietetic Association*. Chicago, Ill: The American Dietetic Association.
6. American Diabetes Association. *The Journey and the Dream: A History of the American Diabetes Association*. Alexandria, Va: American Diabetes Association; 1990.
7. American Dietetic Association. Cost-effectiveness of medical nutrition therapy. *J Am Diet Assoc*. 1995;95:88–91.
8. Beebe CA, Pastors JG, Powers MA, Wylie-Rosett J. Nutrition management for individuals with non–insulin dependent diabetes in the 1990s: a review by the Diabetes Care and Education Practice Group. *J Am Diet Assoc*. 1991;91:196–207.
9. Lyon RB, Vinci DM. Nutrition management of insulin-dependent diabetes mellitus in adults: review by the Diabetes Care and Education Dietetic Practice Group. *J Am Diet Assoc*. 1993;93:309–314,317.
10. Connell JE, Thomas-Dobersen D. Nutritional management of children and adolescents with insulin dependent diabetes mellitus: a review by the Diabetes Care and Education Practice Group. *J Am Diet Assoc*. 1991;91:1556–1564.
11. Fagan C, Erick M, King J. Nutritional management of women with gestational diabetes mellitus (GDM): a review by the Diabetes Care and Education Practice Group. *J Am Diet Assoc*. 1991;91:196–207.
12. American Diabetes Association. Nutrition recommendations and principles for people with diabetes mellitus (position statement). *Diabetes Care*. 1995;18(suppl 1):16–19.
13. Diabetes Control and Complications Trial Research Group. The effect of intensive treatment of diabetes on the development and progression of long-term complications in insulin-dependent diabetes mellitus. *N Engl J Med*. 1993;329:977–986.
14. Powers MA, Wheeler ML. Model for dietetics practice and research: the challenge is here, but the journey was not easy (commentary). *J Am Diet Assoc*. 1993;93:755–757.
15. Diabetes Control and Complications Trial Research Group. Expanded role of the dietitian in the Diabetes Control and Complications Trial: implications of clinical practice. *J Am Diet Assoc*. 1993;93:758–764,767.
16. Diabetes Care and Education Practice Group. Scope of practice for qualified dietetics professionals in diabetes care and education. *J Am Diet Assoc*. 1995;95:607–608.
17. Monk A, Barry B, McClain K, Weaver T, Cooper N, Franz MJ. Practice guidelines for medical nutrition therapy provided by dietitians for persons with non–insulin-independent diabetes mellitus. *J Am Diet Assoc*. 1995;95:999–1006.
18. Diabetes Care and Education Practice Group. Nutrition practice guidelines for type I diabetes mellitus. *J Am Diet Assoc*. In preparation.
19. Wheeler ML. New diabetes nutrition resources available. *Diab Spectrum*. 1995;8:254, 267.
20. Franz MJ, Horton ES, Bantle JP, et al. Nutrition principles for the management of diabetes and related complications (technical review). *Diabetes Care*. 1994;17:490–518.
21. Delahanty LN, Halford BH. The role of diet behaviors in achieving improved glycemic control in intensively treated patients in the Diabetes Control and Complications Trial. *Diabetes Care*. 1993;16:1453–1458.
22. Franz MJ, Splett PL, Monk A, et al. Cost-effectiveness of medical nutrition therapy provided by dietitians for persons with non-insulin-dependent diabetes mellitus. *J Am Diet Assoc*. 1995;95:1018–1024.
23. Polonsky WH, Anderson BJ, Lohrer PA, Aponte JE, Jacobson AM, Cole CF. Insulin omission in women with IDDM. *Diabetes Care*. 1994;17:1178–1185.
24. Diabetes Control and Complications Trial Research Group. Weight gain associated with intensive therapy in the Diabetes Control and Complications Trial. *Diabetes Care*. 1988;11:567–573.
25. Chaturvedi N, Stevens LK, Fuller JH. WHO Multinational Study Group. Mortality and morbidity associated with body weight in people with IDDM. *Diabetes Care*. 1995;18:761–765.
26. Chaturvedi N, Fuller JH. WHO Multinational Study Group. Mortality risk by body weight and weight

change in people with NIDDM. *Diabetes Care.* 1995;18:766–774.

27. Ballard DJ, Melton LJ. Sources of disparity in incidence and prevalence studies of diabetic retinopathy: influence of selective survival on risk factor assessment. *Diabetes Care.* 1986;9:313–315.

28. Knatterud GL, Klimt CR, Goldner MG, et al. Effects of hypoglycemic agents on vascular complications in patients with adult-onset diabetes. *Diabetes.* 1982;31:1–26.

29. Pettitt DJ, Lisse JR, Knowler WC, Bennett PH. Mortality as a function of obesity and diabetes mellitus. *Am J Epidemiol.* 1982;115:359–366.

30. Lissner L, Odell PM, Dagostino RB, et al. Variability of body weight and health outcomes in the Framingham population. *N Engl J Med.* 1991;324:1839–1844.

31. Larsson B, Svardsudd K, Welin L, Wilhelmsen L, Bjorntorp P, Tibblin G. Abdominal adipose tissue, obesity and risk of cardiovascular disease and death: a 13-year follow-up of participants in the study of men born in 1913. *BMJ.* 1984;288:1401–1404.

32. McKeigue PM, Shah B, Marmot MG. Relation of central obesity and insulin resistance with high diabetes prevalence and cardiovascular risk in South Asians. *Lancet.* 1991;337:382–386.

33. Wing RR. Use of very-low-calorie diets in the treatment of obese persons with non–insulin-dependent diabetes mellitus. *J Am Diet Assoc.* 1995;95:569–572.

34. Wing RR, Blair EH, Bononi P, Marcus MD, Watanabe R, Bergman RN. Caloric restriction per se is a significant factor in improvements in glycemic control and insulin sensitivity during weight loss in obese NIDDM patients. *Diabetes Care.* 1994;17:30–36.

35. Henry RR, Scheaffer L, Olefsky JM. Glycemic effects of intensive caloric restriction and isocaloric refeeding in noninsulin-dependent diabetes mellitus. *J Clin Endocrinol Metab.* 1985;61:917–925.

36. Bertelsen J, Christiansen C, Thomsen C, et al. Effect of meal frequency on blood glucose, insulin, and free fatty acids in NIDDM subjects. *Diabetes Care.* 1993;16:3–7.

37. Jones PJH, Leitch CA, Pederson RA. Meal-frequency effects on plasma hormone concentrations and cholesterol synthesis in humans. *Am J Clin Nutr.* 1993;57: 868–874.

38. Jenkins KJA, Ocana A, Jenkins A, et al. Metabolic advantages of spreading the nutrient load: effects of increased meal frequency in non–insulin-dependent diabetes. *Am J Clin Nutr.* 1992;55:461–467.

39. Stern MP, Patterson JK, Haffner SM, Hazuda HP, Mitchell BD. Lack of awareness and treatment of hyperlipidemia in type II diabetes in a community survey. *JAMA.* 1989;262:360–364.

40. American Diabetes Association. Diabetes mellitus and exercise (position statement). *Diabetes Care.* 1992; 15(suppl 2):50–54.

41. Yamacouchi K, Shinozaki T, Chikada K, et al. Daily walking combined with diet therapy is a useful means for obese NIDDM patients not only to reduce body weight but also to improve insulin sensitivity. *Diabetes Care.* 1995;18:775–778.

42. Cusi K, Cunningham GR, Comstock JP. Safety and efficacy of normalizing fasting glucose with bedtime NPH insulin alone in NIDDM. *Diabetes Care* 1995;18:843–851.

43. Harris MI, Hadden WC, Knowler WC, et al. Prevalence of diabetes and impaired glucose tolerance and plasma glucose levels in U.S. population aged 20-74 years. *Diabetes.* 1987;36:523–534.

44. Bourn DM, Mann JI, VcSkimming BJ. Impaired glucose tolerance and NIDDM: does a lifestyle intervention program have an effect? *Diabetes Care.* 1994;17:1311–1319.

45. Silverman BL, Metzger BE, Cho NH, Loeb CA. Impaired glucose tolerance in adolescent offspring of diabetic mothers. *Diabetes Care.* 1995;18:611–617.

46. Long SD, O'Brien K, Swanson M, et al. Weight loss prevents the progression of impaired glucose tolerance to non–insulin-dependent diabetes mellitus: a ten-year longitudinal study (Abstract). *Diabetes.* 1992;21 (suppl 1):72A.

Historical Review of Diabetes Nutritional Management

Date	Scientist or Source	Recommendations
1550 BC	Papyrus Ebers	Wheat grains, fresh grits, grapes, honey berries, sweet beer
5 AD	Aretaeus the Cappadocian	Milk or cereals and starch, with fruits and sweet wines
6th century		Limit rice, flour, and sugar
1675	Thomas Willis	High carbohydrate to replace lost sugar; choices limited to milk and barley water boiled with bread; lime water and opium
1797	John Rollo	Avoid carbohydrates; breakfast was a milk mixture and lime water with bread and butter; lunch was plain blood puddings, made of blood and suet only; supper was game or old rancid meats, and fat; opium
1857	Piorry	Agreed with Willis, 125 g of sugar candy and two portions of meat; fluid restriction
1860	Charles Henry Pile Appollinaire Bouchardat	Strict use of animal food alone High fat, no milk; to break the monotony of the Rollo diet, he added green vegetables that were boiled and the water discarded; encouraged low calories and even periodic fasting
1869	Donkin	Skim milk diet
1880	Bernard Naunyn	Pioneered use of measured diets; limited protein and carbohydrate, restricted calories; 24-hour fasts in less severe cases
1892	Dujardin-Beaumetz/Mosse	Diet high in potatoes
1902	Carl Hanko von Noorden	Oatmeal diet

Date	Scientist or Source	Recommendations
1912	Frederick Allen	"Allen Starvation Treatment": low carbohydrate, high fat, calories restricted
1921		Insulin identified; diminished interest in diet
1929	H. Rawle Geyelin	Attempted to "normalize" the diet; did not find a need to increase insulin with drastically increased amounts of carbohydrate (five times); related effect of carbohydrate to amount of fat that was limited
1930	Israely M. Rabinowitch	Limited fat to less than 50 g/d to help lower cardiovascular-renal disease; patients to be 5 to 10 lb underweight
1935	Sir Harold Himsworth Walter Kempner William F. Van Eck Ernest and coworkers E.P. Joslin	High carbohydrate 90–95% carbohydrate 90% carbohydrate 72% carbohydrate 100-200 g carbohydrate/day; average 110-150 g
1950		Introduction of oral hypoglycemic agents; introduction of exchange diet with precalculated meal plans
1971	American Diabetes Association	Individualization essential; attaining ideal body weight primary objective; avoid simple sugars; most use exchange system
1977	Phyllis Crapo	Presented data showing plasma glucose and insulin responses to complex and simple carbohydrates do not support "common thought"
1979	American Diabetes Association	Pre-printed diets discouraged; carbohydrate up to 50 to 60% total calories, decreased fat; differentiate between IDDM and NIDDM
1980s	David Jenkins James Anderson	Devises glycemic index Recommends high carbohydrate, high fiber intake
1986	American Diabetes Association	Individualization important; carbohydrate up to 55 to 60% total calories; decrease fat and cholesterol
1994	American Diabetes Association	Nutrition assessment by experienced dietitian; no % for carbohydrate and fat to promote individualization

Sources: Nutrition Today. 1972; May/June:4, Copyright 1972, Nutrition Today Inc; *Diabetes Care.* 1981;4:647, Copyright © 1981, American Diabetes Association Inc; *The Diabetes Educator* 1992;18:393–400; *Diabetes Care.* 1994;17:519–522.

Nutrition Practice Guidelines for Type I Diabetes

Identifying Levels of Nutrition Care and Examples of Medical Nutrition Therapy for Self-Management Training/Education Needs

Level of Nutrition Care	Patient Identification	Topics To Discuss	Food/Monitoring Plan	Timing of Therapy	Goals/ Outcomes

Initial	• newly diagnosed
	• no previous nutrition therapy
	• history of poor glycemic control
		• balance of food, insulin, activity
		  –consistent meal times and food intake
		  –timing of insulin in relation to food intake
		  –consistent exercise/ activity
		• need for food plan
		• blood glucose records are guides for developing care plans
		  –when to test, goals, and testing procedure, if needed
		• hypoglycemia signs, symptoms, treatment
		• sick day management
		• documentation of food, activity, insulin, and blood glucose tests
		• life-style issues; support systems; resources
		• other, identified through assessment
			Food Plan
			• consistency in timing of meals
			• consistency in carbohydrate content of meals/snacks
			  –menu ideas, cookbooks, recipes
			• portion control
			  –average servings for individual
			  –measuring, weighing, and/or estimating
			• treatment guidelines for hypoglycemia
			• sick day food intake guidelines
			• adequate calories for growth of children
			• possible replenishment of nutrients lost from untreated diabetes or poor control
			
			Monitoring Plan
			• individualized testing times
			• test 1–4 times/d
				Initiate: over 3 months
				• 3–4 visits
				• 2–3 hours total
				• see patient within 1 week of referral; if newly diagnosed, see within 24 hours
				  –first two visits about 2 weeks apart
				  –third visit 1–2 months later
				  –fourth visit if necessary
				
				Follow-Up, if not appropriate for continuing care
				• 1–2 visits/yr
				• 1/2–1 hour each
					• follows general healthy eating guidelines
					• fairly consistent intake 75% of time; limited food choices
					• knows how to identify and treat hypoglycemia
					• avoids severe hypoglycemia and ketonuria
					• GHb decrease after 3 months
					• blood glucose monitoring results in downward trend

Continuing	• flows progressively from initial therapy • those who have basic understanding of type I diabetes and its therapy components	• previous topics, if necessary • ways to expand food choices • modifying insulin or food for improved blood glucose levels, within context of health team approach	**Food Plan** • individualized management plan to compensate for any schedule variability • carbohydrate or insulin adjustment to improve daily blood glucose control	**Initiate:** over 3 months • minimum 3 visits • 3–5 hours total –at least 1 individual session to develop/ review individualized therapy (meal plan) and to discuss	• greater understanding of food portions; increased variety of food choices; comfortable eating in a variety of settings

Source: Reprinted with permission from Diabetes Care and Education Dietetic Practice Group. Nutrition practice guidelines for type I diabetes mellitus. *Journal of the American Dietetic Association,* in preparation, Copyright © 1995, American Dietetic Association.

continued

Level of Nutrition Care	Patient Identification	Topics To Discuss	Food/Monitoring Plan	Timing of Therapy	Goals/ Outcomes
Continuing *Continued*		• specific influence of the individual's eating habits/choices and activity on blood glucose levels • lipid values and blood pressure • possible errors that prevent achievement of goals • how food (carbohydrate, protein, fat) affects postprandial blood glucose • reinforce behavior changes	• therapeutic plan for lipids, sodium, protein, if needed • adjusting food for exercise • use of alcohol, eating away from home, label reading, grocery shopping, weight management, travel consider-ations, brown bag/ school lunches, birthdays/holidays • using blood glucose monitoring results for problem-solving food-related issues • other content areas per patient need and interest **Monitoring Plan** • individualized testing times • test 2–4 times/d	blood glucose goals and testing times (third visit of initial level could become first visit of continuing care) –other 2 visits could be classes if within 1 month of above visit –telephone appointments, review of faxed information and records will help support/modify therapy –some may need additional 2 visits as individual therapy **Follow-Up** • 4 visits/yr –when life events change –more frequent after therapy (insulin, food, exercise) changes • 1/2–1 hour each	• food portions and timing of meals consistent 75% of time • some adjustment of regular insulin for blood glucose levels, food intake, activity • appropriate growth and development of children • reasonable weight • avoid severe hypoglycemia and ketonuria • GHb decrease after 3 months • blood glucose monitoring results in downward trend • lipids decrease, if elevated • blood pressure normal • if planning a pregnancy or pregnant provide intensive therapy
Intensive	• those who desire more attention to food choices • those on multiple daily injections of insulin • those using an insulin pump • preconception therapy • therapy during pregnancy	• previous topics, if necessary • potential for weight gain and severe hypoglycemia with multiple daily injections or pump • methods to increase life-style flexibility –insulin algorithms –expanded food information –refinement of exercise guidelines • is insulin schedule appropriate and realistic for patient • reinforce behavior changes	• nutrient content of greater variety of food • weight management approaches to use as management intensifies • insulin/carbohydrate ratios at different times of the day • insulin adjustments (algorithms) based on varying food intake and preprandial blood glucose levels • adjusting insulin injection time related to blood	**Initiate:** over 2 months • 3–5 visits • 3–4 hours total –at least 2 individual sessions to develop insulin algorithm followed by frequent telephone contact with dietitian or health care team; often daily contact to discuss food choices, activity, insulin, and resulting blood glucose values	• quite flexible with food choices based on actual composition or estimating composition • food portions and timing of meals consistent 75% of time; other 25% insulin or food adjustments made based on blood glucose level and activity

continued

Level of Nutrition Care	Patient Identification	Topics To Discuss	Food/Monitoring Plan	Timing of Therapy	Goals/ Outcomes
Intensive *Continued*			glucose level • food intake for varying levels of hypoglycemia • adjusting insulin for delayed meals **Monitoring Plan** • individualized testing times • test minimum 4 times/d	–2 weeks later, third visit to discuss food adjustments, individual blood glucose monitoring results from eating certain foods, modify algorithm –some may need 2 additional individual therapy visits –pump therapy requires additional time to become proficient with pump **Follow-Up** • 4–6 visits/yr (plus telephone and fax review of blood glucose monitoring records) –when life events change –more frequent after therapy (insulin, food, exercise) changes • 1/2–1 hour each	• weight gain less than 10% body weight • avoid severe hypoglycemia and ketonuria • appropriate growth and development of children • GHb decrease after 3 months • blood glucose monitoring results in downward trend • lipids decrease, if elevated • blood pressure normal

Nutrition Therapy Intervention for Persons with Type II Diabetes

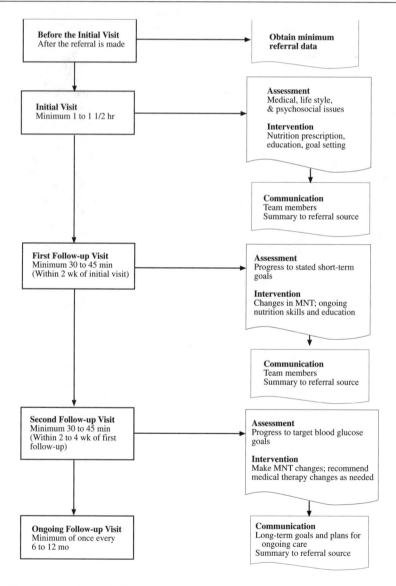

Figure 3-C-1 Nutrition practice guidelines for patients with non–insulin-dependent diabetes mellitus (newly diagnosed or previously diagnosed). MNT = medical nutrition therapy.

Table 3-C-1 Desired Outcomes of Medical Nutrition Therapy (MNT) for Patients with Non–Insulin-Dependent Diabetes Mellitus

Index	Goal	Desired Outcomes 4 to 6 wk after Initial MNT	Desired Outcomes of Ongoing MNT
Glycemic control Fasting/preprandial glucose <115 mg/dL[a]	80–120 mg/dL is acceptable (improvement should be attempted if >140 mg/dL)	Downward trend (~10%) or at target goal; if not, recommend nutrition or medical therapy changes	Maintenance of target goals
Postprandial (2-h) plasma glucose (140 mg/dL is normal)	100–180 mg/dL is acceptable (improvement should be attempted if >200 mg/dL)		
Glycated hemoglobin (HbA$_{1c}$) (<6.0% is normal)[b]	6.0% to 7.5% acceptable	Downward trend (~10%) or at target goal	Maintenance of target goals
Lipids[c] Cholesterol	<200 mg/dL	If cholesterol elevated, a 6% to 12% decrease	If outside the target range after 4 to 6 months of MNT, physician is notified
Low-density lipoprotein-cholesterol	<130 mg/dL		
High-density lipoprotein-cholesterol	>35 mg/dL in men >45 mg/dL in women		
Triglycerides	<200 mg/dL		
Blood pressure	<130/85 mmHg		If no response to life-style changes, physician is notified
Weight change	Maintain reasonable weight[d]; short-term weight loss of 0.2 to 0.5 kg (1/2 to 1 lb)/week; long-term weight loss of 2.5 to 9 kg (5-20 lb)	Weight loss of 1.5 to 3 kg (3 to 6 lb)	Weight loss of 4.5 to 9 kg (10 to 20 lb)
Food/meal planning	Meals and snacks are eaten on a regular basis Appropriate food choices and amounts are made according to the food/meal plan If energy intake exceeds needs, intake is reduced by ~250-500 kcal/d	Positive changes in food selection, amounts, frequency, and timing of meals	Implementation and maintenance of positive changes

continues

Source: Figure 3-C-1 and Tables 3-C-1 through 3-C-6 reprinted with permission from Monk A, Barry B, McClain K, Weaver T, Cooper N, Franz MJ. Practice guidelines for medical nutrition therapy provided by dietitians for persons with non–insulin-dependent diabetes. *Journal of the American Dietetic Association.* 1995;95:999–1006, Copyright © 1995, American Dietetic Association.

Table 3-C-1 continued

Index	Goal	Desired Outcomes 4 to 6 wk after Initial MNT	Desired Outcomes of Ongoing MNT
Exercise	If no medical limitations, physical activity for 10 to 15 min or more, minimum of 3 to 4 times a week	Physical activity level gradually increased or continued	Maintenance of exercise program

[a] To convert mg/dL glucose to mmol/L, multiply mg/dL by 0.0555. To convert mmol/L glucose to mg/dL, multiply mmol/L by 18.0. Glucose of 6.0 mmol/L = 108 mg/dL.

[b] Hemoglobin A$_{1c}$ is referenced to a nondiabetic range of 4.0% to 6.0%.

[c] To convert mg/dL cholesterol to mmol/L, multiply mg/dL by 0.026. To convert mmol/L cholesterol to mg/dL, multiply mmol/L by 38.7. Cholesterol of 5.00 mmol/L = 193 mg/dL.

[d] Reasonable body weight is defined as that level of weight the patient and health care providers acknowledge as achievable and maintainable both short- and long-term. This is in contrast to desirable body weight, which is an ideal body weight for an individual based on height and frame size.

Table 3-C-2 Minimum Referral Data Needed for Medical Nutrition Therapy (MNT) Provided by Dietitians for Persons with Non–Insulin-Dependent Diabetes Mellitus

Factor	Data Needed
Diabetes treatment regimen	MNT alone MNT and oral glucose-lowering agents MNT and insulin or combination therapy
Laboratory values	Glycated hemoglobin Fasting or nonfasting plasma glucose Cholesterol and fractionations Blood pressure Microalbumin
Physician goals for patient care	Target blood glucose levels Target glycated hemoglobin level Method and frequency of self-monitoring of blood glucose levels Plans for instruction and evaluation of self-monitoring of blood glucose levels
Medical history	Dyslipidemia or cardiovascular disease Hypertension Renal disease Automatic neuropathy, especially gastrointestinal
Medications that affect nutrition therapy	Diabetes medications Hypertensive medications Lipid-lowering medications Gastrointestinal medications Others
Guidelines for exercise	Medical clearance for exercise Exercise limitations, if any

Table 3-C-3 Initial Nutrition Intervention

Factor	Interventions
Long-term goals	Identify long-term management goals of patient and health care team; target blood glucose levels and glycated hemoglobin, weight, lipids, blood pressure, and others as appropriate Emphasize healthful life style Review reduction of risk factors and long-term complications
Nutrition prescriptions	Determine nutrition prescription based on nutrition history, treatment modality, treatment goals, and concurrent medical conditions
Food/meal planning and survival skills	Discuss basic nutrition and diabetes nutrition guidelines: what, when, and how much to eat If patient takes insulin or oral agents, emphasize importance of eating meals and snacks consistently, synchronized with medication time actions Review recognition and treatment of hypoglycemia Discuss, depending on interest or readiness: simple definitions and examples of carbohydrate, protein, and fat; guidelines such as for decreasing fat (saturated fat) and using less added sweetener and salt; how to make food choices (eg, grocery shopping tips, restaurant eating guidelines)
Educational tools	Select appropriate meal-planning approach and educational materials Use audiovisual materials (eg, handouts, videos, flip charts, food models, measuring cups and spoons)
Blood glucose monitoring	Teach self-monitoring of blood glucose levels if needed Review target blood glucose goals
Exercise	Discuss exercise recommendations
Short-term goal setting	Address eating, exercise, and blood monitoring behaviors Identify and summarize short-term behavioral goals that are specific, achievable, and short-term (1 to 2 wk) Focus on changing only one or two specific behaviors at a time
Follow-up	Provide record keeping forms (food, exercise, SMBG) to be completed prior to next visit Determine follow-up plans: 2-4 wks

Table 3-C-4 First Follow-Up Visit Intervention

Factor	Interventions
Food/meal planning	Adjust medical nutrition therapy if needed Recommend changes in food and exercise that can improve outcomes (eg, meal spacing; food choices, portions, timing; exercise frequency, duration, type, timing)
Education	Review and reinforce self-management skills and survival-level information Provide new and expanded information about nutrition topics as appropriate
Goal setting	Review and reinforce long-term diabetes management goals Reset short-term behavioral goals based upon assessment
Follow-up	Recommend second follow-up visit within 2 to 4 wk if goals have not been met, changes in therapy are made, patient has difficulty in making life-style changes, patient requires additional support and encouragement, weight loss is the primary focus, further education is needed If goals have been met, recommend ongoing nutrition care in 6 to 12 months Plan for laboratory determination of glycated hemoglobin level before the second follow-up visit

Table 3-C-5 Second Follow-Up Visit Intervention

Factor	Interventions
Therapy changes	Recommend changes in medical therapy if (a) blood glucose levels have not shown a downward trend (~10% decrease) or have not reached the target ranges; (b) glycated hemoglobin has not shown a downward trend; (c) a 2.3- to 4.5-kg (5- to 10-lb) weight loss has occurred with no improvement in blood glucose levels; (d) patient is not willing or able to make additional food and exercise changes; (e) patient is doing well with food plan and exercise and further nutrition intervention is unlikely to result in improved medical outcomes
Education	Follow those in Table 3-C-4
Goal setting	Follow those in Table 3-C-4
Follow-up	Recommend additional follow-up if oral agents or insulin has been added to therapy, follow-up is needed for weight loss, further education is needed If goals have been met, recommend ongoing follow-up in 6 to 12 months

Table 3-C-6 Essential Patient Education Topics for Nutrition Self-Management of Diabetes

Level of Education	*Education Topics*
Basic survival skills for medical nutrition therapy needed by all persons with diabetes	Basic food/meal planning guidelines Exercise guidelines Signs, symptoms, treatment, and prevention of hypoglycemia if taking an oral agent or insulin Nutrition management during short-term illness Self-monitoring of blood glucose levels Plan for continuing care
Essential education for ongoing nutrition self-management. Select topics based on patient's life style, level of nutrition knowledge, and experience in planning, purchasing, and preparing food and meals	Sources of carbohydrate, protein, fat Nutrition labels Grocery shopping guidelines Eating out: restaurant, cafeteria, and fast-food choices Modifying fat intake Use of sugar-containing foods Dietetic foods and sweeteners Snack choices Alcohol guidelines Using blood glucose monitoring for problem solving and identification of blood glucose patterns Adjusting meal times Adjusting food for exercise Behavioral modification techniques Exchanges Recipes, menu ideas, cookbooks Birthdays, special occasions, holidays Brown-bag lunches Travel and schedule changes Vitamin/mineral and other nutrition supplements Working rotating shifts (if needed)

Adjustment in Meal Times and Insulin for Varying Blood Glucose Levels

A. Action of Regular Insulin

		Onset	*Peak*	*Duration*
Based on clinical observation:		20–60 min	90 min–3 hr	5–12 hr
Based on reference data:	• animal	30 min–2 hr	3–4 hr	4–6 hr
	• human	30 min–1 hr	2–3 hr	3–6 hr

B. Target Blood Glucose (BG) Levels (mg/dL)

Testing Time	*Ideal BG*	*"Acceptable" BG*	*Your BG Goals*
Fasting	70–90	70–105	_____
Premeal	70–105	70–130	_____
1-hr postmeal	<140	<180	_____
2-hr postmeal	<120	<150	_____

C. Adjusting Meal Times for Varying Blood Glucose Levels

Usually you eat 30 minutes after you take your insulin. However, if your blood glucose before a meal is less than 80 you may want to eat right away. That way some food has been digested and your blood glucose is beginning to rise by the time the insulin starts to work (onset). If your premeal blood glucose level is high, you may want to wait longer before eating your planned meal. The following are **guidelines**. When you use them, write a note in your record book as to what you did.

If Blood Glucose Level (mg/dL) Is	*Approximate Time Delay before Eating after Taking Premeal Regular Injection or Bolus*
<80	no delay
81–120	wait 20–30 minutes
121–150	wait 45 minutes
151–200	wait 1 hour
201–250	wait 1 hour and 15 minutes
>250	wait 1–2 hours

There are other changes you could also make. They should be discussed with your health care team to determine which method is best for you. Some may take usual insulin dose and decrease the carbohydrate content of their meal. Others may increase their insulin and eat at their usual time. All guidelines need to be developed for you.

D. Guidelines for High Blood Glucose Levels

1. When your blood glucose level is above _____ mg/dL you may need to take extra (supplemental) regular insulin in addition to your usual dose. Give _____ unit per _____ mg/dL that your blood glucose level is above _____ mg/dL. (If you have an algorithm, use it and go to the next step.)

2. Check for ketones if blood glucose level is over _____ mg/dL.
   - With no ketones in urine—use extra regular insulin as calculated above.
   - With trace to small ketones in urine—increase the extra regular by 50%.
   - With moderate to large ketones in urine—double the extra regular.

3. Test blood glucose every hour. If it is still above 150 mg/dL in 3–4 hours, you will need to take more regular insulin. Contact your physician immediately.

Drink (sip) at least 1 cup (8 oz) of noncaloric (diet) beverage per hour during this time. High ketones may make you feel nauseous. If you are vomiting and unable to keep fluids down, call your physician immediately or go to the emergency room.

Note: This educational handout was developed based on clinical observations. It is important that you contact your health care team to be sure they are right for you. Some of the steps in this table require math skills. It is important that you feel comfortable with them before using the guidelines.

Source: Adapted from Diabetes Health Center, Salt Lake City, Utah.

Chapter 4

Nutrition Assessment

Beverly Holt Halford

The dynamic process by which the nutrition professional identifies and evaluates data that reflect or affect an individual's physiologic need for nutrients has been refined in the past decade. Use of computer reporting systems and computer-assisted analysis of food records and/or 24-hour recall information has increased the accessibility of laboratory information and the specificity of the nutritional recommendations made.

Nonetheless, the process of nutrition assessment is also dependent on the skill of the interviewer. The commitment of the professional to gathering unbiased information is paramount. This information will clarify the client's satisfaction with current and future regimens for nutrition and medicinal prescriptions, their socioeconomic status, and life-style factors that may affect the ability and desire of the client to make changes in their diet and daily routine. This chapter surveys the general categories of information that need to be included in a nutritional assessment performed for clients with diabetes mellitus.

PURPOSE AND OVERVIEW

The first purpose of completing a nutrition assessment is to gather adequate data to write the nutrition prescription. The second purpose is to determine intervention and care plans. Ongoing assessments are used to evaluate and update the nutrition prescription and intervention/care plans. Thus the nutrition assessment forms the basis of nutrition therapy and self-management training and is a critical component of diabetes care.

The registered dietitian or other professional collecting information for the nutritional assessment must evaluate data from a data set common to all patients and also individualize the interview and data collection to include components specific to diabetes. This additional information must include insulin or other medication taken, distribution of food intake with attention to both timing and macronutrient distribution, onset of and severity of the diabetic disease process, weight and weight history, lipid abnormalities, and response of blood lipids to alterations in the diet. Sources for this information include:

- medical records
- client interviews
- self-administered client questionnaires
- referral forms
- verbal information from the physician's office
- other team members
- family members and significant others.

The National Standards for Diabetes Self-Management Education Programs state in Standard 17 that the diabetes education assessment should include relevant medical history, present health status, health service or resource use, risk factors, diabetes knowledge and skills, cultural influences, health beliefs and attitudes, health behaviors and goals, support systems, barriers to learning, and socioeconomic factors.[1] All these areas are critical to developing appropriate nutrition intervention and should be included in the nutrition assessment.

Table 4-1 Strategies of Progression to Disordered Eating

Stage	Description
I. Abnormal eating	Eats (or does not eat) in response to dysphasia
	Frequently overeats at meals
II. Compulsive eating	Loses concept of normal eating
	Binges at mealtimes
	Hoards food
	Feelings of being denied food that others are allowed
III. Addictive eating	Manipulation to obtain food
	Denial of eating
	Guilt over eating
	Anxious about not having enough food
IV. Eating disorder	Obsession with weight and food
	Body image disorder
	Binge eating (at meals or nonmeal times)
	Starving
	Purging to relieve guilt or anxiety or to maintain weight (includes skipping insulin)
	Uses food as a weapon

Source: Adapted with permission from Turner M, Davidow DM. Complications of coexisting diabetes mellitus and eating disorders in IDDM, *On the Cutting Edge*. 1994;15(6):8–10, Copyright © 1994, American Dietetic Association.

Nutrition practice guidelines (NPG) for type I and type II diabetes were recently developed, field tested, and shown to improve management outcomes.[2,3] Appendixes 4-A and 4-B identify nutrition assessment content from the NPGs. The practitioner is encouraged to develop a form using this information to assist and enhance the nutrition assessment process. An expanded assessment of potentially disordered eating is described in Table 4-1. Also see Chapter 30 for further discussion of eating disorders and Chapter 10 for assessment of readiness to change. Appendix 4-C is an assessment checklist to use with older persons to determine their nutrition health. It is part of the Nutrition Screening Initiative to promote routine nutrition screening and better nutrition care for older persons.

Type I Diabetes

The NPG for type I diabetes provide an indepth checklist of topic areas and sample questions for the assessment of clients (Appendix 4-A). Particular areas of interest to the practitioner include results of laboratory tests for cholesterol, low-density lipoprotein (LDL)-cholesterol, high-density lipoprotein (HDL)-cholesterol, triglycerides, hemoglobin, glycated hemoglobin, and creatinine.

Integration of knowledge about diet and insulin adjustment is an important indicator of client willingness to change and ability to lower glycated hemoglobin values. Research from the Diabetes Control and Complications Trial indicates three behaviors were associated with lower

Lowers Glycated Hemoglobin

Adherence to prescribed meal plan
Adjusting food in response to hyperglycemia
Adjusting insulin in response to hyperglycemia

Raises Glycated Hemoglobin

Overtreatment of hypoglycemia
Consuming extra snacks beyond meal plan

Figure 4-1 Nutrition Behaviors Associated with Changes in Glycated Hemoglobin. *Source*: Reprinted with permission from Delahanty LN and Halford BN, The role of diet behaviors in achieving improved glycemic control in intensively treated patients in the Diabetes Control and Complication Trial, *Diabetes Care* (1993;16:1452–1458), Copyright © 1993, American Diabetes Association.

glycated hemoglobin values and two with higher values.[4] Adherence to the prescribed meal plan and adjusting food and/or insulin in response to hyperglycemia resulted in lower glycated hemoglobin values, and overtreatment of hypoglycemia and consuming extra snacks beyond the meal plan were associated with higher values[4] (Figure 4-1).

Type II Diabetes

Assessment data necessary to write the nutrition prescription for the client with non–insulin-dependent diabetes are outlined in Appendix 4-B. In addition, the clinical dietitian will need to review referral data (see Appendix 3-C), including, for example, glycated hemoglobin values, cholesterol, LDL-cholesterol, very low-density lipoprotein (VLDL)-cholesterol, HDL-cholesterol, and triglyceride values. Current blood pressure and renal status should also be evaluated. The nutrition assessment for clients with type II diabetes will specify current lipid values, weight and reasonable body weight, blood pressure, and percentage of calories currently consumed as carbohydrate, protein, and fat. It should also identify approximate intake of polyunsaturated and monosaturated and saturated fat as well as sources of trans-fatty acids.

It is easy to assume the person with type II diabetes has been told to modify their food in-

take at some point by a health professional because the person with type II diabetes is frequently overweight and has other chronic medical conditions that require diet modification. This does not mean that the food intake was adequately assessed and an individualized nutrition prescription with proper self-management training was provided. It is imperative that nutrition therapy be treated as any other health consult and begin with a thorough assessment of needs and adequate instruction to carry out the management plan. Persons with type II diabetes can respond positively to adequate health care.

Syndrome X

An assessment may reveal a client with obesity, elevated triglycerides, characteristic deposits of intra-abdominal fat, and elevated blood pressure, along with diabetes. This combination of medical syndromes has been termed syndrome X. The dietitian should evaluate which condition should receive priority in therapy. A thorough assessment should indicate what nutrition change might be best to approach. A discussion with the patient, physician, and dietitian should determine the nutrition and medical priorities for nutrition therapy. Elevation of triglycerides would suggest a trial of diet with moderate carbohydrate content (45% of calories) and a proportionately higher fat intake (40% of calories, with 10% or less coming from saturated fat) content as recommended by some investigators.

Setting Priorities for the Meal Plan

Most nutrition assessments are performed by the dietitian as part of an initial visit. Subsequent interventions provide the opportunity to update and modify the information base. Frequently, the dietitian is concerned that the client will not return for subsequent sessions. The entire health care team should help ensure adequate time is devoted to conducting the nutrition assessment as well as providing intervention and evaluation therapy. The amount of time required will vary. The type I NPGs state that 2 to 3 hours, over 3 to 4 visits are required for initial level of nutrition care (see Appendix 3-B).[7] The type II NPGs state that a minimum of one hour is required for an initial visit with subsequent visits being a minimum of 30-45 minutes (see Appendix 3-C)[3]

PHYSIOLOGIC CHANGES

Diabetes affects the metabolism of all three macronutrients: carbohydrate, protein, and fat. The practitioner should bear in mind that although many nutrition problems encountered by persons with diabetes are related to an elevation in blood glucose, many are caused by lack of insulin. Insulin promotes storage of and prevents the breakdown of carbohydrate, protein, and fat and is therefore necessary for entry of blood glucose into the cell, the clearance of lipids from the bloodstream, and the synthesis of protein. The nutrition assessment includes a review of laboratory and physical data that indicate how the body responds to food intake. Since the response is influenced by exercise patterns, they should also be assessed.

BIOCHEMICAL ASSESSMENT

Measurements of glucose, lipid, and protein metabolism form the basis of nutrition assessment in the person with diabetes. Urine tests such as blood urea nitrogen and creatinine clear-

ance can be used to identify the status of diabetes complications. Table 4-2 gives reference ranges for commonly used blood and urine tests.

Blood Tests

Blood Glucose

Blood glucose can be assessed by several different techniques. A quick assessment of a patient's ability to metabolize food can be obtained by using a 2-hour postprandial blood glucose. The results provide insight into whether an individual would sustain an acceptable blood glucose in a challenged state. Several days of tests can be used to evaluate the current diet, subsequent modifications in the diet, and appropriateness of the current medications.

Fasting blood glucose values can be used as an indication of general diabetes control; however, an isolated fasting blood glucose value may have limited usefulness. A very high value may indicate inadequate insulinization, or it may reflect rebound hyperglycemia caused by a hypoglycemic episode during the preceding night. Each of these situations requires different management interventions, so careful assessment is necessary. Self-monitoring of blood glucose can be performed by the patient at home or work. Fasting and premeal blood glucose values can be used to modify medication, diet, and/or activity to improve overall control. The level of blood glucose over a longer period of time can be measured by the amount of glycosylation occurring in red blood cells. The glycated hemoglobin value may be more meaningful in individuals who have stable diabetes rather than unstable diabetes.

Lipids

The dynamics of cholesterol and triglyceride manufacture and deposition are closely linked with the availability of insulin, diabetes control, and genetic disposition to hyperlipidemias, as well as other metabolic variables. No baseline evaluation of cholesterol or other lipids should be drawn without determining dietary sources of cholesterol, family history of atherosclerotic

Table 4-2 Normal Reference Laboratory Values

Determination	Reference Range	Comment
Blood, Plasma, or Serum Values		
Cholesterol	120–220 mg/100 mL (serum)	Fasting. Children with cholesterol levels between 75th and 90th percentile (170–185 mg/dL)[a] should be counseled.
Triglyceride	40–150 mg/100 mL (serum)	Fasting. Children to age 19 who are above the 90th percentile (104 mg/dL)[b] should be counseled.
Creatinine	0.6–1.5 mg/100 mL (serum)	
Glucose	70–100 mg/100 mL (plasma)	Fasting
Glucose (1 h postprandial)	180 mg/dL (plasma)	Values above this number are considered diagnostic for diabetes and require confirmation by other determinations.[c]
Hemoglobin A_{1c}	3.8–6.4% (plasma)	
Potassium	3.5–5.0 mEq/L (serum)	
Hematocrit	Male: 45–52% Female: 37–48% (blood)	
Ferritin—iron deficiency	0–12 ng/mL 13–20 borderline (serum)	
Albumin	3.5–5.0 g/100 mL (serum)	
Urea nitrogen (BUN)	8–25 mg/100 mL (serum)	
Urine Tests		
Acetone plus acetoacetate Quantitative	0	
Protein Quantitative	<150 mg/24 h	24-h specimen; values less than 150 may require additional evaluation in persons with diabetes
Glucose Quantitative	0	24-h or other timed specimen

[a] Glueck CJ. Pediatric primary prevention of atherosclerosis. *N Eng J Med*. 1986;314:3,175.

[b] Morrison JA, de Groot I, Edwards BK, et al. Lipids and lipoproteins in 1926 school children age 6 to 17 years. *Pediatrics*. 1978;62:990.

[c] Marble A, Ferguson BD. Diagnosis and classification of diabetes mellitus and the nondiabetic melliturias. In: Marble A, Krall LP Bradley RF, Chrislieb AR, Soeldner JS, eds. *Joslin's Diabetes Mellitus*. 12th ed. Philadelphia, Pa: Lea & Febiger; 1985.

Source: Unless noted, the values in this table have been adapted with permission from *New England Journal of Medicine* (1986;314:39), Copyright © 1986, The New England Journal of Medicine.

heart disease, exercise patterns, and level of blood glucose. Cholesterol and triglyceride levels are typically elevated at the time of diagnosis and usually decrease when blood glucose levels are lowered. Lipid tests are routinely recommended for baseline screening of children and adults.

Protein

The level of albumin measures the body's ability to manufacture proteins. It is an adequate indicator for stable patients with a chronic medical condition. Because turnover time for albumin is 14 days, it is less sensitive than other measures. The urinary creatinine height index should be used if the client is being evaluated during an acute illness. Hematocrit and hemoglobin values can be used as a gross indicator of iron status in individuals with diabetes. Low values are generally associated with chronic blood loss, heavy menstrual bleeding, or gastrointestinal bleeding. Diets low in saturated fat and cholesterol that are routinely prescribed for persons with diabetes often contain inadequate supplies of foods high in heme iron. The need for an iron supplement should be assessed.

Protein intake should be monitored in clients at risk for renal disease. Modification of protein intake should become a decision reached by the client, physician, and dietitian.

Sodium and Potassium

The dehydration seen with acute episodes of high blood glucose values may be reflected in abnormal electrolyte values. Hypokalemia, which is often observed with diuretic therapy, may suppress insulin release.[5] Regular measurements of potassium levels should be made in this population.

Urea Nitrogen and Creatinine

Urea nitrogen and creatinine tests evaluate kidney function. The decreased renal function that accompanies nephropathy can be identified by the gradual increase in these laboratory values.

Urine Tests

Protein

Quantitative values for protein may indicate the presence of deteriorating renal function or a urinary tract infection. These infections are more common in persons with diabetes. Microproteinuria is becoming a common test to identify someone in early stages of nephropathy.[6]

Urine Glucose

A urine glucose test provides a gross estimation of diabetes control and is no longer frequently used to indicate degree of diabetes control. Twenty-four-hour urine collection can be used to estimate the number of calories being lost in the urine. If urine and blood glucose values are obtained simultaneously, the renal threshold for an individual can be established.

Urine Acetone

Acetone in the urine indicates breakdown of fatty tissue in uncontrolled diabetes. It is also an indicator that fat is being used in well-controlled diabetes. Pregnant women often are asked to monitor fasting ketones. If ketones are present in the urine and the woman's blood glucose values are within normal range, she should increase her bedtime snack to prevent the occurrence of ketonuria. This state is often referred to as starvation ketosis (or accelerated starvation) as the body is "starved" for glucose and is reverting to fat stores for energy. Individuals with diabetes are also asked to test for urinary ketones when they are ill. Urinary ketones and elevated blood glucose levels can indicate the need for more insulin in those with type I diabetes.

ANTHROPOMETRIC MEASUREMENT AND PHYSICAL EXAMINATION

Actual physical measurements of height, weight, and blood pressure may be readily available in the medical record. If not, the dietitian should obtain them.

Height

In the pediatric patient, serial measurements of growth are a useful determinant of overall nutriture. Short stature or lack of growth may indicate inappropriate insulin dosage or inadequate caloric intake. In the adult client, it is also important to measure height. A height given by the patient may be from early adulthood and may not reflect changes in stature over time. An accurate measure of height assists the dietitian in determining desirable body weight using height/weight charts and various formulas.

Weight

An assessment of a person's weight history can provide valuable information as to what may be a reasonable weight goal for them, their success with weight management, and adequacy of diabetes/nutrition therapy. A family weight history may also be requested. Weight tables and calculations for determining calorie needs are provided in Chapter 19.

Growth Curves

The use of standardized growth curves for children and pregnant women is imperative. To evaluate growth adequately, the pattern of growth in a child after diagnosis needs to be compared with growth before onset. Previous patterns of growth can be used to establish individual norms for the child being evaluated.

The dietitian working with pregnant insulin-dependent diabetes mellitus patients should monitor the pattern and amount of weight gain throughout the pregnancy. Clients with gestational diabetes mellitus should be referred to the dietitian as soon as they are diagnosed. Often these women were obese before conception and have large weight gains during their first months of pregnancy. In the last trimester, weight gains of about 1 lb/wk should follow the slope of a nondiabetic pregnancy when plotted on the growth curve.

Blood Pressure

Untreated hypertension increases the risk of microvascular and macrovascular disease; early detection and treatment are imperative. Because hypertension in the hyperglycemic client can be caused by many mechanisms, the dietitian should recognize the types of hypertension and their physiologic causes. Each type requires an individualized therapeutic treatment.

Xanthomas

Xanthomas are deposits of lipid in the skin, which are characteristically seen in patients with hyperlipidemia or poorly controlled diabetes.[7] There are four types of xanthomas. The most common type is eruptive xanthoma, which forms bright red papules, mottled with a deep rose tint, and usually appear on the buttocks and extremities. Xanthomas may appear on the eyelids and usually begin as one or more pinhead-sized yellow-orange spots. Eventually these spots form irregular plaques that may cover most of the eyelid. Individuals with xanthomas should be screened carefully because these fatty deposits are usually indicative of poorly controlled diabetes mellitus and/or familial hyperlipidemias. Particular attention should be given to percentage of total calories consumed in fats and cholesterol. The patient should be aware that family members should be screened for hyperlipidemias.

Xanthochromia

Xanthochromia (carotemia) is yellowish discoloration of the skin caused by impairment of the patient's ability to convert carotene to vitamin A in the liver. The pigmentation tends to accumulate on the palms, soles, and nasolabial folds. It is accompanied by elevation of blood levels of carotene from a normal range of 140 to 150 mg/100 mL to many times that value. Treatment consists of eliminating carotene-rich foods and improving the hyperglycemic condition. The discoloration experienced by one patient

Table 4-3 Assessment for the Prevention of Foot Ulcers and Infections

Topic	Assess If the Client Does the Following:
Shoes	• Wear well-fitting shoes even if they are not stylish • Change shoes during the day to relieve pressure areas • Try running or walking shoes for everyday wear; select dress shoes of soft leather and have them fitted carefully • Break in new shoes slowly • Shake shoes out and inspect them before wearing for areas that might cause blisters or rubbing
Foot hygiene	• Wash feet daily with mild soap; rinse and dry thoroughly, especially between the toes • Apply moisture-restoring creams once or twice daily except between the toes • Wear clean intact socks appropriate for the shoes being worn • Avoid astringents and all over-the-counter preparations for calluses, corns, nails, etc • Trim nails with a slightly rounded edge • Avoid "self-bathroom surgery"; seek a qualified professional for treatment of all foot problems • Do not use foot soaks • Do not use heating pads or sleep next to space heaters or stoves; hot or cold sensations in the feet result from neuropathy, not poor circulation • Wear socks if feet feel cold • Never go barefoot
Problems to report to physician	• Cuts or breaks in the skin • Ingrown nails • Changes in color or discoloration of the foot • Change in sensation or pain • Change in architecture of the foot

Source: Reprinted from Gibbons GW, Logerfo FW. Foot ulcers and infections. In: HE Lebovitz, ed. *Therapy for Diabetes Mellitus and Related Disorders*. 2nd ed, with permission of the American Diabetes Association, Copyright © 1994.

was noticeably improved after 1 month of treatment (B. Holt Halford, clinical observation).

Feet

The condition of the client's feet and shoes and tolerance of weight-bearing are important elements of the nutrition assessment. Before dietitians can promote regular exercise, they must determine whether the patient can tolerate walking. An examination of the feet reveals any existing problems with foot ulcers and also gives the professional an opportunity to discuss with the patient the importance of appropriate footwear. Shoes worn for walking should feature closed toes and low heels. Once patients develop good foot care habits, exercise requiring use of the feet can be encouraged.

Table 4-3 outlines components of preventing foot ulcers and infections. Patients should be encouraged to ask their health care provider to examine their feet to aid in early detection of possible devastating complications. Although this topic is not typically addressed by dietitians, it is of such critical concern and too frequently neglected that the dietitian should be concerned that it is properly addressed.

Dentition

Good dentition is necessary for proper mastication. Because non–insulin-dependent diabetes mellitus is more common in the elderly, as are missing teeth or poorly fitting dentures, each patient's dentition should be evaluated. Specific assessment questions are outlined in Chapter 33.

COMPUTER-AIDED ASSESSMENTS

Dietitians seeking to reduce the time necessary to produce complete nutrient analysis of their clients' menus or wishing to calculate the macronutrient values of a meal plan have found that personal computers and hand-held computers offer substantial assistance. Reviews of software programs are available.[8,9] Advantages of using computer programs include greater accuracy, availability of graphing functions, and instant nutrient analysis. Judging from the response to surveys of diabetes educators conducted by the Diabetes Care and Education Practice Group, dietitians are using computers to facilitate teaching, to calculate, and to generate shopping lists. Five diet/recipe analysis programs are in common usage; three hand-held computers are available.

REFERENCES

1. American Diabetes Association. National standards for diabetes self-management programs. *Diabetes Care.* 1995;18(suppl):94–96.

2. Kulkarni K. Diabetes Care and Education Practice Group. *Nutrition Practice Guidelines for Persons with Type I Diabetes.* American Dietetic Association, in preparation.

3. Diabetes Care and Education Practice Group. Nutrition Practice Guidelines for Type I Diabetes Mellitus. Chicago, Ill: American Dietetic Association, in preparation.

4. Monk A, Barry B, McClain K, Weaver T, Cooper N, Franz MJ. Practice guidelines for medical nutrition therapy provided by dietitians for persons with non–insulin-dependent diabetes mellitus. *J Am Diet Assoc.* 1995;95(9):999–1006.

5. Delahanty LN, Halford BN. The role of diet behaviors in achieving improved glycemic control in intensively treated patients in the Diabetes Control and Complications Trial. Diabetes Care. 1993;16:1453–1458.

6. Conn JW. Hypertension, the potassium ion and impaired carbohydrate tolerance. *N Engl J Med.* 1985;273:1135.

7. American Diabetes Association. Consensus statement: consensus development conference on the diagnosis and management of nephropathy in patients with diabetes mellitus. *Diabetes Care.* 1994;17(11):1357–1361.

8. Gordon D, ed. Computer use in diabetes nutrition therapy. *On the Cutting Edge.* Chicago, Ill: Diabetes Care and Education Practice Group of the American Dietetic Association; 1994.

9. Lee RD, Nieman DC, Rainwater M. Comparison of eight microcomputer dietary analyses programs with the USDA Nutrient Data Base for Standard Reference. *J Am Diet Assoc.* 1995;95(8):858–867.

Assessment Questions for Type I Diabetes

Content Area*	Minimum Assessment	Sample Questions
Medical history/present health status	✔ ✔ ✔	Do you have any health problems? What medications are you taking? Include over-the-counter medications. Present health status?
Health service or resource use		Where do you go for usual diabetes care (eg, physician's office, public health clinic, hospital)? Who is your primary care physician?
Risk assessment	✔	Determine risk for acute and chronic complications—hypoglycemic unawareness, microproteinuria, etc.
Diabetes knowledge and skills	✔ ✔ ✔	What have you been told about diabetes? Do you do anything differently now that you have diabetes? Has anyone ever taught you anything about diabetes? Food and diabetes? Who have you learned about diabetes from? Do you know anyone with diabetes? What do you think about that person? Have they told you anything about diabetes? Are you using a specific meal planning method? (ie, exchanges, carbohydrate counting, menus, etc)? If in poor control (high glycated hemoglobin—HbA$_1$ or HbA$_{1c}$) assess for errors in care that prevent achievement of goals.

continued

*Content areas correspond with National Standards for Diabetes Self-Management Education Programs from the American Diabetes Association.

Source: Adapted from D. Davis, RD, LDN, CDE, and B. Pratt Gregory, MS, RD, LDN, Vanderbilt Diabetes Research and Training Center, Nashville, Tennessee, Nutrition practice guidelines for type I diabetes mellitus, *Diabetes Care and Education*, practice group of the American Dietetic Association, in preparation.

Content Area*	Minimum Assessment	Sample Questions
		Blood glucose monitoring (BGM)
		Are you presently doing BGM? If yes, when and what do you do with the information?
	✔	Do you understand why BGM is performed?
		When did you last have your technique checked? Assess or refer for assessment.
		Is test data recorded?
		What meter is used?
		Is insulin or food intake adjusted in response to blood glucose tests?
Life-style/cultural influences	✔	Describe to me a typical day.
	✔	How do some days vary from typical?
		What type of activity do you have in a usual day?
	✔	Who lives with you? How do they impact your daily schedule?
		What is your occupation?
		What cultural traditions do you have (celebrations, health beliefs, hierarchy of decision making, food)?
		What do you feel proud of in your life?
		How do you perceive your quality of life?
		What have you accomplished that makes you feel good?
Health beliefs and attitudes	✔	Do you think your diabetes can get better?
		Assess psychosocial factors affecting readiness to change behaviors. Precontemplation/contemplation; preparation/action; action/maintenance. (This will help guide goal setting and intervention. For example, if in the contemplation phase, detailed discussion of problem-solving techniques will be met with resistance.)
		On a scale of 1 to 10, rate your desire to make changes related to your health. (This may have different meanings to different patients; this question can promote more in-depth discussion about "change.")

continued

Content Area*	Minimum Assessment	Sample Questions
Health behaviors and goals		***Goals***
	✔	What are your goals related to diabetes care?
	✔	Do you have target blood glucose goals? If yes, what are they?
	✔	What are your specific nutrition-related goals?
		What do you hope to accomplish as a result of time spent with the registered dietitian?
		Usual eating habits
	✔	Have you changed your eating habits as a result of diabetes?
	✔	How do you decide what you are going to eat?
	✔	What are two typical days of food intake? Are weekends different from weekdays?
		How often do you eat out?
		Who buys and prepares your food? Do they influence these decisions?
		Are you satisfied with the way you currently eat? Do you want to change anything?
		Does stress affect your eating in any way?
		Do you use food as a reward?
		How do you treat insulin reactions?
		Exercise
		What is your current activity/exercise level? Frequency, duration, and intensity? Timing in relation to insulin regimen and food intake?
		Are you willing to continue or expand activity?
		Other
		Do you have any problems chewing your food?
	✔	Do you have a dentist?
		How do you care for your teeth?
		How do you feel about your overall health and health behaviors?

continued

Content Area*	Minimum Assessment	Sample Questions
Support systems		Do your family, friends, babysitters, teachers, coworkers know about your diabetes?
		How do family/friends feel about your diabetes?
		Who helps you with your diabetes? Do they have fears about diabetes?
		Do you have access to a support group?
		How often do you miss school because of diabetes?
Barriers to learning	✔	What difficulties have you had in the past when trying to make changes in your life with diabetes?
		What obstacles have you overcome when caring for your diabetes?
		Has anything happened that prevented you from being able to follow through with your diabetes care?
		Is transportation to medical/nutrition visits difficult?
		Is transportation to obtain food difficult? Does it influence your food supply?
		What obstacles, if any, prevent exercise/activity?
		How do you prefer to learn—reading, doing (experiential), observing, discussing, a combination; with others in a group or individually?
Socioeconomic factors		Do you adjust diabetes care due to lack of financial resources (ie, test less frequently than desired, not schedule nutrition visits)?
		Are finances available to buy necessary supplies and appropriate foods?

Nutrition Assessment for Type II Diabetes

Table 4-B-1 Initial Nutrition Assessment

Factor	*Assessments*
Clinical data	Obtain height and weight (when patient is wearing light clothing and no shoes) Determine a reasonable body weight Estimate daily energy needs Assess minimum referral data, especially medications (type, amount, and timing), and glucose, glycated hemoglobin, and other laboratory data
Nutrition history	Determine usual food intake and pattern of intake Evaluate energy intake, macronutrient composition (types and amounts), nutrient distribution, other nutritional concerns, and frequency and timing of meals Obtain weight history, recent weight changes, and weight goals Assess appetite and eating or digestion problems Determine frequency of and choices in restaurant meals Assess alcohol intake Determine use of vitamin/mineral or nutrition supplements
Exercise history	Determine activity types and frequency Estimate energy expenditure Determine limitations that hinder or prevent exercise Assess willingness and ability to become more physically active
Psychosocial and economic issues	Assess living situation, cooking facilities, finances, educational background, and employment Assess ethnic or religious belief considerations Assess level of family and social support Determine if there are other important issues
Blood glucose monitoring	Assess knowledge of target blood glucose ranges Assess blood glucose testing method and frequency of testing Assess blood glucose records for frequency of hyperglycemia and hypoglycemia and number of target range blood glucose values
Knowledge, skill level, attitudes, and motivation	Assess survival or continuing education knowledge level Assess basic knowledge level Assess attitudes toward nutrition and health and readiness to learn

Table 4-B-2 First Follow-Up Visit Assessment

Factor	Assessments
Follow-up data	Obtain weight (when patient is wearing light clothing and no shoes)
	Review any new or updated laboratory data
	Assess changes in medication (eg, dose of oral agent or dose/frequency of insulin)
	Review blood glucose monitoring records, including frequency of testing, time of day testing was done, and results
	Assess changes in exercise habits
	Review food records completed since initial visit or complete a 24-hour food recall
Blood glucose monitoring	Determine whether there is a downward trend in blood glucose values
	Determine the percentage of blood glucose values within the target range
	Assess whether blood glucose monitoring goals are being met and determine willingness and ability to do additional self-monitoring if needed
	Assess occurrence, causes, and patterns of hypoglycemia
Nutrition progress	Assess understanding of initial nutrition information and food/meal plan
	Determine whether meals and snacks are eaten on a regular basis
	Assess whether food choices are appropriate and portions reasonable
	Determine further improvements that can be made in the quality of the diet
Short-term goals	Assess achievement of short-term behavioral goals
	Determine willingness and ability to make further changes

Table 4-B-3 Second Follow-Up Visit Assessment

Factor	Assessments
Follow-up data	Evaluate glycated hemoglobin and other new or updated laboratory data
	Make other assessments—same as at first follow-up visit (see Table 4-B-2)
Blood glucose monitoring	Make same assessments as at first follow-up visit (see Table 4-B-2)
Nutrition progress	Make same assessments as at first follow-up visit (see Table 4-B-2)
Short-term goals	Make same assessments as at first follow-up visit (see Table 4-B-2)

Source: Reprinted with permission from Monk A, Barry B, McClain K, Weaver T, Cooper N, Franz MJ. Practice guidelines for medical nutrition therapy provided by dietitians for persons with non–insulin-dependent diabetes mellitus. *Journal of the American Dietetic Association*. 1995;95(9):999–1006. Copyright © 1995, American Dietetic Association.

Assessment Checklist

DETERMINE YOUR NUTRITIONAL HEALTH

The Warning Signs of poor nutritional health are often overlooked. Use this checklist to find out if you or someone you know is at nutritional risk.

Read the statements below. Circle the number in the yes column for those that apply to you or someone you know. For each yes answer, score the number in the box. Total your nutritional score.

	YES
I have an illness or condition that made me change the kind and/or amount of food I eat.	2
I eat fewer than 2 meals per day.	3
I eat few fruits or vegetables, or milk products.	2
I have 3 or more drinks of beer, liquor, or wine almost every day.	2
I have tooth or mouth problems that make it hard for me to eat.	2
I don't always have enough money to buy the food I need.	4
I eat alone most of the time.	1
I take 3 or more different prescribed or over-the-counter drugs a day.	1
Without wanting to, I have lost or gained 10 pounds in the last 6 months.	2
I am not always physically able to shop, cook, and/or feed myself.	2
TOTAL	

TOTAL YOUR NUTRITION SCORE. IF IT'S—

0–2   **Good!** Recheck your nutritional score in 6 months.

3–5   **You are at moderate nutritional risk.** See what can be done to improve your eating habits and life style. Your office on aging, senior nutrition program, senior citizens center, or health department can help. Recheck your nutritional score in 3 months.

6 or more   **You are at high nutritional risk.** Bring this checklist the next time you see your doctor, dietitian or other qualified health or social service professional. Talk with them about any problems you may have. Ask for help to improve your nutritional health.

These materials developed and distributed by the Nutrition Screening Initiative, a project of:

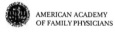 AMERICAN ACADEMY OF FAMILY PHYSICIANS   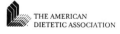 THE AMERICAN DIETETIC ASSOCIATION   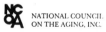 NATIONAL COUNCIL ON THE AGING, INC.

Remember that warning signs suggest risk, but do not represent diagnosis of any condition. See other materials from the Nutrition Screening Initiative for further information, 2626 Pennsylvania Avenue NW, Suite 301, Washington, DC 20037, (202) 625-1662.

Source: Reprinted with permission by the Nutrition Screening Initiative, a project of the American Academy of Family Physicians, the American Dietetic Association and the National Council on the Aging, Inc. and funded in part by a grant from Ross Products Division, Abbott Laboratories.

Chapter 5

Diabetes Medications and Delivery Methods

Susan L. Thom

With the conclusion of the Diabetes Control and Complications Trial (DCCT) in June 1993, the answer was a resounding "Yes" to the question of whether near-normal glycemic control would prevent the onset or delay the progression of the long-term complications of type I diabetes.[1] The results of this ten-year prospective, randomized, clinical trial not only demonstrated the benefits of self-management of diabetes for the subjects, but also expanded the role of the diabetes educators (dietitians and nurses) involved.[2] As health care providers or case managers, registered dietitians need to be knowledgeable about diabetes medications because diabetes care is a balance of food intake, activity, and oral agents and/or insulin (endogenous or exogenous).

TREATMENT WITH INSULIN: INDICATIONS FOR USE

Individuals with insulin-dependent diabetes mellitus (IDDM, type I), regardless of age at onset, will eventually develop ketosis and die if not treated with insulin. For those patients who are at less risk for ketosis, as is most often the case for those with non–insulin-dependent diabetes mellitus (NIDDM, type II), insulin should still be prescribed in the following instances to achieve optimal blood glucose control. These instances may include, but are not limited to, the following scenarios: (1) acute illness, surgery, or trauma in which the production of catecholamines (insulin antagonists) increases dramatically; (2) failure of intensive nutrition interven-

tion (at least four to six visits with a registered dietitian) to promote necessary weight loss or blood glucose control; (3) primary or secondary failure on oral hypoglycemic agents necessitating supplementary insulin (combination therapy) or total replacement of the oral agents; (4) unusual work or life-style schedule impacting mealtimes and food choices; and (5) sensitivity or allergy to sulfa drugs, limiting or negating their potential use.

Insulin is also required in the management of gestational diabetes, when nutrition intervention alone does not result in targeted glucose ranges. Certain patients with a diagnosis of secondary diabetes mellitus may require insulin, as in the case of pancreatitis where ß-cell production of insulin is severely diminished. Insulin, in conjunction with rehydration, is always used in the treatment of diabetic ketoacidosis and occasionally used in the treatment of hyperglycemic hyperosmolar nonketotic syndrome.

Exogenous insulin may be administered to nondiabetic individuals to maintain normal glucose levels during periods of insulin resistance or increased insulin demand. These instances would include surgery, trauma, acute illness, and patients receiving enteral or parenteral nutritional supplements to meet increased intermittent energy needs or treat another condition (malabsorption syndrome, for example).

CHARACTERISTICS OF INSULIN

Insulin exerts a variety of effects on body tissues, but basically it can be categorized as a "storage hormone." Under conditions of adequate insulinization: (1) insulin stimulates the entry of amino acids into cells, enhancing protein synthesis; (2) insulin promotes fat storage (lipogenesis) and prevents the mobilization of fat for energy (lipolysis); (3) insulin stimulates the entry of glucose into cells for utilization as an energy source and promotes the storage of excess glucose as glycogen in muscle and liver cells (glycogenesis).[3]

Exogenous insulin became available in 1921. Since that time injection has been the most convenient method of administration. Insulin cannot be administered orally as the protein chains which comprise the insulin molecule are degraded by digestive enzymes as any other ingested protein would be, thus rendering the insulin nonfunctional. Exogenous insulins have four properties—type, concentration, purity, and source—that determine their time-action profiles.

Type

At present, two pharmaceutical firms produce approximately 20 different insulins. Depending on the onset, peak, and duration of its action, each type is considered to be either short-acting, intermediate-acting, or long-acting insulin. *Regular, or crystalline, insulin* is clear in appearance, is fast-acting, and mimics the insulin produced physiologically by the ß-cells (although its onset, peak, and duration are longer than insulin produced in vivo). It is frequently used in combination with one of the intermediate- or long-acting insulins. However, it is used alone during acute illness (regular insulin is the only type that can be administered intravenously), during pregnancy, with the insulin pump (continuous subcutaneous insulin infusion [CSII]), and in some individualized insulin regimens (multiple daily injection [MDI]).

The intermediate-acting insulins, *NPH* and *lente*, are cloudy in appearance and nearly identical in onset, peak, and duration of action.

Ultralente, a long-acting insulin, is cloudy in appearance and has an action that lasts beyond

36 hours. It is important to note that the extended action of the intermediate-acting and long-acting insulins is attributed to the addition of either zinc and/or protamine suspensions. The addition of these other substances to regular insulin reduces its predictability and potentiates acute complications, such as hypoglycemia.

In 1996, Eli Lilly and Company began distributing an *insulin analog* named lispro. It is an extremely rapid-acting insulin that peaks in 5 minutes and is eliminated from the circulation in less than 2 hours. The advantages of this rapid action are reduced postprandial hyperglycemia (secondary to the rapid peaking) and elimination of delayed hypoglycemia (due to the rapid clearance). This analog of regular insulin was developed by simply reversing the proline-lysine amino acids at the 28th and 29th positions in the

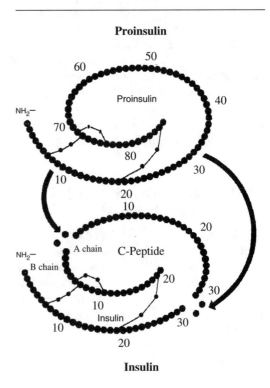

Figure 5-1 Human Insulin Molecule. *Source:* Reprinted with permission from Galloway, JA, ed. *Diabetes Mellitus*, 9th ed. Indianapolis, Ind: Lilly Research Laboratories; 1988:49.

beta chain of the insulin molecule. (See Figure 5-1.)

The rapid action is related to the monomeric form that it achieves once injected. Typically, insulin molecules cluster in hexamers (six molecules) composed of three dimers (two molecules). Dissociation of the hexamer must occur after injection before the insulin molecules can function effectively. With the availability of lispro, persons with diabetes will be able to "dose and eat," thus eliminating the need for injection 30 minutes prior to a meal or snack. Without this time lag, patients will have increased flexibility in food choices and a spontaneity that they were not afforded with regular insulin on injection regimens.

In order to simplify diabetes education and the overall daily regimens of persons with diabetes, the insulin manufacturers have developed *premixed* ratios of NPH and regular insulin. For patients who are elderly, less literate, or learning-challenged, these premixed insulins prevent mixing and dosing errors. Consider that there are some 27 steps involved in learning to draw and inject just one type of insulin (see Appendix 5-C). Imagine how much more complicated this process becomes when two types of insulin must be mixed together.

The most commonly prescribed premixed insulin is 70/30 (70% NPH and 30% regular, a standard based on the two-thirds to one-third guideline). Also available is 50/50 insulin, which can reduce both postprandial hyperglycemia and the risk of subsequent hypoglycemia. Table 5-1 summarizes the characteristics of insulins currently available in the United States.

Concentration

All of the insulin in the United States is of U-100 concentration. The number refers to the concentration of insulin per milliliter; thus, U-100 means 100 U/mL. U-100 was developed to allow most insulin users to take a smaller volume of insulin (due to its greater concentration) than they could with the now obsolete U-80 and U-40 concentrations. In addition, it is easier to convert U-100 to metric values.

For international travelers, the customer service departments of the insulin manufacturers, Eli Lilly and Company (1-800-LILLY-RX or 1-800-545-5979) and Novo Nordisk Pharmaceuticals (1-800-727-6500), can provide availability information on concentrations of insulins in a given country (addresses in Appendix 5-A). For example, U-40 and U-100 insulins are available in over 90 countries worldwide. It is anticipated that streamlining of insulin products will continue into the near future, so that it will be unlikely that persons with diabetes will have to alter their regimen or product use while traveling. It is best when traveling, however, for persons with diabetes to take double the needed quantity of insulin with them in a carry-on bag.

For individuals requiring large doses of insulin (extreme insulin-resistance), U-500 is available as a prescribed insulin by special order from Eli Lilly and Company. U-100 insulin is available in the US without a prescription. However, a prescription is highly suggested, especially when traveling. U-500 is a purified pork product that is administered subcutaneously, like other insulins. For individuals who are extremely insulin-sensitive or for those who require very small doses (as in children), diluents specific to the type of insulin are available from both companies. The diluents are a mixture of the preservatives, buffers, and base for a given type (regular, NPH, lente, ultralente) and, thus, must be matched to the appropriate insulin type. Empty vials are also provided to mix the diluent and insulin. The physician will determine the appropriate dilution (the most common ones are 50% and 25%), and the pharmacist will mix them. Diluents are most often used today with the insulin pump in order to prevent clogging with an increased flow rate.

Purity

The purity of insulin is expressed as parts per million (ppm) of proinsulin, the primary contaminant remaining after extraction from the

Table 5-1 Insulins Available in the United States

Type	Formulation	Species	Concentration	Route of Administration[a]	Appearance
			Characteristics		
Regular insulin injection (Lilly)	Humulin R	Human (bio)	U-100	SQ, IV	Clear
	Regular Iletin I	Beef/pork	U-100	SQ, IV	Clear
	Regular Iletin II	Purified pork	U-100, U-500	SQ, IV	Clear
Regular insulin injection (Novo Nordisk)	Novolin R	Human (bio)	U-100	SQ, IV	Clear
	Velosulin	Human (semi)	U-100	SQ, IV	Clear
	Regular	Purified pork	U-100	SQ, IV	Clear
NPH insulin isophane suspension (Lilly)	Humulin N	Human (bio)	U-100	SQ	Cloudy
	NPH Iletin I	Beef/ pork	U-100	SQ	Cloudy
	NPH Iletin II	Purified pork	U-100	SQ	Cloudy
NPH insulin isophane suspension (Novo Nordisk)	Novolin N	Human (bio)	U-100	SQ	Cloudy
	NPH	Purified pork	U-100	SQ	Cloudy
Lente insulin zinc suspension (Lilly)	Humulin L	Human (bio)	U-100	SQ	Cloudy
	Lente Iletin I	Beef/ pork	U-100	SQ	Cloudy
	Lente Iletin II	Purified pork	U-100	SQ	Cloudy
Lente insulin zinc suspension (Novo Nordisk)	Novolin L	Human (bio)	U-100	SQ	Cloudy
	Lente	Purified pork	U-100	SQ	Cloudy
Ultralente extended insulin zinc suspension (Lilly)	Humulin U	Human (bio)	U-100	SQ	Cloudy
70/30[b] (Lilly)	Humulin 70/30	Human (bio)	U-100	SQ	Cloudy
70/30[b] (Novo Nordisk)	Novolin 70/30	Human (bio)	U-100	SQ	Cloudy
50/50[b] (Lilly)	Humulin 50/50	Human (bio)	U-100	SQ	Cloudy
Lispro (Lilly)	Humalog	Modified human (analog)	U-100	SQ, IV	Clear

[a] IV Intravenous (includes insulin, pump); SQ, subcutaneous.

[b] All 70/30 insulins are a combination of 70% human insulin isophane suspension (NPH) and 30% human insulin (regular) injection. The 50/50 insulin is a combination of 50% human isophane insulin suspension and 50% human insulin injection.

Notes: Any change of insulin should be made cautiously and only under medical supervision. Changes in purity, strength, brand (manufacturer), type (regular, NPH, lente, etc.), species (pork, beef/pork, human), and/or method of manufacture (biosynthetic, semisynthetic, animal-derivation) may result in the need for a change in dosage.

Some individuals with diabetes and many practitioners claim that human insulin peaks faster and is eliminated more quickly from the circulation than animal source insulins. Although research does not support a significant difference in time-action curves when changing from animal to human insulins, personal and clinical experiences may vary. For example, many pediatric endocrinologists prefer to use purified pork insulins in children as they remain in the circulation longer (providing better basal coverage) and they may not peak as quickly, thus avoiding frequent hypoglycemia.

pancreas of cows or pigs or dissolution of the cells used for recombinant DNA reproduction of insulin molecules (refer to Figure 5-1). Concern about purity of insulin is almost a non-issue today, as all insulins are highly purified. This improvement in purity has had several therapeutic benefits. Allergic reactions and lipoatrophy (loss of subcutaneous fat) have virtually disappeared, and improved diabetes control can usually be achieved with a smaller dose of a purified insulin. In addition, there appears to be less antibody formation to these insulins due primarily to species source (pork and human) and purification. Even though information on the adverse long-term effects of insulin antibodies is limited, reducing the formation of antibodies seems to be a desirable goal. Individuals who need to take insulin for just a short period of time, such as those with NIDDM in need of surgery or those who develop gestational diabetes, are less likely to develop antibodies to insulin if they use the purified ones available today.[4]

Source

In 1983, human insulin became clinically available, and it is now the most prescribed source of insulin in the United States.[4] Until 12 years ago, the only available forms of insulin were derived from the cow and pig pancreas. By 1994, all standard insulin products of beef source only were discontinued by the two major insulin manufacturers in the United States. Standard products derived from a combination of beef/pork pancreases are still available, although it is projected that most animal insulins may become obsolete by the year 2000.

Human insulin is now produced synthetically by two laboratory methods. The first method is *recombinant DNA technology* (biosynthetic), which capitalizes on the fermentation of a micro-organism that can reproduce rapidly. The micro-organisms used are bacteria (*Escherichia coli*) or fungal cells (*Saccharomyces cerevisiae*), which have the appropriate DNA coding for human proinsulin inserted into their genetic strand. The second process involves chemical conver-

sion of pork insulin to human insulin (*semisynthetic*) because it is so similar in structure to human insulin. In this method, threonine is substituted for alanine at the B-30 site on the ß-chain of pork insulin to convert it to human insulin (refer to Figure 5-1). Both methods produce insulin shown to be identical to the hormone occurring naturally. Table 5-2 compares the differences between various insulin species.

Studies have shown that human insulin is comparable to purified pork insulin when used clinically. There have been some reports, however, that absorption is faster and the duration of action is shorter with biosynthetic human NPH, lente, and ultralente insulins when compared with animal-derived insulins. For this reason, purified pork insulins are used by many diabetes centers that treat children.[4] Human insulin can be used with individuals who are allergic to beef or pork insulin, in those who develop insulin resistance to animal insulin, and in those whose religious beliefs or value systems influence their choice of pharmaceuticals (Muslims, Orthodox Jews, Hindus, vegetarians). In addition, individuals requiring intermittent insulin therapy, those who are pregnant, and those who are newly diagnosed with IDDM may benefit from using human insulin due to its lower immunogenicity. In most cases of newly diagnosed type I diabetes and in all cases of initiation of insulin therapy in type II diabetes, human insulin is recommended.[4]

It is important to remember that each person who takes insulin will respond individually to the insulin dose. The information presented in Table 5-3 represents averages in onset, peak, and duration of action. The type, concentration, purity, and source of insulin can each be changed, if necessary, to provide the individual with optimal glucose control. The diabetes educator should discuss such options with the physician when indicated.

INSULIN ADMINISTRATION

Insulin administration encompasses a number of topics: storing insulin, mixing insulins, insu-

Table 5-2 Amino Acid Sequence Difference between Various Insulin Species

	A-Chain		B-Chain
Species	A-8	A-10	B-30
Bovine	Alanine	Valine	Alanine
Porcine	Threonine	Isoleucine	Alanine
Human	Threonine	Isoleucine	Threonine

Source: Adapted with permission from Galloway JA. Chemistry and clinical use of insulin. In: Galloway JA, ed. *Diabetes Mellitus.* Indianapolis, Ind: Lilly Research Laboratories; 1988.

Table 5-3 Human Insulin

			Approximate Timing of Action[a]		
Type	Name[b]	Appearance	Onset (hours)	Maximum Effect (hours)	Duration (hours)
Fast-acting	Regular				
	Humulin R	Clear	0.5	2–4	6–8
	Novolin R	Clear	0.5	2–5	6–8
Intermediate-acting	NPH				
	Humulin N	Cloudy	1–1.5	6–12	24
	Novolin N	Cloudy	1–1.5	4–12	24
	Lente				
	Humulin L	Cloudy	1–1.5	4–12	22–24
	Novolin L	Cloudy	1–1.5	4–12	22–24
Premixed (70% intermediate + 30% fast)	70/30				
	Humulin 70/30	Cloudy	0.5–1	2–12	22–24
	Novolin 70/30	Cloudy	0.5–1	2–12	22–24
(50% intermediate + 50% fast)	50/50				
	Humulin 50/50	Cloudy	0.5–1	2–12	22–24
Long-acting	Ultralente				
	Humulin U	Cloudy	4–6	6–16	24–36

[a] The timing of action varies greatly among individuals and at different times within the same individual, depending on the source, dose, injection site, exercise of the injected area, ambient temperature, insulin antibodies, and the route of administration. IV insulin works most rapidly; only regular insulin can be given IV.

[b] Eli Lilly and Company human insulins are called Humulin; Novo Nordisk Pharmaceuticals human insulins are called Novolin. Both Lilly and Novo Nordisk use biosynthetic processes to manufacture human insulins; Lilly uses *Escherichia coli* and Novo Nordisk uses *Saccharomyces cerevisiae.*

lin delivery methods, factors affecting insulin absorption and glucose response, and complications of insulin therapy. Each of these topics needs to be covered thoroughly with the patient and reviewed periodically; feedback demonstrations should be requested, where appropriate. Treatment of each topic must also address development of problem-solving abilities to prevent the occurrence of complications of therapy and to preserve target blood glucose control. Successful administration of insulin requires correct supplies, adequate preparation, and consistent application of proper technique.[5]

Storing Insulin

Insulin needs to be stored properly to ensure its full potency. If refrigerated (36 to 46°F, 2 to 8°C), *unopened* insulin will remain potent until its expiration date, which is found on both the product box and the bottle label. If refrigerated, *opened* insulin will retain up to 90% of its potency for 90 days, but beyond this 90 days changes will probably need to be made in dose to accommodate the loss of potency. *Opened* insulin may be kept at controlled room temperature (59 to 68°F, 15 to 20°C), if the entire contents of the vial will be used within 1 month. Vials should be dated when opened and discarded after 30 days. Insulins stored at room temperature beyond 1 month deteriorate, with a loss of potency, especially if stored at temperatures over 86°F (30°C). Exposing insulin to temperature extremes (ie, storing it in the glove compartment of the car, near a radiator, on top of the refrigerator, in the bathroom, or on a windowsill) should be avoided to prevent loss of potency.[5–8]

Penfills and disposable pen storage guidelines differ.[5,6] Penfills are cartridges containing 150 U each of insulin that can be used with the NovolinPen (available with Novolin R, Novolin N, or Novolin 70/30). Penfill regular insulin can be stored at room temperature for 30 days after puncture of the cartridge when it is inserted into the barrel of the NovolinPen; penfills 70/30 and NPH can be stored at room temperature for 7 days after puncture.

Prefilled syringes of either single formulations or mixtures of insulins should be kept refrigerated and used within 3 to 4 weeks.[7–9] Often, these prefilled syringes are prepared by family members for elderly relatives or by home health care professionals who only see clients one to two times per week.

The appearance of the insulin should be examined for sediment or other visible changes before withdrawing into a syringe. Cloudiness or discoloration of clear (regular) insulin, clumping of insulin suspensions (NPH, lente, ultralente), or flocculation (frosting) of insulin suspensions indicates an alteration in the pharmacologic effects of the insulin. These insulins should be discarded and fresh vials obtained prior to administration. Although a rare occurrence, frosting can be minimized with temperature stabilization through refrigeration and refraining from shaking or agitating the vial.

Mixing Insulins

Organizing materials prior to insulin injection limits errors. Preplanning makes administration more routine for traveling purposes also. Five general rules of thumb for mixing insulins are: (1) both insulins should be made by the same manufacturer, (2) the recommended order for mixing insulins is "clear before cloudy" (regular insulin is drawn first, followed by the intermediate-acting insulin), (3) semisynthetic human insulin (Velosulin) should not be mixed with lente insulins, (4) the concentration of each insulin should be the same, and (5) within the guidelines of compatibility (same concentration and same manufacturer), human and animal species insulins may be mixed, although there are no rational advantages for this combination.[8] Exhibit 5-1 summarizes mixing and prefilling guidelines.[9] Commercially prepared premixed insulins (70/30 and 50/50) are manufactured and stabilized by using different buffering agents from those used with the individual insulins.

Insulin Delivery Methods

Needles of disposable syringes, disposable and regular pen devices, and insulin pump tubing sets are extremely thin and sharp (27- to 30-gauge), causing minimal discomfort during injection/insertion.

Disposable Syringes. The oldest and most convenient form of insulin delivery is injection using *disposable syringes.* To accommodate the

Exhibit 5-1 Guidelines for Mixing Insulin and/or
                Prefilling Syringes

Regular and NPH
Mixture stable in any ratio
Mixture of choice, if rapid and intermediate
combination
   is needed
Extemporaneously prepared syringes that are
refrigerated
are stable for at least 1 month
Prefilling is acceptable

Regular and lente
Binding of regular begins immediately, reducing its
   action
Binding continues for 24 hours
Activity of regular is blunted
Velosulin should not be mixed with lente insulins
If mixed or prefilled, the interval between mixing the
   insulins and administering the insulin should be
   standardized

Commercially prepared premixed insulins
Prefilling is acceptable

Lente and ultralente
Mixture stable in any ratio
Mixture stable for 18 months
Prefilling is acceptable

Source: Adapted with permission from White JR, Campbell
RK. Guide to mixing insulins. *Hosp Pharm.* 1991;26:1046–
1048.

---

amount of the dose, 1 mL (100 U), $^1/_2$ mL (50 U),
$^3/_{10}$ mL (30 U), and $^1/_4$ mL (25 U) syringes are
available. All are made for U-100 concentration
insulin. Four different companies in the United
States manufacture disposable syringes.[10]

For those taking more than one injection per
day, reuse of syringes can be done safely in
order to save costs. Syringe reuse may carry an
increased risk of infection for some individuals.[5]
If the dilemma for a patient is skipping an injection due to cost versus reusing a syringe, there is
no doubt that the latter alternative is preferred.
The patient should be advised that the needle
will dull after repeated use and that the markings
on the plastic barrel may rub off with repetition,
making dosing errors more likely. After use, pa-

tients should wipe the needle with alcohol, re-
cap, and store in the refrigerator until ready to
reuse.

Injection Aids. These serve two different purposes: (1) to make the injection with a syringe
easier and more comfortable and (2) to provide
an alternative to syringes. Before making the decision to use one of these products, the patient
should sample it first because some require considerable dexterity and skill to execute and
maintain.[10]

Insertion aids are devices that accelerate
needle insertion into the skin; some aids even
push the plunger into the skin. Most are spring-
loaded devices and hide the needle from view.
These products are useful for those who are
needle-phobic or who hesitate during the injection.

Syringe alternatives include infusers, insulin
pens, and jet injectors. Infusers create "portals"
into which the insulin is injected. A needle is inserted into subcutaneous tissue (usually the abdomen) and remains taped in place for 48 to 72
hours. The insulin is injected into it, rather than
directly through the skin into the fatty tissue.
Some individuals are prone to infections with
infusers, so diabetes education must include a
review of sterile techniques and cleaning procedures with the patient.

Insulin pens are becoming more popular with
the standard of care shifting to multiple injections of short-acting insulins. An insulin pen is
much like an old-fashioned cartridge pen but,
instead of a writing point, there is a needle and,
instead of an ink cartridge, there is an insulin
cartridge. The NovolinPen uses 150-U cartridges of Novolin R, N, or 70/30. The use of a
pen can save on supplies because syringes do not
have to be purchased, just the needle tips (which
can be reused following the same precautions for
reuse of syringes). In fact, the needle remains
sharper because it does not have to penetrate the
rubber stopper on the insulin vial. With the pen
device insulin does not have to be drawn; the
patient simply dials to the correct dose.

Novo Nordisk also manufactures a prefilled
disposable plastic pen with prefilled Novolin

70/30, R, or N cartridges. Once the cartridge is emptied, the entire pen is appropriately discarded. These pen devices are preferred by travelers, business people, and those with impaired coordination.

Jet injectors release a tiny jet stream of insulin, which is forced through the skin under high pressure; there is not a puncture of the skin surface. While there are no needles with these devices, there can be problems with bruising, hypertrophy (overgrowth of subcutaneous fat), and thus, insulin absorption rates. Jet injectors are expensive and can involve a complicated cleaning procedure, but many insurance companies appear to offer coverage. Those patients who seem to fare the best with these injectors are slim older women who may have insulin absorption problems; in some cases, their insulin doses may be reduced.[11]

Insulin Pump. Continuous subcutaneous insulin infusion (CSII) devices, or insulin pumps, are the last type of insulin delivery devices. Based on the results of the DCCT, the application and function of these devices are worth reviewing. During the DCCT, subjects in the experimental study group (followed an intensive management protocol) had the option of using either multiple daily injections, consisting of three or more injections per day, or CSII.[1]

The insulin pump is a small computerized device that delivers regular insulin via a plastic catheter that is attached to a metal needle or teflon infusion set that is inserted subcutaneously in abdominal tissue. Doses of insulin, often as little as 0.1 U, can be delivered with accuracy. An insulin pump is an open-loop system. That is, the pump can neither measure nor control blood glucose levels independently; it is programmed by the individual to deliver insulin from information gained through blood glucose monitoring.[13]

In a nondiabetic pancreas, the ß-cells release precise amounts of insulin to cover two needs. First, the pancreas releases a background flow of insulin into the blood when a person is not eating (during periods of fasting; for example, overnight or between meals). This *basal insulin* directs the release and uptake of glucose and, to some extent, fat as fuels. An insulin pump mimics this background flow of insulin with its basal rate.

Second, short bursts of insulin are released by the normal pancreas into the bloodstream to match the rise in glucose produced primarily by carbohydrate in foods eaten. This larger, quicker release of insulin is mimicked by the insulin pump via *bolus doses*.[12,13]

The insulin pump allows a more precise match between insulin delivery and the body's need for insulin. When an insulin pump is used well, it can be the most physiologic tool for achieving blood glucose control and promoting a freer life style. To control blood glucose levels well in diabetes, the pump matches three needs: (1) the basal rate covers background insulin requirements; (2) the bolus doses cover carbohydrate content of foods eaten, and (3) extra insulin delivered via bolus and/or increased basal rate brings high blood sugars back to normal range.

Another advantage of the insulin pump is that it allows more reliable insulin absorption because it delivers minute amounts of regular insulin slowly and steadily over time.[14] NPH, lente, and ultralente insulins work over longer periods of time than regular. When injected, a large pool or depot of insulin forms under the skin and is absorbed from the injection site over the next 24 to 36 hours. Unfortunately, these pools of insulin affect the absorption of insulin into the bloodstream, resulting in wide variations in insulin uptake—as much as 25% from one day to the next.[15]

There are many reasons why an insulin pump might be selected over other methods. Exhibit 5-2 summarizes personal reasons that might influence a patient with diabetes to consider pump therapy, as well as clinical situations that would demand the precision and flexibility the insulin pump offers. It is important to realize, however, that an insulin pump is not a panacea for poorly controlled diabetes. It requires a substantial investment in terms of time and resources to derive maximum benefit for the patient. Exhibit 5-3 lists those criteria that should be considered

Exhibit 5-2 Reasons To Consider Pump Therapy

Clinical indications for pump therapy
- Metabolic instability
- Early neuropathy or nephropathy
- Planning for pregnancy or pregnant
- Post renal transplant

Personal indications for pump therapy
- Shift work
- Unpredictable workloads/hours
- Frequent travel
- Extremely active in sports (amateur or professional level)

Exhibit 5-3 Personal Attributes Predictive of Patient Success with Pump Therapy

---

- Desire for glycemic control and/or flexibility
- High degree of motivation
- Realistic expectations
- Intellectual, physical, and technical ability to operate the pump
- Adequate financial resources/reserves
- Good support system
- Psychological stability including, but not limited to:
  –expectations of pump therapy
  –body image
  –privacy issues
  –dependence on a mechanical device
- Demonstrated ability to perform intensive therapy with frequent self-monitoring of blood glucose

---

when judging candidacy for pump therapy; the relative absence of any of these factors may be a contraindication to pump therapy and should be explored with the patient during the selection process.[16]

Implantable insulin pumps are undergoing clinical trials. The Programmable Implantable Medication System (PIMS) is under investigation by MiniMed Technologies (Sylmar, California). This disc-shaped pump, which is about the size of a hockey puck, is surgically implanted in an abdominal pocket. The reservoir holds approximately 3 months' supply of U-500

insulin which is delivered using programmed radio signal commands from a simple transmitter. While the device holds promise for the future, there are problems with fascitis and other infections arising from its use, as well as a finding of tissue proliferation around the device that may affect its function. These problems must be addressed before the pump can be approved as a marketable device.

There is a wide variety of devices available for insulin administration. Industry is encouraged to continue upgrading current technologies (syringes and pen devices) and to develop new administration tools that will enhance the lifestyle needs of persons with diabetes.

Many inexpensive devices are available for persons with visual impairments to aid in drawing their insulin dose, measuring their insulin dose, or magnifying the syringe barrel. Articles detailing the features of these many products are regularly updated in journals on diabetes.[10]

Factors Affecting Insulin Absorption and Glucose Response

In many individuals, a period of remission or a "honeymoon phase" occurs shortly after the diagnosis of type I diabetes (IDDM) is made. A large reduction in insulin requirements may occur, or glucose tolerance may even return to normal. The explanation is a "last-ditch" effort by the pancreas to secrete endogenous insulin. Often, cases of type I diabetes in older patients (> 40 years old) are misdiagnosed with type II diabetes (NIDDM) because these individuals may be placed on oral agents for the first few months and achieve relatively well-controlled blood glucose levels due to the "honeymoon phase." The length of the remission can vary from several weeks to as long as a year. These individuals need to understand this phenomenon so that they do not mistakenly believe that their diabetes has been "cured." Dietary intervention is still of paramount importance in control of blood glucose levels, regardless of whether insulin therapy diminishes or ceases during this phase.

Individuals who present with fasting hyperglycemia in the wake of increasing insulin doses and worsening diabetes control may be experiencing the Somogyi Effect. In this condition, hypoglycemia in the middle of the night is unrecognized and the counterregulatory hormones that increase blood glucose as a protective mechanism—cortisol, growth hormone, glucagon, and catecholamines—induce a rebound hyperglycemia. Generally the recommendation is to increase the insulin dose to combat early morning hyperglycemia, which actually exacerbates the problem. This effect can be documented by self-monitoring of blood glucose at 3 A.M.

Another condition that is relatively more rare in individuals with diabetes is the Dawn Phenomenon. Sensitivity to insulin may diminish between 4 A.M. and 9 A.M.—probably due to a surge of growth hormone that is released during the early morning hours—resulting in fasting hyperglycemia. Again, to document this phenomenon, blood glucose monitoring at 3 A.M. is required. Exhibit 5-4 presents the differential diagnosis of Somogyi Effect and Dawn Phenomenon.

The registered dietitian needs to understand the time-action curves of all insulin preparations, individually and in combinations. The DCCT utilized 38 different insulin regimens, employing unusual combinations, such as ultralente with NPH or NPH three times per day, in order to achieve specified blood glucose targets.[1] Figures 5-2 through 5-3 visually depict the time-action curves of various combination insulin regimens. Information on these time-action curves is essential to appropriate meal planning efforts, which are aimed at achieving the appropriate combination of foods (what to eat) in calculated amounts (how much to eat) to be eaten at the best times (when to eat) in order to prevent glycemic excursions (wide fluctuations in blood glucose levels). Working with the medication information allows the registered dietitian to

---

Exhibit 5-4 Differential Diagnosis: Somogyi Effect and Dawn Phenomenon

	Somogyi Effect	*Dawn Phenomenon*
Characteristics	Rebound hyperglycemia following unrecognized and untreated hypoglycemia (frequently nocturnal)	Exaggeration of a normal physiologic process producing a surge of growth hormone during sleep (3 to 5 A.M.) resulting in a high fasting glucose
Occurrence	Seen less with tid or qid insulin dose than with bid	Rare; varies from day to day
Identification	3 A.M. blood glucose	3 A.M. blood glucose
Blood glucose level	Low between 2 to 4 A.M.	Normal or elevated between 2 to 4 A.M. With further elevation in FBG despite overnight fast
Ketones	May be present in A.M.	Absence of ketones
Treatment	Increase bedtime snack; decrease before-supper insulin (N or L) or move to bedtime; do not increase A.M. insulin	Decrease bedtime snack; increase before-supper insulin (N or L) or change to bedtime, based on frequency of Dawn Phenomenon; do not increase A.M. insulin

Note: tid, three times a day; qid, four times a day; bid, twice a day.

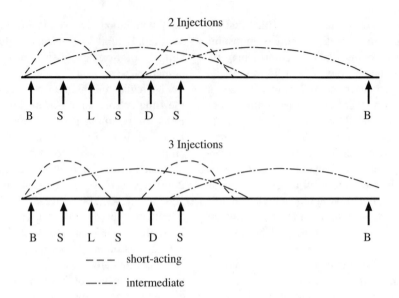

Figure 5-2 Time Actions Insulin Regimen. *Source:* Reprinted with permission from *Physician's Guide to Insulin-Dependent (Type I) Diabetes*, 1988. Copyright © 1994 by American Diabetes Association. All rights reserved.

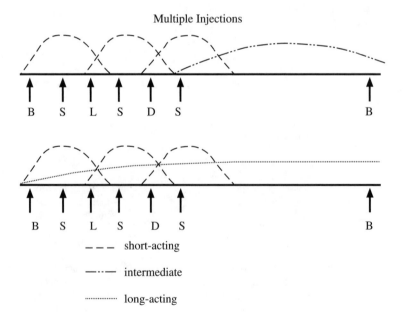

Figure 5-3 Time Actions Insulin Regimen. *Source:* Reprinted with permission from *Physician's Guide to Insulin-Dependent (Type I) Diabetes*, 1988. Copyright © 1994 by American Diabetes Association. All rights reserved.

maintain a strategic position on the diabetes management team. Problem solving for common blood glucose patterns is summarized in Table 5-4, providing a generic basis for alterations in meal composition, amounts, and timing.

A number of factors can influence the blood glucose response to a single dose of insulin. The technique used in preparing a dose of insulin can determine its effect on blood glucose; for example, neglecting to roll a bottle of cloudy insulin in order to mix the contents prior to drawing it up may decrease the effectiveness of the insulin. Upon injection, the site will have a major impact on the consistency and rate of absorption of the insulin (abdomen > arm > thigh > buttocks).[17] In addition, absorption occurs more rapidly if the insulin is injected into an area that is about to be exercised (eg, the thigh before jogging). Rotation of injection sites is critical to maximizing the rate of absorption. If the same site is used repeatedly, the rate of absorption will gradually decrease. However, to ensure consistency in absorption it is recommended that individuals rotate within the same area (eg, the right side of the abdomen) for 2 to 3 weeks before changing to another area, such as the right arm. Or, individuals with diabetes may find that the morning injection is best absorbed when given abdominally, affording better blood glucose levels after breakfast, and that the evening injection is best administered in the thigh because a walk will be taken after dinner. See Figure 5-4 for a rotation guide for insulin site determination.

How the insulin is injected also has an effect on the rate of absorption. Whether the injection enters the skin at a 45° or 90° angle will determine its rate of absorption. Insulin is more rapidly absorbed intravenously, less rapidly intramuscularly, and least rapidly subcutaneously. Rate of absorption of insulin will increase with increasing temperature and with massage of the site after injection.

The registered dietitian must be informed of all of these possibilities in order to assess the reason(s) for erratic blood glucose values. The best way to evaluate the effectiveness of an individual insulin dose regimen is through self-monitoring of blood glucose (SMBG). The frequency of testing may be determined by the frequency of insulin administration and the eating schedule. Because insulin is not the only factor affecting blood glucose, an adjustment in the meal plan may be a more desirable alternative than a change in the insulin regimen. Thus, dietitians must be adept at interpreting blood glucose values in order to recommend appropriate modifications in an individual's meal plan (refer to Table 5-4 and Chapters 6 and 8).

Complications of Insulin Therapy

Complications or side effects of insulin treatment include insulin allergy (localized or systemic reactions), lipodystrophy (lipoatrophy, hypertrophy), insulin resistance, insulin antibodies, hypoglycemia, and weight gain. With the advent of human insulin, decreased utilization of animal source insulins, and the highly purified nature of insulin preparations today, these problems have been virtually eliminated.

Before insulin preparations were purified, nearly half of all individuals taking insulin had *local or skin reactions* at the injection site. The area would become hardened, red, and itchy 3 to 6 hours after the injection. The discomfort could last for several days. Because the incidence of local reactions has decreased since the advent of highly purified insulins, it has been assumed that the impurities (proinsulin) were the cause. Treatment includes using as highly purified an insulin as possible and, if necessary, an antihistamine locally or systemically.

A rarer complication of insulin treatment is *insulin allergy*. It tends to occur in people who have stopped taking insulin for a while and then resume insulin treatment. This allergy is less frequently seen in patients who remain on insulin uninterrupted.

The allergic response usually appears within a week or two after insulin treatment is resumed. The first sign is a local skin reaction at the injection site within 30 to 60 minutes of administration. The individual's body is soon covered with

Table 5-4 Common Problem Patterns Found from Blood Glucose Monitoring

Problem	Potential Cause*	Potential Solutions
High fasting glucose	Insulin resistance,† insufficient insulin available overnight, rebound hyperglycemia overnight (Somogyi effect), Dawn Phenomenon	Adjust P.M. intermediate- or long-acting insulin dose or time Weight reduction to reduce insulin resistance
High glucose after breakfast	Inadequate insulin produced or injected to cover breakfast, peak insulin action not at anticipated time	Adjust time or dose of short-acting A.M. insulin Decrease size of breakfast or adjust amount of breakfast carbohydrate or divide breakfast into two smaller morning meals
Insulin reactions (hypoglycemia) before lunch	Insufficient breakfast for A.M. short-acting insulin or peak action later than anticipated time	Adjust time, type, or dose of A.M. short-acting insulin Add morning snack or increase breakfast
Insulin reactions (hypoglycemia) in afternoon	Excessive A.M. intermediate-acting insulin, skipping or inadequate lunch	Adjust time, type, or dose of A.M. intermediate-acting insulin Decrease or omit afternoon snack or decrease lunch
High glucose in afternoon	Inadequate insulin produced or intermediate-acting A.M. insulin is insufficient for need, or excessive snack or lunch	Adjust time or dose of P.M. insulin Decrease or omit afternoon snack or decrease lunch carbohydrate
High glucose at night after evening meal	Inadequate insulin produced or insufficient insulin to cover dinner, or evening meal too large	Adjust time or dose of P.M. insulin Reduce size of meal or alter meal composition (↓ carbohydrate)
Insulin reactions (hypoglycemia) at night	Excessive amount of insulin or insufficient dinner meal or evening snack	Adjust time, type, or dose of evening or bedtime insulin Increase dinner and/or snack carbohydrate

* In addition to food and insulin, other factors may affect blood glucose (eg, exercise, sick days, infection).

† Insulin resistance associated with obesity is likely to result in high glucose levels throughout the day.

Source: Adapted from Powers MA, Barr P, Franz M, Holler H, Wheeler ML, Wylie-Rosett J. *Nutrition Guide for Professionals: Diabetes Education and Meal Planning.* Chicago, II: American Dietetic Association/American Diabetes Association, 1989, p. 6.

hives, and he or she may be in danger of developing anaphylactic shock if treatment is not begun. Desensitization is the only effective treatment for insulin allergy. The affected individual is given small but increasing doses of insulin at frequent intervals. The desensitization should occur with the species of insulin that the individual will use daily. This process is successful in most people experiencing this complication. These individuals should not have their insulin

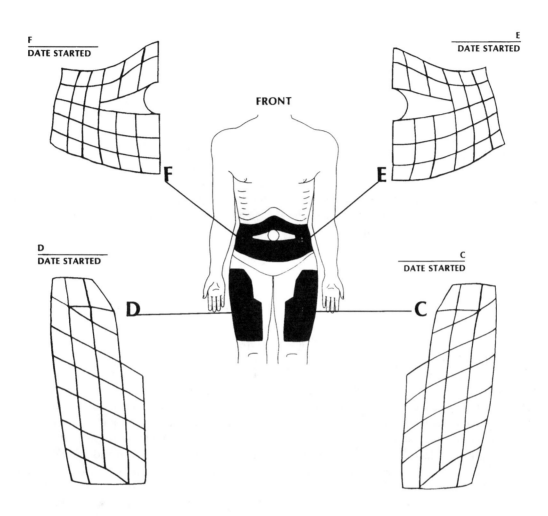

FRONT

This body map is designed to help you record your insulin injections. Write down the date that you start an area. Place an X in the space on the map to show which site you used. One suggested pattern for using the map is to rotate your injections in one area for 1 week or until you have used each site in the area once.

This system will help you rotate insulin injection sites over the 12 body areas and avoid using any one area or site too often. Choose a site one knuckle's width away from the previous site as you rotate within a given area.

Figure 5-4 Injection Log. *Source:* Eli Lilly and Company, Indianapolis, Indiana.

---

treatment interrupted. Some people may require repetition of the desensitization process over time.[18]

Some insulin users develop *lipoatrophy*, a loss of subcutaneous fat, at the site of the injection; an indented area results. Although this condition is benign, there can be a psychologic re-sponse to the cosmetic effect of the fat loss. Although the cause of lipoatrophy is unknown, it may be due to contaminants in the insulin. Changing to a more purified form of insulin and injecting around the periphery of the affected area can encourage reaccumulation of the fat tissue. Continuation with a highly purified form of insulin and use of the affected site will prevent further loss of fat tissue.

Lipohypertrophy, an enlargement or overgrowth of subcutaneous fat, occurs in some insulin users at the site of injection. This condition results in bumps or knots that are sometimes visible through clothing. It has been assumed that repeated injections in the same area are responsible for this problem. Individuals tend to use the same sites for injection because, as the depot of fat increases, the discomfort on injection decreases. Again, cosmetic changes in the area result, but may be compounded with the problem of decreased insulin absorption. In some individuals, the extra fat tissue will eventually disappear if the area is no longer used for injections. The key to both of these complications is stressing the importance of proper site rotation.

Insulin resistance is the need for more than 200 U of insulin daily for more than 2 days. This complication is often associated with other medical conditions as described in the text that follows.[3] In Cushing's syndrome, the excessive action of glucocorticoids accounts for the insulin resistance that occurs. Glucocorticoids increase gluconeogenesis and interfere with insulin's ability to enhance glucose uptake by peripheral tissues. Acromegaly is caused by an excessive secretion of growth hormone from the pituitary gland. Growth hormone antagonizes insulin action, which may or may not manifest in development of diabetes. Individuals who develop hemochromatosis, a disorder of iron metabolism in which excessive iron deposits appear in the liver, pancreas, and other body tissues, are prone to develop diabetes. Many of these individuals develop insulin resistance. Many people diagnosed with acanthosis nigricans, a disorder of the prickle-cell layer of the epidermis in which a gray to black pigmentation develops in body folds, also become insulin-resistant. A probable mechanism is a serious defect in the ability of the receptor cell to bind insulin, or to antibodies that block the insulin receptor. People requiring more than 200 U of insulin per day are candidates for U-500 insulin. Because of its greater concentration, a smaller volume is needed.

All people who receive exogenous insulin develop some *insulin-binding antibodies*, regardless of the purity or source of the insulin used. For the majority of insulin users, these antibodies never become a problem. For those patients who develop antibody-mediated insulin resistance, the use of a more concentrated form of insulin is recommended (U-500). Self-monitoring of blood glucose is essential as there is rarely a clear-cut indication that insulin sensitivity is returning. To prevent serious hypoglycemia as the sensitivity is restored, SMBG must be done regularly.

Hypoglycemia is the most common risk of insulin treatment. In those who are intensively managed, as demonstrated by the DCCT, severe hypoglycemia (requiring assistance by another) was threefold higher than in individuals on more conservative conventional insulin regimens.[1] Hypoglycemia results from too much insulin, not enough food, a delayed meal, extra activity, and certain forms of stress. Ingestion of propranolol and alcohol, liver or kidney failure, hypopituitarism, and adrenal insufficiency can cause hypoglycemia in people taking insulin. The signs and symptoms of hypoglycemia, although different for each individual, begin with an adrenergic response to a falling blood glucose, resulting in trembling, sweating, tachycardia, and visual changes. Left untreated, hypoglycemia progresses to neuroglycopenic symptoms, such as drowsiness, headache, disorientation, behavior changes, and irritability. Prompt treatment with 15 g of a fast-acting carbohydrate is the recommended course of action. Monitoring of blood glucose should be done after 15 minutes to confirm that the blood glucose has risen to within normal range. If not, another 15 g of carbohydrate should be administered, followed by a protein-containing food. If the hypoglycemia progresses to unconsciousness, nothing should be given by mouth. Instead, injectable glucagon (available by prescription) should be administered. Glucagon will only work if there are stores of glycogen in the liver to stimulate. In individuals with frequent hypoglycemia, glucagon may not be effective be-

Table 5-5 Characteristics of Hypoglycemia and Hyperglycemia

	Hypoglycemia	*Hyperglycemia*
Also known as	Low blood sugar Insulin reaction	High blood sugar Diabetic acidosis
Onset	Rapid—minutes	Slow—days
Causes	Too much insulin Not enough food Delayed/skipped meal Unusual amount of exercise	Lack of knowledge/understanding Intercurrent disease Infection, fever Stress Neglect of therapy: diet or medication
Symptoms	Perspiration Light-headedness Weakness, dizziness Trembling Heart pounding Nausea and vomiting Headache Sudden hunger Nervousness, anxiousness, irritability Drowsiness Confusion Lack of concentration Difficulty verbalizing Impaired vision: double, blurred Numbness of tongue and mouth Personality change Inappropriate behavior	Increased thirst Frequent urination Hunger (in some) Weight loss Abdominal pain Nausea and vomiting Headache Anorexia Vision change
Signs	Pallor Shallow respiration Perspiration Pulse normal Eyeballs normal	Ruddy, flushed Kussmaul air hunger Dehydration Pulse rapid Eyeballs soft Acetone breath
Urine	Glucose usually negative Acetone negative	Glucose positive Acetone positive
Blood	Glucose usually <60 mg/dL CO_2 usually normal Leukocytes usually normal	Glucose >250 mg/dL CO_2 <20 vols.% (53–64) Leukocytes may be high
Treatment	Carbohydrate (take by mouth, instant product) Nothing by mouth if unconscious (glucagon) Call physician Rarely hospitalized	Call physician Give fluids without sugar if able to swallow Continue to take insulin Monitor urine for ketones May need hospitalization
Response	Usually rapid—minutes	Slow—days

cause their stores of glycogen may be sparse. If frequent episodes of hypoglycemia are occurring, adjustments in activity, food, and/or insulin are in order. Table 5-5 compares characteristics of hypoglycemia and hyperglycemia (which is also a complication of inadequate insulin therapy).

Intensive management of diabetes via an insulin pump or even multiple daily injection therapy is associated with two adverse events, as demonstrated by the DCCT: (1) a threefold greater incidence of severe hypoglycemia, and (2) weight gain.[1] The weight gain was attributed to several different causes: frequent treatment of hypoglycemia due to its increased rate of occurrence, improvement of blood glucose control (remember, insulin is a storage hormone when adequate amounts are available to metabolize food), and use of more flexible dietary regimens on intensive therapy.[1]

SITUATIONS IN WHICH INSULIN REQUIREMENTS MAY CHANGE

Stress, acute illness, menstruation, other medications, changes in food intake, and changes in activity level all have an effect on insulin requirements. Stress can refer to the tension of daily living and working or it can be an unusual traumatic experience, such as the death of a friend. Depending on the type of stress or excitement that occurs, an individual on insulin may require more or less insulin. The reaction to a particular type of stress can only be determined through self-monitoring of blood glucose levels. Insulin needs are generally higher during acute illness (colds, flu, infections) and, although nausea and decreased appetite may be present, continuation of the insulin is essential. The body becomes extremely insulin-resistant during acute illness due to the overproduction of catecholamines. Self-monitoring of blood glucose and monitoring of urine ketone levels are recommended more frequently during illness. Changes in food intake (type, amount, or timing) will affect insulin requirements. The best way to note

Exhibit 5-5 Drugs That May Increase and Decrease Blood Glucose Levels

Drugs That Increase Blood Glucose Levels
- Caffeine (in large, irregular doses)
- Calcium channel blockers
- Corticosteroids
- Diazoxide
- Estrogen
- Furosemide
- L-asparaginase
- Niacinamide
- Nicotine
- Phenobarbital
- Rifampin
- Thiazide diuretics
- Thyroid replacements

Drugs That Decrease Blood Glucose Levels
- Alcohol
- Allopurinol
- Anabolic steroids
- Bishydroxycoumarin
- Cimetidine
- Clofibrate
- Monoamine oxidase inhibitors
- Phenylbutazone
- Potassium salts
- Probenecid
- Propranolol (beta blockers)
- Salicylates (large doses)
- Sulfonamides

the effect of any change in food intake is to test preprandially and, again, 2 hours postprandially. Changes in types and duration of activity will affect blood glucose levels and thus insulin dosages. Determining the "drop value" of any form of exercise is done by testing prior to the onset of the activity and again upon completion of the exercise period. Either a decrease in medication or an increase in food (or both) can adjust for an alteration in exercise.

Menstruation in approximately 30% of women with diabetes can dramatically increase insulin resistance during the luteal phase (1 to 1-1/2 weeks prior to menstruation). As a result, insulin requirements may increase by as much as 30 to 50% prior to the initiation of the menstrual flow. Once the menstruation begins, however, insulin will immediately need to be readjusted downward to prevent hypoglycemia.

Individuals with diabetes are frequently on many other medications for various other conditions or complications of their disease. It is important to consider the possible effect of these medications on blood glucose levels. Exhibit 5-5 lists drugs that can increase or decrease blood glucose, possibly necessitating a change in insulin dosages to optimize control.

DETERMINING INSULIN DOSES AND REGIMENS

Choosing the kind and amount of insulin to use depends on the type of diabetes and the medical targets established for the individual. The optimal goal is a near-normal blood glucose value most of the time, while avoiding extremes of hypoglycemia and hyperglycemia.

As discussed earlier in this chapter, there are many insulin types and, therefore, many possibilities for combining insulins to achieve metabolic control. A regimen involving three or more injections daily is called multiple daily injection therapy, and this type of therapy is considered to be more intensive. Use of an insulin pump is also considered more intensive management. Self- monitoring of blood glucose values remains a critical element in determining the effectiveness of any particular insulin prescription and the appropriate dosages.

The total requirement for insulin in a 24-hour period (i.e., the total daily dose [or TDD]) is initially based on body weight and subsequently adjusted according to metabolic needs (see Appendix 5-D). In general, 0.5 to 0.6 U/kg of body weight is usually the starting point. Adolescents may require two to three times the usual dose when they reach puberty due to the production of growth hormone and catecholamines. Practitioners need to consider overinsulinization when dosages reach 1.5 to 2.0 U/kg, which can start a vicious cycle of Somogyi reactions. Although it is important to achieve metabolic control by having the correct amount of insulin on board, it is frustrating to deal with the phenomenon of "feeding the insulin" when too much is present in the circulation.

Appendix 5-B lists some tips and thoughts that registered dietitians will want to keep in mind when helping patients with diabetes to problem solve to reach target blood glucose levels. Changes in insulin dosages should not be made in a reactionary fashion, but should be based on patterns that are observed over several days' time.[19]

TREATMENT WITH ORAL AGENTS

Unlike type I diabetes (IDDM) in which metabolic abnormalities are thought to result primarily from absolute insulin deficiency caused by loss of ß-cell mass, type II diabetes (NIDDM) is recognized as a heterogeneous disorder with at least three defects.[20] These defects are abnormalities in insulin secretion, reduced sensitivity to insulin (peripheral resistance), and excessive hepatic glucose production in the basal state (glycogenolysis). Awareness of these defects, their interaction, and their natural history is necessary to understand the pathogenesis and treatment of type II diabetes mellitus (see Chapter 1).

Approximately 90% of the individuals with type II diabetes are obese. It is believed that a state of insulin resistance is created in the presence of obesity and that the eventual diagnosis of type II diabetes is a natural progression that is simply a matter of time.[21] Most individuals with type II diabetes can be treated with a healthy diet and regular exercise, but these two facets of care present the greatest challenges due to the issue of patient compliance.

Nutrition practice guidelines define a systematic approach for the medical nutrition therapy (MNT) provided by dietitians; these guidelines are based on scientific evidence and expert opinion.[22] Nutrition practice guidelines can be implemented for those with newly diagnosed or previously diagnosed NIDDM at the time of the first visit to the dietitian for initial or ongoing MNT (see Chapter 3). The guidelines apply to patients treated with MNT alone, MNT and glucose-lowering agents, or MNT and insulin.

MNT accompanied by regular physical activity is the preferred initial treatment for NIDDM. Various authors disagree on the appropriate length of the initial course of nonpharmacologic therapy. It has been suggested, for example, that the initial course last 4 to 6 weeks, 4 to 12 weeks, 3 to 6 months, and 4 to 6 months.[23] The middle ground appears to be 3 to 4 months at a minimum, individualized according to symptoms and blood glucose level.

An estimated 40 to 60% of newly diagnosed patients with NIDDM will not adequately respond after 3 months of treatment by diet alone. Many who are initially responsive fail subsequently, primarily due to poor adherence.[23] Pharmacologic intervention with either oral glucose-lowering agents or insulin is added to the initial therapy if adequate metabolic control is not achieved. This action should not be viewed as a "diet failure"; instead, it means that as ß-cell function becomes progressively impaired, the insulin secretory response becomes deficient. In fact, experience shows that most individuals with NIDDM will be taking the maximum dose of an oral agent within 5 to 6 years of diagnosis with eventual progression to complementary insulin with the oral agent or insulin alone as the primary medication.

Table 5-6 Oral Hypoglycemic Agents (oral sulfonylureas)[2]

Drug	First Generation			Second Generation	
	Orinase	Tolinase	Diabinese	DiaBeta Micronase Glynase PresTab[a]	Glucotrol Glucotrol XL[a]
Generic name	Tolbutamide	Tolazamide	Chlorpropamide	Glyburide	Glipizide
Daily dosage range (mg)	250–3000 divided	100–1000 single or divided	100–750 single dose	1.25–20 0.75–12[a] single, divided	2.5–40 5.0–20[a] single, divided
Maximum dose (g)	2–3	0.75–1.0	0.5	0.02	0.04
Metabolism	Liver	Liver	Liver	Liver	Liver
Excretion	Urine	Urine	Urine	50% urine 50% bile	Urine
Half-life (hours)	4–6	7	36	10 4[a]	2–4 2–24[a]
Duration of activity (hours)	6–12	24	24–72	24	12–24

[a] Half-life and daily dosage ranges are different for Glynase PresTab and Glucotrol XL.

Note: Glucophage (generic name: Metformin) is considered an antihyperglycemic agent vs. an oral hypoglycemic agent because it does not affect normal blood glucose levels (see text). Metformin is not metabolized in man and is rapidly excreted in the urine unchanged. Metformin should be given in divided doses along with meals. Initial regimens are typically one 500-mg tablet twice daily. It is also available in 850-mg tablets. Doses can be escalated weekly in increments of 500 mgs. Maximum doses consist of 2500 mgs/day of 500-mg tablets or 2550 mgs/day of the 850-mg tablets, taken three times daily. Taking metformin with food minimizes the gastrointestinal side effects. Metformin binds negligibly to plasma proteins and its plasma half-life is approximately 6 hours.

Exhibit 5-6 Factors in Choosing an Oral Agent

Drug Characteristics
- Inherent hypoglycemic potency
- Duration of action
- Half-life
- Site (organ) in which drug is chiefly metabolized
- Nature and severity of potential side effects

Patient Characteristics
- Risk of hypoglycemia (age; hepatic/renal function; adherence to prescribed diet, medications, exercise)
- Drugs being taken for conditions other than diabetes
- Hyperlipidemia

Characteristics

Oral agents fall into two chemical categories: sulfonylureas and biguanides. They have different mechanisms of action and effects on the body (see Table 5-6). Sulfonylureas are actually hypoglycemic drugs (hypoglycemia is a severe side effect), while biguanides are simply considered antihyperglycemic in their effect because they do not affect normal blood glucose levels.[24] Therefore, the patient with diabetes is not at risk for hypoglycemia while on biguanides. Biguanides do not exacerbate hyperinsulinemia, and they prevent insulin resistance, unlike the sulfonylureas. The biguanides also have possible vasoprotective effects and improve dyslipidemia.[25] The beneficial lipid changes noted with sulfonylurea treatment most likely result from improved glycemic control rather than a direct effect of the drug itself.[26]

Indications for Use

As with all successful drug therapy, optimal use of oral agents requires matching a compound's pharmacologic properties with the patient's metabolic needs and biologic limitations. Factors to consider in choosing an oral agent are summarized in Exhibit 5-6. Because most patients with NIDDM are likely to require treatment with other drugs at one time or another, awareness of possible drug interactions is necessary for managing these patients.

Generally, the second-generation sulfonylureas are less likely to cause drug interactions because of nonionic binding to albumin, which renders them less susceptible to displacement from albumin binding sites and therefore drug interaction. All sulfonylurea drugs are metabolized by the liver, so patients with any degree of liver impairment or a history of alcoholism are not acceptable candidates for sulfonylurea therapy.

The reputed advantages of second-generation over first-generation sulfonylurea agents include increased therapeutic effectiveness, fewer side effects, reduced possibility of interactions with other drugs, and biliary as well as urinary excretion. Satisfactory responses to sulfonylurea treatment can be expected in 60 to 70% of patients whose diabetes was diagnosed after age 40 and is of less than 5 years' duration. Several studies have established that the secondary failure rate with sulfonylurea agents is 3 to 5% per year.[27,28]

The biguanide metformin is indicated as an alternative to sulfonylureas in patients with NIDDM after diet and exercise therapy has failed. Glycemic control improves in more than 90% of patients taking metformin, and it is tolerated by over 95% of patients. Metformin has a failure rate of 5 to 20%.[25]

Decreased hepatic and renal function drastically increases the risk of lactic acidosis developing while the patient is on metformin. Lactate blood levels greater than 3 mmol/L also are associated with a greater chance of lactic acidosis. Metformin should be discontinued if these events occur. Other conditions that increase the risk of biguanide toxicity include pulmonary disease, hypoxia, alcohol toxicity, use of tetracycline, and increased age. Contraindications for metformin use include renal failure, hepatic disease, history of lactic acidosis, cardiac insufficiency, and hypoxic conditions.[25]

Pharmacologic Effects

The hypoglycemic effect of oral sulfonylureas is achieved, at least initially, via stimulation of insulin secretion, which results from the interaction of the drug with specific high-affinity membrane receptors on ß-cells. Sulfonylureas also increase ß-cell sensitivity to glucose. The second-generation sulfonylureas appear to increase both insulin secretion and tissue sensitivity to the insulin.

The three major mechanisms of action of metformin include reduced hepatic glucose output, improved glucose utilization, and decreased glucose absorption. Relative to the first, studies have demonstrated that metformin does not consistently reduce hepatic glucose output, but dramatically reduces basal glucose levels leading to moderate reduction in gluconeogenesis.[29] Regarding the second mechanism of action, metformin increases glucose utilization in tissues requiring insulin for glucose uptake such as in smooth and skeletal muscles. The tremendous improvement in glucose utilization occurs during hypoglycemic conditions. Metformin has no effect on glucose utilization during euglycemia.

The third mechanism of action is decreased glucose absorption. In patients with NIDDM, concentrations of metformin in the intestinal wall increase to a level that reduces the rate of glucose uptake by the intestinal ring. However, metformin does not decrease the amount of glucose absorbed in the intestine.

Metformin has a beneficial effect on the plasma lipid profile. The specific mechanism of this effect is unknown, but significant reductions in total cholesterol and low-density lipoprotein cholesterol occur with doses of 1 to 2 g/day. Elevated triglyceride levels are reduced by 50% while normal triglyceride levels decrease 10 to 20%. Because metformin does not cause weight gain in patients with NIDDM, stored triglyceride levels do not increase.[24]

Positive vascular effects are associated with metformin therapy. Arterial blood flow increases, as does fibrinolytic activity. Metformin decreases platelet sensitivity to platelet aggregation agents. Metformin does not increase insulin levels while decreasing the glucose concentration, thus reducing the risk of arterial vascular disease. For the registered dietitian, metformin can enhance dietary efforts directed at weight management and lowering lipids.

Side Effects

The frequency of adverse events reported during treatment with sulfonylurea agents ranges from approximately 3 to 6%, with most events occurring within the first 2 months of therapy.[3] Hypoglycemia and cardiovascular events deserve special mention.

In a review of 473 cases of drug-induced hypoglycemia, 47% were found to be due to sulfonylurea agents.[30] Factors contributing to the development of hypoglycemia included excessive doses of the sulfonylurea, omission of meals, advanced age, impaired renal function, and interaction of the sulfonylurea with other hypoglycemia-potentiating drugs, such as alcohol. The possibility of prolonged hypoglycemia (7 to 14 days) with sulfonylurea agents is frequently overlooked. Patients need to be followed closely after initiation to prevent this condition.

Specific cardiovascular toxicity of the sulfonylurea agents has not been established. However, cardiovascular safety has been questioned in view of the results of the university group diabetes program, a multicenter trial involving 12 university centers in the United States and over 1,000 patients with NIDDM.[31] The current consensus appears to be that this study contained several design flaws, most relating to the fact that different study groups displayed different baseline characteristics for cardiovascular risk.

Other common complaints related to sulfonylurea use are rashes and gastrointestinal symptoms. These symptoms include nausea, vomiting, anorexia, heartburn, and gas. Frequently the symptoms disappear with a decreased dosage.

A disulfiram (antabuse-like) reaction has been reported in patients who consume alcoholic beverages while on chlorpropamide.[32] The symptoms mimic a heart attack and can include headache, nausea, vomiting, thirst, sweating, flushing, a feeling of warmth, syncope, palpitations, chest pain, confusion, vertigo, difficulty breathing, and/or hypotension. The severity of symptoms, which can last anywhere from 30 minutes to several hours, depends on the amount of alcohol consumed. People on oral agents, particularly chlorpropamide, need to be counseled on discontinuation or moderation of alcohol intake.

About 20% of patients on metformin experience side effects during therapy. The more common mild side effects are diarrhea, abdominal discomfort, metallic taste, nausea, and anorexia. These side effects are dose related, transient, and minimized by taking metformin with food and slowly increasing the dose. Long-term metformin therapy has been associated with decreased absorption of vitamin B_{12} and folate.[25]

The rare severe side effect of therapy with metformin and other biguanides is lactic acidosis. The incidence of lactic acidosis is 0 to 0.084 cases per 1,000 patients per year, and 80% of these cases are fatal.[25] Nearly 100% of the cases of lactic acidosis associated with metformin therapy have been secondary to contraindications or suicide risk. Factors that increase the blood concentration of lactic acid, and thus increase the risk of lactic acidosis, are hepatic disease, peripheral hypoxia, chronic lung disease, and alcohol abuse. The only known drug interaction that results in lactic acidosis is the concurrent use of alcohol and metformin.

Combination Therapies

Because metformin and sulfonylureas have different mechanisms of action, combination therapy with the two different agents is possible. This treatment approach synergizes the oral antihyperglycemic therapy, prolonging or preventing the need for insulin, and decreases the necessary dose of each drug, reducing the incidence of adverse drug reactions. Additional improvements in lipid profile occur in patients with NIDDM when metformin is added to their sulfonylurea regimen. Studies have demonstrated a 20% greater reduction in basal glucose with combination metformin and sulfonylurea therapy than with sulfonylurea monotherapy.[33] Combination therapy may be effective only in select patients, however, such as those with fasting blood glucose concentrations below a particular level.[33] The advantages of this combined therapy result from enhanced total body glucose metabolism and improved glycemic control through a reduction in basal hepatic glucose production.[34]

Another combination therapy is the use of an intermediate-acting insulin with a sulfonylurea. Often referred to as BIDS (bedtime insulin, daytime sulfonylurea) therapy, it is designed to lower fasting blood glucose levels that are elevated secondary to nocturnal basal hepatic glucose production. With many sulfonylureas, the patient often experiences approximately 80% of the effectiveness of the medication at half the maximum dose. Increasing to the maximal dose may not afford much more benefit in terms of blood glucose control. Initiating insulin sooner in combination with the sulfonylurea is effective in improving some of the metabolic abnormalities of NIDDM, such as high fasting plasma glucose levels, decreased peripheral glucose disposal, and high basal hepatic glucose production.[35]

With self-monitoring of blood glucose and the availability of several types of insulin, individuals can be given algorithms by which to adjust their insulin dose based on blood glucose readings and food intake (see Appendix 5-B and Table 5-4). More often than not, it is the bolus doses of regular insulin that are adjusted to make short-term corrections in control. This type of flexibility in medication choices and administration makes diabetes a relatively controllable chronic disease.

REFERENCES

1. The Diabetes Control and Complications Research Group. The effect of intensive treatment of diabetes on

the development and progression of long-term complications in insulin-dependent diabetes mellitus. *N Engl J Med.* 1993;329:977–986.

2. The DCCT Research Group. Expanded role of the dietitian in the Diabetes Control and Complications Trial: implications for clinical practice. *J Am Diet Assoc.* 1993;93:758-767.

3. Galloway JA, ed. *Diabetes Mellitus.* 9th ed. Indianapolis, Ind: Lilly Research Laboratories; 1988.

4. Skyler J, Erkelens W, Becker D, eds. Human insulin: a decade of experience and future developments. *Diabetes Care.* 1993;16(suppl 3):1–165.

5. American Diabetes Association. Position statement: insulin administration. *Diabetes Care.* 1995;18(suppl 1):29–32.

6. Product information and recommendations. Indianapolis, Ind: Eli Lilly and Company; 1994.

7. Product information and recommendations. Princeton, NJ: Novo Nordisk Pharmaceuticals Inc; 1993.

8. Anderson JH, Campbell RK. Mixing insulins in 1990. *Diabetes Educator.* 1990;16:380–387.

9. White JR, Campbell RK. Guide to mixing insulins. *Hosp Pharm.* 1991;26:1046–1048.

10. American Diabetes Association. 1996 buyer's guide to diabetes products. *Diabetes Forecast.* 1995;48(10):43–88.

11. Jovanovic L, Biermann J, Toohey B. *The Diabetic Woman.* Los Angeles, Calif: Tarcher/St. Martin's Press; 1987.

12. White JR, Hartman J, Campbell RK. Drug interactions in diabetic patients. *Postgrad Med.* 1993;93:131–139.

13. Walsh J, Roberts R. *Pumping Insulin.* San Diego, Calif: Torrey Pines Press; 1994.

14. Lauritzen T, et al. Pharmacokinetics of continuous subcutaneous insulin infusion. *Diabetologia.* 1983;24:326–329.

15. Binder C, et al. Insulin pharmacokinetics. *Diabetes Care.* 1984;7:188–199.

16. Brackenridge B, D'Almeida B, Fredrickson L, Swenson K. *The Pump Trainer Manual.* Sylmar, Calif: MiniMed Technologies; 1993.

17. Albisser AM, Sperlich M. Adjusting insulins. *Diabetes Educator.* 1992;18(3):211–219.

18. Pulini M. Insulin allergy in clinical practice. *Pract Diabetol.* 1983;2:1.

19. Powers MA, ed. *Nutrition Guide for Professionals: Diabetes Education and Meal Planning.* Chicago, Ill: American Dietetic Association/American Diabetes Association; 1988.

20. Olefsky JM. Diabetes mellitus. In: Wyngaarden JB, Smith LH, eds. *Cecil's Textbook of Medicine.* 17th ed. Philadelphia, Pa: WB Saunders; 1985.

21. Felber J-P, Acheson KJ, Tappy L. *From Obesity to Diabetes.* West Sussex, England: John Wiley & Sons, Ltd; 1993.

22. Monk A, Barry B, McClain K, Weaver T, Cooper N, Franz MJ. Practice guidelines for medical nutrition therapy provided by dietitians for persons with non-insulin-dependent diabetes mellitus. *J Am Diet Assoc.* 1995;95:999–1006.

23. Williams G. Management of non-insulin-dependent diabetes mellitus. *Lancet.* 1994;343:95–100.

24. Tanya JJ, Langlass TM. Pharmacy update: Metformin: a biguanide. *Diabetes Educator.* 1995;21:509–514.

25. Bailey CJ. Biguanides and NIDDM. *Diabetes Care.* 1992;15:755–772.

26. Groop LC. Sulfonylureas in NIDDM. *Diabetes Care.* 1992;15:737–754.

27. Feldman JM. Glyburide: a second-generation sulfonylurea hypoglycemia agent: history, chemistry, metabolism, pharmacokinetics, clinical use, and adverse effects. *Pharmacotherapy.* 1985;5:43–62.

28. Lebovitz HE. Glipizide: a second-generation sulfonylurea hypoglycemic agent: pharmacology, pharmacokinetics and clinical use. *Pharmacotherapy.* 1985;5:63–77.

29. Perriello G, Misericordia P, Volpi E, et al. Acute antihyperglycemic mechanisms of metformin in NIDDM. *Diabetes.* 1994;43:920–982.

30. Seltzer HS. Drug-induced hypoglycemia: a review based on 473 cases. *Diabetes.* 1982;31:890–896.

31. Meinart CL, Knatteraud GL, Prout TE, Klimt CR. The university group diabetes program: a study of the effects of hypoglycemic agents on vascular complications in patients with adult-onset diabetes. II. Mortality results. *Diabetes.* 1970;19(suppl 2):789–930.

32. Wiles PG, Pyke DA. The chlorpropamide alcohol flush. *Clin Sci.* 1984;67:375.

33. Hermann LS. Biguanides and sulfonylureas as combination therapy in NIDDM. *Diabetes Care.* 1990;13(suppl 3):37–41.

34. Hermann LS, Schersten B, Bitzen PO, Kjellstrom T, Lindegarde F, Melander A. Therapeutic comparison of metformin and sulfonylurea, alone and in various combinations. *Diabetes Care.* 1994;17:1100–1109.

35. Longnecker MP. Insulin and the sulfonylurea agent in non–insulin-dependent diabetes mellitus. *Arch Intern Med.* 1986;146:673.

Drug Company Addresses

Bristol-Meyers-Sqibb
777 Scudders Mill Road
Plainsboro, NJ 08536

Eli Lilly and Company
Lilly Corporate Center
Indianapolis, IN 46285
800-545-5979

Hoechst-Roussel Pharmaceuticals, Inc.
Route 202–206 North
Somerville, NJ 08876

Novo Nordisk Pharmaceuticals Inc.
100 Overlook Center, Suite 200
Princeton, NJ 08540-7810
800-727-6500

Pfizer Inc.
US Pharmaceuticals Group
235 East 42nd Street
New York, NY 10017
212-573-2323

Upjohn Company
7000 Portage Road
Kalamazoo, MI 49001

Adjusting Insulin

There are several tips and thoughts that registered dietitians will want to keep in mind as they help patients with diabetes to problem solve to reach target blood glucose values.

1. Make sure target blood glucose ranges have been set or negotiated with the patient. Otherwise, the patient has no idea what is to be accomplished. An old saying applies: "If you don't know where you're going, any road will you get you there!"

2. Fix the fasting first. Because blood glucose levels will stay in about the same range or elevate throughout the day for those with NIDDM, getting the fasting blood glucose level normalized sets the tone for the rest of the day, provided the patient continues to eat appropriately.

3. Look to the previous medication dose when solving a problem time of day. For example, if there is a high midafternoon blood glucose pattern and the morning shot of NPH/regular insulin was the last administration, perhaps more NPH is required then.

4. Do not be reactionary. Observe patterns of blood glucose levels versus responding to one or two isolated values. Practitioners may want to discard the lowest and highest values as outliers when perusing blood glucose logs. Allow a new regimen (an increase or decrease in food, medications, or activity) to be tried for at least 3 days before considering another change.

5. Do not automatically blame the diet. Just because you are a dietitian does not mean that diet is the only aspect of diabetes care you must consider. Timing of meals and medications, poor fluid intake, site selection and rotation for insulin administration, activity changes, acute stress, illness, or other medications can account for out-of-range blood glucose values.

6. Change only one or two things at a time when modifying the diet so that the effectiveness of each change can be documented separately. If too many components are altered at once, the cause cannot be determined because it is confounded by other variables.

7. Correct the basal rates first. For those on intensive therapy (MDI or CSII), boluses of regular insulin can only be accurately determined if basal insulin (lente, NPH, ultralente, or basal rate on an insulin pump) is correct. Similarly, insulin-to-carbohydrate ratios cannot be refined unless basal rates have been correctly adjusted. Basal rates are correct when the individual with diabetes can skip a meal and the blood glucose remains stable (hypoglycemia or hyperglycemia does not occur).

The 27 Steps to Injecting Insulin

Drawing up Insulin: Step-by-Step

Check each new bottle for:

Type of insulin _____

Strength of insulin _____

Expiration date _____

Record and adjust as needed:

	B	L	D	S
Dose of insulin _____				_____
Time to take insulin _____				_____
Time to eat _____				_____

1. Wash your hands thoroughy.

2. Check bottle of insulin for above information (type, strength, expiration date).

3. Mix cloudy insulin gently by rolling sideways between hands and tipping bottle upside down (to check for any remaining white particles/sediment). DO NOT SHAKE THE BOTTLE!

4. Remove cap on top of new bottle of insulin.

5. Wipe white rubber area on top of bottle with alcohol swab.

6. Remove cap from plunger of syringe.

7. Pull plunger back to _____ units to draw air into syringe equal to your current dose: _____ units of insulin.

8. Remove cap over needle of syringe.

9. Insert needle into bottle (leave bottle upright on table).

10. Push plunger in. The air injected into the bottle will allow insulin to be easily withdrawn.

11. Turn bottle upside down, leaving syringe and needle in the bottle.

12. Pull out plunger beyond your dose of _____ units.

13. Check for air bubbles as these can decrease the amount of the dose. If air bubbles are present, push plunger to push insulin back into the bottle.

14. Redraw insulin again by pulling plunger out to beyond the correct dose of _____ units of insulin.

15. Push plunger back up to the line of the correct dose of _____ units of insulin.

16. Pull needle out of insulin vial.

17. Place cap loosely over needle until ready to inject.

continues

18. Choose a site for injection (see Figure 5-4, Injection Log)
    a. Place subsequent injections in the same area about $^1/_2$ inch apart OR one knuckle's width apart.
    b. Rate of absorption is best from the abdomen > arm > thigh > buttock.

19. Make sure skin is clean and dry at site for injection.

20. Remove cap from needle.

21. Hold syringe in one hand as if it were a dart.

22. Spread skin with other hand (be gentle). You may pinch the skin if you are thin or feel more comfortable doing this.

23. Dart needle quickly into skin.

24. Push down plunger until all insulin is injected.

25. Release skin (if pinching) or relieve pressure (if spreading skin).

26. Pull out needle. Apply pressure with swab to the site of injection. Count to 10 while applying pressure.

27. Discard syringe according to local department of health policy. (Use a sharps disposal container OR empty bleach bottle or 2-liter soda bottle).

Note: Several more steps are involved when a patient needs to draw up two different types of insulin into the same syringe. A simple rule-of-thumb is "clear before cloudy." The clear insulin must be drawn up before the cloudy insulin so that the clear (short-acting) insulin is not contaminated with longer-acting insulin that could severely blunt its action. However, air must be injected first into the cloudy insulin equal to the appropriate dose of longer-acting insulin; then, air is injected into the clear insulin vial and that insulin is drawn up; finally, the syringe is removed and placed into the cloudy insulin vial again to draw out the dose of longer-acting insulin.

Calculating Insulin Dosages/Algorithms

Initial Dosing:
- start with approximately 0.5 to 0.6 units insulin/kilogram/day based on current weight
- administer about $^2/_3$ of total daily dose (TDD) in A.M. and about $^1/_3$ of TDD in P.M.
- multiple daily injections (MDI) or pump therapy: approximately $^1/_2$ of the TDD will serve as the background or basal (long-acting or intermediate-acting) insulin and approximately $^1/_2$ will serve as the bolus doses of insulin to cover meals and snacks
- for those on split/mixed dosages of intermediate short-acting insulin, administer a ratio of 2:1 (NPH:Regular) in A.M. and a ratio of 1:1 (NPH:Regular) in P.M.
- adolescents may require two to three times the normal amount of insulin they need during puberty
- toddlers and children, very thin, active, or fit individuals may have considerably lower insulin requirements (TDD)

Example: Split/mixed dose of insulin:
175 lbs = 79.5 kgs
79.5 x 0.5 units = 40 units TDD
$^2/_3$ x 40 units = 27 units in A.M.
$^1/_3$ x 40 units = 13 units in P.M.
A.M. ratio of 2:1 = 18 units NPH/9 units regular
P.M. ratio of 1:1 = 7 units NPH/6 units regular

Example: Insulin pump therapy
155 lbs = 70.5 kgs
70.5 x 0.5 units = 35 units TDD
$^1/_2$ x 35 units = 17.5 units basal dose
17.5 units basal dose/24 hours = 0.7 units/hour
$^1/_2$ x 35 units = 17.5 units total bolus doses
17.5 units boluses/3 meals - 5.8 units/meal if all meals contain approximately same number of grams of carbohydrate

Complementary Dosing:
- use the 1500 Rule to determine the amount of insulin an individual must take to lower pre-meal blood glucose levels into target ranges before calculating insulin coverage for carbohydrate consumption
- 1500/TDD = number of points blood glucose will drop with administration of one unit of Regular insulin
- 1500 Rule can accurately be used if blood glucose levels are already fairly well-controlled

Example: Split/mixed dose of insulin:
1500/40 units TDD = 37.5 mg/dL drop per unit of insulin

Example: Insulin pump therapy:
1500/35 units TDD = 43 mg/dL drop per unit of insulin

Algorithm Dosing:

- based solely on blood glucose monitoring using constant carbohydrate diet for at least two to three weeks so that basal and bolus insulin can be correlated to preprandial and postprandial blood glucose levels

Chapter 6

Exercise Benefits and Guidelines for Persons with Diabetes

Marion J. Franz

The positive role of exercise in the management of diabetes, especially for persons with non–insulin-dependent diabetes mellitus (NIDDM), is frequently underemphasized by health professionals; emphasis tends to be placed on the balance of food intake and insulin action, ignoring the third side of the triad of food, insulin, and exercise. Dietitians need to take an active role in encouraging and educating persons with diabetes to initiate or to continue a safe and enjoyable exercise program.

Through modulation of the body's sensitivity to insulin and increasing peripheral glucose use, exercise can have a role in improved metabolic control for those with diabetes. The goals of an exercise program for individuals with diabetes are (1) to maintain or improve cardiovascular fitness to prevent or minimize the long-term cardiovascular complications of diabetes; (2) to improve flexibility, which is impaired as muscle collagen becomes glycated; (3) to improve muscle, which may deteriorate as a result of neuropathy and which uses glucose as fuel; (4) to allow people with insulin-dependent diabetes mellitus (IDDM) to participate safely in and enjoy physical or sport activities; (5) to assist in glucose management and weight control in people with NIDDM; and (6) to allow individuals with diabetes to experience the same benefits and enjoyment that people without diabetes gain from a regular exercise program.

PHYSIOLOGY OF EXERCISE

To evaluate the benefits versus the risks of an exercise program in persons with diabetes mellitus, it is necessary to understand the metabolic and hormonal effects of sporadic periods of exercise as well as physical training (exercise performed on a regular basis for extended periods of time) on glucose homeostasis. Understanding the alterations in fuel metabolism during exercise in both persons with and without diabetes assists both professionals and individuals with diabetes problem-solve situations that arise with exercise.

Fuel Metabolism during Exercise in Persons Who Do Not Have Diabetes

Euglycemia is achieved during exercise through the precise regulation of hepatic glucose production and the use of glucose at the cellular level. In persons who do not have diabetes, blood glucose fluctuates very little, even during intense exercise, despite what can be a 20-fold increase in glucose uptake by exercising muscles. The regulatory mechanism involves a hormonal balance between an inhibition of insulin release and an increase in the counterregulatory hormones: glucagon, cortisol, epinephrine, norepinephrine, and growth hormone.[1]

An orderly sequence of fuel usage takes place during prolonged exercise. When exercise is of a short duration, fuel availability is seldom a limiting factor. But when muscle is required to contract continuously for longer than 1.5 hours, some of the fuels critical for performance may be depleted.

Energy, in the form of adenosine triphosphate (ATP), for exercise is generated from a variety

Table 6-1 Sequence of Fuel Use

Exercise Duration	Source of Fuel	Substrate
First 5–10 minutes	Intramuscular	Glycogen (Triglycerides)
10–40 minutes	Circulating substrates	Glucose and NEFA
~40 minutes and longer	Tissue stores Liver Adipose tissue	Glucose from glycogenolysis and gluconeogenesis Triglyceride NEFA

of substances. At the beginning of exercise, intramuscular fuel—primarily glycogen—is the primary source. These stores are depleted rapidly. The initial rapid breakdown of muscle glycogen stores is stimulated by activation of the sympathetic nervous system. Muscle glycogen is of use in meeting the energy requirements of muscle fibers in which it is contained but does not contribute to the maintenance of blood glucose homeostasis, except via the Cori cycle.[2]

In a short time, local glycogen stores become depleted and substrates—glucose and nonesterified fatty acids (NEFA)—carried in the bloodstream assume a more important role. Increased glucose uptake and use by muscle cells require the presence of insulin, although the amount required is low. As exercise progresses, circulating substrates are also limited, requiring mobilization of substrate from tissue stores (ie, glycogen from the liver and fat in the form of triglycerides stored in adipose tissue).

As exercise continues and the availability of muscle glycogen declines, blood glucose becomes responsible for 75 to 90% of the total carbohydrate consumed during approximately the first 40 minutes of exercise.[2] Beyond 40 minutes of exercise, the rate of glucose use by working muscles increases progressively to a peak at 90 to 180 minutes, after which it declines slightly in parallel with a gradual fall in the blood glucose level. Thus, blood glucose is a quantitatively important substrate for contracting muscles during brief as well as prolonged work (Table 6-1).

The increase in glucose uptake by muscle that characterizes exercise requires a parallel increase in glucose production by the liver. Approximately 75% of the glucose output comes from hepatic glycogenolysis, with the remaining 25 to 30% from gluconeogenesis. Lactate, pyruvate, alanine, and other gluconeogenic amino acids released from muscle, along with glycerol released from adipose tissue, are extracted by the liver and used for gluconeogenesis. Gluconeogenesis becomes more important during prolonged exercise and may account for 40 to 50% of hepatic glucose output.

As exercise progresses, NEFAs are used by the muscle cells as substrate. However, the oxidation of fat-derived fuels cannot fully replace the use of glucose, even during prolonged endurance exercise. When the supply of carbohydrate is limited, the oxidation of fat is incomplete, resulting in the production of ketone bodies. These ketone bodies can later be reused in the fatty acid oxidation cycle of skeletal musculatures but may also be excreted in the urine, resulting in a net energy loss.

In response to exercise, NEFA uptake by muscle increases with time, and after 40 minutes of mild exercise, it may account for 25 to 35% of the oxygen consumed. NEFA use continues to increase during prolonged exercise, and between 1 to 4 hours the uptake of NEFA rises approximately 70%.[2] Thus, after 4 hours the relative contribution of NEFA to total oxygen use is twice that of blood glucose. For a summary of the stages of fuel use in prolonged exercise, see Figure 6-1.[3]

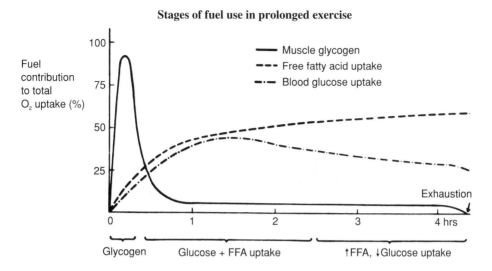

Figure 6-1 Relative Contribution of Muscle Glycogen and Blood Glucose and Nonesterified Fatty Acids to Oxidative Energy during Various Time Periods of Exercise. *Source:* Reprinted from Felig P and Koivisto VA. Metabolic response to exercise. Implications for exercise. In: Lowenthal DT, Bhradwaua K, and Oaks WW, eds. *Therapeutics through Exercise*; with permission of Grune & Stratton, Copyright © 1979.

Carbohydrate is the fuel of choice for short-duration, high-intensity exercise. Its glucose structure contains more oxygen molecules than other nutrients, which allows for rapid oxidation and, therefore, release of energy. Glucose is the main substrate used in anaerobic glycolysis. The major problem with glucose as the primary fuel source is its limited storage capacity. Untrained persons store only enough carbohydrate for 1 day of sedentary activity (about 15 g/kg of muscles). In a 70-kg person, approximately 1500 kcal are stored as glycogen—300 to 400 g in the form of muscle glycogen and 80 to 90 g as liver glycogen. With training, the ability to store and use carbohydrate is enhanced; however, even in trained athletes only about 2000 kcal are stored in the body as blood glucose and as liver and muscle glycogen. If carbohydrate were the only fuel used during exercise, sports events longer than 2 hours would be impossible, because overwhelming fatigue occurs when the glycogen content becomes depleted.[4]

In persons with proper amounts of body fat, however, 90,000 to 100,000 kcal can be stored as fat. Availability of this fat requires a substantial amount of oxygen to be metabolized. To meet this oxygen requirement, exercise intensity must be reduced and some carbohydrate made available.

To the endurance athlete, the most important function of fat metabolism is glycogen sparing. With training, the body develops the ability to sustain long periods of muscle contraction by deriving between 50 to 85% of energy needs from fat. When this happens, limited glycogen stores are conserved. The state of training also influences the proportion of substrate used by allowing greater oxidation (aerobic) metabolism via the Krebs' cycle and oxidation phosphorylation pathways. With the increased ability to use oxygen, the trained individual can produce the same amount of energy (ATP) without having to rely as much on anaerobic pathways. Because ATP levels are maintained by oxidizing more fatty acids, less carbohydrate is oxidized, and the overall contribution of carbohydrate to both anaerobic and aerobic metabolism is diminished.[5]

Glucose Regulation

Despite the increase in glucose uptake by muscles during moderate-intensity exercise, glucose levels change very little. Hepatic glycogenolysis and gluconeogenesis closely match the uptake increase. Muscular work causes a fall in plasma insulin and a rise in glucagon. This balance is the major determinant of hepatic glucose production. The fall of insulin is necessary for the complete increase in hepatic glycogenolysis, and the increase in glucagon is necessary for the complete increase in both hepatic glycogenolysis and gluconeogenesis.[6,7] By contrast, epinephrine plays only a minor role in regulating hepatic glucose production and appears to occur only during the latter stage of prolonged exercise.[8]

The response of the liver to high-intensity exercise differs from the response to moderate exercise. Glucose production no longer matches but instead exceeds the rise in glucose use.[9] This results in an increase in glucose levels that extends into the postexercise state. It has been hypothesized that during exercise of high intensity there may be a shift in the control of glucose production away from pancreatic hormones to the catecholamines.[10] Norepinephrine and epinephrine can increase by 10- to 20-fold, whereas the increase in the glucagon to insulin ratio is considerably less.[9]

Exercise leads to a workrate-dependent increase in muscle glucose use. Moderate-intensity exercise (<50% maximum oxygen uptake) increases glucose uptake by 2 to 3 mg/kg per minute above usual daily requirements. This means that when a 70-kg person exercises, an added 140 to 210 mg of glucose for every minute of moderate exercise or an added 8.4 to 12.6 g for every hour is needed.[1] During high-intensity exercise (80 to 100% maximum oxygen uptake), glucose uptake may increase by 5 to 6 mg/kg per minute above usual needs. As a result, 350 to 420 mg of glucose is extracted from the blood and used every minute. Despite the increased rate of glucose use, the demand on glucose stores and the risk of hypoglycemia is less because exercise of this intensity cannot be sustained for long intervals.

Regulation of Fat Mobilization

NEFA levels are also increased gradually by exercise. This increase is due to both an increase in lipolysis and a decrease in NEFA re-esterification and is regulated by insulin and the catecholamines.[11] The increase in ketogenesis that occurs with prolonged exercise results from increased NEFA mobilization from adipose tissue and delivery to the liver. In addition to hepatic NEFA delivery, the exercise-induced rise in glucagon stimulates hepatic fat oxidation and is necessary for the full ketogenic response. In contrast to glucose whose uptake is closely regulated by hormonal and nonhormonal mechanisms, muscle NEFA use is primarily determined by its availability to muscle.[1]

Postexercise Fuel Regulation

The glucoregulatory hormones play a role in the more sustained effects of exercise and accelerate the transition of the body into a more fasted state. Liver and muscle glycogen become depleted, and hepatic gluconeogenesis is accelerated. The extent this occurs depends on the level of the exercise intensity and the duration. Muscle glycogen depletion is a potent stimulus for glycogen synthesis and facilitates repletion of glycogen stores after exercise.[1]

Glycogen resynthesis is primarily influenced by the provision of carbohydrate. Without feeding, muscle glycogen stores are replenished rather slowly. With feeding, muscle glycogen stores are replenished rapidly, reaching normal levels within 12 to 24 hours postexercise.[12] The repletion of muscle glycogen after exercise occurs in two phases. In phase 1, glycogen synthetase activity is elevated, and muscle glycogen is rapidly restored. The amount replenished is dependent on carbohydrate intake; thus, the importance of carbohydrate intake during this time period. This occurs immediately after exercise and does not require insulin. The second phase is characterized by a marked and persistent increase in insulin action. The added insulin-stimulated glucose disposal after exercise is solely attributable to an increase in nonoxidative glucose metabolism (glucose being stored as glycogen).[13]

Alterations with Exercise in Persons with Insulin-Dependent Diabetes Mellitus

Considering the complexity of fuel flux during exercise and the important regulatory role played by insulin and the counterregulatory hormones, it is not surprising that persons with diabetes have management problems when exercising. Persons with IDDM, because of their use of exogenous insulin, are especially susceptible to these problems. The intensity, duration, and type of exercise, fitness level, nutritional state (glycogen stores), relationship to when food was last eaten, and the calories and content of the meal are all factors that influence the response to exercise. Furthermore, in persons with IDDM, state of metabolic control, timing, type of insulin, and possibly the sites of insulin injections are other considerations.

Acute (Short-Term) Effects of Exercise

Because of the time action of exogenous insulin, persons with IDDM commonly experience fluctuations from states of insulin excess to insulin deficiency. When insulin deficiency is present, for example, in persons who are ketotic or who have blood glucose levels greater than 250 to 300 mg/dL, exercise can cause an increase in plasma glucose and an acceleration of ketone body production. These conditions occur because exercise-mediated muscle glucose uptake is insulin-dependent, and with insulin deficiency, the usual increase in muscle glucose uptake during exercise is diminished. Insulin deficiency and high concentration of counterregulatory hormones also enhance gluconeogenesis, resulting in an exaggerated increase in hepatic glucose production and circulating plasma glucose concentrations[14] (Figure 6-2). Persons with IDDM in poor metabolic

control may also have diminished glycogen stores and increased lipid stores within muscle, which also results in a decrease and an increase, respectively, in the use of these intramuscular stores.

Insulin deficiency results in increased NEFA mobilization and accelerated ketone formation in the liver. Because insulin inhibits NEFA mobilization, NEFAs are released in response to decreased levels of insulin in the blood. Uptake of NEFA by muscle is dependent on serum NEFA concentration and is not insulin-dependent; it is increased because of the higher arterial concentration, insulin deficiency, and inhibition of glucose uptake by the decreased insulin and constant pressure of high levels of NEFA. In the ketotic diabetic patient, the abnormally increased uptake of NEFA already exists at rest and is accelerated with exercise, resulting in an even greater percentage being converted to ketone bodies[14] (Figure 6-3).

The metabolic and hormonal response to exercise therefore varies with degree of metabolic control at the onset of exercise and, more specifically, the availability of insulin. A minimal level of insulin is necessary for glucose uptake by the muscles, as well as for regulation of the production of glucose by the liver. In the person with IDDM under moderately poor control, exercise also induces an abnormally increased secretion of the glucoregulatory hormones—catecholamines, glucagon, cortisol, and growth hormone.

Exercise is therefore not always effective in decreasing elevated blood glucose levels and is not a replacement for insulin. In persons with hyperglycemia (blood glucose > 250 to 300 mg/dL) and ketosis (small, moderate, or large urine ketones or blood ketones 2 to 3 mmol/dL), exercise is accompanied by a significant rise in blood glucose concentration. For these individuals, exercise is not recommended until ketones are no longer present and blood glucose control has improved.[1] This precaution is of particular concern for individuals whose diabetes has been in poor control for a period of time—several days or longer.

High-intensity exercise can be more deleterious to metabolic control than moderate exercise of the same duration. Even persons well-controlled may have an increase in blood glucose and NEFA levels after high-intensity exercise.[15] This may be due to the increase in counterregulatory hormones during this type of exercise or because insulin fails to rise as it would normally with heavy exercise in persons without diabetes.

This response to exercise with hyperglycemia and insulin deficiency can be contrasted with the more commonly associated situation with diabetes—hyperinsulinemia and hypoglycemia. In persons who do not have diabetes, insulin levels decrease with exercise, thereby allowing increased glucose production by the liver. Blood glucose levels may remain unchanged or may even be slightly elevated during approximately the first 40 minutes of exercise because the ini-

tial increase of catecholamines causes a temporary increase in available hepatic blood glucose. But depending on the available glycogen stores, blood glucose levels then begin to decrease (but not below normal) along with the decrease in insulin in all individuals during exercise. However, with a relative excess of insulin in the circulation, such as usually occurs in individuals with diabetes, plasma glucose levels predictably decrease dramatically during exercise, resulting in exercise-induced hypoglycemia. Persons on insulin therapy may experience serum insulin levels two to three times above the level needed because injected insulin does not respond to physiologic lowering effects of exercise. The elevated insulin levels cause an inhibition of hepatic glucose output, preventing the increase in glucose delivery that normally matches augmented muscle glucose uptake during exercise. Muscle glucose uptake increases with exercise,

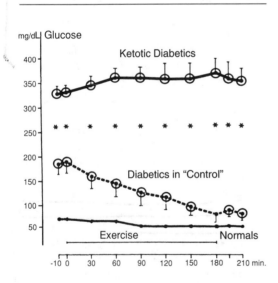

Figure 6-2 Effect of Prolonged Exercise on Blood Glucose Levels in Healthy Control Subjects (Normals), Persons with Diabetes in Moderate Control (Diabetics in "Control"), and Persons with Diabetes and Ketotic (Ketotic Diabetics). (Encircled values are significantly different from corresponding values of the control group at p < .05.) *Source:* Reprinted with permission from *Diabetologia* 1977;13:355, Copyright © 1977, Springer-Verlag.

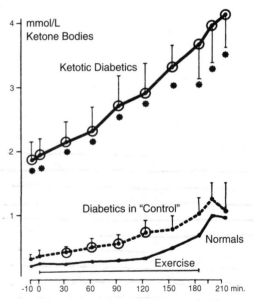

Figure 6-3 Effect of Prolonged Exercise on Blood Levels of Ketone Bodies. (Stars indicate statistical differences between the corresponding values and the two groups of persons with diabetes at p < .05.) *Source:* Reprinted with permission from *Diabetologia* 1977;13:355, Copyright © 1977, Springer-Verlag.

and the liver is unable to increase its production of glucose to replenish the loss of glucose from the circulation.[15] Hypoglycemia can result.

Hypoglycemia can be prevented by increasing food intake before and/or after exercise or by reducing the dosage of insulin acting during the time of exercise. Hypoglycemia can occur during exercise and for up to 24 hours after strenuous or prolonged exercise. The most common times for hypoglycemia to occur are reported to be 6 to 15 hours after exercise.[16,17] After exercise, the exercise-induced fall in muscle glycogen content is corrected through prolonged stimulation of glycogen synthetase for glycogen resynthesis, leading to prolonged increased glucose uptake. Replenishment of muscle and liver glycogen stores can occur for up to 24 to 40 hours.[2] During this time, there is improvement in glucose tolerance and diminished insulin requirements. For this reason, insulin adjustment and/or increased food may be required on the day after exercise, as well as on the day of exercise. Monitoring of blood glucose levels is crucial.

In persons with diabetes, the amount of stored carbohydrate is related to the degree of glycemic control, because insulin availability determines the extent of liver and muscle glycogen storage and depletion. Therefore, a person experiencing frequent bouts of hypoglycemia or hyperglycemia will have depleted hepatic and muscle glycogen stores available for energy during exercise and should avoid exercise until blood glucose control is improved. In insulin-deprived persons, the rate of glycogen use during exercise is no different from normal. However, resynthesis of muscle glycogen during the second phase of postexercise recovery is an insulin-dependent process. In persons with poorly controlled diabetes, muscle glycogen repletion is minimal, whereas with adequate insulin the rate of repletion is the same as is seen normally.

Long-Term Effects of Exercise Training

A few studies have been performed on the effect of exercise training on long-term metabolic control in IDDM. Most studies of diabetes and exercise have focused on metabolic short-term responses to exercise in persons with diabetes compared with normal controls. These studies suggest that physical training can increase insulin sensitivity and improve lipoprotein concentrations. However, a long-term effect on improving blood glucose control as measured by glycated hemoglobin in exercise has not been demonstrated.[18,19] Because of the increased risks of exercise, it has been debated whether exercise should be recommended for all persons with IDDM. The goal should be to encourage exercise for those who do not have any significant contraindications and who wish to participate. With adequate education, careful blood glucose monitoring, appropriate adjustments in insulin and food intake, and the observation of exercise's effects, many persons with IDDM can learn to exercise safely and receive the same benefits of exercise that individuals who do not have diabetes receive.

Alterations with Exercise in Persons with Non–Insulin-Dependent Diabetes Mellitus

NIDDM is characterized by insulin resistance, hyperinsulinemia, and impaired insulin secretion. Upper body obesity, dyslipidemia, and hypertension are commonly associated with glucose intolerance.[20] Medical nutrition therapy (MNT) continues to be the primary therapy along with oral hypoglycemic agents (OHAs) or insulin if needed to attain and maintain near-normal blood glucose levels. Regular activity or exercise can be an important adjunct in the management of NIDDM.

Short-Term (Acute) Effects of Exercise

The improved insulin sensitivity in persons who exercise regularly helps decrease the insulin resistance many persons with NIDDM have. More important, after acute exercise, insulin sensitivity is increased for 24 to 72 hours in most individuals. This does not appear related to effects on insulin receptors but is probably mediated by increases in glucose transport proteins in skeletal muscle allowing circulating insulin to more efficiently transport glucose intracellularly.[21]

Acute exercise in untrained persons is associated with increased insulin sensitivity and glucose metabolism that persist for several hours after exercise. Exercise has been shown to enhance peripheral glucose use in muscles whereas hepatic glucose production does not rise proportionally to the increased use; therefore, plasma glucose declines. Glucose has been shown to drop 30 to 40 mg/dL during 45 minutes of moderate exercise in persons treated with MNT alone or with MNT plus an OHA. Because persons with NIDDM are often mildly hyperglycemic, moderate exercise can be beneficial in restoring glucose homeostasis in this group.[5] Because many of the benefits of exercise are of a short duration, it is especially important that exercises be prescribed or suggested that can be repeated frequently and can be continued for a lifetime.[22,23]

Bogardus et al.[24] compared obese NIDDM persons before and after treatment on a hypocaloric diet, either alone or in combination with a physical training program. The major effect of training, compared with treatment by diet alone, was to increase peripheral use of glucose during hyperinsulinemia; the improved glucose disposal was due primarily to an increase in nonoxidated pathways of glucose metabolism resulting in increased glycogen synthesis.

Training Effects of Exercise

Several well-controlled studies[25,26] have demonstrated that insulin sensitivity and glycemic control improve in persons with NIDDM when they regularly (a minimum of three to four times per week) increase their physical activity. Most studies show that glycated hemoglobin (HbA$_{1c}$) levels decrease between 10 and 20% within 6 to 10 weeks of initiating an exercise program. This can be maintained as long as the individual exercises regularly.

With more intensive long-term exercise, insulin sensitivity and glucose control can improve even more, due to increases in lean body composition. The effects on blood glucose control are greatest in those with mild NIDDM and more severe insulin resistance.

Training in persons who do not have diabetes has been shown to cause beneficial adaptation in lipid metabolism, including decreased levels of serum triglycerides, very low-density lipoprotein-cholesterol, and low-density lipoprotein-cholesterol. Training that may lead to a decreased risk of coronary heart disease has been shown to increase levels of high-density lipoprotein-cholesterol.

Large epidemiologic studies in the general population suggest that individuals who increase their physical activity decrease their risk for premature coronary artery disease. Although such studies have not been conducted specifically in persons with diabetes, the cluster of cardiovascular risk factors that may predispose persons to premature atherosclersosis improves significantly with regular physical activity. This is related to improved insulin sensitivity that occurs in all persons with exercise. Therefore, with regular exercise, the risk of atherosclerosis in persons with diabetes may also decrease.[27]

Prevention of NIDDM

Improving insulin sensitivity through exercise may also help prevent NIDDM. Insulin resistance often occurs decades before overt, clinically evident NIDDM develops. Because regular exercise can reverse insulin resistance, it can also prevent the sequence of events that result in clinical disease. Three large studies, two in men and one in women, have shown that individuals at increased risk of developing NIDDM who maintain high levels of physical activity significantly decrease their risk of developing diabetes. Helmrich et al[28] in a study of 5990 males over a 14-year period reported the risk of developing NIDDM fell by 6% for every 500 kcal of exercise performed each week. In the Nurses Health Study, 8 years of information from 87,253 women, aged 34 to 59, showed risk for developing NIDDM was 33% lower among women who did vigorous physical activity at least once a week compared with women less active.[29] The same group reported that in 22,271 male physicians between 1982 and 1988 regular exercise decreased the incidence of NIDDM. Men who exercised greater than five times per week had a 42% reduction in risk compared with a 23% drop in men who exercised only once a week.[30]

INSULIN-DEPENDENT DIABETES MELLITUS AND EXERCISE

The role of exercise as a therapeutic measure for improving metabolic control in IDDM is not supported by experimental evidence. Mechanisms of glucoregulation indicate that the therapeutic role of exercise cannot be put into practice because the glycemic responses to exercise depend on too many inter- and intraindividual variables, such as state of nutrition, training, metabolic control, and intensity, duration, and time of exercise performed. Instead all persons with IDDM should be strongly encouraged to exercise whenever they want in order to maintain their physical fitness and for recreational purposes. Furthermore, regular exercise can be beneficial to the person with IDDM for the following reasons:

- Risk factors for coronary heart disease are reduced. Exercise, when regular (three to four times a week) and aerobic, has been shown to reduce the incidence of coronary heart disease in nondiabetic persons. Training is related to a reduction in the low-density lipoprotein-cholesterol and an increase in the high-density lipoproteins. This is particularly important for persons with IDDM because the risk of coronary heart disease is increased in this population. Evidence of significant coronary heart disease has been found in IDDM persons on whom autopsies were performed at ages 19 to 38 when onset of diabetes was before age 15.[31] Epidemiologic data from the Framingham Study confirmed this finding and indicated that diabetes is an independent risk factor for coronary atherosclerotic disease. The Framingham Study also demonstrated that risk factors are additive; thus, the importance of a "low-risk" profile—lean, normotensive, nonsmoking, exercising, and low serum cholesterol values for persons who have diabetes.[31]

Significant changes in cardiovascular function consistent with a decrease in mortality rate have been shown to occur with regular exercise that causes an increment in energy expenditure of 1500 kcal/wk (or 5 hours of walking per week).[32] Fitness can be achieved by exercising 4 to 7 d/wk at 50 to 70% predicted maximum heart rate for a minimum of 20 minutes per exercise session or by physical activity every day (walking, taking the stairs, housework, etc) at moderate intensity (equivalent to a brisk walk) for an accumulated 30 minutes or more over each day.[33] In general, it seems that persons with IDDM show the same improvement in coronary risk factors in response to regular exercise as nondiabetic subjects.[1]

- Improved glucose tolerance results from increased glucose use and increased sensitivity to insulin. A smaller amount of insulin is needed to stimulate glucose uptake in exercising muscles than at rest.[34] Perhaps more important than this acute effect of exercise is its more prolonged effect on glucose metabolism. This results from the replenishment of muscle and liver glycogen during the 24 to 48 hours after exercise. The exercise-induced fall in the glycogen content of liver and muscles causes a prolonged stimulation of glycogen synthetase and glucose use in these tissues. As a result, glucose tolerance improves and insulin requirements diminish.[2] This increase in the storage and use of glucose results in less extreme fluctuations in blood glucose over a 24-hour period.

- Exercise increases work capacity and increased percentage of lean body mass in nondiabetic persons and in persons with IDDM.
- Exercise causes participants to feel an improvement in the quality of their life, an enhancement of self-image, and an increased sense of well-being.[1]

Precautions

It is important that persons with diabetes who want to exercise be encouraged to participate in exercise activities both at a recreational and professional level. However, several precautions should be emphasized. Before an exercise program is initiated, a detailed medical evaluation should be performed if persons are older than age 40 or have had diabetes for longer than 15 years.[1]

Some chronic complications can be worsened by strenuous exercise. With exercise, blood pressure may rise higher in persons with IDDM than in nondiabetic individuals. For these patients, strenuous exercise should be avoided. There are also renal changes. Exercise had been shown to result in proteinuria in persons with diabetes but not in nondiabetics; however, the consequences of this are unknown. Persons with neuropathy should avoid activities with a significant potential for joint or bone injury.

Individuals who complain of such symptoms as chest pain, palpitations, or unexplainable exercise-related fatigue need to be referred for a noninvasive workup for coronary heart disease. Individuals should be counseled that symptoms of chest pain, dizziness, unusual fatigue, visual disturbances, or nausea should alert them to stop exercising and to consult their physician.

In general, if before exercise, blood glucose levels are less than 80 mg/dL, the risk of hypoglycemia is significant and exercise should not be begun without the ingestion of carbohydrate. If fasting blood glucose is greater than 250 mg/dL and ketone bodies are present in the urine or if the fasting blood glucose is greater than 300 mg/dL, irrespective of whether ketones are present, it is generally advisable to improve metabolic control before beginning to exercise.[1]

Guidelines to Safe Exercise[35]

Blood glucose monitoring is essential. Ideally, the person would expend approximately the same amount of energy at the same time each day. For practical reasons, this is rarely possible. Blood glucose levels often are harder to control with exercise, but for most persons with diabetes the benefits of exercise far exceed the risks. It is imperative that individuals use the results of blood glucose monitoring to learn how to handle exercise safely.

Depending on the time of day that exercise is performed, various changes in blood glucose levels can occur. For example, exercising late in the afternoon may cause a greater drop in blood glucose values than if the same exercise were performed before or after breakfast. When possible, individuals should be encouraged to schedule exercise to improve postprandial hyperglycemia. If exercise can be anticipated, it should ideally occur 1 to 3 hours after a meal when starting blood glucose is greater than 100 mg/dL. After breakfast may be the most ideal time, because blood glucose levels tend to be the highest during this time. Blood glucose monitoring before, during, and after exercise can allow the person with diabetes to determine his or her particular pattern of response to exercise, especially as it relates to the time of day at which the exercise is performed. Records of blood glucose levels and exercise duration and intensity must be kept so patterns can be used to adapt food or insulin requirements to the time and amount of exercise that is planned.

Adequate metabolic control is important. When insulin deficiency results in poor diabetes control (blood glucose >300 mg/dL), especially with ketonuria, the production of glucose and the breakdown of fat to ketones exceed the ability of the muscles to use them. This is of particular concern when diabetes regulation has been suboptimal over several days or more.

Precautions to avoid hypoglycemia should be taken, especially when engaged in over an extended period. Exercising when insulin is at peak effect can result in a precipitous fall of blood glucose, and additional carbohydrate may be needed to prevent hypoglycemia. Decreasing insulin acting during the times of exercise may also be important.

Exercise can accelerate insulin absorption from the injection site in exercising limbs when it is begun immediately after an insulin injection. However, the absorption of regular insulin is unaffected by exercise when at least 40 minutes have elapsed between the insulin injection and the onset of exercise.[36] This is because by 40 minutes postinjection more than half of the administered regular insulin has already been mobilized. Likewise, intermediate-acting insulin absorption remains unaffected when exercise is initiated 1.5 hours after the subcutaneous injection. Thus, it seems unnecessary to advise diabetic persons with diabetes to rotate the sites of insulin injection to parts of the body that are not involved in the physical activity, unless exercise is begun immediately after an insulin injection. In that case, the client should be advised to inject into a nonexercising area, such as the abdomen, to minimize the effect of exercise on insulin absorption.

Food intake may need to be increased. In general, individuals with IDDM tend to overeat before exercise. Increased calorie intake on exercising days has been shown to reduce the long-term benefit of training with regard to overall glucose control.[18,19] See Table 6-2 for suggested food adjustments for exercise. The meal plan should be developed only after consideration of the person's exercise pattern. Well-trained individuals who regularly exercise at about the same time each day usually need less additional food than people who exercise only occasionally. The best way to determine how much extra food is needed is to monitor blood glucose levels before, during, and after exercise, especially in the planning stages of developing the meal plan.

Fluid intake is essential. In addition to increasing their food intake, exercisers must remember the need for increased fluid intake.

Individuals whose diabetes is less well controlled are particularly prone to dehydration when exercising on warm days.[37] One-half cup of fruit juice (15 g CHO) diluted with 1/2 cup of cold water, for a total of 1 to 2 cups/h, or as often as needed, can be an excellent way to take in both carbohydrate and fluid while exercising. It is imperative that an adequate amount of fluids be consumed before, during, and after exercise. Persons with IDDM often become so preoccupied with replacing carbohydrate that they forget the most important nutrient during exercise: water. For every 1 lb of weight loss during exercise, 2 cups of fluid are needed for replacement. Cool water is absorbed faster than warm.

Exercise may require a decrease in insulin dosages. A conservative recommendation is to begin by decreasing the insulin or insulins acting during the time of the activity (morning or afternoon) by 10% of the total insulin dose. If the person is doing an activity lasting the entire day, both the short-acting and intermediate-acting insulin would be decreased 10%, for a total of a 20% decrease in insulin dosage. See Exhibit 6-1 for suggested adjustments in insulin for exercise.

For persons on intensive therapy (multiple injections of insulin or infusion pump therapy), the regular insulin can be decreased by approximately 30 to 50% before exercise. In one study, subjects with IDDM maintained on intensive insulin therapy became hypoglycemic over the course of 45 minutes of moderate-intensity exercise conducted 2 hours after the usual insulin injection and 90 minutes after the standard meal.[38] Hypoglycemia was avoided by reducing the regular insulin dose by 30 to 50% (Figure 6-4).

More prolonged exercise may require a greater reduction in insulin dosage. Individuals with IDDM in whom the regular insulin dosage was reduced by 80% were able to exercise in the postabsorptive state for nearly 3 hours without becoming hypoglycemic compared with 90 minutes when the dosage was reduced by 50%.[39]

Because blood glucose continues to decrease after exercise, it is important to continue testing blood glucose after exercise is completed. It can

Table 6-2 Suggested General Guidelines for Making Food Adjustments for Exercise for Persons with IDDM[a]

Type of Exercise and Examples	General Guidelines		
	If Blood Glucose Is:	Increase Food Intake by:	Suggestions of Food to Use:
Exercise of short duration and of low-to-moderate intensity (walking a half mile or leisurely bicycling for < 30 minutes)	<100 mg/dL	10 to 15 g of carbohydrate	1 fruit or 1 starch exchange
	≥100 mg/dL	Not necessary to increase food	
Exercise of moderate intensity (1 hour of tennis, swimming, jogging, leisurely bicycling, golfing, etc)	<100 mg/dL	25 to 50 g of carbohydrate before exercise, then 10 to 15 g/h of exercise	1/2 meat sandwich with a milk or fruit exchange
	100–180 mg/dL	10 to 15 g of carbohydrate	1 fruit or 1 starch exchange
	180–300 mg/dL	Not necessary to increase	
	≥300 mg/dL	Do not begin exercise until blood glucose is under better control	
Strenuous activity or exercise (about 1–2 hours of football, hockey, racquetball, or basketball; strenuous bicycling or swimming; shoveling heavy snow)	<100 mg/dL	50 g of carbohydrate, monitor blood glucose carefully	1 meat sandwich (2 slices of bread) with a milk and fruit exchange
	100–180 mg/dL	25 to 50 g of carbohydrate depending on intensity and duration	1/2 meat sandwich with a milk and fruit exchange
	180–300 mg/dL	10 to 15 g of carbohydrate	1 fruit or 1 starch exchange
	≥300 mg/dL	Do not begin exercise until blood glucose is under better control	

[a] Self-blood glucose monitoring is essential for all persons to determine their carbohydrate needs. Persons with NIDDM usually do not need an exercise snack. During periods of exercise, all individuals need to increase fluid intake.

Source: Reprinted from *Diabetes and Exercise: Guidelines for Safe and Enjoyable Activity* (p 16) by MJ Franz and B Barry with permission of the International Diabetes Center, Copyright © 1993.

take the body up to 24 hours to replace the glycogen stores used during exercise. By monitoring blood glucose levels at 1- or 2-hour intervals after especially strenuous exercise, the individual can assess how he or she responds to the blood glucose-lowering effects of the exercise and make the necessary adjustments in insulin and food intake. It is often more important to eat a small snack after exercising than before exercise. ***All individuals should carry adequate identification and a source of readily available carbohydrate.*** Exercise goals should be realistic and practical. It is wise to have several exercise options in case weather, scheduling, or interest

Exhibit 6-1 Adjusting Insulin for Extended Exercise

- **Decrease insulin acting during the extended exercise time by 10% of the total insulin dose.**

For example:
Insulin dose before breakfast: 10 regular + 20 NPH
Insulin dose before supper: 5 regular + 5 NPH
Total: 10+30 = 40 U of total insulin
10% of 40 = 4 U

For morning extended activity, decrease morning regular by 4 U.
   Insulin dose before breakfast: 6 regular (10 minus 4) + 20 NPH

For afternoon extended activity, decrease morning NPH by 4 U.
   Insulin dose before breakfast: 15 regular + 16 NPH (20 minus 4)

- **For extended activity lasting the entire day,** decrease both regular and NPH by 10%.
   For example, using the example above:
   Insulin before breakfast: 6 regular (10 minus 4) + 16 NPH (20 minus 4)

- **Insulin dose at suppertime** may also need to be decreased to prevent hypoglycemia from occurring after exercise.

- **Blood glucose monitoring before and after physical activities** is essential to allow persons with diabetes to make adjustments in these general guidelines.

Source: Reprinted from *Diabetes and Exercise: Guidelines for Safe and Enjoyable Activity* (p 17) by MJ Franz and B Barry with permission of the International Diabetes Center, Copyright © 1993.

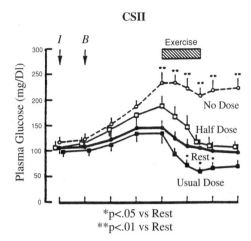

CSII

*p<.05 vs Rest
**p<.01 vs Rest

Figure 6-4 Plasma Glucose Levels in Persons with Diabetes Treated with Intensive Insulin Therapy in the Form of Continuous Subcutaneous Infused Insulin (CSII) during Rest and Exercise. (*I* indicates insulin administration and *B* indicates start of breakfast. Breakfast and exercise without prior insulin administration resulted in a significant increase in plasma glucose. Breakfast, exercise, and one-half the usual insulin dose resulted in an increase of plasma glucose similar to that observed during rest. Breakfast, exercise, and usual dose of insulin resulted in a significant drop in plasma glucose after exercise.) *Source:* Reprinted with permission from *Diabetes Care* 1985;8:339, Copyright © 1985, American Diabetes Association.

does not permit the usual activity to take place. See Appendix 6-A for a case study on exercise and IDDM.

NON–INSULIN-DEPENDENT DIABETES MELLITUS AND EXERCISE

Life-style changes that include a combination of improved nutrition, safe and enjoyable exercise, moderate weight loss, and blood glucose monitoring have been shown to be the best initial approach to therapy for NIDDM. Studies

have demonstrated diminished circulating insulin levels in the presence of normal or impaired glucose tolerance, indicating that increased insulin sensitivity is associated with physical training.[40,41] Overall increased physical activity will improve insulin sensitivity and glucose tolerance and reduce cardiovascular risk factors in persons with NIDDM. Also, the following benefits can be outlined:

- Working muscles use glucose more effectively, thereby helping improve blood glucose control. The overall effect of training is enhanced body sensitivity to insulin; therefore, carbohydrate and lipid metabolism and metabolic control are improved. Even a single bout of glycogen-depleting exercise has been shown to increase glucose disposition for at least 12 to 14 hours in obese subjects with insulin resistance.[42] More important, improvements in glucose metabolism may persist for hours to days, more than likely as a result of the increased insulin sensitivity in muscle and other tissues.[43] Exercise is especially effective in people with impaired glucose tolerance or mild-to-moderate diabetes (fasting glucose levels <200 mg/dL) who are also hyperinsulinemic.[44]

- If persons use insulin or an OHA, the dosage can frequently be reduced and in some cases eventually eliminated as a result of regular exercise and weight control.

- Training may lower the risk of coronary heart disease by improving serum lipid and lipoprotein profiles. Regular exercise also lowers blood pressure. Persons with diabetes have an increased propensity to all types of vascular disease, and cardiovascular mortality in patients aged 40 to 73 is roughly twice that of the general population. Furthermore, people with diabetes who have myocardial infarction are less likely to survive.[37]

- Exercise may be a helpful adjunctive therapy to MNT for weight loss. Attempts to substitute exercise for nutrition therapy to produce weight loss have been less than successful. Although weight loss may not occur, the main benefit may be changes in body composition. When formerly sedentary persons start exercise programs, their body fat decreases as muscle mass increases, but the individual may not lose weight.

Exercise may have an added benefit in obese persons with NIDDM because it may be particularly effective at reducing intra-abdominal fat stores and related metabolic abnormalities. Decreasing calorie intake and adding activity are the most efficient ways to control weight. Because individuals with NIDDM who are not on OHAs or insulin are not likely to become hypoglycemic with exercise, as is the problem with persons taking insulin or OHAs, it usually is not necessary or recommended to increase food intake before exercise.

However, it is important for professionals to guard against giving unrealistic expectations of quick or easy weight loss to individuals beginning an exercise program. Although exercise appears to be at least partially protective of lean body mass when energy restriction is implemented, it does not significantly increase the resting metabolic rate nor the rate of weight loss seen. This may be because the intensities of exercise possible in individuals at the initiation of exercise programs are not significant enough to lead to the oft promised benefits of exercise programs for weight loss.[45,46]

Precautions

If individuals use insulin or an OHA, they must follow the same precautions as persons with IDDM. However, because they are still producing endogenous insulin, their blood glucose levels are not as unstable with exercise as the person who produces no endogenous insulin.

Blood glucose regulation during exercise in NIDDM is not significantly different from that in persons without diabetes. During mild-to-moderate exercise, elevated blood glucose concentrations fall toward normal but do not reach hypoglycemic levels. Exercise-induced hypoglycemia rarely occurs, except in individuals using insulin or OHAs who have higher-than-normal insulin concentration during exercise, which may inhibit hepatic glucose production sufficiently to result in hypoglycemia. For persons being treated by MNT alone, there is no need for supplementary food before, during, or after exercise, except when exercise is exceptionally vigorous and of long duration. In this case, extra food may be beneficial, just as it is in persons who do not have diabetes. Individuals treated with OHAs or insulin may need supplementary food to prevent hypoglycemia, and a decrease in insulin dose may be needed. However, care must be taken not to overeat at these times.

Silent coronary ischemia can be common in patients with diabetes. A stress test to uncover occult coronary artery disease is especially important if patients have been previously sedentary or have had years of poorly controlled diabetes. Patients with cardiac autonomic neuropathy are at risk for arrhythmias; postural hypotension, especially after intense exercise; and sudden death. Patients with autonomic neuropathy do not tolerate intense exercise. More moderate levels of exercise should be encouraged.

Individuals should check with their physician to be sure they do not have medical problems that prohibit or restrict exercise. An exercise-stress electrocardiogram is recommended in all persons older than 35 years old.[23] This test is also helpful for identifying patients who have an exaggerated hypertensive response to exercise or develop postexercise orthostatic hypotension. An evaluation of peripheral sensitivity and circulation should be performed, and individuals with peripheral neuropathy or decreased circulation should avoid forms of exercise that involve trauma to the feet.

Guidelines to Safe Exercise[35]

It is important that individuals be encouraged to start with a mild exercise program, such as walking or riding a stationary bicycle, and be urged to rest if they feel out of breath. Because many individuals with NIDDM may have been sedentary for many years, they are frequently deconditioned and unable to exercise continuously for any period of time. A program of gradually increasing exercise sessions is most successful and safest for this group. It is important to encourage any increase in activity and to help the individual continue exercising during the sometimes lengthy period before improvement is actually evident.

Present physical activity levels should be assessed, and the individual should be encouraged to increase this level. The activity need not necessarily be as intense as physical training or

Table 6-3 Exercise Intensity Based on Perceived Exertion Scale

Rating	Description
0	Nothing at all
0.5	Very, very weak
1	Very weak
2	Weak
3	Moderate
4	Somewhat strong
5	Strong
6	
7	Very strong
8	
9	
10	Very, very strong
	Maximal

Source: Reprinted from Borg G. Subjective effort in relation to physical performance and working capacity. In: Pick HL, ed. *Psychology: From Research to Practice.* (pp 333–361), with permission of Plenum Publishing, Copyright © 1978.

aerobic activity. Physical training of milder intensity may be sufficient to improve metabolic parameters.[47] Because many of the metabolic effects of exercise on blood glucose control are of short duration, it is more important that physical activity be repeated frequently. Persons with NIDDM may have lower maximum oxygen uptake levels and need a more gradual program of increasing exercise than persons without diabetes. Autonomic neuropathy or some blood pressure medications may not allow for doing target heart rates. For these persons, learning to use a perceived exertion scale[48] is especially important (Table 6-3).

Furthermore, multiple short bouts of moderate-intensity exercise training have been shown to increase peak oxygen uptake significantly.[49] Therefore, it is recommended that adults should accumulate 30 minutes or more of moderate-intensity physical activity over the course of most days of the week. For many individuals, short bouts of exercise training may fit better into a busy schedule than a single long session.

Exercise should be low-impact to prevent injury to bones and joints. Low-impact exercises are performed with at least one foot touching the floor at all times. There should be no jumping or jarring, which causes stress on the joints. Exercises recommended for weight loss include brisk walking, jogging, swimming, bicycling, and low-impact aerobic dance. Most important, exercise sessions must gradually increase in length.

Muscle strengthening exercises can also be useful for improving glucose levels. Resistance exercise (ie, weight lifting) may also lead to improved glucose disposal and plasma lipid profiles.[50,51] Properly designed resistance exercise can be safe and more effective than previously thought.[52]

For weight management, persons are encouraged to exercise for 25 to 30 minutes five to six times a week. They should begin gradually with sessions of exercising lasting 5 to 10 minutes. The goal is to burn 250 to 300 kcal per exercise session for a total of 2000 kcal in a week. See Appendix 6-B for a case study on exercise and NIDDM.

PREGNANCY IN DIABETES AND EXERCISE

Pregnant diabetic women have been typically denied the option of exercising during pregnancy primarily due to fear of affecting the fetus. However, women who were doing regular exercise before becoming pregnant can usually continue their exercise program during pregnancy, with appropriate timing of exercise to balance insulin action and food intake. Exercise can be another tool to facilitate the maintenance of optimal blood glucose levels.[53]

It would seem prudent to advise women who wish to exercise during pregnancy to exercise at a lower intensity than nonpregnant diabetic women. Target heart rates for exercise prescription are not available for pregnancy; however, heart rates at 50% target rate are believed to be of adequate intensity to stimulate the training effect necessary to improve glucose use. The significant increase in glucose use during exercise is accompanied by simultaneous increases

in glucose production, but hypoglycemia remains the major clinical problem during and after exercise. At this time, it is not known if pregnancy is a contributing factor to exercise-related hypoglycemia.

For women with gestational diabetes, mild aerobic exercise does not seem to have an adverse effect on the pregnant woman or her fetus. Available evidence indicates that women with an active life style may continue a program of moderate exercise. For many women with gestational diabetes, an exercise program of three to four times weekly at a low intensity could be sufficient to attain improved glucose control and reduce the need for insulin. It is postulated that low-level exercise would increase the sensitivity of insulin receptors to the high levels of circulating insulin and partially reverse their glucose tolerance.[54]

The safest form of exercise would be that type of exercise that does not cause either fetal bradycardia, uterine contractions, or produce maternal hypertension. Exercises that do not cause uterine activity are those that use the upper body muscles or place little mechanical stress on the trunk region during exercise. Possibilities include recumbent bicycles or upper-arm ergometers. Women can be taught to palpate their own uteruses during exercise and stop the exercise if they detect a contraction.[55]

NUTRITIONAL CONSIDERATIONS FOR ATHLETES WITH DIABETES

Adequate and appropriate nutrition is important for any person engaging in physical activity or fitness programs; however, for the person with diabetes it takes on added importance. Not only can adequate nutrition help with athletic performance, but nutrition also plays a pivotal role in the regulation of blood glucose levels before, during, and after physical activities.

Fatigue that causes anybody to stop exercising can result from deficiencies of oxygen, water, or fuel, which can occur separately or in combination. The ability to take in and process an adequate supply of oxygen is related to physical training, whereas fluids and fuel are related to nutrition. Dehydration leads to fatigue, heat cramps, heat exhaustion, and even heat stroke. For exercise to continue, muscles must also have a source of fuel. Although all athletes will eventually need fuel replacements to continue exercising, individuals with diabetes may need replenishment of fuel, especially carbohydrates, sooner.[56] Total energy requirements as well as the source of energy are important considerations for the person with diabetes.

Energy Needs

Persons participating in regular physical activity programs have increased energy needs, ranging from 2000 to 6000 kcal/d or more.[57] The lower caloric density of the recommended high-carbohydrate/low-fat diet often makes it difficult to provide sufficient food to meet high energy requirements. High-carbohydrate food choices in a pattern of more frequent eating with planned snacks are often necessary. Liquid meal supplements for the athlete wanting to gain weight or maintain a high weight may be helpful, as they provide a high-carbohydrate meal in an easily ready-to-consume form.[57]

Men may require up to 50 kcal/kg or more during periods of regular heavy physical activity. This is in contrast to 40 kcal/kg for more moderate physical activity and 30 kcal/kg for very light physical activity. Women may require greater than 44 kcal/kg compared with 37 kcal/kg for more moderate activity and 30 kcal/kg for very light physical activity.[58] For exercisers with diabetes, the best way to determine caloric needs is to begin with a detailed nutrition history. Compare current intake with an estimate of caloric needs and calculate a meal plan based on the nutrition assessment. Weight can be monitored and used to evaluate caloric adequacy.

Carbohydrate

In general, it is recommended that approximately 60% of total energy for exercisers should come from carbohydrate.[58] A threshold of 500 to 800 g (2000 to 3200 kcal) carbohydrate, regardless of energy intake, may be necessary to maintain maximal muscle glycogen stores in athletes.[59,60] However, for the athlete with diabetes, blood glucose control is also essential. Consuming additional carbohydrate and then losing it through glycosuria is futile.

Carbohydrate during Daily Training

For individuals training 1 hour or less per day, 6 g of carbohydrate per kilogram body weight per day is needed to replenish muscle glycogen stores on a regular basis. For most individuals, this is approximately 60% of total daily calories. For individuals training 2 hours or more per day, 8 g of carbohydrate per kilogram body weight per day or approximately 70% of the total daily calories may be needed. For endurance activities, this is increased to 10 g carbohydrate per kilogram body weight per day.[59]

Because average intake is generally 4 to 5 g of carbohydrate per kilogram body weight per day (46% of calories), increasing carbohydrate requires effort and concentration on the part of the athlete. Chronic low intake of carbohydrate leads to progressive depletion in liver glycogen stores. If liver and muscle glycogen is not replenished on a day-to-day basis, chronic fatigue is the result.

Carbohydrate loading is a technique used by athletes doing events of long duration to increase glycogen stores. With high levels of muscle glycogen at the onset of exercise, athletes do not work at a faster pace but are able to maintain a high intensity of exercise for a longer time.[60] However, carbohydrate loading is effective only for maximizing exercise of long duration and endurance (more than 90 minutes) or for multiple events. Each extra gram of glycogen stored carries approximately 3 g of water, which causes some weight gain, stiffness, cramps, and early fatigue. Individuals with diabetes who carbohydrate-load must monitor blood glucose levels carefully and adjust insulin doses appropriately.

Carbohydrate Feedings before Exercise

Recommendations of not eating during the 3 hours before exercise or to avoid sugar intake 30 to 45 minutes before exercise no longer apply. Pre-exercise carbohydrate feedings do not impair athletic performance and may, in fact, improve athletic performance. Eating a meal 3 to 4 hours before activities or pre-exercise carbohydrate feedings 1 to 4 hours before exercise have been shown actually to improve performance. Intakes in the range of 1.1 g carbohydrate per kilogram 1 hour before exercise are reported to lead to carbohydrate oxidation and adequate blood glucose levels.[61]

Depending on the time of day that exercise is performed, 1 to 4 g carbohydrate per kilogram body weight in an easily digested meal 1 to 4 hours before the event is recommended.[60] For example, 1 g carbohydrate per kilogram 1 hour before an event might be toast, jam, or juice. Four grams carbohydrate per kilogram 4 hours before an event might be pancakes or potatoes, bread, and fruit. For an event early in the day (early morning), athletes can eat 1 hour before exercise. This will enhance performance compared with exercising in a fasting state. After exercise, morning insulin should be taken and breakfast eaten. For events later in the day, a small meal may be eaten 3 to 4 hours before the event.

Athletes with diabetes can eat a snack before or after exercising, depending on what is most convenient for them. Nathan et al.[62] reported that a simple pre-exercise snack, 15 to 30 minutes before exercise of short duration (<45 minutes), prevented postexercise hypoglycemia. Thirteen grams of carbohydrate was an adequate amount. Foods containing carbohydrate and low in fat (such as crackers, muffins, yogurt, or soups) rather than sugary sweets are good choices. Other nutritious snacks include peanut butter and crackers, fig bars, oatmeal raisin cookies, dried fruit, bread sticks, and granola bars. Fruits such as apples, fruit juices, peaches, plums, and pears have not only natural sugars, vitamins, and minerals but are 85% water as well. Self-blood glucose monitoring can provide valuable information to document and maximize the benefits of nutrition.

Carbohydrate Intake during Exercise

Carbohydrate is also needed during exercise to maintain carbohydrate oxidation for fuel use over exercise of long duration. As muscle glycogen becomes depleted, blood glucose supplies the carbohydrate oxidation fuel source. There are two ways to maintain blood glucose levels: by pre-exercise snacks or by carbohydrate during exercise. Particularly for the exerciser with diabetes whose blood glucose levels may drop sooner, faster, and to lower levels, carbohydrate during exercise takes on added importance.

Exercisers receiving a carbohydrate feeding of 1 g/kg at 20 minutes and 0.25 g/kg every 20 minutes maintained blood glucose levels better and exercised longer compared with exercisers receiving no carbohydrate. Muscle glycogen was depleted in both groups at the same rate, but the exogenous carbohydrate source allowed exercise to proceed for a longer time.[63]

Either a solid or liquid appears to work equally well. Athletes consuming 25 g carbohydrate every 30 minutes of either a solid or liquid performed equally well. The advantage of the liquid is that it provides hydration, whereas solids may prevent hunger. In general, 30 to 60 g carbohydrate every hour should be consumed over 15- to 30-minute intervals.

Fluids with carbohydrate are recommended for exercise lasting longer than 90 minutes. It is important to speed gastric emptying and get fluids to the cells as quickly as possible. Gastric emptying is affected by temperature, volume, osmolarity, and sugar content. As volume increases, so does the rate of gastric emptying. The higher the sugar content, the slower the rate of emptying. Cold fluids pass through the stomach more quickly than warm ones.[64]

Five percent and 7% solutions containing water, polymerized glucose, fructose, and electrolytes empty from the stomach as quickly as plain water.[65] Up to 70 g of carbohydrate, along with trace minerals, can be made available to the athlete without compromising rehydration.[66] As the sugar absorption increases, the athlete requires more water to facilitate absorption. For the athlete with diabetes, these beverages can provide fluids and a source of carbohydrate.

The sugar content of "sports drinks" should not exceed 10%. Concentrated drinks can cause gastrointestinal upset such as cramps, nausea, diarrhea, or bloating.[67] Fruit juice and most regular soft drinks contain approximately 12% carbohydrate and so need to be diluted with an equal amount of water.

Carbohydrate after Exercise

Combining carbohydrate before and during events increases performance ability, but of equal importance is carbohydrate intake after exercise. Carbohydrate should be consumed as soon as possible after exercise. Eating carbohydrate immediately compared with waiting 2 hours has been shown to replete carbohydrate stores more efficiently. One and a half grams carbohydrate per kilogram within 30 minutes after exercise with continuing feeds at 2-hour intervals is recommended.[68] This is the time in which high-carbohydrate feedings may be most useful. When muscle glycogen is depleted, a carbohydrate-rich diet will restore glycogen to its pre-exercise levels within 24 hours.[69] For a woman weighing 50 kg (110 lb), that means 2 cups of apple juice or 1 cup of corn flakes with 1 medium banana and 1 cup of skim milk. Replacing carbohydrate after exercise is absolutely essential for the athlete with diabetes who is at great risk for late-onset hypoglycemia.[16]

Fluids

During exercise, water should be consumed on a set schedule. Because the thirst mechanism is blunted with exercise, it is essential for athletes and trainers to monitor and meet fluid needs. Cool, plain water is the recommended beverage for fluid replacement in short-term moderate exercise and should be drunk before, during, and after exercise. Athletes should note

weight changes from fluid losses during exercise and drink 2 cups of water for every pound lost. If body weight has not returned to within 1 to 2 lb of pre-exercise weight, exercise should be moderated and fluid intake continued.

Nutrition Guidelines for the Athlete with Diabetes

Guidelines for increasing food intake should be based on blood glucose levels before and after exercise, on how close exercise is to scheduled meals and snacks, and on how often the person exercises. The more regular the exercise, the more the body adapts. As a result, it does not require as much extra food. If exercise is performed on a regular basis, the snacks should be part of the usual meal plan.

It is prudent for athletes with diabetes to eat additional carbohydrate after or before a short period (about 1 hour) of exercise, although care must be taken not to overeat. Fifteen grams of carbohydrate (60 kcal) may be enough to prevent hypoglycemia while not adding excessive calories. Ten to 15 g of carbohydrate should be consumed for every hour during a long event. For very intense or competitive activities, such as a marathon, athletes may need 10 to 15 g of carbohydrate every 30 minutes. Reduction in the dose of insulin before exercise (and possibly after) may also be required.

Up to about 1 hour, plain water is usually the best replacement beverage. For exercise lasting longer than 1 hour, water and extra carbohydrate may be needed. Fruit juices (diluted with water) and sports drinks are good sources of fluids and carbohydrate.

After exercise, blood glucose levels should be monitored at 1- or 2-hour intervals to assess the response to exercise and to make the necessary adjustments in insulin and food intake.

If possible, exercise should be performed 1 to 3 hours after a meal, with a starting blood glucose value greater than 100 mg/dL. If exercise is not performed after a meal, the exerciser should take care not to overeat. Extra food before or after exercise is in addition to the usual meal plan.

Although guidelines can help exercisers get started, each athlete is an individual. Everyone varies in their responses to training and physical stress. Adjustments that work for one person may not work for another. Persons with diabetes need to be aware of the signals their body provides and become experts at interpreting these signals.

EXERCISE PRESCRIPTION

The goal of exercise training is to achieve optimal cardiovascular, muscular, and metabolic benefits. Aerobic exercises are endurance exercises that require increased oxygen use for prolonged periods. Aerobic exercise improves cardiovascular and pulmonary function and tends to burn a significant number of calories. Examples are walking, swimming, jogging, cycling, and dancing and usually involve movement of many large muscles.

Anaerobic exercise involves resistance. They are muscle-building, strengthening exercises that are brief and intense and not associated with increased oxygen use. This type of exercise usually results in lower total caloric expenditure because fatigue occurs more quickly. Examples are weight lifting and sprinting. Resistance exercises increase muscle mass and decrease fat mass. Because muscle is the major site of glucose deposition, increasing muscle mass improves glucose disposal. Resistance exercise is also associated with reduced blood pressure,

improved lipid profiles, and better weight maintenance. In general, persons with uncomplicated diabetes can safely participate in resistance exercise sessions.

In determining the exercise prescription, the following steps need to be taken: (1) determine if medical clearance has been obtained; (2) establish with the client his or her goals for the duration of the exercise program in time (minutes) per week; (3) take an activity inventory to determine activities that the client enjoys and are considered appropriate for training, providing the proper intensity level is reached; and (4) suggest exercise intensity based on exercising heart rate or rating of perceived exertion.[70]

An effective exercise prescription clearly specifies type, intensity, duration, and frequency of the activity in days per week. Three essential ingredients are needed to achieve training: intensity, duration, and frequency.

With aerobic exercises, individuals should start slowly and increase the frequency and intensity as endurance improves. Exercise training intensity can be estimated either by heart rate (heart rate = beats per minute) or by rating of perceived exertion (RPE). Many individuals can base their exercise intensity on their heart rate; the eventual target heart rate should be 60 to 80% of maximal heart rate. However, lower intensities should be used for certain high-risk patients, such as those with severe exercise-related hypertension. The American Diabetes

Table 6-4 Target Heart Rates during Exercise: Heart Beats per 10 Seconds for Years of Age

Intensity (%)	Age (y)											
	15	20	25	30	35	40	45	50	55	60	65	70
50	17	17	16	16	15	15	15	14	14	13	13	12
60	20	20	19	19	18	18	17	17	16	16	15	15
75	25	25	24	23	23	22	22	21	20	20	19	19
85	29	28	27	27	26	25	25	24	23	22	22	21

Source: Reprinted from *Diabetes and Exercise: Guidelines for Safe and Enjoyable Activity* (p 26) by MJ Franz and B Barry with permission of the International Diabetes Center, © 1993.

Association's recommendations for patients with diabetes are to exercise aerobically at 50 to 70% of maximum oxygen uptake.[23]

One method to calculate target heart rate is to determine a percentage of the maximum heart rate (subtract current age in years from 220) and divide by 6 for target heart rate for 10 seconds (Table 6-4). However, for many individuals with diabetes, perceived exertion should be used instead; their heart rate may not increase as it does in persons without diabetes, perhaps as a result of autonomic neuropathy. RPE was developed by Borg[48] to help individuals estimate how intense they feel the work is. Individuals rate the degree of perceived exertion (total amount of exertion and physical fatigue) by how they feel on a scale from 6 to 20. Table 6-3 shows an adaptation of RPE using a scale of 0 to 10.

Workouts should begin with a 5- to 10-minute warm-up session. This allows blood pressure, pulse, and metabolic changes to occur more gradually. Furthermore, these exercises also increase flexibility. Persons with diabetes frequently complain of muscle stiffness, which may be related to muscle protein glycation. Stretching exercises can help relieve this stiffness.

Individuals should exercise for 20 to 45 minutes, although shorter sessions spread throughout the day may also be helpful. Exercise for longer than 60 minutes is associated with a higher incidence of musculoskeletal injury.

To achieve cardiovascular and lung conditioning, an exercise program should be performed at least three to four times each week. For weight control, the exercise program should be performed five to six times per week. To reduce chances of injury, different activities that use different muscle groups should be chosen. Cessation of exercise in highly trained, nondiabetic athletes leads to decrease in insulin sensitivity within 3 days. The duration of glycemic improvements after the last bout of exercise for persons with NIDDM is longer than 12 but shorter than 72 hours.[22]

The exercise session should end with a cool-down period of 5 to 10 minutes, which consists of cardiovascular cool-down, specific muscle strengthening exercise, and exercises for flexibility and relaxation. The cool-down period allows the body to return gradually to the resting state. Sudden cessation of exercise can cause problems to the individual.

Persons with diabetes should be encouraged to exercise but not without careful evaluation and information about the benefits and risks of exercise. With proper advice, most persons with diabetes can enjoy the benefits of regular exercise.

REFERENCES

1. Wasserman DH, Zinman B. Exercise in individuals with IDDM (American Diabetes Association Technical Review). *Diabetes Care*. 1994;17:924–937.

2. Wahren J, Felig P, Hagenfeldt L. Physical exercise and fuel homeostasis in diabetes metabolism. *Diabetologia*. 1978;14:213–222.

3. Felig P, Koivisto VA. Metabolic response to exercise: implications for exercise. In: Lowenthal DT, Bhradwaua K, Oaks WW, eds. *Therapeutics through Exercise*. New York, NY: Grune & Stratton; 1979.

4. Bergstrom J, Hermansen L, Hultman E, et al. Diet, muscle glycogen, and physical performance. *Acta Physiol Scand*. 1967;71:140–150.

5. Zinman B, Vranic M. Diabetes and exercise. *Med Clin North Am*. 1985;69:145–157.

6. Wasserman DH, Lacy DB, Goldstein RE, William PE, Cherrington AD. Exercise-induced fall in insulin and hepatic carbohydrate during exercise. *Am J Physiol*. 1989;256:E500–E508.

7. Wasserman DH, Spalding JS, Lacy DB, Colburn CA, Goldstein RE, Cherrington AD. Glucagon is a primary controller of the increments in hepatic glycogenolysis and gluconeogenesis during exercise. *Am J Physiol*. 1989;257:E108–E117.

8. Moates JM, Lacy DB, Cherrington AD, Goldstein RE, Wasserman DH. The metabolic role of the exercise-induced increment in epinephrine. *Am J Physiol*. 1988;255:E428–E436.

9. Marliss EB, Simantirakis E, Purdon C, Gougeon R, Field CJ, Halter JB, Vranic M. Glucoregulatory and hormonal responses to repeated bouts of intense exercise in normal male subjects. *J Appl Physiol*. 1991;71:924–933.

10. Marliss EB, Purdon C, Halter JB, Sigal RJ, Vranic M. Glucoregulation during and after intense exercise in control and diabetic subjects. In: Devlin J, Horton ES, Vranic M, eds. *Diabetes Mellitus and Exercise*. London: Smith-Gordon; 1992:173–188.

11. Wasserman DH, Lacy DB, Goldstein RE, Williams PE, Cherrington AD. Exercise-induced fall in insulin and the increase in fat metabolism during prolonged exercise. *Diabetes*. 1989;38:484–490.

12. Hultman E, Bergstrom J, Roch-Norland AE. Glycogen storage in human skeletal muscle. In: Pernow B, Saltin B, eds. *Muscle Metabolism during Exercise*. New York, NY: Plenum; 1971:273–388.

13. Garetto LP, Richter EA, Goodman MN, Ruderman NB. Enhanced muscle glucose metabolism after exercise in the rat: the two phases. *Am J Physiol*. 1984;246:E471–E475.

14. Berger M, Berchtold P, Cuppers H, et al. Metabolic and hormonal effects of exercise in juvenile type diabetes. *Diabetologia*. 1977;13:355–367.

15. Mitchell TH, Abraham G, Schiffrin A, Leiter LA, Marliss EB. Hyperglycemia after intense exercise in IDDM subjects during continuous subcutaneous insulin infusion. *Diabetes Care*. 1988;11:311–317.

16. MacDonald MJ. Postexercise late-onset hypoglycemia in insulin-dependent diabetic patients. *Diabetes Care*. 1987;10:584–588.

17. Campaigne BN, Wallberg-Henriksson H, Gunnarsson R. Glucose and insulin responses in relation to insulin dose and caloric intake 12 h after acute physical exercise in men with IDDM. *Diabetes Care*. 1987;10:716–721.

18. Zinman B, Zuniga-Guajaido S, Kelly D. Comparison of the acute and long-term effects of exercise in glucose control in type I diabetes. *Diabetes Care*. 1984;7:515–519.

19. Wallberg-Henriksson H, Gunnarsson R, Henriksson J, et al. Increased peripheral insulin sensitivity and mitochondrial enzymes but unchanged blood glucose control in type I diabetics after physical training. *Diabetes*. 1983;31:1044–1050.

20. DeFronzo RA, Ferrannini E. Insulin resistance, a multifaceted syndrome responsible for NIDDM, obesity, hypertension, dyslipidemia, and atherosclerotic cardiovascular disease. *Diabetes Care*. 1991;14:173–194.

21. Goodyear LJ, King PA, Hirshman MF, Thompson CM, Horton ED, Horton ES. Contractile activity increases plasma membrane glucose transporters in the absence of insulin. *Am J Physiol*. 1990;258:E667–E672.

22. American Diabetes Association Technical Review. Exercise and NIDDM. *Diabetes Care*. 1990;13:785–789.

23. American Diabetes Association. Diabetes mellitus and exercise (position statement). *Diabetes Care*. 1992;15 (suppl 2):50–54.

24. Bogardus C, Ravussin E, Robbins DC, et al. Effects of physical training and diet therapy on carbohydrate metabolism in patients with glucose intolerance and non-insulin dependent diabetes. *Diabetes*. 1984; 33:311–318.

25. Schneider SH, Khachadurian AK, Amorosa LF, Clemow L, Ruderman NB. Ten year experience with an exercise-based outpatient lifestyle modification program in the treatment of diabetes mellitus. *Diabetes Care*. 1992;15(suppl 4):1800–1810.

26. Krotkiewski M, Lonnroth P, Manrwoukas K, et al. Effects on physical training of insulin secretion and effectiveness and glucose metabolism in obesity and type 2 (non-insulin dependent) diabetes mellitus. *Diabetologia*. 1985;28:881–890.

27. Schneider SH, Vitug A, Ruderman NB. Atherosclerosis and physical activity. *Diabetes Metab Rev*. 1986;1:513–553.

28. Helmrich SP, Raglund DR, Leung RW, Paffenbarger RS. Physical activity and reduced occurrence of non–insulin-dependent diabetes mellitus. *N Engl J Med*. 1991;325:147–152.

29. Manson JE, Rimm EB, Stampfer MJ, et al. Physical activity and incidence of non–insulin-dependent diabetes mellitus in women. *Lancet*. 1991;338:774–778.

30. Manson JE, Nathan SM, Krolewski AS, et al. A prospective study of exercise and incidence of diabetes among US male physicians. *JAMA*. 1992;268:63–67.

31. Stein R, Goldberg N, Kalman F, et al. Exercise and the patient with type I diabetes mellitus. *Pediatr Clin North Am*. 1984;31:665–673.

32. Paffenbarger RS, Wing AL, Hyde RT. Physical activity as an index of heart attack risk in college alumni. *Am J Epidemiol*. 1978;108:161–175.

33. Pate RR, Pratt M, Blair SN, et al. Physical activity and public health, a recommendation from The Centers for Disease Control and Prevention and The American College of Sports Medicine. *JAMA*. 1995;273:402–407.

34. Yki-Jarvinen H, DeFronzo RA, Koivisto VA. Normalization of insulin sensitivity in type I diabetic subjects by physical training during insulin pump therapy. *Diabetes Care*. 1984;7:520–527.

35. Franz MJ, Barry B. *Diabetes and Exercise: Guidelines for Safe and Enjoyable Activity*. Minneapolis, Minn: CHRONIMED Publishing; 1993.

36. Berger M, Cuppers HJ, Hegner H, et al. Absorption kinetics and biologic effects of subcutaneously injected insulin preparation. *Diabetes Care*. 1982;5:79–91.

37. Richter EA, Rudemman NB, Schneider JH. Diabetes and exercise. *Am J Med*. 1981;70:201–209.

38. Schiffrin A, Parikh S. Accommodating planned exercise in type I diabetic patients on intensive treatment. *Diabetes Care*. 1985;8:337–343.

39. Kemmer A, Berger M. Therapy and better quality of life: the dichotomous role of exercise in diabetes mellitus. *Diabetes Metab Rev*. 1986;2:53–68.

40. Koivisto VA, Yki-Jarvinen H, DeFronzo RA. Physical training and insulin sensitivity. *Diabetes Metab Rev*. 1986;1:445–481.

41. Horton ES. Role and management of exercise in diabetes mellitus. *Diabetes Care*. 1988;11:201–211.

42. Devlin JT, Horton ES. Effects of prior high-intensity exercise on glucose metabolism in normal and insulin-resistant men. *Diabetes.* 1985;34:973–979.

43. Kemmer FW, Berger M. Exercise and diabetes mellitus: physical activity as a part of daily life and its role in the treatment of diabetic patients. *Int J Sports Med.* 1983;4:77–88.

44. Minuk HL, Vranic M, Marliss EB, Hanna AK, Albisser AM, Zinman B. Glucoregulation and metabolic response to exercise in obese non-insulin dependent diabetes. *Am J Physiol.* 1981;240:E458–464.

45. Broeder CE, Burrhus KS, Svanevik LS, Wilmore SH. The effects of aerobic fitness on resting metabolic rate. *Am J Clin Nutr.* 1992;55:795–801.

46. Horton TJ, Geissler CA. Effect of habitual exercise on daily energy expenditure and metabolic rate during standardized activity. *Am J Clin Nutr.* 1994;59:13–19.

47. Schneider SH, Khachadurian AK, Amorosa LF, Gavras H, Fineberg SE, Ruderman NB. Abnormal glycoregulation during exercise in type II diabetes. *Metabolism.* 1986;36:1161–1167.

48. Borg G. Subjective effort in relation to physical performance and working capacity. In: Pick HL, ed. *Psychology: From Research to Practice.* New York, NY: Plenum Publishing; 1978:333–361.

49. DeBusk RF, Stenestrand U, Sheehan M, Haskell WL. Training effects of long versus short bouts of exercise in healthy subjects. *Am J Cardiol.* 1990;65:1010–1013.

50. Miller WJ, Sherman WM, Ivy JL. Effect of strength training on glucose intolerance and post-glucose insulin response. *Med Sci Sports Exerc.* 1984;16:539–543.

51. Yki-Jarvinen H, Koivisto VA. Effects of body composition on insulin sensitivity. *Diabetes.* 1983;32:965–969.

52. Goldberg AP. Aerobic and resistive exercise modify risk factors for coronary heart disease. *Med Sci Sports Exerc.* 1989;21:669–674.

53. Artal P, Wiswell R, Romem Y. Hormonal response to exercise in diabetic and nondiabetic pregnant patients. *Diabetes.* 1985;34:78–80.

54. Metzger BE and Organizing Committee. Summary and recommendations of the Third International Workshop-Conference on Gestational Diabetes Mellitus. *Diabetes.* 1991;40(suppl 2):197–201.

55. Jovanovic-Peterson L, Peterson CM. Is exercise safe or useful for gestational diabetic women? *Diabetes.* 1991;40:179–181.

56. Franz MJ. Nutrition: can it give athletes with diabetes a boost? *Diabetes Educ.* 1991;17:163–172.

57. Horton E. Metabolic fuel, utilization, and exercise. *Am J Clin Nutr.* 1989;49:931–932.

58. The American Dietetic Association and The Canadian Dietetic Association. Nutrition for physical fitness and athletic performance for adults. *J Am Diet Assoc.* 1993;93:691–696.

59. Sherman WM, Doyle JA, Lamb DR, Strauss RH. Dietary carbohydrate, muscle glycogen, and exercise performance during 7 d of training. *Am J Clin Nutr.* 1993;57:27–31.

60. Sherman WM, Costill DL, Fink WJ, Miller JM. The effect of exercise and diet manipulation on muscle glycogen and its subsequent use during performance. *Int J Sports Med.* 1981;2:114–118.

61. Costill DL. Carbohydrate nutrition before, during, and after exercise. *Fed Proc.* 1985;44:364–368.

62. Nathan DN, Madnek S, Delahanty L. Programming pre-exercise snacks to prevent post-exercise hypoglycemia in intensively treated insulin-dependent diabetics. *Ann Intern Med.* 1985;4:483–486.

63. Coyle EF, Hagberg JM, Hurley BF, Martin WH, Ehsani AA, Holloszy JO. Carbohydrate feeding during prolonged strenuous exercise can delay fatigue. *J Appl Physiol.* 1983;55:230–235.

64. Ivy JL, Miller W, Dover V, et al. Endurance improved by ingestion of glucose polymer supplement. *Med Sci Sports.* 1983;56:466–471.

65. Seiple RS, Vivian VM, Fox EL, Bartels RL. Gastric-emptying characteristics of two glucose polymer-electrolyte solutions. *Med Sci Sports Exerc.* 1983;15:366–369.

66. Davis JM, Lamb DR, Bursess WA, Bartoli WP. Accumulation of deuterium oxide in body fluids after ingestion of D2O-labeled beverages. *J Appl Physiol.* 1987;63:2060–2066.

67. Lamb DR, Brodowicz GR. Optimal use of fluids of varying formulations to minimize exercise-induced disturbances in homeostasis. *Sports Med.* 1986;3:247–274.

68. Ivy JL, Katz SL, Cutler CL, Sherman WM, Coyle EF. Muscle glycogen synthesis after exercise: effects of time of carbohydrate ingestion. *J Appl Physiol.* 1988;64:1480–1485.

69. Zachwieja J. Influences of muscle glycogen depletion on the rate of resynthesis. *Med Sci Sports Exerc.* 1991;23: 44–48.

70. Cunningham LW, Barr P. Developing an endurance exercise program for the diabetic patient. *Diabetes Educ.* 1982;8:11–16.

Case Study for Exercise and IDDM

Christine, 35 years old, has well-controlled IDDM of 20 years duration. She wants to change her evening running to the morning. She currently takes 6 U of regular and 12 U of NPH insulin before breakfast, 5 U of regular at supper, and 5 U of NPH at bedtime. She usually monitors her blood glucose two to three times a day, and her most recent HbA$_{1c}$ was 7.6% (normal 4 to 6%). She usually takes her insulin and eats breakfast between 7 and 7:30 A.M. each morning. She would like to be able on some days to run at 6 A.M. as her work schedule is from 8:30 A.M. to 5:00 P.M. and she often has other activities to do after work. She is in for her regularly scheduled team visit with her endocrinologist, dietitian, and nurse. What should the dietitian do?

ASSESSMENT

Before making recommendations to Christine, begin with the following steps:

1. Determine if medical clearance has been obtained. Christine's physician is very supportive of her exercise program, as are the other team members.
2. Establish her exercise goals. Christine would like to be able to exercise safely either before going to work or after work. She generally runs for approximately 30 to 45 minutes, 4 to 5 days a week.
3. Take an exercise inventory. She does warm-up and cool-down exercises before and after running along with some muscle strengthening exercises, usually push-ups and curl-ups, three to four times a week.
4. Determine exercise intensity. When Christine began her running program a year ago, she would monitor her target heart rate, keeping it between 20 to 25 beats for 10

seconds. She now tries to keep her perceived intensity level at somewhat strong.

PLAN

The following guidelines will be given to her:

1. Review the effects of exercise. Exercise can both lower and raise blood glucose levels.
- Exercise is more likely to lower blood glucose levels after exercise than during exercise (especially in persons who are untrained or do sporadic exercise). Christine should be aware of her blood glucose levels late in the morning if she exercises before breakfast or during the evening and at bedtime if she exercises late in the afternoon.
- Exercise of high intensity can cause blood glucose levels to be higher after exercise than at the start due to the effects of "stress" hormones.
- If blood glucose is greater than 250 to 300 mg/dL with urine ketones, exercise can also cause blood glucose levels to remain elevated. Control should be improved before continuing to exercise.
2. Review the following general guidelines for exercise of about 1 hour:
- If blood glucose is less than 100 mg/dL before exercise, eat a pre-exercise snack of 15 g of carbohydrate. Monitor blood glucose after 10 to 15 minutes. Be sure blood glucose is greater than 100 mg/dL before beginning to exercise.
- If blood glucose is 100 to 150 mg/dL, go ahead and exercise and, if necessary, eat a snack or meal afterward depending on the time of day when exercising.

- If blood glucose is greater than 250 mg/dL with ketones or greater than 300 mg/dL, do not exercise until control is improved.

3. General guidelines based on timing of exercise:

- To exercise before breakfast: test blood glucose level; if 100 mg/dL or higher, eat or drink 15 g of carbohydrate (as a safety precaution). If blood glucose is less than 100 mg/dL, eat or drink 30 g of carbohydrate instead of 15, wait 10 to 15 minutes, and test again. When greater than 100 mg/dL, go ahead and exercise. After exercise, do another blood glucose test, take morning insulin, eat breakfast, and enjoy the rest of the day. Take usual insulin dose at supper and bedtime. Monitor blood glucose to see if there is a pattern (such as pattern of low A.M. blood glucose values) that suggests decreasing insulin acting at that time (evening NPH).

- To exercise late in the afternoon: do a blood glucose test before exercise. If blood glucose is 100 to 180 mg/dL, eat or drink 15 g of carbohydrate and exercise. If less than 100 mg/dL, eat or drink 30 to 50 g of carbohydrate before exercise. If blood glucose is 180 to 300 mg/dL, it may not be necessary to eat any extra carbohydrate; eat or drink usual afternoon snack.

- To exercise after supper: take evening injection of insulin, eat supper, and exercise. Test blood glucose before evening snack. Extra food may need to be added to the evening snack depending on the type and amount of exercise performed and blood glucose level. If there is a pattern of low blood glucose levels after exercise and before evening snack, consider decreasing regular insulin before supper by 10% of the total insulin dose.

MONITORING

After 1 week of exercise, Christine will call one of the team members to discuss the effects of her exercise program on her blood glucose tests. At that time, additional changes in her diabetes management may need to be made.

Case Study for Exercise and NIDDM

Sylvia, aged 44, has had NIDDM for 3 years and has progressively gained weight. She now weighs 185 lb and is 64 in. tall. She usually monitors her blood glucose two or three times a day, 2 or 3 days a week. Her HbA₁c level is 8.3% (normal 4 to 6%). She agrees with the dietitian to decrease her caloric intake by 500 calories per day, achieved by changing from whole milk to 1% milk and from juice to diet soft drinks and by moderating her evening snacks. She states she is ready to increase her physical activity and her physician has provided medical clearance for Sylvia to begin an exercise program. If after 3 months these lifestyle changes have not allowed Sylvia to meet her target blood glucose levels (80 to 140 mg/dL before meals; HbA₁c ≤7.5%), an OHA will be added to her diabetes management. What should the dietitian do?

ASSESSMENT

For Sylvia to safely begin an exercise program, begin with the following steps:

1. Determine if medical clearance has been obtained. In this case, it has.

2. Establish with Sylvia her exercise goals. She is willing to exercise 10 or 15 minutes 3 or 4 days a week.

3. Take an activity inventory. Sylvia prefers to begin walking around her block. On days when the weather is inclement, she can walk in a shopping mall, and she is interested in purchasing a video with exercises she can do at home.

4. Determine exercise intensity. Sylvia should monitor intensity by using perceived exertion. She should think her exercise is of moderate exertion. She can deter-

mine this by being sure she experiences no shortness of breath and can always talk while she is exercising.

PLAN

The following guidelines will be given to her:

1. Sylvia should start with mild and gradually increasing exercise sessions. She can begin by walking 10 to 15 minutes, 4 to 5 days a week. This should gradually be increased to 20-minute walks, 5 to 6 days a week.

2. She will be given information on how she can purchase appropriate exercise videos.

3. She should be sure that she does not experience any shortness of breath while exercising. She should be able to talk while exercising; otherwise the intensity at which she is exercising is too high for her.

4. Before beginning her exercise program, she should do a few warm-up exercises. Exercises such as shoulder rolls, waist bending or stretching, and calf stretching would be appropriate for her. After her walk, she should repeat the same exercises and add some muscle strengthening exercises, such as curl-ups and arm push-ups off the wall.

5. The goal of the exercise program is to improve Sylvia's blood glucose control. This can be done by increasing her exercise level and making better food choices (even without weight loss). However, losing 10 to 20 lb may also lead to improved glycemia.

MONITORING/EVALUATION

A follow-up visit with Sylvia should be scheduled in about 3 months. Some patients may need additional therapy to support change. At that point if she has not achieved her target blood glucose levels or experienced a 10% decrease in blood glucose levels or HbA$_{1c}$, the physician should be notified that the addition of an OHA is needed.[1] Blood glucose control should continue to be emphasized rather than weight loss as the main benefit from life-style changes. Encourage Sylvia to continue with her life-style changes. If she does need to add an OHA, once blood glucose control improves and if she continues with her exercise program she may be able to discontinue the OHA in the future.

REFERENCE

1. Monk A, Barry B, McClain K, Weaver T, Cooper N, Franz MJ. Practice guidelines for medical nutrition therapy by dietitians for persons with non–insulin-dependent diabetes. *J Am Diet Assoc.* 1995;95: 999–1006.

Chapter 7

Comprehensive Monitoring for Evaluating Diabetes Therapy

Judith Wylie-Rosett
Elizabeth A. Walker
Samuel S. Engel

The purpose of monitoring patients with diabetes is to identify treatment needs, evaluate the effectiveness of treatment, and help patients to avoid extremes in blood glucose levels and to achieve treatment goals. The 1994 American Diabetes Association (ADA) nutrition recommendations focus on balancing food intake with exercise and medical management (if any) to achieve an as near-normal blood glucose as possible and optimal serum lipid levels.[1] The absence of an "ADA diet" as a formulated prescription places greater emphasis on monitoring and adjusting dietary composition-related metabolic outcome goals. The nutrition treatment goal is not limited to achieving an ADA-prescribed macronutrient distribution. Monitoring is used to evaluate the influence of food intake and life style on metabolic control. Monitoring is also needed to make dietary adjustment related to the treatment of diabetes complications and related risk factors. This chapter provides an overview of monitoring tests and methods that are used to assess nutrition-related problems and to evaluate the success of nutritional intervention in diabetes. Clinical cases are presented to illustrate how information obtained from monitoring can be used to improve the quality of nutritional care.

PATIENT MONITORING OF PHYSIOLOGIC PARAMETERS

Patient monitoring of various physiologic parameters between medical/nutritional visits can provide valuable information for self-care of diabetes. In some cases, patients may use the information to adjust therapy at home using guidelines developed with their health care team. In other cases, the information may be an indication that the patient needs to initiate contact with the health care team.

Regardless of the type of diabetes the person has, some monitoring of glucose levels between medical/nutritional visits can be beneficial (see Chapter 8). Patients with diabetes are increasingly adjusting therapy based on monitoring. More data are available today than ever before to assist health care professionals in managing diabetes mellitus. All health professionals involved in diabetes management should be aware of how clinical parameters are influenced by intervention. The extent to which each member of the health care team is involved in adjusting medical therapy in relation to insulin depends on issues related to licensure, institutional, and regulatory policy. Physicians may assume responsibility for overseeing the case management; dietitians and nurses may adjust therapy using agreed-on guidelines or algorithms for day-to-day management. The primary responsibility for case management involves frequent patient contact, and which discipline assumes this role is highly variable. When weight or other nutritional problems are the primary treatment issues, the dietitian may coordinate other aspects of monitoring care as well. Nurses likewise may be involved in nutrition-related monitoring and may use dietitians in a consultative role for day-to-day management and by referral for periodic assessment/intervention. Across disciplines, collaboration is needed to use monitoring effectively to refine the physiologic goals of diabetes therapy.

Capillary Blood Glucose Testing

Until the late 1970s, urine glucose determinations were used for patient monitoring of glycemic control between medical visits. Although some patients still monitor their glycemic control using a dipstick, tablet, or testing tape for urine glucose, the limitations of the information gained from these methods make capillary blood glucose testing a preferable monitoring technique. Limitations of urine glucose testing include retrospective versus current glycemic control information; semiquantitative (eg, 1%, 2%) versus quantitative (eg, 154 mg/dL) data; and dependence of the result on the person's renal threshold for glucose.

The 1994 ADA consensus statement on self-monitoring of blood glucose (SMBG) proposed several indications for SMBG.[2] These include achievement and maintenance of a targeted goal for glycemic control, prevention and detection of hypoglycemia, avoidance of severe hypoglycemia, and regimen adjustments for lifestyle changes in persons taking hypoglycemic agents.[2] Insurance coverage for SMBG supplies has not been consistent among third-party payers. The cost of SMBG is of concern to users, as the consumable parts of the process (eg, the reagent strips and the fingersticking lancets) are often not fully covered by health insurance.[3]

Capillary blood glucose testing, often referred to as SMBG, is used by patients at home or wherever it is that they test. Because of their familiarity with different monitoring devices, diabetes educators can assist a patient in matching his or her needs with the various features of various options for measuring capillary glucose level.[4] Promotional materials may promise "free" or very inexpensive monitors, when the continuing costs of the reagent strips may be the real economic challenge. Choosing a monitoring system that is compatible to the patient will likely increase the accuracy of the results, as well as the patient's adherence to a schedule of testing. Traditionally, reagent strips determine blood glucose levels using a glucose oxidase reaction that can be read visually by virtue of a color change or by a reflectance meter. Many products for SMBG are available. Although material from reagent strip and meter manufacturers provides extremely useful information, product comparisons are usually found in diabetes magazines for consumers such as the annual Buyer's Guide in the October issue of *Diabetes Forecast*. As the number of products increases and products are reformulated, such an overview can provide useful information.

Achieving Accurate Results

"Follow the manufacturer's directions" cannot be emphasized too strongly! Steps for determining a blood glucose level may vary with each method of testing, and certain variables may affect the results with certain testing procedures. Environmental conditions, such as extremes of temperature and humidity and high altitude, may affect instrument or strip performance. Or there may be interferences from medical conditions, such as extremes of the hematocrit range, edema at the puncture site, hypotension, or certain medications. Packaging inserts and instructions for blood glucose testing devices must be read and understood by both patient and health care professional when choosing a new device.

The blood sample should be obtained from a clean finger near the tip. Using the sides of the finger, rather than the pad, is recommended because there is (1) less discomfort because of fewer nerve endings found on the side of the finger and (2) less subsequent contact with hard surfaces that may cause tenderness long after the test is performed. Whenever possible, wiping the first drop of blood away and using the second drop may enhance accuracy by decreasing the chances that the sample contains excess tissue fluid or alcohol if alcohol is used to clean the finger. (Accurate results may also be obtained using the first drop of blood if the drop obtained is large enough to cover the entire pad to ensure accuracy when read either visually or by reflec-

Exhibit 7-1 General Guidelines for Capillary Blood Glucose Testing

- Collect testing supplies (eg, testing device/meter, reagent strips, disposable latex gloves if performing test for a patient, lancet, spring-loaded lancet holder).
- Perform calibration, as required by device may include matching a code number from strip container to the device (this ensures that the meter is adjusted to slight differences in strip batches). Use this meter-specific check strip to assess meter electronics.
- Prepare the site for puncture (preferably, wash with warm water and soap or use alcohol to wipe site). Dry skin before skin puncture. Hold finger downward to pool blood supply or milk the finger by gently rubbing downward.
- Use a new lancet for skin puncture. Wipe off first drop of blood. Obtain a second drop of blood from the puncture site.
- Apply amount of blood indicated by manufacturer onto reagent strip.
- Allow designated length of time for the test.
- Record results immediately or store results in device memory for future recall.

tance meter and is not diluted by water or alcohol.) Although gentle rubbing of the finger to increase blood flow is acceptable, squeezing of the fingertip to produce a drop of blood may cause inaccuracies from either excess tissue fluid or hemolysis. Once the blood specimen is obtained, the procedure followed to analyze it varies according to the product used.

Types of Blood Glucose Tests

Visually Read. SMBG can be performed using visually read reagent strips, which gives the patient an estimate of the blood glucose level in increments (eg, 20 mg/dL, 40 mg/dL, 80 mg/dL). When this visually read test is performed as described by the manufacturer, good results can often be achieved by patients who do not need the specificity of an "exact" number. Because the blood glucose level is assessed through color changes on the reagent pad, the patient must be able to discriminate color changes and have access to well-lit areas to per-

form the test. Patients must also be encouraged to record the result they see, as opposed to the result they *hope* to see.

Meters. Although there are more than 15 different monitoring devices for patients to choose from, each has features that make it more or less valuable to individual patients. Examples of characteristic features of monitoring devices to assess when determining which one may be a better match for a particular client include

- a nonwipe versus a wipe system for reagent strips
- size and portability of the monitoring device
- length of test time
- ability to store data (ie, a memory)
- size of LCD display
- simplicity of test procedure for accurate results
- ability to accommodate for various hematocrit levels

Attention to the details of the test procedure is of the utmost importance, in particular, providing an adequate drop of blood, proper timing of the test, and correct wiping of the strip when appropriate. See Exhibit 7-1 for general guidelines about capillary blood glucose testing.

Potential for New Technology. More than 50 corporations/manufacturers are pursuing a noninvasive technology to assess blood glucose levels without puncturing the skin. Most of these devices use near-infrared beams to assess the blood glucose. The extent to which having a "noninvasive" method to assess blood glucose will affect patient monitoring behavior and quality of life remains to be determined. However, the risk of transmission of blood-borne diseases would be eliminated. Implantable sensors also offer the hope of assessing blood glucose levels without obtaining a capillary blood sample and can potentially obtain samples as often as once a minute using a needle-type sensor probe.[5] If technological advances allow the implantable sensor to be used in combination with an insulin infusion pump, a closed loop system could be developed that would be truly an artificial pancreas. These alternatives to capillary glucose testing are considered to be experimental at the present time.

Quality Assurance for Patient and Health Professional

Quality assurance for capillary blood glucose monitoring for either patient or health care professional is the entire process of steps to achieve reliable results for good patient outcomes. This process may involve quality control procedures, training in proper testing procedures, cleaning and upkeep of the instrument, documentation of results, and problem solving.[6] Health care facilities using blood glucose testing devices have specific guidelines to follow under the Clinical Laboratory Improvement Amendments of 1988, as well as state and institutional regulations, and those from other laboratory regulatory agencies and accrediting bodies.

Patients using blood glucose testing devices must be taught and strongly encouraged to perform the instrument-specific quality assurance activities in the home setting that are required for them to achieve reliable results. One way for health care professionals to assess the clinical significance of error in the blood glucose monitoring results is to use the error grid analysis system (Figure 7-1). Clarke and associates[7] formulated this grid for the comparison of capillary blood glucose test results (on the Y axis) compared with reference or laboratory blood glucose values (on the X axis). Five zones (A through E) have been designated by the authors as follows:

- Zone A: blood glucose values that deviate no more than 20% from the reference values.
- Zone B: blood glucose values that deviate more than 20% of the reference values, but decisions based on the SMBG values would not compromise the patient.
- Zones C, D, E: blood glucose values deviate from the reference values by either over- or underestimation, and these errors could adversely affect the patient.

This error grid for SMBG has been used to analyze both individual patient or provider errors, as well as to evaluate larger groups of data for individual blood glucose testing devices. Its value lies in its use in assessing clinical significance of user error.

Patients' testing skills should be evaluated on a regular basis; this evaluation can include a venous sample obtained simultaneously for laboratory comparison with the capillary blood glucose results.[8,9] Plasma glucose from the laboratory is usually 10 to 15% higher than values obtained from capillary testing because the red blood cells are removed from the plasma. Comparison is best on fasting samples, as postprandial venous values will be less than capillary values.

Prevention of Blood-Borne Diseases

Blood-borne infections to be considered in setting up guidelines are hepatitis B virus and human immunodeficiency virus. Potential for cross-infection exists with multiple patient use of the monitoring device, the fingersticking device and lancet, or any parts that can be contaminated with blood. General guidelines include

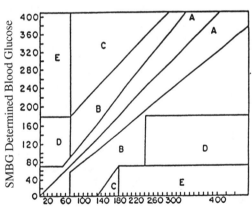

Figure 7-1 Error Grid Analysis System. *Source*: From Clarke WL, Cox D, Gonder-Frederick LA, et al. Evaluating clinical accuracy of systems for self-monitoring of blood glucose. *Diabetes Care*. 1987;10:622-628, 1987; Copyright © 1987, The American Diabetes Association, Inc; with permission.

Table 7-1 Glycemic Control for People with Diabetes

Biochemical Index	Nondiabetic	Goal	Action Suggested
Preprandial glucose (mg/dL)	<115	80–120	<80 >140
Bedtime glucose (mg/dL)	<120	100–140	<100 >160
Hemoglobin A₁c (%)	<6	<7	>8

These values are important for nonpregnant individuals. "Action suggested" depends on individual patient circumstances. Hemoglobin A₁c is referenced to a nondiabetic range of 4.0–6.0% (mean 5.0%, standard deviation 0.5%).

Source: Reprinted with permission from the American Diabetes Association. Standards of medical care for patients with diabetes mellitus (position statement). *Diabetes Care.* 1995;18(suppl):8–15.

disposal of used supplies in puncture-resistant containers; cleaning contaminated parts and areas with a solution of 1 part hypochlorite (household bleach) to 10 parts water; and the wearing of new latex gloves when health professionals perform tests for patients.[10,11]

Use of Glucose Data

The patient and the health care team need to determine how monitoring will be used to help achieve treatment goals.[12] Dietitians are increasingly involved in this process because the nutrition assessment reveals data critical to individualizing monitoring times and therapy goals. The choice of monitoring method and testing frequency are largely based on the treatment goals. The upper limits for various levels of blood glucose control have been established by the ADA. (See Table 7-1). In establishing target goals or ranges, one must consider carefully the risk of severe hypoglycemia and the patient's quality of life.

Quality of life issues must also be considered and include personal food choices and occasional use of sweets. A patient with insulin-dependent diabetes mellitus (IDDM) or who is pregnant may perform SMBG seven to ten times a day to obtain data to adjust therapy. Once blood glucose values are within agreed-on ranges, patients usually test four times a day. Some patients with non–insulin-dependent diabetes mellitus (NIDDM) may test only 2 or 3 days a week if glucose values are stable; the frequency may need to increase if glucose levels

fluctuate because of illness or change in therapy. Blood glucose determinations may be performed before meals, 1 to 2 hours postprandially, predawn, or other times when glucose values are likely to change. If the patient exercises, blood glucose determinations before and after exercise can help assess its impact on control. Some health care providers think patients need to check blood glucoses routinely before exercise to avoid exercise-induced hyperglycemia, which can occur when glucose values are greater than approximately 250 to 300 mg/dL.

The impact of exercise on glucose should be based on three or more determinations. Some practitioners also use blood glucose monitoring to reinforce nutrition therapy, especially for weight reduction in NIDDM patients. Patients are instructed to test before a meal and then 1 to 2 hours after completing the meal to observe the glucose excursion and return to the premeal level.

Blood glucose data can help patients with IDDM, NIDDM, or gestational diabetes identify foods that they need to omit or limit in their diets. The dietitian can use postmeal glucose testing to reinforce both qualitative and quantitative goals for food intake. Maintaining a log of glucose monitoring results is essential to facilitate use of the results by both the patient and provider. Forms to record the time of test, values obtained, foods eaten, and medication taken are typically found in most diaries and logbooks specially designed for recording SMBG results,

Exhibit 7-2 Food Diary

Time _____   Date _____
Before eating BG _____
Diabetes Medication _____
Activity _____

Day (Mon Tue Wed Thur Fri Sat Sun)

Meal (Breakfast Lunch Dinner Snack)

Place (Home Work Restaurant Other)

People (Family Friend Alone Other)

Mood (Negative Neutral Positive)

Overate (Yes No)   Planned (Yes No)

Food/Amount	*Calories/CHO*

Total _____
After eating BG _____   **Time** _____
Starch _____   **Veg** _____   **Milk** _____
Meat _____   **Fruit** _____
High-Fat Food/Added Fat (Yes No)
Sweets (Yes No)

Source: Adapted with permission from *Behavior Research Methods, Instruments, and Computers* (1987;19:215–223), Copyright © 1987, Psychonomic Society Inc.

Exhibit 7-3   Framework for Interpreting Self-Monitoring Blood Glucose Logs

SMBG records are used to evaluate the diabetes triad (food, insulin, and activity) as well as other factors that affect diabetes care—stress, sick days, change in schedule, cause and treatment of hypoglycemia, etc. Asking the following three questions will provide guidance in interpreting the records. Involve the patients with each question to obtain their perspective.

1. Is ADDITIONAL DATA needed?
- Is food intake consistent from day to day?
- Is regular eating noted?
- How are low blood glucose levels treated? Are they really low blood glucose levels?
- Are changes in activity noted?
- Are stressful situations noted?
- Has the patient made medication adjustments?
- Are possible reasons for glucose excursions written in the comment column?
- Do you need more blood tests?
- Can the patient provide answers to your questions or other insights regarding schedule or life-style variations?

2. Are all POSSIBLE INTERPRETATIONS considered?
- Is there a trend to the results or are fluctuations isolated?
- Could meals be spaced more appropriately?
- Is one meal too large or too small?
- Is the diet understood and followed?
- Is activity irregular?
- Is there improper insulin coverage for meals?
- Consider the influence of food, activity, and insulin (endogenous and/or exogenous).

3. Are all POSSIBLE MANAGEMENT CHANGES considered?
- What changes would the patient choose to make?
- Should the foods be distributed differently?
- Should weight reduction be the priority?
- Should changes in carbohydrate, amount, alcohol intake, etc, be made?
- Should activity be more regular, increased, decreased?
- Should the medication regimen be adjusted?
  –Would multiple insulin injections help?
  –Would a larger/smaller oral agent dose be helpful?

Source: © 1987 Margaret A. Powers.

although calendars and regular notebooks can also be used. Exhibit 7-2 is a sample diary that may be used for weight control or to monitor the effect of meals. Exhibit 7-3 provides a framework for interpreting SMBG results and evaluating the triad of diabetes therapy: food, insulin (endogenous or exogenous), and activity. Some logbooks contain graphs on which values can be plotted for easy visualization. Also, reflectance meters with memory capacity and computer software are being developed to enhance visualization of blood glucose values. Being able to see the rises and falls in the blood glucose values at different times of the day and different days of the week can help both the patient and the provider make therapy changes as needed.

When negotiating with a patient about a schedule for capillary blood glucose monitoring, explain why the times and frequency have been suggested to enhance adherence to the testing schedule. Patients should be involved in making decisions about goals for frequency of monitoring. Teaching patients what to do with the values they obtain can also enhance adherence. For example, patients on split doses of insulin who mix an intermediate-acting insulin with a short-acting insulin and who test four times a day can be taught to adjust their insulin dose.

Urinary Ketone Testing

Episodic monitoring of urinary ketones is needed for most patients with IDDM to assess for developing ketosis. Urinary ketone monitoring can provide valuable information that is used in patient management during illness and stress when blood glucose levels are likely to be elevated. The most commonly available tests are based on a nitroprusside reaction to assess urinary levels of ketones, acetone, acetoacetate, and α-hydroxybutyrate. The presence of acetone and acetoacetate causes a positive result, but if the proportion of α-hydroxybutyrate is high, the reading may be falsely depressed. Patients with IDDM should be instructed to test for ketones whenever their blood glucose monitoring indicates a blood glucose level greater than 240 mg/dL). The tablets used for testing acetone can also be used to test blood serum. However, patients are rarely taught to test blood ketones because they do not separate blood to obtain serum. Dipsticks are also available for testing urinary ketones.

Patients with NIDDM are not usually taught to test for ketones because, by definition, these patients are not ketosis-prone. However, during severe caloric deprivation or during severe stress, a NIDDM patient may be asked to test for ketones. When the calorie or carbohydrate level is low, pregnant women may have starvation ketosis, which can adversely affect the fetus.[13] This occurs when blood glucose is low and the body reverts to breaking down fat for energy. (In diabetic ketoacidosis, blood glucose levels are elevated along with ketones, indicating the need for insulin.) Therefore, most pregnant women with diabetes are asked to test for ketones. Starvation ketosis may also account for ketosis that may occur in a patient with IDDM who has blood glucoses of less than 240 mg/dL and is not pregnant.

Blood Pressure Monitoring

Many patients with diabetes who are concerned about blood pressure may monitor their blood pressure at home. Dietitians are beginning to measure blood pressure as part of their routine care, especially those in private practice. When a dietitian obtains a blood pressure level during nutrition consultation, the importance of nutritional modification to control blood pressure is reinforced.

The accuracy of various techniques has been reviewed extensively.[14] Many blood pressure monitoring devices can be easily used at home. Self-inflating arm cuffs or finger devices have made home evaluation of blood pressure much easier. Blood pressure changes continually throughout the day. Frequently, patients are instructed to measure their blood pressure soon after they arise, but this value may be considerably lower than other values obtained during the day. Caffeine can increase catecholamine levels, and blood pressure may be higher for up to 1 hour after consuming coffee or other products high in caffeine. Patients with diabetes may record their blood pressure values in their monitoring log for glucose levels, dietary intake, etc. Usually no adjustments in therapy are made based on home determination of blood pressure. However, these determinations may provide useful information if a patient appears to have falsely low or high readings during medical visits. Blood pressure monitoring skills should be assessed annually using the device that is used at home just as blood glucose monitoring skills are reassessed annually.

Weight Monitoring

Cosmetic and health concerns about excess body weight as well as the availability of bathroom scales make body weight at home the most widely used home monitoring technique. The desired frequency for monitoring body weight at home is highly individual. Weekly weights are usually recommended while a patient is trying to lose weight. Weighing more frequently can be a source of frustration and can encourage crash-dieting behavior. After a patient has achieved a goal weight, weighing several times a week may be helpful in maintaining a 3 to 5 lb range, which can signal when more careful attention to dietary and exercise habits is needed. Poor glycemic control often results in a decrease in body weight. Therefore, caution is needed to avoid placing greater emphasis on weight than metabolic control goals.

LABORATORY TESTS

Laboratory tests can focus on specific times and circumstances and also provide more long-term assessments of metabolic control and the presence of chronic complications of diabetes.

Blood Glucose

A blood glucose level is frequently obtained by physicians as part of the routine blood chemistries that are monitored in patients with diabetes, as well as in patients with other medical problems. Because the test is actually performed on serum or plasma rather than whole blood, values will probably vary from the whole blood glucose determinations performed on capillary blood in the fingerstick method. Laboratory values are usually 10 to 15% higher than capillary values.

Fasting blood glucose measurements are performed after an overnight fast of 8 to 12 hours. Patients are usually instructed not to take their morning insulin or oral hypoglycemic agent (OHA) until after the blood sample is obtained. The fasting blood glucose level measures the endogenous production of glucose by the patient's liver during the overnight period; in general, the glycemic excursions due to food consumed more than 8 hours earlier have resolved and thus do not influence this measurement. In patients with IDDM, this measurement is an indicator of the adequacy of the overnight insulization and can be used to adjust the dosage of the intermediate-acting or long-acting insulin given in the evening. In patients with NIDDM, the fasting glucose level is a measure of the patient's own overnight insulin secretion and can indicate the need for further improvement in metabolic control, either by weight reduction, initiation/adjustment of an OHA dose, or initiation/adjustment of insulin therapy. Because the fasting blood glucose level tends to be a more stable measurement in patients with NIDDM than in those with IDDM, it is a more reliable measure of overall metabolic control in those patients.

Nonfasting blood glucose measurements may be performed randomly or at specified times. Random blood glucose measurements may be more difficult to interpret than fasting or specified-time measurements because the influence of such factors as the timing of insulin action, the postprandial rise in glucose levels, and exercise may not be readily apparent. Thus, they cannot be precisely used to make specific adjustments in therapy. However, they are easily obtained in an office setting and have been shown to correlate roughly with other glycemic measurements.

Specified-time measurements can be used more precisely as an indicator of the need for therapeutic changes. Preprandial blood glucose measurements are performed immediately before a meal or, when insulin is being taken before the meal, immediately before the insulin injection. Postprandial blood glucose measurements are often performed 1 to 2 hours after meals. The one-hour result represents the peak of the glycemic excursion after a meal. The two-hour value should return to a level close to the glucose level before the meal. The two-hour measure is sometimes used to assess persons who are at high risk for developing diabetes in lieu of a glucose tolerance test, but an oral glucose load is considered to be diagnostic. Although laboratory postprandial glucose determinations were traditionally used to help synchronize insulin with carbohydrate (CHO) intake, patient-performed capillary postprandial determinations are generally used now (see Case 3). For patients who are unable or unwilling to monitor their own blood glucose levels, a 4 P.M. glucose laboratory determination may be used to assess the "peak" action of intermediate-acting insulin that was injected at 8 A.M. In patients who are treated with single large daily doses of an intermediate-acting insulin, hypoglycemia may occur in the late afternoon. The 4 P.M. glucose may indicate the need for adjustment of the insulin dose or the addition of a midafternoon snack. Adjustment in therapy should be on the basis of patient's capillary determinations whenever possible, because this provides a more realistic view of day-to-day glycemic patterns (see Chapter 8).

Glycated Hemoglobin

Measurement of the glycated hemoglobin concentration can provide an assessment of the degree of hyperglycemia over a prolonged time. Glucose binds to hemoglobin in a biochemical reaction that is not enzymatically mediated but rather is dependent on the degree of hyperglycemia.

Hemoglobin + Glucose → Glycated Hemoglobin

Because the average lifespan of the red blood cell and thus the hemoglobin contained within the red blood cell is 120 days, measurement of the amount of hemoglobin that has been glycated provides an index of the average blood glucose over the preceding 2 months; the measurement includes both "new" hemoglobin that has recently been synthesized and has not been exposed to glucose and "old" hemoglobin that has been exposed to glucose for up to 120 days. Thus, the "average" duration of glycosylation is 60 days.

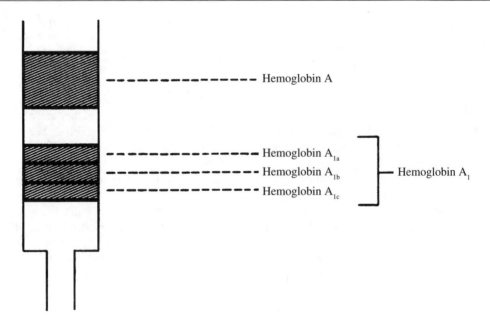

Figure 7-2 Glycosylated Forms of Hemoglobin

Table 7-2 Typical Normal Ranges for Glycosylated Hemoglobin Assays

Test Name	Test Method	Normal Range (%)
Hemoglobin A_{1c} (HbA_{1c})	Cation exchange	3–6
Hemoglobin A_1 (HbA_1)	Cation exchange	5.5–8.5
Glycohemoglobin (Gly-Hb)	Boronate affinity	4.0–8.0

Source: Isolab Inc, Akron, Ohio.

Glycated hemoglobin should be evaluated every 2 months to provide an assessment of control. This test can be used to help identify various types of problems. If the fasting plasma glucose level is normal and glycated hemoglobin is elevated, blood glucose rise during the day is likely. If patient monitoring indicated normal glucose levels and the glycated hemoglobin is consistently elevated, the self-monitoring may not be properly performed or may be inaccurately recorded.

However, the diagnosis of diabetes is not based on glycated hemoglobin; there are no standards established for using it for this purpose, and there can be overlap with the normal range even in patients with diabetes.

There are several different forms of glycated hemoglobin.[15] Hemoglobin A, the predominant type of hemoglobin within the red blood cell, can be glycated at several different positions. The glycation of hemoglobin A causes it to migrate more quickly through a chromatographic column. The forms of hemoglobin that migrate most quickly through the "cation exchange resin" chromatographic column are referred to as "fast hemoglobins," or hemoglobin A_1 (HbA_1). There are actually three different forms of glycated hemoglobin in the fast hemoglobin, or HbA_1, fraction: HbA_{1a}, HbA_{1b}, and HbA_{1c} (Figure 7-2). HbA_{1c} is the form that is most directly increased in relation to increases in average blood glucose levels.

Thus, measurement of either the HbA_{1c} or the total HbA_1, which includes HbA_{1c}, can provide an assessment of overall glycemic control over the preceding 2 months. Because the HbA_1 fraction contains other hemoglobins in addition to HbA_{1c}, the actual numerical values for the normal range will vary, depending on the technique used. Glycated hemoglobin can be measured in several ways, and assessment kits are available for use in the office or small clinic laboratories. The normal range of several different methods of measurement is shown in Table 7-2.

Several factors may affect the accuracy and reliability of the HbA_1 measurements. The test may be sensitive to changes in temperature, so the laboratory performing the test must be careful to control the environmental temperature. Also, some older assay techniques also measure what has been termed the *labile component* of HbA_1; this is a glycated hemoglobin molecule that is caused by the temporary binding of glucose to hemoglobin. Labile component levels may rise acutely in response to recent hyperglycemia, giving a false weight to recent hyperglycemia that may not reflect the longer period of diabetic control. Fortunately, methods are available and are widely used to eliminate the labile component before performing the actual measurements. Another potential source of confusion in the interpretation of HbA_1 levels arises in patients with various hemoglobinopathies, such as sickle cell anemia or sickle cell trait. Anything that alters the lifespan of the red blood cell may affect the results because the time for glycosylation of hemoglobin is varied.

Other glycated proteins besides hemoglobin may sometimes be used to provide an assessment of diabetic control. Fructosamine measurements and glycated albumin measurements are based on the same principle as glycated hemoglobin measurements. However, due to the shorter half-life of these proteins, these measurements provide a shorter-term assessment of glycemic control—2 to 3 weeks, as opposed to the 2 to 3 months measured by HbA₁ methods.

Lipids

Patients with diabetes often have abnormalities of fat metabolism, as well as carbohydrate metabolism. These are not only a consequence of the abnormalities in insulin secretion and insulin action that are seen in the disease but are also due to the frequent coexistence of obesity. Nutrition counseling addresses these metabolic derangements, both through modification of the quantity and quality of dietary fat intake and through the promotion of the maintenance of reasonable body weight. Monitoring the various lipid fractions in the patient's plasma provides a method of assessing the accomplishment of these goals. The total cholesterol concentration is now routinely obtained as part of multichannel automated testing, such as the SMA 20 or chemistry screen.

The National Cholesterol Education Program has established moderate and high-risk cardiovascular risk categories based on the total cholesterol level[16] (see Chapter 18). This measurement includes several different subfractions of cholesterol, each of which has different prognostic implications. Cholesterol is transported in blood in association with several different lipoproteins. The fraction of cholesterol that is bound to the low-density lipoproteins (LDL) has been found to be correlated with the risk of developing atherosclerosis and coronary artery disease[16]; patients with high LDL-cholesterol concentrations have greater risks of atherosclerotic vascular disease. By contrast, patients with high levels of cholesterol bound to the highdensity lipoproteins (HDL), or HDL-cholesterol, have low risks of atherosclerotic vascular disease.

Another lipid that is often measured on routine chemistry screens is the serum triglyceride concentration. Triglycerides are also transported in the blood in association with various lipoproteins. The very low-density lipoproteins carry most of the circulating triglycerides. Hypertriglyceridemia is often seen in uncontrolled diabetes, as well as in isolated lipid disorders. Marked elevations of the serum triglyceride concentrations (> 500 mg/dL) are associated with an increased risk of pancreatitis, and according to the National Institutes of Health, triglyceride levels between 250 and 500 mg/dL are associated with increased cardiovascular risks.[17]

HDL-cholesterol measurements are now readily available from many commercial laboratories and from some of the capillary lipid testing machines. The LDL-cholesterol level, although not easily measured, can be approximated by the following formula:

LDL-cholesterol =

$$\text{Total cholesterol} - \text{HDL-cholesterol} - \frac{\text{Triglycerides}}{5}$$

The risk of atherosclerosis steadily increases with increasing LDL-cholesterol levels; thus there is no clearly defined "normal" range. Furthermore, the level of LDL-cholesterol that is high risk varies with increasing age. If triglycerides are greater than 500 mg/dL, this method will not give a reliable estimate of LDL-cholesterol.

Renal Function Tests

Patients with diabetes are at increased risk for the development of renal insufficiency. The dietitian needs to be familiar with the interpretation of a variety of assessments of kidney function, both to recognize the potential need for dietary modifications and to monitor the effects of such modifications on the progress of renal complications. Serum creatinine and blood urea nitrogen (BUN) levels are both routinely obtained as part of automated chemistry screens. Patients who develop renal failure are not able to excrete urea or creatinine efficiently, and thus the levels in the blood rise. The elevation of the serum creatinine or BUN level occurs at a rather late phase, however, in the development of renal insufficiency.

Urinary studies provide a better assessment of kidney dysfunction in its earlier stages. The creatinine clearance is a measure of the ability of the kidney glomerulus to filter creatinine and thus is an indicator of the glomerular filtration rate. This rate is calculated by measuring the serum creatinine and the amount of creatinine excreted in the urine over a 24-hour period. However, the serum creatinine level can remain normal despite a significant reduction in creatinine clearance and thus is not very sensitive for detecting early stages of renal failure. The development of diabetic kidney disease can also be monitored by the detection and quantitation of urinary protein excretion. Normally, no protein is excreted in the urine. With the onset of glomerular dysfunction, small amounts of protein begin to "leak" and can be measured in the patient's urine using a dipstick for measuring protein excretion. Another method for monitoring proteinuria is to measure the total 24-hour urine collection for protein creatinine; this method is frequently used as a yearly measure of kidney function even in patients without obvious renal disease. It becomes particularly important in patients who have diabetes for longer than 10 years.

Recently, sensitive radioimmunoassays have been developed that can detect very minimal amounts of protein in the urine (microproteinuria or microalbuminuria). Microalbuminuria measurements can be performed on a random urine specimen or on a timed collection, making it more convenient for outpatient testing. Thus, microalbumin assessment is replacing previously described urinary protein measurements for the routine detection of early renal insufficiency in diabetes. Normal values for renal function tests are:

Test Name	Normal Range
• blood urea nitrogen	7–25 mg/dL
• serum creatinine	0.7–1.4 mg/dL
• creatinine clearance	>100 mL/h
• urinary protein	0 mg

Traditionally, up to 150 mg of protein in a 24-hour urine collection was considered a normal result (see Chapter 28). However, concerns about microalbuminuria as a possible indicator of early renal complications warrants a more in-depth evaluation of values even less than 150 mg per 24-hour period. A urine collection during one's menstrual period or after intensive exercise may produce a false-positive test result.

NUTRITIONAL MONITORING

The goals and methods of nutritional monitoring vary according to individual needs and type of diabetes. The parameters that are to be monitored should reflect treatment goals and may need to be changed as treatment priorities change.

A baseline evaluation is necessary to assess an individual's specific nutritional needs and priorities. It may be accomplished through a variety of nutritional history techniques, such as food frequency, 24-hour recall, or patient food records. Pertinent information should include goals for dietary intake, measurement of body weight, weight history, assessments of glycemic control, level of blood lipids, presence of complications, other health problems, and level of physical activity. The target nutrients that will be monitored depend on the treatment goals. Both the quantity and the quality of macronutrients may need to be evaluated (eg, type and amount of CHO or polyunsaturated versus saturated fats). Intake of micronutrients, such as sodium or potassium, may need to be monitored. The focus of monitoring may vary for different types of diabetes. For example, weight control may be a method to reduce insulin resistance and achieve glucose control for a patient with NIDDM; decreasing caloric and fat intake, and increasing physical activity are likely to be addressed in monitoring. For individuals with a history of binge eating, monitoring behavior related to episodes of binge eating rather than actual food intake may be desirable. With IDDM patients, synchronization of food and insulin is a major focus area. Pregnant women with diabetes must have their weight gain regulated in conjunction with prevention of starvation ketosis and postprandial hyperglycemia. Table 7-2 lists

Table 7-2 Common Monitoring Parameters for People with Diabetes

	IDDM	NIDDM	Gestational
Dietary intake			
Calories	M	H	M
Carbohydrate	M	L	M
Fat	M	M	M
Other nutrients[a]	L	L	L
Patient testing			
Urinary ketones	H	L	M
Premeal blood glucose	H	M	H
Postmeal blood glucose	H	M	H
Testing blood for hypoglycemia	H	L	H
Urinary glucose[b]	L	L	L
Physical factors			
Weight	M	H	H
Blood pressure	M	H	M
Laboratory tests			
Glycated hemoglobin	H	H	M
Fasting glucose[c]	H	M	H
Postprandial glucose[c]	H	M	H
Glucose tolerance test[d]	L	M	H
4 P.M. glucose[c,e]	M	L	M
Lipids	M	H	L

Note: H = high priority
         M = moderate priority
         L = low priority

[a] Other nutrients may be monitored in the presence of diabetic complications or other health problems.
[b] This test may be needed to evaluate calorie loss or to monitor control in NIDDM if capillary testing is not used.
[c] This may be done by capillary testing by the patient.
[d] This is used to establish the diagnosis of diabetes.
[e] For the patient taking insulin, 4 P.M. represents the peak effect of intermediate-acting insulin that is injected at 8 A.M.

monitoring tests and their relative importance for the three major classifications of diabetes.

Non–Insulin-Dependent Diabetes Mellitus

When weight reduction is the primary treatment modality, a patient diary focusing on eating behaviors, physical activity, and mood should be used. Urinary or blood glucose tests can be recorded with the food intake to help the patient and the health care provider see the relationship between food and glucose levels. SMBG after meals may help control the size of meals and serve as a motivating force for dietary change. Because blood glucose levels tend to be fairly stable in NIDDM, testing of blood glucose

may be limited to a few days a week or performed in the medical office at the time of routine visits. Urinary ketones do not usually need to be tested because ketosis is relatively infrequent. However, urinary ketones may be found if a patient is encountering metabolic stress or has an insufficient CHO or a very low calorie intake. Clinical visits may focus on monitoring lipids and/or blood pressure, as well as glycemic control, because the obese patient with NIDDM may also have hyperlipidemia or hypertension.

Insulin-Dependent Diabetes Mellitus

When the focus of monitoring is on the synchronization between dietary intake and insulin therapy, such variables as timing of insulin injections, food intake, activity, and glucose levels are important. Because the person with IDDM is ketosis-prone, testing for urinary ketones is important whenever the blood glucose is greater than 240 mg/dL.

Pregnancy and Gestational Diabetes

The target range for blood glucose in pregnancy and gestational diabetes is lower than in other forms of diabetes because normal blood glucose is lower in pregnancy. Because blood glucose control is so critical, patients usually measure capillary blood glucose levels seven times a day. Urinary ketones should also be monitored to evaluate for starvation ketosis, which is accelerated in pregnancy. See Chapter 26 for further discussion.

Food Diaries

The use of a diary is extremely helpful in targeting the nutritional interventions. A diary is a data base used to analyze the relationship among food intake, diabetes medication, activity, glucose results, lipid levels, body weight, and blood pressure.

The amount and quality of information recorded in a patient's diary are highly variable, depending on the personal preferences of the provider and the patient. Some patients strongly prefer a small diary that can be easily carried; others are willing to use a somewhat larger diary that can graphically illustrate the relationship between blood glucose tests and other variables.

The complexity of the method used may be influenced by the patient's sophistication and motivation. For some patients, keeping a diary of food intake for 1 or 2 days may be all that is realistic. Other patients may monitor food intake, calculate amount of macronutrients consumed, and record blood glucose levels on a daily basis.

CASE ILLUSTRATIONS

The dietitian involved with diabetes care and education needs to understand the technique that patients use to monitor control and to be able to use monitoring results to provide nutritional counseling. Dietitians should be able to help patients make dietary adjustments based on SMBG results. Familiarity with all laboratory tests is needed to assess the appropriateness of dietary prescriptions, to provide counseling that addresses the needs of patients with diabetes, and to communicate clearly with patients and other health professionals.

Case 1

A 45-year-old woman was diagnosed with NIDDM 3 weeks ago. She had seen her physician after losing 15 lb without any caloric restriction and was noted to have a fasting blood glucose of 238 mg/dL. Her cholesterol was 245 mg/dL, and her triglycerides were 232 mg/dL. She was 5 ft 3 in. tall and weighed 162 lb. She was initially treated with an OHA, which was discontinued 1 week ago when her fasting glucose fell to 183 mg/dL. At that time, she had a HbA$_1$ of 10.2%. Her current therapy includes a 1200-calorie diet that was started 1 week ago. Her diary indicates that all her capillary blood glucose measurements are less than 200 mg/dL, with a 25 to 50 mg/dL difference between the levels before meals and those 1 to 2 hours after meals. During the past week, she has not lost any weight despite being on a restricted diet. She is somewhat confused by her earlier weight loss without calorie restriction and her failure to lose weight on a 1200-calorie diet. She returns to the dietitian for answers to questions about her weight.

Comment

The dietitian is able to determine that the patient's calorie intake is, in fact, approximately 1600 calories. Her CHO intake conformed to the outlined plan, and blood glucose measurements reinforced the patient's food choices. However, her diet contained more protein and fat than had been prescribed. The patient had anticipated losing weight rapidly and was unaware that when she was in poor diabetic control she had been losing calories through the excretion of urinary glucose. She was also unaware that protein and fat were making a major contribution to her calorie intake. The dietitian provided a reassessment of the dietary plan, and the patient was then able to set realistic goals for rate of weight loss. Her plan included more precise measurement and monitoring of her food intake, as well as testing of her blood glucose four times a week. In the 3 months after this intervention, she lost 15 lb and reduced her plasma cholesterol to 218 mg/dL, her triglycerides to 158 mg/dL, and her HbA$_1$ to 7.3%.

Case 2

A 29-year-old woman was diagnosed with gestational diabetes in the 26th week of pregnancy. Her weight was within the normal range before conception, and there had been 14-lb increase during the pregnancy. She was taught to monitor her capillary blood glucose and began testing it seven times a day. Her premeal glucose levels were between 70 and 80 mg/dL and her 2-hour postprandial blood glucose level ranges between 90 and 95 mg/dL. Preliminary nutritional counseling was provided by her physician. During the 30th week of gestation, she was referred to the dietitian of the high-risk pregnancy unit for nutritional evaluation. Examination of her diary indicated that her postprandial glucose levels were between 125 and 140 mg/dL on three occasions when she had eaten large meals. The dietitian recommended redistribution of caloric intake, and postprandial glucoses subsequently remained between 90 and 106 mg/dL. She was gaining approximately 1 lb/wk. However, during the 35th week of gestation, she was found to have lost 1 lb and had ketones in her urine. The dietitian was asked to reassess her intake, and the patient indicated that she decreased her food intake to avoid taking insulin.

Comment

A detailed nutritional assessment indicated that the patient's caloric intake had fallen below the prescribed amount by 400 calories in an at-

tempt to prevent postprandial hyperglycemia. She had developed starvation ketosis, ketonuria, and weight loss. The decrease in caloric intake resulted in inadequate nutrition for mother and fetus. Monitoring weight gain and urinary ketones was critical in ensuring detection of the potential complication of caloric restriction. The dietitian explained the physiology of gestational diabetes and the need for quality nutritional intake. A meal plan was designed to include frequent small meals in an attempt to avoid postprandial hyperglycemia.

Case 3

A 24-year-old woman with IDDM has been managed for several years on conventional therapy with a dose of 56 U of NPH insulin at 8 A.M. and an injection of 22 U of NPH at 6 P.M. She has noted a 26-lb weight gain in the 3-year period since initiation of the second daily injection. Her height is 64 in., and her current weight is 146 lb. She reports frequent night-time binges, typically at 2 A.M., which she associates with stress induced by her job. She states that she eats three meals and two snacks daily, that she tries to be consistent in regard to both timing and composition of meals, and that she tests blood glucose twice a day. If meals or snacks are delayed by more than 30 minutes, she experiences severe hypoglycemic reactions, the frequency of which has recently increased. She is referred for dietary counseling and is advised to test her blood glucose more often to obtain a fuller glycemic picture. Self-monitoring reveals low blood glucose levels at 2 A.M., as well as occasional preprandial hypoglycemia. It becomes apparent that the peaks of insulin action are not synchronous with food intake, and when questioned she reports that since a job change 3 years ago, her schedule has been erratic.

Comment

Recording food intake and blood glucose values can provide a comprehensive assessment of problems with achieving synchronization between food intake and the peak action of exogenous insulin. Monitoring data were used to adjust her insulin therapy to "match" her food intake and current life style. Weight gain was partially attributed to the need to eat in response to the insulin peaks and insulin-induced hypoglycemia.

Case 4

A 28-year-old graduate student with IDDM is found to be proteinuric on routine urinalysis. He is 5 ft 11 in. tall and weighs 176 lb. Blood pressure is 145/90. A glycated hemoglobin of 10% shows fair diabetes control on his regimen of 18 U NPH and 6 U regular insulin before breakfast and 10 U NPH and 6 U regular before dinner. Urines are always negative for glucose and ketones. Routine urine dipstick reveals I + proteinuria. A 24-hour urine collection reveals 2.3 g of protein. Some months before, the patient began to test blood glucose and noted that many values were in the 180- to 225-mg/dL range. In an attempt to improve glucose control, he put himself on a low-carbohydrate, high-protein diet. When the patient was referred to a dietitian for evaluation of sodium and protein intake, it was found that his diet included large quantities of cured meats and cheese. Sodium intake was estimated to be in excess of 7 g/d.

Comment

This patient shows evidence of early renal insufficiency. Data that the dietitian obtained about dietary sodium and protein intake can be used to help target his nutritional therapy. The effect of any therapeutic changes will be monitored by assessing blood pressure, creatinine clearance, urinary protein, sodium excretion, and blood glucose.

REFERENCES

1. American Diabetes Association. Position statement: nutrition recommendations and principles for people with diabetes mellitus. *Diabetes Care.* 1994;17:519–522.

2. American Diabetes Association. Consensus statement: self-monitoring of blood glucose. *Diabetes Care.* 1994;17:81–86.

3. Harris MI, Cowie CC, Howie LJ. Self-monitoring of blood glucose by adults with diabetes in the United States population. *Diabetes Care.* 1993;16:1116–1123.

4. Davis M, Walker EA. Capillary blood glucose monitoring for clinical decision making. *Lab Med.* 1992;23:591–595.

5. Hashiguchi Y, Sakkida M, Nishida K, Uemura T, Kajiwara K-I, Shichiri T. Development of a miniaturized glucose monitoring system by combining a needle-type glucose sensor with a microdialysis sampling method. *Diabetes Care.* 1994;17:387–396.

6. National Committee for Clinical Laboratory Standards. *Ancillary (Bedside) Blood Glucose Testing in Acute and Chronic Care Facilities: Tentative Guidelines.* Villanova, Pa; 1991. NCCLS Document C30-T.

7. Clarke WL, Gonder-Frederick LA, Carter W, Pohl SL. Evaluating the clinical accuracy of systems for self-monitoring of blood glucose. *Diabetes Care.* 1987; 10:622–628.

8. Walker EA. Quality assurance for blood glucose monitoring: the balance of feasibility and standards. *Nurs Clin North Am.* 1993;28:61–70.

9. National Steering Committee for Quality Assurance in Capillary Blood Glucose Monitoring. Proposed strategies for reducing user error in capillary blood glucose monitoring. *Diabetes Care.* 1993;16:493–498.

10. Centers for Disease Control. Update: universal precautions for the prevention of transmission of human immunodeficiency virus, hepatitis B virus, and other blood-borne pathogens in health care settings. *MMWR.* 1988;37:377–382.

11. American Association of Diabetes Educators' Task Force. Infection control guidelines for patient education as a means of preventing blood-borne disease transmission during diabetes self-care procedures. *Diabetes Educ.* 1991;17:259.

12. American Diabetes Association. Standards of medical care for patients with diabetes mellitus. *Diabetes Care.* 1994;17:616–623.

13. American Diabetes Association. *Medical Management of Pregnancy Complicated by Diabetes.* Alexandria, Va: American Diabetes Association; 1993.

14. Appel FJ, Statson WB. Ambulatory blood pressure monitoring and blood pressure self-measurement in the diagnosis and management of hypertension. *Ann Intern Med.* 1993;118:867–882.

15. Goldstein D. Understanding GHb assays: a guided tour for clinicians. *Clin Diabetes.* 1986;4:1.

16. Expert Panel on Detection, Evaluation and Treatment of Blood Cholesterol in Adults. Summary of the second report of the National Cholesterol Education Program (NCEP) expert panel on detection, evaluation, and treatment of high blood cholesterol in adults (adult treatment panel II). *JAMA.* 1993:269:3015–3023.

17. National Institutes of Health. Treatment of Hypertriglyceridemia: Consensus Development. Conference Summary. *JAMA.* 1984;251:1196–1200.

Chapter 8

Blood Glucose Monitoring for Nutrition-Focused Care

Linda M. Delahanty
Maryanne Grinvalsky Richardson

When we think about the role of diet in improving blood glucose (BG) control or attaining normoglycemia, many nutrition issues come to mind. For clients with insulin-dependent diabetes mellitus (IDDM), these issues include diet consistency, insulin adjustment for changes in food intake, appropriate treatment of hypoglycemia, snacks for exercise, and meal and insulin timing.[1] Whereas, for most clients with non–insulin-dependent diabetes mellitus (NIDDM), meal spacing, exercise, and weight loss are important strategies.[2] Our challenge is to help persons with diabetes to manage these issues by showing them how they affect the entire management plan for better BG control. This necessitates a more extensive use of self-monitoring BG (SMBG) results to evaluate the impact of dietary factors and to tailor nutrition therapy to achieve these goals.[3]

In the Diabetes Control and Complications Trial (DCCT), dietitians demonstrated the important role of nutrition in achieving target BG levels in clinical practice and through research.[1,4] To do this, they changed their approach in nutrition counseling sessions. They tailored nutrition interventions to each patient's life style, motivation, and capabilities and used each patient's SMBG results as a basis for meaningful discussions of nutrition issues.[5] In the process, dietitians expanded and redefined their role in such a way that they were viewed differently by both patients and the treatment team. They became the providers who taught flexibility with food by explaining food–BG relationships instead of the providers who taught diet restric-

tions by limiting food choices. When dietitians are included as integral members of the treatment team, instead of ancillary providers to refer to when patients are not doing well, they can develop the relationships that are necessary to empower patients in diabetes self-management.

In this chapter, we demonstrate through case studies the dramatic impact that ongoing nutrition management can have on BG control. We discuss a problem-solving approach to explore the effects of food, insulin, and activity on pre- and postprandial BG levels and BG excursions for persons with IDDM and NIDDM. In each case situation, the dietitian uses knowledge about the glycemic impact of foods and the patient's predetermined BG goals to establish guidelines for interpreting BG patterns and to tailor self-management training.

DIET CONSISTENCY

Nutrition education has traditionally focused on the importance of diet consistency through adherence to an exchange system-based meal plan. This type of meal planning strategy requires consistency with carbohydrate, protein, and fat components of the diet and involves careful monitoring of all food consumed. Problems with achieving long-term diet adherence have been cited as the most common explanation for poor diabetes control.[6,7] Consequently, dietitians have often been in the position of trying to improve diabetes control. Because efforts to simplify treatment regimens can improve adherence,[8] shifting to a focus on carbohydrate consistency may improve adherence and at the same time emphasize the nutrient that has the greatest impact on 2-hour postprandial BG levels.[5] We use this method in our case studies.

Currently, dietitians have the exciting opportunity to use SMBG results to show clients how diet consistency impacts BG control. In this capacity, dietitians can help clients become empowered about diabetes management by teaching them to interpret the effect of carbohydrate consistency versus variability on BG patterns.[4]

Case example: Patient SM tells the dietitian that his goal is to stabilize his blood sugars. He says that he does not understand why his blood sugars are so erratic because he eats the same meals. A diet recall reveals the following carbohydrate (CHO) comparisons:

Meal 1	CHO (g)	Meal 2	CHO (g)
Breakfast			
3/4 cup cereal	15	2 slices toast	30
4 oz juice	15	4 oz juice	15
1 banana	30	margarine	0
4 oz milk	06		
	66		45
Lunch			
3/4 cup cereal	15	2 slices bread	30
4 oz milk	6	tunafish	0
1 banana	30	mayonnaise	0
kiwi	15		
	66		30
Supper			
6 oz chicken	0	2 cups pasta	60
large potato	30	1 cup sauce	10
1 cup beets	10	2 slices bread	30
1 slice bread	15	margarine	0
margarine	0	1 cup canned fruit	30
	55		130

Discussing this client's meals using CHO counting allows the dietitian to translate food intake into one number that can be related to BG results. By comparing breakfast 1 and breakfast 2, this client can begin to predict which breakfast will have a greater impact on subsequent BG readings he obtains before lunch. By comparing lunch 1, which contains 66 g CHO, with lunch 2, which contains 30 g CHO, this client can see why his presupper BG level was lower after lunch 2. By comparing supper 1 to supper 2, the client can see that the CHO variations are even more dramatic and can see the effects on bedtime BG readings and/or fasting BG readings the next day. This evaluation process involves the client in problem solving and fosters his ability to relate food intake to BG results, thus reinforcing the importance of diet consistency in stabilizing BG patterns.

Once clients establish a framework of diet consistency, insulin needs can be tailored to a client's usual food intake (CHO profile), and improvements in BG patterns can be seen via SMBG and glycated hemoglobin results. For the NIDDM patient on diet alone or diet plus an oral hypoglycemic agent (OHA), SMBG can be used to show the impact of CHO variability on postprandial BG values or on BG excursions. In some patients, documenting pre- and postprandial BG excursions with similar preprandial BG ranges will demonstrate the impact of CHO variability.

Case example: DB was a 16-year-old male with type I diabetes with a HbA$_1$ of 11.8 (normal range, 5 to 7.3). His height was 5 ft 10.5 in., and his weight was 165 lb. His insulin regimen was 31 U lente with 9 to 12 U regular (sliding scale by BG range) before breakfast and 22 U lente with 8 to 12 U regular before dinner. Review of his SMBG records revealed fasting BG 55 to 271 mg/dL; predinner BG 48 to 323 mg/dL; and bedtime BG levels 44 to 311 mg/dL. Diet review revealed wide variations in CHO intake at all meals (see Table 8-1), which contributed to erratic BG results.

Once the client was able to see and understand the relationship of variations in CHO intake to fluctuating BG patterns, he was more receptive to trying to streamline CHO intake, especially because he had experienced several unpleasant episodes of severe hypoglycemia in the past. DB

Table 8-1 DB's CHO Intake before and after Dietary Intervention

	CHO Intake (g)	
	Before Dietary Intervention	After Dietary Intervention
Breakfast	66–99	80
Lunch	54–99	84
Afternoon snack	0–30	30[a]
Dinner	44–84	69
Bedtime snack	15–30	27

[a]Pre-exercise only.

selected his own goals (also referred to as quotas) for CHO intake at meals and snacks with some coaching from the dietitian. Three months later, his HbA$_{1c}$ was 5.97 (normal range, 4.0 to 6.4), and he felt much more in charge of his diabetes control.

INSULIN ADJUSTMENTS FOR CHANGES IN FOOD INTAKE

Once clients realize that diet consistency is helpful in establishing appropriate insulin regimens and improving BG control, they often have greater motivation to strive for this goal. However, realistically clients need to acquire additional self-management skills so that when their eating habits deviate from their usual intake, they know how to manage insulin doses accordingly to maintain BG targets. The first step in learning to manage variations in food intake is to collect data. Food records that include CHO content of meals and snacks, insulin doses, activity/exercise information, hypoglycemic episodes, and pre- and postprandial BG (90 to 120 minutes after meals) levels are necessary. Accurate documentation of the time food is consumed and the time insulin is injected is critical to proper evaluation of the data.

Once it has been collected, the dietitian can help the client analyze the data. Clients can learn to evaluate individual glycemic impact of meals and snacks and develop insulin-to-CHO ratios for meals. Estimates of insulin-to-CHO ratios

need to be based on BG goals,[9] which need to be individualized. An example of BG goals for the nonpregnant individual would be a premeal (30 minutes before meal starts) BG of 70 to 120 mg/dL, an excursion goal of 40 mg/dL minimum, and a postprandial (90 minutes from meal end) BG of 180 mg/dL maximum. Glucose excursion goals can be used to warn the patient that they are more susceptible to hypoglycemia if their postprandial BG at 90 to 120 minutes is not sufficiently elevated. Caution is necessary in using excursion goals if the patient uses variable time frames between their injection of insulin and the start of a meal. This is explained in more detail in the section on importance of appropriate food-to-insulin timing in this chapter.

Table 8-2 shows some of the data that the client, DC, collected. DC had 55 g of CHO for lunch and took 5 U of regular insulin, which is an insulin-to-CHO ratio of 1 U for every 11 g CHO. His pre- and postprandial BG levels were within target ranges. However, his BG excursion was only 30 mg/dL, which is less than the minimal goal. Because DC's BG excursion was too small, he risked hypoglycemia later on. Indeed, at 2:30 P.M. his BG level was 50 mg/dL. Therefore the next time DC has a 55-g CHO lunch and his preprandial BG is in the target range, he may need 4 U regular, which would be an insulin-to-CHO ratio of 1 U for 14 g CHO.

At 6:00 P.M., DC had supper, which contained 45 g CHO. His premeal BG level was 80 mg/dL and he took 5 U regular and 15 U ultralente insulin. His postprandial BG level was 140 mg/dL, and his glucose excursion was 60 mg/dL. Because his BG results were in the target range, the dietitian then discussed that an insulin-to-CHO ratio of 1 U regular insulin to 9 g CHO seemed appropriate for supper meals.

If DC repeats this process for at least 3 days and patterns of insulin-to-CHO ratios are consistent, then DC can use this information to make decisions about adjusting insulin doses for more or less food at a particular meal. DC realized through this problem-solving exercise that he may have different insulin-to-CHO ratios at each meal. With practice, he will feel more com-

may differ depending on time of day, etc.

Table 8-2 DC's Data Collection

Time	Meals and Snacks	CHO (g)	BG (mg/dL)	Insulin (U)
11:30 A.M.			70	5 regular
12:00 P.M.	4 oz fish	0		
	1 cup chickpeas	45		
	1 cup green beans	10		
	Diet soda			
	Total CHO	55		
1:30 P.M.			100	
2:30 P.M.	Large apple	30	50	
4:00 P.M.			110	
5:30 P.M.			80	5 regular
				15 ultralente
6:00 P.M.	1 cup pasta	30		
	6 oz steak	0		
	1 1/2 cup carrots	15		
	Total CHO	45		
7:30 P.M.			140	
10:00 P.M.	6 oz milk	9	80	
	2 crackers	5		
	Peanut butter	(<5)		
	Total CHO	17		
11:30 P.M.			115	

(handwritten annotation: excursion of 30 mg/dl (should be 40 or more))

fortable adjusting insulin doses for any desired modifications in food intake. DC can also use his data on SMBG and food intake to learn the glycemic impact of different snacks. The dietitian can point out to DC that both his afternoon and evening snacks resulted in similar BG responses. At 2:30 P.M. he had 30 g CHO and a 60-mg/dL BG excursion. At 10:00 P.M., he consumed 17 g CHO and had a 35-mg/dL BG excursion. Both excursions were two times the amount of CHO consumed. DC can make note of this pattern and monitor food–BG relationships on other days to see if this pattern repeats. This type of information can be helpful in deciding whether insulin is necessary to cover a particular snack and in tailoring appropriate hypoglycemia management.

HYPOGLYCEMIA MANAGEMENT

Use of SMBG results is also important in teaching prevention of and appropriate treatment for hypoglycemia. SMBG can be used to detect trends in BG patterns, especially when there is a change in regimen related to food, insulin, or exercise. Symptoms of hypoglycemia can change and become more subtle as BG control improves, contributing to hypoglycemic unawareness. Therefore clients should pay attention to subtle symptoms they experience at the time they detect low BG levels and potentially improve symptom recognition.

Therapeutic goals for management of hypoglycemia are to treat promptly, use an appropriate CHO source, minimize overtreatment, and individualize treatment guidelines. Dietitians can use SMBG as a tool to help clients see and understand the importance of these goals in improving BG control.

It is important for dietitians to discuss a strategy for hypoglycemia management in initial counseling sessions when addressing issues of meal timing and consistency and in follow-up sessions when reviewing BG data. The standard hypoglycemia treatment guidelines are to take 10 to 15 g simple CHO when blood glucose is less than 70 mg/dL, wait 10 to 15 minutes, and retest BG. If repeat BG is less than 70 mg/dL, treatment should be repeated.

These guidelines are a helpful starting point and may need to be individualized based on several factors. These factors include (1) degree of hypoglycemia—the lower the BG level, the higher amount of simple CHO needed (to avoid overtreatment of hypoglycemia, more rapidly absorbed forms of carbohydrate [simple carbohydrate] are preferred), (2) time of day—at certain times, it may not need to be treated as aggressively, (3) cause of hypoglycemia—varying amounts of CHO may be necessary for hypoglycemia due to skipped meals versus less food, versus exercise induced, (4) past experience with hypoglycemia—consider what the client has learned about his or her own individual glycemic responses to foods, and (5) history of severe hypoglycemia—health care providers should consider setting higher thresholds for treatment of low BG (eg, treat for BG <80 mg/dL instead of 70 mg/dL).

Case example: PF has had a history of severe hypoglycemia and not surprisingly a tendency to overtreat hypoglycemia. Therefore, PF and the dietitian worked out a plan to document level of BG, food used to treat the hypoglycemia, and the BG response 15 minutes and 1 hour after treatment. Table 8-3 shows the results of PF's record keeping.

Reviewing this type of data helped PF deal with hypoglycemia management from a more objective viewpoint. He was able to see a quicker BG response to a set amount of simple CHO compared with a larger amount of CHO in a mixed meal containing protein and fat. He also noted the delayed effect of overtreatment versus appropriate treatment. He also began to see that in a different situation such as hypoglycemia related to extra exercise that a different amount of CHO may be necessary, especially when BG is as low as 30 mg/dL.

SNACKS FOR EXERCISE

General guidelines are available for adjusting food intake for exercise based on varying levels of BG.[10] (Also see Chapter 6 for additional guidelines.) The guidelines in Exhibit 8-1 or other guidelines can be used as a *beginning* for individualizing snacks for unplanned exercise.

Table 8-3 PF's Record Keeping Related to Hypoglycemia

Day/Time/Cause	BG (mg/dL)	Food Intake	C:P:F	BG Response 15 min	BG Response 1 hr
Monday—11:00 A.M. Smaller A.M. snack	45	3 glucose tablets *5 gm CHO each*	15 g CHO 15:0:0	80	100
Saturday—6:00 P.M. Delayed meal	40	12 oz juice 2 slices bread 2 tablespoons peanut butter	75 g CHO 75:14:16	70	250
Sunday—4:00 P.M. Extra exercise	30	3 glucose tablets	15 g CHO 15:0:0	45 (retreated with additional 15 g CHO)	75

Note: C:P:F = carbohydrate:protein:fat.

Exhibit 8-1 Guidelines for Adjusting Food Intake for Exercise by Intensity of Activity and BG Level in Insulin-Requiring Individuals (IDDM or NIDDM)

Intensity	Duration (min)	Starting BG (mg/dL)	Food Compensation
Low to moderate (eg, walking)	<60	<80	No exercise until >80
		80–120	10–15 g CHO. Check BG after exercise and supplement 10–15 g CHO if <100
		121–250	No food, recheck BG after 30 min and after exercise and supplement 10–15 g CHO if BG <100
		>250	No food. Check urine for ketones. If positive, follow medical team guidelines for ketonuria. If negative, exercise and check BG after. If >250, check for ketonuria and follow medical team guidelines if positive
	>60	<80	No exercise until BG >80
		80–120	15 g CHO, check BG after 30 min and then hourly. Supplement 15 g CHO if <120
		121–250	No food, check BG after 30 min and then hourly. Supplement 15 g CHO if <120
		>250	No food. Check urine for ketones. If positive, follow medical team guidelines for ketonuria. If negative, exercise and check BG hourly. If BG remains >250, recheck urine for ketones. If positive, follow medical team guidelines for ketonuria
Moderate (eg, jogging)	<30	<80	No exercise until BG >80
		80–150	15 g CHO. Recheck BG after exercise and supplement 15 g if <100
		151–250	No food, recheck BG after exercise and supplement 15 g if <100
		>250	No food. Check urine for ketones. If positive, follow medical team guidelines for ketonuria. If negative, exercise and recheck BG after. If >250, recheck urine for ketones. If positive, follow medical team guidelines for ketonuria
	>30	<80	No exercise until BG >80
		80–150	15–30 g CHO. Recheck BG after 30 min and then hourly. Supplement any BG <120 with 15–30 g CHO

continues

Exhibit 8-1 continued

Intensity	Duration (min)	Starting BG (mg/dL)	Food Compensation
		151–250	No food. Recheck BG after 30–60 min and then hourly. Supplement any BG <120 with 15 g CHO
		>250	No food. Check urine for ketones. If positive, follow medical team guidelines for ketonuria. If negative, exercise and recheck BG after 30–60 min, and then at least hourly. Supplement any BG <120 with 15–30 g CHO. Check urine for ketones if any BG >250. If positive, stop exercising and follow medical team guidelines for ketonuria
High (eg, running)	<30	<80	No exercise until BG >80
		80–150	15–30 g CHO. Recheck BG after exercise and supplement 15 g CHO if <120
		150–250	No food. Recheck BG after exercise and supplement 15 g CHO if <120
		>250	No food. Check urine for ketones. If positive, follow medical team guidelines for ketonuria. If negative, exercise and recheck BG afterward. If >250, recheck urine and follow guidelines if positive
	>30	<80	No exercise until BG >80
		80–150	15–30 g CHO. Recheck BG after 30 min and resupplement 15–30 g CHO for any BG <120
		150–250	No food. Recheck BG after 30 min and then hourly. Supplement 15–30 g CHO if BG <120
		>250	No food. Check urine for ketones. If positive, stop exercise and follow medical team guidelines for ketonuria. If negative, exercise, but recheck BG and urine after 30–60 min. Supplement any BG <120 with 15 g CHO, and follow medical team guidelines for any ketonuria

Source: Reprinted from *Stepping Out: A Diabetes Exercise Starter Kit* with permission of the American Diabetes Association, © 1992.

Even before that, medical clearance for exercise should be obtained, and there should be discussion of the particular client's reasons for exercise and the benefits they anticipate. When the goal is weight loss, lower-calorie snacks and/or reducing insulin dose (where applicable) should be

Table 8-4 DC's Exercise Data Collection

Exercise	Time	BG (mg/dL)	Food	Exchanges
	5:00 P.M.	76	33 g CHO	1 1/2 milk
			12 g protein	1 fruit
Moderate-intensity biking for 1 hour	6–7 P.M.			
	7:30 P.M.	163	Usual supper	

pursued rather than adding higher-calorie snacks.

Factors to consider when individualizing snacks for exercise include (1) exercise type, (2) intensity, (3) duration, (4) pre-exercise BG, (5) time of day related to meals and snacks, (6) peaking insulin, (7) insulin injection site, (8) level of conditioning, (9) past experience with exercise, and (10) whether there is potential for dehydration. Regarding past experience, it is possible that a person who exercises competitively or intensely may experience *hyper*glycemia. We have seen clients require more insulin on days when they are involved in competition. Caution must be used to prevent severe hypoglycemia postexercise in anyone with diabetes, but especially in these individuals.

Also, a patient's usual BG patterns without exercise should be taken into account. For example, a patient who is usually hyperglycemic predinner and wants to exercise in the late afternoon may need a less substantial snack, or no snack at all.

As you can see in Exhibit 8-1, guidelines for exercise can be overwhelming (also see Table 6-2). To simplify these for the beginner, we suggest selecting a specific form of exercise and its expected intensity for that individual. Specific snacks can then be discussed, and the client can be given an opportunity to collect data, which can then be reviewed and discussed with the dietitian. The dietitian should help the patient understand the effect of different sources of CHO and the addition of protein or fat in preventing hypoglycemia, dependent on the BG level, duration and intensity of exercise, and insulin kinetics. For example, an individual starting to jog with a pre-exercise BG of 90 mg/dL may want to add protein and fat to his or her snack for more

than 30 minutes of exercise. Because the starting BG is 90 mg/dL, a quickly absorbed form of CHO may be preferred. In this case, 8 oz milk would be ideal, with the option of following it with an additional 15 g of a more complex carbohydrate.

Individuals also need to be aware that the physical effects of exercise can be similar to the symptoms of hypoglycemia. For example, an increased heart rate, perspiration, or fatigue may signal hypoglycemia. When in doubt, SMBG should be used to ensure safety. They also need to know that the effects of exercise can last well into the next day, and they should be on guard against hypoglycemia, especially overnight. Nocturnal SMBG is advisable when this is a concern.

Case example: DC evaluated the use of these exercise guidelines for an hour of biking at moderate intensity in the late afternoon when his morning intermediate-acting insulin was at peak action. Table 8-4 shows the results of his data collection.

DC's past experiences with planning snacks for exercise had resulted in postexercise hypoglycemia. Therefore, he had developed a habit of snacking before, during, and after exercise to prevent hypoglycemia. When he was able to see that implementing these general guidelines did not result in hypoglycemia, he was more comfortable in continuing to evaluate the recommendations for varying intensity and durations of activity.

IMPORTANCE OF APPROPRIATE FOOD-TO-INSULIN TIMING

The use of appropriate food–insulin timing is important in the management of type I diabetes and insulin-requiring type II diabetes. Although often overlooked, appropriate timing can prevent weight gain by preventing the use of excess insulin. SMBG can demonstrate the value of using timing for the client.

Perhaps the most common error individuals make is failure to wait an adequate amount of time between taking regular insulin and beginning a meal. For most individuals, this interval should be a half hour, during which the insulin is absorbed but does not have an effect on the preprandial BG. Individuals who begin eating within the first half hour will have higher postprandial BG levels and ultimately require more insulin to achieve optimal control. If hypoglycemia occurs during the half hour after regular insulin, it is usually due to insulin overlap from a previous meal, an intermediate-acting insulin, or in the case of continuous subcutaneous insulin infusion, an excessive basal rate. Extra activity, or exercise resulting in a higher than usual metabolic rate, may necessitate abbreviating this half-hour time frame. Likewise, a low but not hypoglycemic BG may also mean that

waiting less time is appropriate. A hypoglycemic premeal BG should be treated as such, and the BG retested to ensure safety, before additional mealtime insulin is given. Above all else, individual experience should dictate what guidelines are used in these situations. This experience should be based on BG data accumulated over time and the insulin regimen currently in use.

Case example: KR has been beginning her meals right after her injection of regular and NPH in the morning and regular before dinner. She had been working with the dietitian to achieve a consistent carbohydrate intake at breakfast. The dietitian explained the concept of timing and requested that KR keep 2 weeks of detailed food and BG records, the first week continuing her usual habits and the second week attempting to use timing. Table 8-5 summarizes some of the data she collected at breakfast.

In reviewing the data with KR, the dietitian pointed out that two of the glucose excursions in week 2 were less than week 1. Even when KR consumed 60 g CHO (30 g extra) without adjusting her insulin scale on day 14, the excursion

---

Table 8-5 KR's Breakfast Data Collection

Day	CHO (g)	BG (Pre) Regular Insulin [a] (U)	BG (Post) (mg/dL) [b]	Excursion (mg/dL) [c]	(mg/dL) [d]
Week 1 (Food consumed 5 min after insulin injection)					
1	30	5	153	302	149
2	30	4	90	200	110
3	30	8	262	431	169
Week 2 (Food consumed 30 min after injection)					
8	30	7	213	302	89
10	30	5	135	200	65
14	60	4	75	200	125

[a] Regular insulin dosage based on BG before meal. For breakfast:
   4 U—70–100 mg/dL
   5 U—101–180 mg/dL
   7 U—181–240 mg/dL
   8 U—>240 mg/dL

[b] BG 5 minutes before meal (week 1) or 30 minutes before meal (week 2), at time of injection.

[c] BG 90 minutes after meal began.

[d] Difference between pre- and post-BG.

was less than two of the days in week 1 and only 15 mg/dL higher than the excursion on day 2, when the starting BG was similar. This exercise made it clear to KR that less insulin would be needed if she used appropriate timing, which was adequate motivation for her to try and integrate these concepts into her daily management.

There are some situations in which waiting more than 30 minutes may be beneficial to the postprandial BG. In pregnancy or obesity, insulin absorption from the injection site may take more than 30 minutes because of extra adipose tissue. Therefore, waiting more than 30 minutes will allow the premeal regular insulin to lower a high (ie, above the designated target) preprandial BG. Caution must be taken to prevent subsequent hypoglycemia from waiting too long, especially in individuals who are using sliding-scale insulin coverage. Individuals with renal or gastrointestinal complications have an even greater need for the individualization of timing guidelines.

There are always occasions when the individual is unable to wait between an injection and the start of the meal. Some strategies that will help control postprandial hyperglycemia are (1) eating the noncarbohydrate portion of the meal first, (2) beginning the meal with a salad or noncarbohydrate appetizer, or (3) selecting a portable carbohydrate source that can be consumed at a later time.

MEAL SPACING: NIDDM

For clients with NIDDM, meal spacing is an important strategy that can be used to improve glycemic control.[2] Use of SMBG results can help clients see the potential benefit of spacing nutrients over the day on BG patterns.

Case example: PG presented with a HbA1c of 10.21% (average BG, 254 mg/dL) and random BG of 228 mg/dL. He was started on 2.5 mg glyburide per day (one pill per day). Diet recall reveals an eating pattern of coffee in the morning, no breakfast or lunch, and then a large dinner at 6:00 P.M., which contained 2100 calories. After distributing his food intake into three

meals per day, PG was able to discontinue glyburide pills and maintain fasting BG levels between 70 to 140 mg/dL and predinner BG levels between 80 to 120 mg/dL. Because PG's weight was stable during this time and he maintained the same level of exercise, he was able to see the impressive effect of meal spacing on BG control. His follow-up HbA1c was 6.93 (average BG of 145) 6 months later despite a weight gain of 15 lb. His weight gain highlights the potential for weight gain in some individuals when the frequency of exposure to food increases. The positive impact of nutrition counseling on diabetes control may encourage the client to seek further follow-up to focus on portion control and low-fat food choices.

WEIGHT LOSS: NIDDM

Mild-to-moderate weight loss (10 to 20 lb) has also been shown to improve diabetes control even if desirable body weight is not achieved.[2] When clients use SMBG results to assess the impact of calorie reduction and weight loss, they can see the benefits of their efforts.

Case example: DT was a 69-year-old woman who presented to nutrition services saying "I'm very motivated to lower my BG and avoid insulin." Her height was 5 ft 5 in., and her weight was 231 lb. Random BG was 231 mg/dL, and HbA1c was 9.09%. A diet history revealed three meals per day and an afternoon snack. After four monthly follow-up visits in 5 months, her weight was 222 lb. This weight loss was attributable to emphasis on low-fat eating and behavioral management strategies. DT was able to see her HbA1c drop from 9.09 (average blood sugar, 217) to 6.9 (average blood sugar, 144). More important, she was able to see the downward trend in her BG patterns as she lost weight. Initially, fasting BG values were 137 to 185 mg/dL, and bedtime BGs were 195 to 298 mg/dL (post-supper readings). After 1 month and a 3-lb weight loss, fasting BG values were 107 to 124 mg/dL, and bedtime BG values were 184 to 209 mg/dL. DT kept food records to watch fat and calorie intake and was able to see BG excursions

Table 8-6 BJ's Cheese Pizza Data Collection

Other Food	Source	Portion	Regular Insulin (U)	BG: 30 Min Before/ 1 Hour Post	Timing Insulin– Food (min)
Diet Coke	Pepe's	3 slices of 16-in.-diameter pie cut in 1/8's	6	100/250	30
Diet Coke	Sam's	same	6	105/192	30
Diet Coke	Sam's	same	6	88/169	30

that occurred when she consumed larger amounts of food at meals. This process enabled her to take charge of her diabetes and have a collaborative relationship with the dietitian.

FOODS WITH A LESS PREDICTABLE BLOOD GLUCOSE IMPACT: IDDM AND NIDDM

Many foods are consumed containing unknown ingredients or carbohydrate content. These foods present extra challenges for the individual taking insulin and even more for those on oral agents or diet alone. Many individuals omit foods such as pizza and bagels after several incidents of postprandial hyperglycemia. However, with accurate documentation and experimentation with various foods and/or insulin doses, and/or exercise, these foods can be integrated into the meal plan.

Experimentation should consider the following:

1. Food and amount consumed.

2. Source: brand name or restaurant.

3. Any additional foods consumed in that meal need to be identical in composition and portion size from one experiment to the next.

4. If applicable, insulin dose and BG before and either 90 or 120 minutes after the food or meal. The choice of 90 versus 120 minutes may be based on convenience for the patient, as long as whichever time frame chosen is used consistently.

5. Consistent time frame between the insulin injection or OHA and the start of the meal. Individuals taking insulin should use a consistent injection site.

6. If clients choose to take extra insulin to cover a food, caution must be exercised to prevent hypoglycemia. This may mean an extra snack, a larger snack than usual, and/ or more BG monitoring.

Through careful experimentation and data collection, individuals will be left with choices to decide how to incorporate these foods into their meal plan. These choices include taking more insulin, eating smaller portions of the food in question or the accompanying foods, or trying different brands or restaurants. The dietitian can help the client set up these experiments and then assist in the data review and decision-making process.

There are several important points to consider in data review. First, in a mixed meal, clients can blame the wrong food for an exaggerated BG response. The dietitian can assist the client in assessing food composition or obtaining ingredient specifics from the source. Second, there is often a tendency to jump to conclusions. It usually takes several attempts with adjustments to assess how to best integrate these less predictable foods. Third, some foods are best omitted from the meal plan. These are usually foods with such a high sugar content that insulin alone cannot be used to prevent an exaggerated BG excursion. These foods might, however, be incorporated if consumed in association with exercise.

Case example: The dietitian worked with BJ to find a pizzeria near his apartment that would not result in postprandial BGs as high as 400, which had happened on more than one occasion. She reminded him to take his injection in the same site and the same amount of time before eating for each experiment and that it would be easier to evaluate his data if the premeal BG was similar each time. The data BJ collected is in Table 8-6.

In reviewing these data, it appeared Pepe's pizza had a higher sugar or CHO content. The dietitian and BJ decided to try it again before settling on a strategy to incorporate it in his meal plan, because BJ liked that pizza much better than Sam's.

When he obtained similar results, they outlined three options. First, have two slices from Pepe's instead of three, or second, take more premeal regular insulin, or third, try exercising after eating the pizza. BJ decided on the second choice and found that 2 extra U of regular insulin worked well and did not cause hypoglycemia later on.

The following categories list some foods that may have a less predictable impact on BG and a possible reason for their unpredictability:

- Foods that may have hidden sugar, or sugar in several forms that increase the total CHO content: bagels, baked beans, barbecue sauce, bran products, croissants, coleslaw, potato products, especially french fries, pizza, soups, tomato sauces, and marinated or pickled foods.
- Ethnic foods in which one or more ingredients are unknown: Japanese, Chinese
- Foods with a CHO content that people tend to underestimate: bagels, muffins

CONCLUSION

Quality nutrition management of diabetes requires use of SMBG results. Dietitians need to use a problem-solving approach to help their clients understand food–insulin–activity–BG relationships so that they can feel empowered and positive about nutrition-focused care.

REFERENCES

1. Delahanty L, Halford B. The role of diet behaviors in achieving improved glycemic control in intensively treated outpatients in the Diabetes Control and Complications Trial (DCCT). *Diabetes Care.* 1993;16(11): 1453–1458.

2. American Diabetes Association. Position statement: nutrition recommendations and principles for people with diabetes mellitus. *Diabetes Care.* 1994;17:519–522.

3. American Diabetes Association. Consensus statement: self monitoring of blood glucose. *Diabetes Care.* 1994;17:81–86.

4. DCCT Research Group. The expanded role of the dietitian in the Diabetes Control and Complications Trial (DCCT): implications for clinical practice. *J Am Diet Assoc.* 1993;93:758–764,767.

5. DCCT Research Group. Nutrition interventions for intensive therapy in the Diabetes Control and Complications Trial (DCCT). *J Am Diet Assoc.* 1993;93:768–772.

6. Stone DB. A study of the incidence and causes of poor control in patients with diabetes mellitus. *Am J Med Sci.* 1961;241:436–442.

7. Lockwood D, Frey ML, Gladish NA, et al. The biggest problem in diabetes. *Diabetes Educ.* 1986;12:30–33.

8. Meechenbaum D, Turk DC. *Facilitating Treatment Adherence.* New York, NY: Plenum Press; 1987.

9. Brackenridge BP. Carbohydrate gram counting: a key to accurate mealtime boluses in intensive diabetes therapy. *Practical Diabetology.* 1992;11:22–28.

10. American Dietetic Association. *Stepping Out: A Diabetes Exercise Starter Kit.* Chicago, Ill:1992.

Chapter 9

Preparing and Evaluating Diabetes Education Programs

Melinda Downie Maryniuk

A critical function of the dietitian who works with people with diabetes is to communicate effectively the message of nutrition and diabetes care. Whether the dietitian is called a diabetes educator, a nutrition consultant, a counselor, a behavior change agent, a self-management trainer, or a diabetes management specialist, the importance of communicating a message that is not only understood by the patient but is acted on is essential to overall diabetes control. The process of intervention, education, and counseling is called diabetes self-management training.*

This chapter covers a broad spectrum of topics including looking at access to education, general principles of learning, the content of diabetes education, the process of diabetes education, promoting behavior change, program development, and the special needs patient.

This chapter can be read in its entirety or in segments that seem valuable to your practice. The five main messages of this chapter are as follows:

- Be prepared for the dietitian's expanded role. The dietitian who becomes more trained in diabetes management has an exciting opportunity for an expanded role on a diabetes team or in private practice. No longer are dietitians just teaching meal planning, but they are involved in a variety of other areas including blood glucose monitoring training, hypoglycemia preven-

tion and treatment, insulin adjustments, sick day management, and exercise. Enhance your credentials by becoming a certified diabetes educator (CDE).

- Communicate effectively. The likelihood that what is taught to a patient will be learned and acted on may be related to how carefully one listens to the patient, personalizes the message to their individual needs, and communicates using the ten principles of education.

- Set priorities. It is important to make the most of the time available. In the ideal world, we can describe a comprehensive diabetes education program with multiple follow-up visits and frequent phone contact. However, in reality, cost constraints and lack of reimbursement may limit the access a patient has to a diabetes educator. The diabetes educator must resist temptation to teach too much, so the patient ends up walking away overwhelmed and confused. It is better to focus on one or two behavioral changes the patient can make that will lead to improved metabolic control. This approach may actually enhance follow-up.

- Behavior change is key to metabolic control. Having extensive knowledge about diabetes will not ensure that healthy behav-

---

* *This terminology (self-management training) is recommended for reimbursement purposes as are medical nutrition therapy, nutrition treatment, therapy, and management.*

iors will be incorporated into a patient's daily routine. Many studies have found that knowledge either is not or is only weakly associated with other outcomes.[1,2] A critical role of the diabetes educator is not as much to impart information, but to help the patient set behavioral goals that will specify how that information will be used to ultimately lead to improved short-term and long-term health outcomes.

• Evaluate your efforts. Collect outcomes data to evaluate and justify your education program. Ideally, outcomes measurements should look at indicators in addition to changes in knowledge and glycohemoglobin. Research has only just begun to evaluate the effectiveness of nutrition intervention in diabetes care, but the results are positive. Nutrition intervention does yield improvements in metabolic control.[3] Data need to continue to be collected to document the improved outcomes and cost savings.

ACCESS TO SELF-MANAGEMENT TRAINING

One of the objectives listed in *Healthy People 2000: National Health Promotion and Disease Prevention Objectives* is to have, by the year 2000, 75% of people with diabetes receiving diabetes education.[4] Access to patient education has become more of a challenge in the 1990s because many of the traditional inpatient teaching programs and diabetes treatment units are no longer available due to stricter standards for admitting patients to hospitals. Because of lack of reimbursement, patients are less likely to seek out ambulatory education services in which they will likely have to pay out of pocket.

A nationwide survey administered to 2405 individuals with diabetes older than age 18 revealed that only 35.1% had attended a class or program about diabetes at some time during the course of their disease.[5] Persons who were insulin-treated were more likely to have received

education versus only about 24% of persons with non–insulin-dependent diabetes mellitus (NIDDM) who were not treated with insulin. Factors in persons with NIDDM that were associated with having had diabetes education include younger age, black race, residence in the midwest section of the United States, higher level of education, and presence of diabetes complications. This same study also discovered that when asked, "Where have you obtained your information about diabetes?" more people are likely to get their diabetes information from a relative or a friend (14%) than from a diabetes education class (12%).

The findings of this national study showed only a slight improvement from a statewide study in Michigan, which revealed that only 32% of diabetic individuals had received some sort of formal education when assessed in 1983 to 1984.[6] The Michigan study also revealed that almost half of the persons with NIDDM had never seen a nutritionist, despite the importance of weight management and diet control in this type of diabetes. Clearly, if the Healthy People 2000 objective is to be met, great changes need to be made in access to educational services.

There is also the perception that patient education is not effective.[7] This belief seems to persist despite several separate, comprehensive meta-analyses that have demonstrated the effectiveness of patient education in improving knowledge, behavior, and metabolic control of patients with diabetes.[8,9]

In a National Institutes of Health publication, *Metabolic Control Matters. Nationwide Translation of the Diabetes Control and Complications Trial: Analysis and Recommendations*, a set of six recommendations were made regarding diabetes education.[10] These recommendations are based on the implications of the Diabetes Control and Complications Trial (DCCT) and an analysis of pertinent education literature. The expert panel that authored the publication also identified barriers to implementing the recommendations as well as strategies to overcome the barriers. A summary of these key points is shown in Exhibit 9-1.

Exhibit 9-1 Metabolic Control Matters: Six Education Recommendations

Recommendations	Barriers	Strategies To Overcome Barriers
1. Patients with diabetes and the general public should know that diabetes is a serious disorder and that "metabolic control matters."	• Many believe that diabetes (particularly NIDDM) is a relatively mild disorder • It is estimated that half the people with diabetes remain undiagnosed	• Initiate a broad-based national media campaign to disseminate the "metabolic control matters" message to professionals, patients, and the public
2. Diabetes patient education should be a fundamental treatment for diabetes and be provided at the time of diagnosis and ongoing throughout the patient's life.	• Lack of coordination of services • Lack of adequate preparation of physicians and educators • Lack of interest and commitment of administration	• Adopt national guidelines that include mandatory patient education for diabetes care • Educate the physicians/educators • Activate the patient to demand education
3. Patient education should enable and activate patients to practice self-care behaviors that are effective in achieving the best possible metabolic control.	• Lack of behavioral models specifically applicable to empowering patients with diabetes to make informed self-care decisions	• Empower patients to make responsible self-care decisions through patient education programs • Conduct behavioral research in approaches to empowerment
4. Patient education should be tailored to the characteristics of individual patients.	• Barriers to following a diabetes regimen include knowledge, beliefs, family support, economic factors, language barriers, and cultural differences	• Develop and test useful behavioral models that address the cultural, socioeconomic, and motivational aspects of patient self-care behavior
5. Diabetes patient education should be paid for as any other health care.	• Coverage of diabetes education varies from state to state, is inconsistent, and is generally minimal	• Restructure the way in which diabetes care is financed
6. The content of diabetes patient education should be appropriate to the patient's metabolic characteristics.	• Educational needs will vary based on metabolic characteristics (type of diabetes mellitus); however, little information is available on this	• Conduct research into the educational requirements of patients with different metabolic characteristics

Source: Reprinted from *Nationwide Translation of the Diabetes Control and Complications Trial: Analysis and Recommendations,* US Department of Health and Human Services, Metabolic Control Matters, 1993.

PRINCIPLES OF LEARNING

A favorite comic strip of educators depicts two young boys talking together. One boy, who is holding his dog exclaims, "I taught Spot how to whistle!" The other replies, "Let me hear him." The boy responds, "I said I *taught* him, I didn't say he *learned* it."

This simple message serves as an important reminder for diabetes educators. Even though we may have the knowledge about a subject such as nutrition and diabetes, it takes more than knowledge to communicate it in such a manner that it will result in the desired behavior change. Educators need to be aware of the three variables that may affect learning. Also, an understanding of the ten basic principles of effective learning is essential. In this way, the educators can more effectively assess their patients' needs and communicate in a style that will enhance learning.

Exhibit 9-2 Key Variables Affecting Learning

Dietitian/Educator	Patient/Learner	Setting

• Knowledge of diabetes
• Knowledge of nutrition
• Experience
• Style of communicating
• Time available
• Personal experience with diabetes
• Individualization of the message
• Appropriate teaching tools:
  –cultural sensitivity
  –reading level
  –level of detail
  –specific to patient needs
• Detail and complexity of the message
	• Interest and motivation
	• State of health/wellness
	• Previous instruction
	• Current knowledge and skills/
	  behaviors
	• Family involvement
	• Educational/literacy levels
	• Degree of self-efficacy or self-
	  confidence
	• Belief in the benefits of learning/
	  making a change
	• Learning style preference
		• Privacy
		• Distracting noises
		• Visual aids and teaching tools
		• Temperature
		• Comfort

Variables Affecting Learning

For learning to take place most effectively, three main categories of variables all need to be in harmony with each other: dietitian (the educator), patient (the learner), and setting. The dietitian educator may not be able to control all the variables, but it is important to have an awareness of those factors that will affect what should be taught and what may, in fact, be learned. In completing an education assessment, the educator needs to review those learner characteristics that will affect the learner's receptivity to the material. Exhibit 9-2 summarizes some of the key variables for the educator, the learner, and the content, which all have a role in determining how well the learner actually learns. Assessing the patient's readiness to learn involves evaluating all these areas—or at least identifying quickly which ones may present the biggest barriers and therefore may need to be addressed.

Ten Principles of Effective Learning

Effective communication skills are critical in facilitating the learning process. Adult learners have special learning characteristics that the educator needs to be aware of to design the most effective intervention. The following are ten important principles of effective learning and describes their application to diabetes education.

1. *Learning is facilitated when the learner feels the need to know.* When a patient wants to learn, particularly when they come to a diabetes educator on their own initiative, the success of learning is enhanced. One study found that individuals who initiated contact with a diabetes education program were more likely to participate than individuals who were contacted by the program.[11] The educator must balance what the patients say they *want* to know with what is determined they *need* to know. (Sometimes patient wants must be filled before needs can be addressed.) At the same time, the educator must avoid teaching those topics that may not be needed by particular patients—such as reviewing guidelines for travel for the person who never leaves his or her hometown.

2. *Learning is enhanced when it is related to what the learner already knows.* It is important that the educator assess what the patient already knows, as well as their behaviors (what they do; their diabetes skills) and their attitudes (how they feel about it). Understanding their past experiences with diabetes and education can help clarify misconceptions, identify barriers to learning, and help the educator fit what is being taught into the patient's frame of reference.

3. *Learning is improved when what is taught is personally relevant.* Educators should minimize teaching of abstract and theoretical information and emphasize knowledge and skills that will be personally useful to the patient. A good way to begin a class or a counseling session is to simply ask, "What are your questions?" By doing this, you immediately identify what may be on the patient's mind. It also functions as a quick needs assessment. The importance of personal goal setting cannot be overemphasized. For changes to occur, the educator and patient must identify and document realistic goals that can be measured at a later date.

4. *Learning is facilitated when the person has self-confidence and a desire to learn.* Part of the educator's role is to reinforce continually the idea that the patient can master the skills and knowledge needed to control diabetes. A patient's self-efficacy, their confidence at making and maintaining changes, can be very predictive of their success in making change. This process is enhanced when the education program builds on a series of carefully planned success experiences that leads to successfully achieving short-term goals. Guide the patient with poor confidence in making positive self-talk statements such as "I can do it."

5. *Learning is more effective when it is active rather than passive.* Patients will acquire and retain knowledge and skills better if they are given opportunities to be active participants in the learning process rather than passive recipients of information. It has been said that we remember about 10% of what is read, 20% of what is heard, 30% of what is seen, 50% of what is seen and heard, 70% of what is said and written, and 90% of what is said and done or applied.[12] It has also been suggested that during a counseling session, the educator should only be delivering information for 20% of the time, and the patient should be talking for 80% of the time. This principle of active learning is easy to apply when teaching skills such as blood glucose monitoring or insulin injection in which the patient must demonstrate a skill. Teaching nutrition behaviors in an active manner may require a bit of creativity and planning, but it will yield great results. For example, when teaching portion control, demonstrate with real food by having the patient pour out a 4-ounce glass of juice or by shaking three-quarters of a cup of cereal in a bowl. A simulation of food, such as using clay to estimate a 3-oz meat portion, could also be used. Having a patient point to a plastic food model is much less effective. Nutrition teaching could also involve role playing and problem solving to be more active. Take the patient "shopping" by browsing through a notebook filled with food labels and discuss good choices. Bring the patient to a "restaurant" by dressing up your counseling table with a tablecloth and a variety of menus and have the patient select a meal.

6. *Learning is reinforced when it can be applied immediately.* Patients will retain knowledge and skills longer if they have opportunities for frequent application and repetition. Practice and rehearsal also increase the retention of knowledge and skills. There may even be value in offering "homework" assignments, such as looking for a particular food label, so the patient can practice this new knowledge.

7. *Learning should be staged and short-term goals set.* Only deliver one or two main messages at a time. Staging the learning and setting priorities to not go into more detail than is needed will help enhance the learning. Remember the KISS principle of education: "Keep It Short and Simple." Weight control is a good example for goal setting. The initial goal should not be pounds lost but perhaps just keeping a food diary for 3 days or controlling intake during the after-dinner hours. When a patient accomplishes a small goal (and that goal is

acknowledged and praised by the educator) self-confidence will increase, and it is more likely that further goals will be set and met.

8. *Periodic plateaus occur in learning.* Patients do not always learn at a constant rate. Occasionally, educators need to adjust the pace at which they teach to accommodate the variations in the patient's ability to absorb and retain information.

9. *Learning should be fun.* A warm smile and a good sense of humor on the part of the educator can go a long way in enhancing learning. Think about your patient as a "customer." If they do not find the education session somewhat enjoyable, do you think they will come back? Can you offer a recipe of the month? A coupon and free samples display table? Waiting room contests that offer inexpensive prizes for guessing the number of calories in a sample meal—or some other simple educational game? A computer analysis of their 24-hour recall? A little bit of what you do is "marketing"—so make sure you are offering activities that are fun and enjoyable as well as educational.

10. *Knowledge and skills need to be reviewed, reinforced, and repeated.* Remember these three R's of education: review, reinforce, and repeat. People forget what they have learned as time passes. The length of time someone has diabetes is no predictor of how much they know. A system should be in place to ensure that diabetes knowledge and skills are reviewed and updated at least annually. The checklist in Appendix 9-A provides a model for how this can be carefully followed and documented. Throughout the year, reviews and reinforcement should occur in a variety of ways through usual diabetes care.

CONTENT OF DIABETES EDUCATION

Since their initial development in 1983, The National Standards for Diabetes Patient Education Programs have set the standard for diabetes education. In 1993, the National Diabetes Advisory Board charged the American Diabetes Association to appoint a task force to review and revise the standards (Appendix 9-B). Goals for diabetes education have been defined by the American Diabetes Association, and the National Diabetes Advisory Board has identified 15 content areas that people with diabetes should master as part of a recognized diabetes program[13] (Exhibit 9-3). The standards emphasize the importance of the assessment to determine what is taught to the patient. In addition, educators may stage the objectives in two or three levels (eg, survival, continuing, intensive). Not all patients need to go through all levels.

The skilled diabetes educator knows how to stage the education to offer just the right amount of information to not overwhelm the patient and to make the patient recognize the need to return for more. An important, but often overlooked survival level objective should be for the patient

---

Exhibit 9-3 National Standards: Content Areas

15 Content Areas

- Diabetes overview
- Stress and psychosocial adjustment
- Family involvement and social support
- Nutrition
- Exercise and activity
- Medications
- Monitoring and use of results
- Relationships among nutrition, exercise, medication, and blood glucose levels
- Prevention, detection, and treatment of acute complications
- Prevention, detection, and treatment of chronic complications
- Foot, skin, and dental care
- Behavior change strategies, goal setting, risk factor reduction, and problem solving
- Benefits, risks, and management options for improving glucose control
- Preconception care, pregnancy, and gestational diabetes
- Use of health care systems and community resources

to verbalize that nutrition care and diabetes self-management training is an ongoing process and that not everything is taught in one session. It has been estimated that it may take up to 7 hours during the first year after diagnosis to teach just the nutrition information.[14]

The dietitian who is a CDE should be comfortable teaching a wide variety of diabetes education topics, not just meal planning. More and more diabetes nutrition educators have expanded duties including teaching blood glucose monitoring and discussing insulin actions, prevention and treatment of hypoglycemia, and exercise recommendations, to name a few. Dietitians are well suited to work with the physician and patient in recommending insulin adjustments based on a review of the blood glucose records because the dietitian is most familiar with the food-related factors that may be having an effect on the blood glucose.

There is currently active discussion regarding what the scope of practice should be for a dietitian CDE. The Scope of Practice Statement of the Diabetes Care and Education Practice Group includes such skills as teaching general diabetes information, blood glucose monitoring, and insulin adjustment.[15] A summary of these skills divided according to level of practice can be found in Table 3-2 (Chapter 3). There is also discussion within the American Association of Diabetes Educators to define an advanced level of practice beyond the CDE. Although it is recognized that all CDEs, no matter what their discipline, have a certain core knowledge, the question remains regarding how unique each discipline should remain.

Appendix 9-C is an example of a typical teaching checklist that can be used by the diabetes education team in assessing current knowledge and skills and then documenting changes after education.

The importance of imparting all these skills and knowledge to persons with diabetes, however, should not be overemphasized. Up-to-date diabetes education programs should have an emphasis on empowerment and self-management skills training. Diabetes education must include training in problem solving and coping skills. Outcomes measurements should go beyond assessing knowledge and mechanical skills (such as insulin or monitoring techniques) and focus on self-efficacy and perceived sense of control.[16]

PROCESS OF DIABETES EDUCATION

The process of diabetes education must be thought of as a partnership. The success of the DCCT was not about physicians or diabetes educators effectively managing the care of their patients. It was about how patients and health care providers worked together for the best care.

Empowerment is the term applied to this philosophy of practice. Empowerment means being in control of one's life and taking responsibility for self-care. Training programs based on empowerment have been designed to help patients with diabetes develop the psychosocial skills necessary for effective diabetes self-care, including goal setting, problem solving, coping, and stress management.[17] Research has even shown that patients who participate in empowerment training have improved blood glucose control.[18]

Research has shown that just by training patients to become more active participants in their care, they are able to improve blood glucose control. Patients who were more assertive (those who asked more questions, expressed opinions, brought up topics of concern), who expressed more positive and negative emotion, and who were more adept at eliciting information from their doctors experienced better metabolic control.[19] It is important to remember that patients can and should be trained to be more active consumers of health care—not to take the victim or passive role and sit back waiting for the health care provider.

The teaching process should follow a four-step sequence: assessment, goal setting, intervention, and evaluation. Currently, nutrition practice guidelines are being defined by the American Dietetic Association for type I and type II diabetes to best guide dietitians through the process of diabetes education (see Appendixes 3-B and 3-C in Chapter 3).

Assessment

The assessment phase involves gathering important information that will help clarify the therapeutic goals. Knowledge, skills, and attitudes regarding health, diabetes care, and nutrition must be assessed. Also, life style (eg, family, work, and exercise habits) must be reviewed to identify barriers as well as positive influences for behavior change. The assessment will also identify other risks associated with diabetes as well as readiness to change.

This information may be gathered in a variety of ways, including forms completed by the patient before the visit, pretests, review of the medical record, and interviews with the patient and referring physician. Some dietitians may need to be cautioned to not spend too much time on an assessment but to focus on identifying what the patient perceives as the primary problem. It is an important skill of an experienced dietitian to be able to focus the assessment quickly on some key issues and to continue collecting assessment data at subsequent visits.

Several nutrition behaviors have been identified in a study done of DCCT patients that were associated with a lowering of glycohemoglobin levels. They are (1) adherence to the meal plan, (2) adjustment of insulin dose on the basis of expected meal/snack, (3) appropriate treatment of hypoglycemia, (4) prompt response to hyperglycemia, (5) consistency of bedtime snacks, and (6) avoidance of extra bedtime snacks.[20] It is recommended that the diabetes educator pay particular attention to these behaviors as part of the assessment as they will have an important impact on outcomes. (See Appendixes 3-B and 3-C in Chapter 3).

Goal Setting

Both short-term and long-term goals for therapy are to be mutually determined by the patient and the educator. Involving the patient by asking a few key questions will help the dietitian determine the patient's understanding, willingness, and interest in making the necessary behavior changes. The following are some questions that can be asked to elicit valuable information about the patient's goals and help facilitate the establishment of a cooperative nutrition education plan.[14]

- What do you expect from nutrition counseling?
- What is the most important goal for you in managing your diabetes and the way you eat?
- What are some changes you could make to your present plan of eating to follow more closely the diabetes nutrition goals that we discussed?
- How would you make these changes in your eating patterns?

Patient-centered behavioral goals are an important component of diabetes management and education. Written goals should be a component of documentation, and the American Diabetes Association requires that the patient's success at meeting goals be assessed and documented at some time after the goals were established. Goals are measurable and realistic. The written goal will include an action verb such as demonstrate, identify, choose, or state, not verbs like know or understand. The patient should be given a copy of the goals that have been agreed on. Generally, not more than three goals should be set at each visit. Several examples of patient-centered behavioral goals are as follows:

I agree to:

- record food intake in a daily food record for 5 days during the next 2 weeks
- walk for 15 minutes after supper three times a week
- select only snack foods from the snack list the dietitian gave me for my bedtime snack
- measure my fruit juice every morning for 1 week
- eat only 5 carbohydrate servings (starch/bread, milk, fruit) at supper each night and measure my blood sugar before bed for 1 week

Intervention

Intervention refers to the diabetes educator's activities that enable, facilitate, or support the patient's diabetes management plan. Effective nutrition intervention requires the dietitian to function both as a provider of information and a counselor.

Based on the assessment and patient goals, the dietitian educator will determine which meal planning approach may best fit the patient's needs: general guidelines, menu-planning systems, counting systems (such as carbohydrate or fat gram counting), or an exchange system. Appropriate teaching methods and tools will also be used to complement the patient's learning style.

As stated earlier, it is not enough to be able to teach information about diabetes and nutrition but to be able to teach it in such a way that it is acted on. Research has revealed that there are several components of effective instruction, regardless of the content or setting. The mnemonic "DR. FIRM," which uses the first letter of each component, serves as a reminder of these essential teaching functions, which are as follows[21]:

- **D**emonstrations, presentations, problem solving
- **R**ehearsal of content by patients, evaluation of performance
- **F**eedback and correctives given to patients
- **I**ndependent practice of new learnings by patients on their own
- **R**eview and reassessment at periodic intervals
- **M**otivation to persevere with new behaviors

Evaluation

There are many components to diabetes education evaluation. In its most basic form, evaluation refers to the activities of both the diabetes educator and the patient that enable them to determine the effect of the self-care plan. At a follow-up visit, the educator evaluates if the behavioral goals that were set were met and if there are improvements in specific clinical outcomes such as glycohemoglobin, lipids, or weight.

Listed below are four reasons for doing an evaluation. There is overlap between the type of information that may be collected for these different evaluations.

- *To assess the patient(s):* it is important to determine if the nutritional care plans or teaching program had any measurable impact on patients as individuals or as a group. Factors to evaluate include knowledge, skills or behavior changes, and laboratory changes. Feedback not only enables the instructor to see how well the patient is doing, but it is also motivating for patients to receive feedback about their progress.

- *To assess the program or service:* many aspects of the program itself should be examined, such as length of each class and the total program, time of the class, number and types of participants, location, cost, handouts and audiovisual aids, and other factors that may influence the patients' satisfaction with the program and ultimately their learning. It is also important to assess if the program is reaching those persons who need it most and if referral procedures are working appropriately. The program may be evaluated by patients and by the instructors and/or administration.

- *To demonstrate program effectiveness:* With the rising costs of health care, careful documentation of services and the benefits of nutritional intervention becomes essential. When the need for dietetic services and diabetes education is being questioned, results from careful evaluations can illustrate why nutritional education and counseling is a needed and cost-beneficial service and should be reimbursable. Program effectiveness is demonstrated by a combination of all the above evaluations, and the results are useful to share with a variety of parties, including other team members, the patients, referring physicians, the community (for marketing the program), insurance companies, and actual or potential funders.

- *To assess yourself (the dietitian):* In addition to the objectives we write to guide patient learning, we should write teaching and performance objectives for ourselves so that we may better evaluate our practice. Sometimes, as counselors, we assume that what worked for one patient or group will work for another. Doing frequent evaluations of ourselves can help keep us fresh and able to meet the needs of our clients.

Generally, a diabetes education program includes both formative and summative evaluations. *Formative* evaluations provide feedback to the patient and educator during the process of the program. Examples include keeping regular track of patient's anthropometric measures and laboratory values, doing brief knowledge assessment measures during each class or teaching contact, and having patients complete satisfaction evaluations on a particular class. A *summative* evaluation, also referred to as an outcome evaluation, is performed after the program is completed. It may include a final knowledge test, a demonstration of skills, a summary of the patient's medical status, and/or the patient's overall evaluation of the program. Another type of summative evaluation measures the knowledge, skills, behavior, and/or attitudes demonstrated by the patient several weeks or months after the conclusion of the program. This is also referred to as an impact evaluation.

Evaluation of diabetes education material is another component of a diabetes program. Materials should be reviewed for their reading level by using a scale such as a SMOG Readability Formula (Appendix 9-D). It is also helpful to keep a written record of diabetes education material that may be reviewed for use at your worksite. A sample evaluation tool is included in Appendix 9-E. Also, there are other helpful resources that review educational materials for diabetes and nutrition education.[22]

The critical question to continually ask is, "Does what we do make a difference?" Whether it is medical nutrition therapy or diabetes self-management training, diabetes educators need to measure and document outcomes of their care. As a result of our interventions, do patients have decreased hospitalizations or shorter lengths of stay? Do they have lower serum lipids, which may contribute to reduced risks for cardiovascular disease? Are their glycohemoglobins improved, which may lead to reduced risks of complications? Is their quality of life better? Are they more satisfied with their care? Do they save money? Outcome measures must be assessed as a part of the total evaluation process.[23]

With the emphasis on having the patient take on more responsibility for self-care, a yearly planner or management guide is helpful in organizing what topics and tests the patient should keep track of at each visit. A very useful guidebook, *Take Charge of Your Diabetes: A Guide for Patients*, includes sample charts for patients to use in tracking their diabetes care.[24] Appendix 9-A includes some of this summary information.

PROMOTING BEHAVIOR CHANGE

The four-step approach to nutrition intervention (assessment, goal setting, intervention, and evaluation) was designed to maximize the likelihood of making and maintaining behavioral changes. In addition to making sure that the nutrition care plan is designed according to this model, there are several additional elements the educator should be aware of that may help promote behavior change. In this section, the following three topics will be addressed: teaching problem-solving skills, tips to enhance motivation, and the transtheoretical model of change.

Teaching Problem-Solving Skills

Effective diabetes management requires the patient know how to deal with the wide variety of decisions and problems that may be encountered on a daily basis. To empower the patient with those skills necessary to make good decisions, it may take some practice. The diabetes educator will help the patient identify potential barriers to diabetes management or problems and obstacles that may arise so that the patient may think through ahead of time what a good plan of action might be. A problem-solving framework has been designed that is applicable to diabetes education.[21] It is suggested that the patient learn the IDEAL problem-solving process and that the educator be prepared to raise some potential problems or obstacles in management so that the patient can practice problem-solving skills. The following steps should be taken:

- **I**dentify the problems.
- **D**efine the problems.
- **E**xplore possible solutions or coping strategies.
- **A**ct on a strategy.
- **L**ook at the effects and learn from them.

Motivation

The diabetes educator does not necessarily have a role to "motivate" patients toward behavioral change. Rather, the educator's role is to help patients discover how they are motivated and to help them use their motivation so that they can bring about positive changes in eating behavior.

To increase the likelihood that patients will be able to adhere as closely as possible to their meal plans, the educator can consider using a variety of behavioral strategies. Although these approaches have not proved overwhelmingly successful in large groups, they have been very useful in individual cases.[25] When faced with adherence problems, dietitians should consider using one or more of the following strategies[21]:

- Increase attention and contacts. Schedule frequent follow-up visits and have phone contacts as necessary.

- Suggest changes and substitutions in the patient's habits and environment so that reminders to follow the plan are present and cues to abort the plan are absent. For example, rearranging the kitchen cabinets or refrigerator so that the high-calorie snack foods are not easily accessible and visible can help decrease unplanned snacks.

- Paint a picture of the positive and negative short- and long-term consequences of adherence and nonadherence. Keep this picture objective and avoid scare tactics.

- Use self-monitoring, including detailed food records that can collect information on what, where, when, and in which mood one eats.

- Obtain signed contracts. Suggest that the patient be rewarded with something positive for meeting the agreed-on goals.

- Provide models and reinforcers. Encourage patients to join a support group or meet others who have been successful.

- Make referrals. Be able to recognize that a patient's problem may not be dietary at all but may require the services of a counselor such as a psychologist or social worker.

Transtheoretical Model of Change

An understanding of the transtheoretical model that is based on research on how people change behaviors is important in aiding our ability to help people make change. The transtheoretical model postulates that cessation of high-risk behaviors (such as smoking) and acquisition of heath-enhancing behaviors (such as exercise) involve the progression through five stages of change. This model, which has been successfully researched and applied in the area of smoking cessation, is now being explored in diabetes management, which involves a variety of behavior changes.[26]

The five stages include (1) precontemplation, not thinking about making changes; (2) contemplation, considering change in the foreseeable future; (3) preparation, seriously considering change in the near future; (4) action, in the process of changing behavior; and (5) maintenance, continued change for an extended period. People go through each of these stages for changes to be made and maintained. Progression through the stages is not linear, because most individuals relapse and recycle back through earlier stages. Individuals may cycle through the stages several times before they succeed in their efforts to change behavior.

The diabetes educator has an important role in helping patients progress through each of the stages of readiness. In the early phases, the educator may assist the patient's decisional balance by helping the patient weigh the benefits against the disadvantages of changing a particular behavior. For example, the dietitian may have the patient list the pros and cons of weight loss as an early step of moving toward the decision to actually make behavior changes that would result in weight loss. The educator can also help enhance the patient's self-efficacy, the individual's situational confidence in making and maintaining a behavior change. Currently, this model is being tested in diabetes. Exhibit 10-1 in Chapter 10 outlines this model.

PROGRAM DEVELOPMENT

Since 1986, the American Diabetes Association has had a program to recognize diabetes education programs that are comprehensive and meet certain basic criteria. The content of the comprehensive program must cover all 15 content areas as described by the American Diabetes Association in Exhibit 9-3. Programs that are administered to groups as well as individuals, in both outpatient and inpatient settings, may become recognized (see Appendix 9-B). The manual, *Meeting the Standards*, which was developed by the American Diabetes Association for use in completing the application for recognition, is very helpful.[27]

To apply for recognition, a diabetes education program has to be operating for at least 1 year. Outcomes data that evaluate how well patients are able to meet their behavioral goals after the program are also documented.

THE SPECIAL NEEDS PATIENT

The message that teaching and meal planning should be individualized should be clear. But attention must be given to those groups of people who may require special individualization.

This chapter has dealt primarily with the adult learner. However, a very important and challenging group to teach is the family when a child is diagnosed with diabetes. The topic of diabetes and the pediatric population is covered in Chapter 25, but a few teaching points are highlighted here:

- Teach the whole family, not just the child and the mother. Fathers, grandparents, caregivers, siblings, and close friends must also be involved in the process.

- When offering diabetes education classes, avoid including a parent of a child with diabetes in a group of older adults with diabetes. Their needs and issues are very different. The parent may end up coming away from the education session more confused, scared, and frustrated.

- If doing groups for children, remember that the needs, interests, and abilities vary greatly. A grouping that usually works fairly well is 4- to 7-year-olds, 8- to 11-year-olds, and 12 and older.

- If at all possible, go to the child's school to spend time teaching the teacher, the school nurse, and the child's classmates. This can be a great experience for the child with diabetes to "show-off" his or her own new skills and knowledge as the child helps to teach the class.

When working with other special needs populations, make sure you have access to available resources and teaching aids that will enhance the delivery of the message. There are resource guides and materials for the visually impaired,[28–30] persons with limited reading skills,[31] and persons from culturally diverse groups who require an understanding not only of food habits but of family dynamics, cultural influences on behavior change, and attitudes toward health and disease. Some available diabetes nutrition education resources for specific population groups include Jewish, Navajo, Chinese, Hmong, Alaska Native, Hispanic, Southern/Soul, and Filipino.[32,33]

THE HOSPITALIZED PATIENT

Traditional inpatient diabetes education programs have been disappearing from the hospital setting. However, there is good evidence that employing the team approach (MD, RD, RN) for hospitalized patients with a principal diagnosis of diabetes significantly reduces length of stay when compared to patients who receive just an endocrine consult. This also results in obvious cost savings.[34]

EDUCATION FOR THE DIABETES EDUCATOR

It is an exciting time to be a dietitian working in the area of diabetes care and education. There are many opportunities to further one's education and to expand one's scope of practice. Consider pursuing one of more of the following ideas, which will enhance your own skills and knowledge as well as potentially expand your practice.

- *Become a CDE or a certified specialist.* A dietitian may sit for the CDE examination after at least 2000 hours of direct patient education in no less than 2 years is documented. Contact the American Association of Diabetes Educators for information on the National Certification Exam at 1-800-338-3633. The American Dietetic Association also has a program that credentials dietitians who may specialize in one of the

following three areas: pediatrics, renal, or metabolic nutrition care. Contact the Commission on Dietetic Registration for more information at (800) 877-1600.

- *Learn from your team and expand your skills.* If you are fortunate enough to work with a team including a physician, nurse, and possibly an exercise physiologist and mental health counselor, plan for these team members to teach each other and not only the patients. Develop cross-training checklists that may be used as a guide for annual skills and knowledge assessments. For example, the nurses might make sure the dietitians are able to teach one or two of the blood glucose meters, and the dietitians might make sure the nurses are able to estimate a patient's usual caloric intake. Many dietitians are becoming more involved in broader aspects of diabetes management and education, including teaching home blood glucose monitoring, insulin injections, sick-day and well-day insulin adjustments, and basic foot care. With the support and backing of the physician with whom you work most closely, it may be helpful to make sure you are comfortable with teaching these skills and knowledge.

- *Take advanced courses in diabetes.* There are many opportunities available for continuing education programs in diabetes care. There is a program within the American Association of Diabetes Educators called ASIDE, Advanced Studies Institute in Diabetes Education, which administers advanced level courses that lead to further recognition. Currently, there is discussion within this organization regarding the development of an advanced level practice credential that would be beyond the CDE level. An excellent resource for the process of education and group program planning continues to be *You've Got to Get through the Outside Layer: A Handbook for Diabetes Educators Using Diabetes As a Model.*[35]

- *Live with diabetes for a few days.* If you do not have diabetes, try living with it. Follow a meal plan for a week. Learn to inject yourself with saline, measure your blood glucose up to seven times a day, and inspect your feet at the end of each day. You can never know exactly what it feels like to have diabetes, but putting yourself in a simulation model will certainly help you appreciate the many decisions that must be faced on a daily basis—and give you a better appreciation for what your patients go through.

- *Strengthen your business skills.* Learn more about marketing, business development, managed care, coding and reimbursement, outcomes management, and evaluation. Even though we may think of ourselves only as clinicians and educators, it is essential that we can also be involved with these other areas, as they ultimately affect our jobs. We need to market our services to other physicians, communicate our outcomes and effectiveness data to managed care groups, and understand how to maximize our reimbursement potential by using the correct codes.

- *Become active with a diabetes organization.* An excellent way to learn more is to learn by doing. Volunteering time with organizations such as the American Diabetes Association is usually very rewarding as it brings together health professionals from a variety of settings as well as people with diabetes. Involvement with the Diabetes Care and Education Practice Group offers the opportunity to network with dietitians across the country.

REFERENCES

1. Benny LJ, Dunn SM. Knowledge improvement and metabolic control in diabetes education: approaching the limits? *Patient Educ Counsel.* 1990;16:217–229.
2. Dunn SM. Rethinking the models and modes of diabetes education. *Patient Educ Counsel.* 1990;16:281–286.
3. Franz MJ, Monk A, Barry B, et al. Effectiveness of medical nutrition therapy provided in the management of non-insulin dependent diabetes mellitus: a randomized, controlled clinical trial. *J Am Diet Assoc.* 1995 (September):1009–1017.
4. Department of Health and Human Services. *Healthy People 2000: National Health Promotion and Disease Prevention Objectives. Full Report, with Commentary.* Washington, DC: US Government Printing Offices; 1990.
5. Coonrod BA, Betschart J, Harris MI. Frequency and determinants of diabetes patient education among adults in the U.S. population. *Diabetes Care.* 1994;17:852–858.
6. Halpern M. The impact of diabetes education in Michigan. Abstract. *Diabetes.* 1989;38(suppl 2):151A.
7. Lipetz MJ, Bussigel MN, Bannerman J, Risley B. What is wrong with patient education programs? *Nurs Outlook.* 1990;38:184–189.
8. Brown SA. Effects of educational interventions in diabetes care: a meta-analysis of findings. *Nurs Res.* 1988; 37:223–230.
9. Padgett D, Mumford E, Hynes M, Carter R. Meta-analysis of the effect of educational and psychological interventions on management of diabetes mellitus. *J Clin Epidemiol.* 1988;41:1007–1030.
10. Department of Health and Human Services. *Metabolic Control Matters. Nationwide Translation of the Diabetes Control and Complications Trial: Analysis and Recommendations.* Washington, DC: US Government Printing Offices; 1993.
11. Glasgow RE, Toobert DJ, Hampson SE. Participation in outpatient diabetes education programs: how many patients take part and how representative are they? *Diabetes Educ.* 1991;17:376–380.
12. Wiman RV, Mierhenry WC. *Educational Media: Theory into Practice.* Columbus, Ohio: Charles Merrill; 1969.
13. American Diabetes Association. National Standards for diabetes self-management education programs and American Diabetes Association review criteria. *Diabetes Care.* 1995;18:737–741.
14. Pastors JG, Holler HJ. *Meal Planning Approaches for Diabetes Management.* 2nd ed. Chicago, Ill: American Dietetic Association; 1994.
15. American Diabetes Association. Scope of practice for qualified professionals in diabetes care and education. *J Am Diabetes Assoc.* 1995;95(5):607–608.
16. Glasgow RE, Osteen VL. Evaluating diabetes education: are we measuring the most important outcomes? *Diabetes Care.* 1992;15:1423–1432.
17. Funnell MM, Anderson RM, Arnold MS, et al. Empowerment: an idea whose time has come in diabetes education. *Diabetes Educ.* 1991;17:37–41.

18. Anderson RM, Funnell MM, Butler PM, Arnold MS, Fitzgerald JJ, Terste CC. Patient empowerment: results of a randomized controlled trial. *Diabetes Care.* 1995;18:943–949.

19. Greenfield S, Haplan S, Ware J, Yano EM, Frank HJL. Patients' participation in medical care: effects on blood sugar control and quality of life in diabetes. *J Gen Intern Med.* 1988;3:448–457.

20. Delehanty LM, Halford BN. The role of diet behaviors in achieving improved glycemic control in intensively treated patients in the Diabetes Control and Complications Trial. *Diabetes Care.* 1993;16:1453–1458.

21. Pichert JW. Teaching strategies for effective nutrition instruction. In: Powers MA, ed. *Handbook of Diabetes Nutritional Management.* Gaithersburg, Md: Aspen Publishers; 1987:465–479.

22. Diabetes Care and Education Practice Group. *Selected Diabetes and Nutrition Education Resources: For the Person with Diabetes.* Chicago, Ill: American Dietetic Association; 1994.

23. Maryniuk MD. Measuring outcomes in diabetes care and education. On the cutting edge. In: Maryniuk MD, ed. *Diabetes Care and Management.* Chicago, Ill: American Dietetic Association; 1995;16:1–27.

24. Department of Health and Human Services, Public Health Service. *Take Charge of Your Diabetes: A Guide for Patients.* Atlanta, Ga: Centers for Disease Control, Division of Diabetes Translation; 1991.

25. Wing RR, Epstien LH, Nowalk MP. Dietary adherence in patients with diabetes. *Behav Med Update.* 1984;6:17.

26. Ruggiero L, Prochaska JO. Application of the transtheoretical model to diabetes. *Diabetes Spectrum.* 1993;6:21–60.

27. American Diabetes Association. *Meeting the Standards: A Manual for Completing the American Diabetes Association Application for Recognition*, 4th ed. Alexandria, Va: ADA; 1995.

28. ADEVIP Task Force. Guidelines for the practice of adaptive diabetes education for visually impaired persons (ADEVIP). *Diabetes Educ.* 1994;20:111–118.

29. Williams AS. Recommendations for desirable features of adaptive diabetes self-care equipment for visually impaired persons. *Diabetes Care.* 1994;17:451–452.

30. Cleary ME. *Diabetes and Visual Impairment: An Educator's Resource Guide.* Chicago, Ill: American Association of Diabetics Educators; 1994. (This 300-page comprehensive book may be purchased from AADE for $75.00.)

31. Barr P, ed. *Diabetes Educational Resources for Minority and Low Literacy Populations.* Southfield, Mich: Coalition for Diabetes Education and Minority Health; 1991. (Available from the ADA, Michigan Affiliate, Inc., Clausen Building, North Unit, Suite 400, 23100 Providence Drive, Southfield, MI 48075.)

32. National Diabetes Information Clearinghouse. *Diabetes in Hispanic Americans: Current Research and Education Programs.* Bethesda, Md; 1994. (Available from NDIC, Box NDIC, 9000 Rockville Pike, Bethesda, MD 20892.)

33. American Dietetic Association. *Ethnic and Regional Food Practices: Jewish, Navajo, Chinese, Hmong, Alaska Native, Mexican American, Southern/Soul.* (Available through the American Dietetic Association by calling (800) 877-1600 x5000.)

34. Levetan CS, Salas JR, Wilets IF, Zumoff B. Impact of endocrine and diabetes team consultation on hospital length of stay for patients with diabetes. *Am J Med.* 1995;99:22–28.

35. Tupling H, Webb K, Harris G, Sulway M. *You've Got to Get through the Outside Layer: A Handbook for Health Educators Using Diabetes as a Model.* Sydney, Australia: Diabetes Education and Assessment Programme of The Royal North Shore Hospital of Sydney and The Northern Metropolitan Health Region of the Health Commission of New South Wales; 1981. (Available for $15.00 through Outside Layer, PO Box 802, South Bend, IN 46624.)

GLOSSARY

ADA Recognized Program—The American Diabetes Association (ADA) has established a national voluntary process that formally identifies patient education programs that meet the National Standards for Diabetes Patient Education Programs. Program staff complete a self-evaluation that is submitted for review by the ADA. Programs that meet the standards become a recognized program.

Certified Diabetes Educator—a credential that is awarded to health professionals (such as a registered nurse or a registered dietitian) who have more than 2000 hours experience working with persons with diabetes and pass a national certification examination. The credential (CDE) is good for a 5-year period. For more information, contact the American Association of Diabetes Educators.

Empowerment—a process whereby people gain mastery over their affairs. Empowerment education stresses a mutual partnership between provider and patient in which the patient is responsible for his or her own self-care decisions, with the provider serving as a resource.

Outcome—the effect or result of a particular treatment or intervention. Outcomes are measured to document the effectiveness, value, and benefit of a particular treatment. In the DCCT, the outcomes measured included incidence and severity of microvascular changes, frequency of hypoglycemia, and the costs of the interventions. Although glycohemoglobin is commonly measured to evaluate the impact of an intervention, this, in and of itself, is not a true outcome.

Self-Efficacy—the perception of one's capacity to change an outcome by adopting a new pattern of behavior. It is the confidence in one's ability to achieve a behavioral change. People with higher levels of self-efficacy are better able to manage their diabetes care.

Self-Management Training—the instructional interaction between the patient, physician, and other health care professionals providing services incidental to those of the physician; to train the patient to effectively carry out self-management practices to maintain the best possible level of daily diabetes control. (This term is preferred over the term *education* when describing services provided to a third-party payer.)

Transtheoretical Model—This is a readiness-for-change model that is based on a theory that intervention should be matched to the individual's readiness to make a change. It provides a framework for assessing readiness for changes using the following stages: precontemplation, contemplation, preparation, action, and maintenance.

Take Charge of Your Diabetes

At each visit, discuss these points with your health care provider.

Major Points	Dates of Discussions			
Meal Plan	_____	_____	_____	_____
Activity	_____	_____	_____	_____
Self-Monitoring Blood Sugar	_____	_____	_____	_____
High and Low Blood Sugar Problems	_____	_____	_____	_____
Medicines	_____	_____	_____	_____
Birth Control and Family Planning	_____	_____	_____	_____

At each visit, have your health care provider do these tests.

Major Points	Dates and Results			
Blood Sugar Test	____mg/dL	____mg/dL	____mg/dL	____mg/dL
Glycohemoglobin Test	____%	____%	____%	____%
Weight	____lbs	____lbs	____lbs	____lbs
Blood Pressure Test	____/____ mm Hg	____/____ mm Hg	____/____ mm Hg	____/____ mm Hg
Foot Check	_____	_____	_____	_____

Source: Adapted from *Take Charge of Your Diabetes: A Guide for Patients*, US Department of Health and Human Services, Public Health Service, Centers for Disease Control, 1991.

Write down the questions you want to discuss with your health care provider, so you don't forget.

_____

_____

_____

At least once a year, discuss these major points with your health care provider.

Major Points	**Dates of Discussions**			
Feelings about Diabetes	_____	_____	_____	_____
High Blood Sugars (knowing and treating)	_____	_____	_____	_____
Low Blood Sugars (knowing and treating)	_____	_____	_____	_____
Dental Care	_____	_____	_____	_____
Foot Care	_____	_____	_____	_____

At least once a year, have your health care provider do these tests.

Major Points	**Dates and Results**			
Kidney Tests				
creatinine	____mg/dL	____mg/dL	____mg/dL	____mg/dL
protein or albumin	____mg	____mg	____mg	____mg
Cholesterol, total	____mg	____mg	____mg	____mg
LDL	____mg	____mg	____mg	____mg
HDL	____mg	____mg	____mg	____mg
EKG	_____	_____	_____	_____
Eye Exam	_____	_____	_____	_____
Foot Exam (blood flow and nerves)	_____	_____	_____	_____

Standards and Review Criteria, National Standards for Diabetes Self-Management Education Programs and American Diabetes Association Review Criteria

American Diabetes Association

In 1993, the National Diabetes Advisory Board charged the American Diabetes Association to coordinate a task force of representatives of diabetes and other organizations to review, and revise if indicated, the National Standards for Diabetes Patient Education Programs. The task force consisted of representatives from the following organizations: The American Association of Diabetes Educators, The American Diabetes Association, The American Dietetic Association, the Centers for Disease Control and Prevention, the Department of Defense, the Department of Veterans Affairs, the Diabetes Research and Training Centers, the Indian Health Service, and the Juvenile Diabetes Foundation, Inc. The task force decided to revise the standards to reflect recent research and current health care trends. Thus, the standards were revised and are now termed the National Standards for Diabetes Self-Management Education Programs. These revised standards have been endorsed by the organizations involved in their development.

NATIONAL STANDARDS FOR DIABETES SELF-MANAGEMENT EDUCATION PROGRAMS AND AMERICAN DIABETES ASSOCIATION REVIEW CRITERIA

Diabetes mellitus is a chronic metabolic disorder. Individuals affected by diabetes must learn self-management skills and make lifestyle changes to effectively manage diabetes and avoid or delay the complications associated with this disorder. For these reasons, self-management education is the cornerstone of treatment for all people with diabetes. These National Standards, which were developed in collaboration with diabetes organizations, will provide guidance for the establishment and maintenance of quality diabetes self-management education programs.

The process whereby people with chronic diseases, such as diabetes, learn to take care of these disorders has traditionally been termed "patient education." However, over time, this designation has changed and is currently termed "self-management training" and "self-management education," as well as patient education. This document will use the term self-management education to refer to the process whereby individuals learn to manage their diabetes.

These standards provide:

1. Diabetes educators with the means to:
   - develop quality self-management education programs
   - assess the quality of their education programs
   - identify areas in their programs where changes and improvements are needed

2. People with diabetes with the means to:
   - assess the quality of the diabetes-related services they receive

Source: Reprinted from American Diabetes Association, National Standards for Diabetes Self-Management Education Programs and American Diabetes Association Review Criteria, *Diabetes Care.* 1995;18(5):737–744, with permission of the American Diabetes Association.

- gain an understanding of the skills needed for self-management
3. Referral sources, insurers, employers, government agencies, and the general public with:
- a description of quality self-management education services for people with diabetes
- an awareness of the importance of comprehensive self-management education to enable people with diabetes to effectively manage this disorder

Quality diabetes self-management education programs can be measured in terms of structure, process, and outcomes. Each of these program components includes one or more elements with specific standards. The broad outline of the National Standards for Diabetes Self-Management Education programs is as follows:

Structure
- Organization
- Needs assessment
- Program management
- Program staff
- Curriculum
- Participant access

Process
- Assessment
- Plan and implementation
- Follow-up

Outcomes
- Program outcome evaluation
- Participant outcome evaluation

STRUCTURE

The structure necessary to provide quality diabetes self-management education consists of the human and material resources and the management systems needed to achieve program and participant goals. Such structure includes the support and commitment of the organization that is sponsoring the program, the program administration and management systems, the qualifications and diversity of the personnel involved in the program, the curriculum and instructional methods and materials, and the accessibility of the program.

Organization

The sponsoring organization must provide the support and structure within which the program functions. Organizational commitment to self-management education including operational support, adequate space, personnel, budget, and materials must be clearly evident. Since multiple health care professionals from a variety of disciplines are involved in diabetes care, clear lines of authority and efficient communication systems should be established.

Standard 1. The sponsoring organization shall have a written policy that affirms education as an integral component of diabetes care.

Review criterion

1–1. There is a written statement from the sponsoring organization to reflect that self-management education is an integral component of diabetes care.

Standard 2. The sponsoring organization shall identify and provide the educational resources required to achieve its educational objectives in terms of its target population. These resources include adequate space, personnel, budget, and instructional materials.

Review criterion

2–1. For both individual and group instruction, resources (including space, staff, budget, and educational materials) are adequate to support the programs offered and the participants served.

Standard 3. The organizational relationships, lines of authority, staffing, job descriptions, and operational policies shall be clearly defined and documented.

Review criteria

3–1. The sponsoring institution's organizational chart delineates the placement of the diabetes program, staff, and advisory committee.

3–2. There is a description of the following for the coordinator and each instructional staff member:

- role in the program
- teaching responsibilities
- other program responsibilities
- amount of time spent in the program

3–3. There are written policies approved by the advisory committee concerning the operation of the program.

Needs Assessment

A successful program is based on the needs of the population that the program is intended to serve. Because diabetes populations vary, each organization should assess its service area and match resources to the needs of the defined target population. Needs assessments should guide program planning and management. Periodic reassessment should be done to allow the program to adapt to changing needs.

Standard 4. The service area shall be assessed in order to define the target population and determine appropriate allocation of personnel and resources to serve the educational needs of the target population.

Review criterion

4–1. The target population is defined (specifically the potential number to be served, types of diabetes, age range, language, ethnicity, unique characteristics, and special educational needs) based on an assessment of the service area.

Program Management

Effective management is essential to implement and maintain a successful program and to ensure that resources are adequate for the defined tasks. To ensure that management policies and program design reflect broad perspectives relevant to diabetes, the organization should designate a standing advisory committee that includes health care professionals and people with diabetes to assist staff with program planning

and review. Involvement and support from the medical community are also necessary. At times resources outside the sponsoring institution may be required to enable individuals affected by diabetes to maximize their health outcomes.

Standard 5. A standing advisory committee consisting of a physician, nurse educator, dietitian, an individual with behavioral science expertise, a consumer, and a community representative, at a minimum, shall be established to oversee the program.

Review criteria

5–1. The advisory committee members specified above attend at least two meetings a year.

5–2. The health professional members include at least one physician, one nurse educator, and one dietitian, each with expertise in diabetes.

5–3. The individual with behavioral science expertise is any professional with academic preparation in the behavioral sciences: e.g., counseling, health behavior, psychology, social work, sociology.

5–4. The consumer is any individual with diabetes or the caretaker thereof.

5–5. The community representative is any individual not employed by the institution.

5–6. There is written policy concerning the membership and responsibilities of the advisory committee.

5–7. The advisory committee minutes document that the committee is fulfilling its responsibilities to approve the program plan, recommend and approve policy, and review the program annually.

Standard 6. The advisory committee shall participate in the annual planning process, including determination of target audience, program objectives, participant access mechanisms, instructional methods, resource requirements (including space, personnel, budget, and materials), participant follow-up mechanisms, and program evaluation.

Review criterion

6–1. The advisory committee minutes document the approval each year of a written program plan which includes the items specified above.

Standard 7. Professional program staff shall have sufficient time and resources for lesson planning, instruction, documentation, evaluation, and follow-up.

Review criterion

7–1. The instructors' available hours and resources are adequate to meet the needs of the program and the participants.

Standard 8. Community resources shall be assessed periodically.

Review criterion

8–1. There is a list (including name, address, and telephone number) of community resources within the service area that serve the target population and their families. This list is updated yearly.

Program Staff

Qualified personnel are essential to the success of a diabetes self-management education program. The sponsoring organization should identify the program personnel, which must include a program coordinator who has overall responsibility for the program. Because diabetes is a chronic disorder requiring lifestyle changes, instructors need to be skilled and experienced health care professionals with recent education in diabetes, educational principles, and behavior change strategies.

Standard 9. A coordinator shall be designated who is responsible for program planning, implementation, and evaluation.

Review criteria

9–1. The job description for the program coordinator includes his/her responsibility for:

- acting as a liaison between the program staff, the advisory committee, and the administration of the institution
- providing and/or coordinating the orientation and continuing education for the professional staff
- participating in the planning and review of the program each year
- participating in the preparation of the program budget

- evaluating program effectiveness
- serving as the chair or member of the advisory committee

9–2. The program coordinator is a Certified Diabetes Educator (CDE) or has completed at least 24 hours of approved continuing education that includes a combination of diabetes, educational principles, and behavioral strategies.

Standard 10. Health care professionals with recent didactic and experiential preparation in diabetes clinical and educational issues shall serve as the program instructors. The staff shall include at least a nurse educator and a dietitian who collaborate routinely. Certification as a diabetes educator by the National Certification Board for Diabetes Educators (NCBDE) is recommended.

Review criteria

10–1. Program instructors are professional staff who routinely teach in the diabetes self-management education program and include at least one nurse educator and one dietitian.

10–2. Program instructors are health care professionals with a valid license, registration, or certification and who are CDEs or have completed at least 16 hours of approved continuing education that includes a combination of diabetes, educational principles, and behavioral strategies.

Standard 11. Professional program staff shall obtain education about diabetes, educational principles, and behavioral change strategies on a continuing basis.

Review criterion

11–1. The program coordinator and all instructors complete at least 6 hours per year of approved continuing education that includes a combination of diabetes, educational principles, and behavioral strategies.

Curriculum

A quality diabetes self-management education program should provide comprehensive instruction in the content areas relevant to the target population and to the participants being served. The curriculum, instructional methods, and materials should be appropriate for the specified target population, considering type and duration of diabetes, age, cultural influences, and individual learning abilities.

Standard 12. Based on the needs of the target population, the program shall be capable of offering instruction in the following content areas:

a. Diabetes overview

b. Stress and psychosocial adjustment

c. Family involvement and social support

d. Nutrition

e. Exercise and activity

f. Medications

g. Monitoring and use of results

h. Relationships among nutrition, exercise, medication, and blood glucose levels

i. Prevention, detection, and treatment of acute complications

j. Prevention, detection, and treatment of chronic complications

k. Foot, skin, and dental care

l. Behavior change strategies, goal setting, risk factor reduction, and problem solving

m. Benefits, risks, and management options for improving glucose control

n. Preconception care, pregnancy, and gestational diabetes

o. Use of health care systems and community resources

Review criteria

12–1. There is a written curriculum that includes educational objectives, content outline, instructional methods and materials, and the means for evaluating achievement of the objectives for each content area or session of the program.

12–2. The curriculum is current and includes all 15 content areas as appropriate for the identified target population.

Standard 13. The program shall use instructional methods and materials that are appropriate for the target population and the participants being served.

Review criterion

13–1. Instructional methods and materials are appropriate for the target population and participants in terms of cultural relevance, age, language, reading level, and special education needs.

Participant Access

Quality programs must be readily accessible to those in need of education. The sponsoring organization should facilitate access to self-management education for the target population identified in the needs assessment. Access is promoted by a commitment to routinely inform referral sources and the target population of the availability and benefits of the program.

Standard 14. A system shall be in place to inform the target population and potential referral sources of the availability and benefits of the program.

Review criterion

14–1. The program informs its identified target population and potential referral sources about the program at least once a year.

Standard 15. The program shall be conveniently and regularly available.

Review criterion

15–1. Program utilization, attrition rates, and waiting periods are assessed yearly.

Standard 16. The program shall be responsive to requests for information and referrals from consumers, health care professionals, and health care agencies.

Review criterion

16–1. There is written policy and procedure that stipulates that all requests for information and referrals receive a timely response.

PROCESS

Process refers to the methods or means by which resources are used to attain stated goals. The process of providing diabetes self-management education involves the integration of an individual assessment, goal setting, education plan development, implementation, evaluation, and follow-up. Each component requires documentation that can be evaluated.

Assessment

Because individuals are unique, their educational needs will vary with age, disease process, culture, and lifestyles. Effective instruction can only be accomplished by a collaborative effort between educators and participants to identify individualized educational needs.

Standard 17. An individualized assessment shall be developed and updated in collaboration with each participant. The assessment shall include relevant medical history, present health status, health service or resource utilization, risk factors, diabetes knowledge and skills, cultural influences, health beliefs and attitudes, health behaviors and goals, support systems, barriers to learning, and socioeconomic factors.

Review criteria

17–1. An initial assessment of the items specified above is documented in the education record and updated as needed.

17–2. The participant's pre-program knowledge of and skill level in each of the appropriate content areas of the National Standards is documented in the education record and updated as needed.

Plan and Implementation

For the educational experience to meet the participant's needs, an individual assessment should be used to develop the educational plan. All information about the educational experience should be documented in the participant's permanent medical or education record. Since different health care professionals may be involved in the provision of the educational experience, effective communication and coordination is essential.

Standard 18. An individualized education plan, based on the assessment, shall be developed in collaboration with each participant.

Review criterion

18–1. An education plan, developed in collaboration with the participant and based on the educational needs identified in the initial assessment, is documented in the education record.

Standard 19. The participant's educational experience, including assessment, intervention, evaluation, and follow-up, shall be documented in a permanent medical or education record. There shall be documentation of collaboration and coordination among program staff and other providers.

Review Criteria

19–1. The participant's progress through the program is documented in the education record and includes:

- the initial assessment and education plan as specified above

- an indication of the content taught, dates of instruction, and the instructors

- post-program assessment of the participant's knowledge and skill level of each of the appropriate content areas of the National Standards

- behavior change goals

- a plan for follow-up

- communication of participant's progress and any follow-up recommendations to the primary care provider

- follow-up assessment and any resulting interventions

19–2. Each program instructor documents his/her own interventions with the participants.

19–3. Communication and collaboration among program staff are facilitated by and documented in the education record.

19–4. There is a written policy that the education record is made available to external health care providers with permission from the participant.

19–5. There is a written policy that participants are given a copy or summary of their education record, if requested.

Follow-Up

Because diabetes is a chronic disorder requiring a lifetime of self-management, follow-up services will be needed. Participant's lifestyles, knowledge, skills, attitudes, and disease characteristics change over time, so that ongoing education is necessary and appropriate. Programs should be able to offer periodic reassessment and education as part of comprehensive services.

Standard 20. The program staff shall offer appropriate and timely educational interventions based on periodic reassessments of health status, knowledge, skills, attitudes, goals, and self-care behaviors.

Review criteria

20–1. There is a written policy for the provision of follow-up assessment of the items specified above and any resulting interventions.

20–2. At least one follow-up assessment of the items specified above and any interventions are documented in the education record.

20–3. Participant achievement of behavior change goals is assessed and documented 1–3 months after goal setting.

OUTCOMES

Outcomes are the desired results for the program and participants. For programs, the desired results include achievement of stated objectives, reaching the defined target population, and helping participants improve their health outcomes. For participants, outcomes include the knowledge and skills necessary for self-management, desired self-management behaviors, and improved health outcomes. Assessing outcomes and using the assessments in regular program evaluation and subsequent planning are essential to maintain quality programs.

Program Outcome Evaluation

The advisory committee should periodically review the program to ascertain that the program continues to meet the National Standards for Diabetes Self-Management Education Programs. The results of this review should be documented and used in subsequent program planning and modification.

Standard 21. The advisory committee shall review program performance annually, including all components of the annual program plan and curriculum, and use the information in subsequent planning and program modification.

Review criteria

21–1. The advisory committee minutes document the results of an annual review of the program including:

- program objectives
- the curriculum, instructional methods, and materials
- actual audience compared to the target population
- participant access and follow-up mechanisms
- program resources (space, personnel, and budget)
- program effectiveness/participant outcomes

21–2. The results of the annual review are reflected in the next annual program plan.

Participant Outcome Evaluation

Participant outcomes, such as success in incorporating self-management into their lifestyles, should be periodically reviewed. The specific outcomes evaluated will vary with the program, but the program's effectiveness in helping participants improve their health outcomes should be documented and used for future program planning and modification.

Standard 22. The advisory committee shall annually review and evaluate predetermined outcomes for program participants.

Review criteria

22–1. Participants' outcomes are measured and evaluated, specifically, the degree to which the participants achieve their behavior change goals and one other outcome measure (e.g., monitoring for complications, lost work or school days, metabolic control, or others).

22–2. The program's effectiveness at improving outcomes is evaluated by the advisory committee and the results of this evaluation are reflected in the next annual program plan.

Patient Education Materials Review Form

Category: ___Print
    ___Video
    ___Slides
    ___Other

Title: _____

Date of publication: _____ Cost: _____

Author / distributor: _____

Address: _____
_____

Length (pgs/min): _____
_____

Brief overview: _____
_____
_____
_____
_____

SMOG readability rating: _____

Educational level: ___Survival   ___Continuing   ___Intensive

Target audience: (*check any that apply*)

___children   ___parents   ___public

___adults—type I   ___newly diagnosed   ___parents/family

___adults—type II   ___elderly   ___large print/easy to read

Technical accuracy/content adequacy: _____
_____
_____

Format:

Graphics/use of color: _____

Attractiveness: _____

Overall rating:

___very good   ___good   ___satisfactory   ___unsatisfactory

Reviewer: _____ Date: _____

Source: Courtesy of Joslin Diabetes Center, Boston, Massachusetts.

SMOG Readability Formula

Readability ratings are performed to ensure that an item can be read and comprehended by individuals who will be using them. Sentence and word length and complexity are important factors in assessing readability.

The SMOG formula is one of a number of readability formulas and is a relatively recently developed one. It is quick to perform, ensures 90% comprehension (ie, a person with a 10th grade reading level will comprehend 90% of the material rated at that level), and is relatively reliable and respectable.

1. Count 10 consecutive sentences near the beginning of the text to be assessed, 10 in the middle, and 10 near the end. Count as a sentence any string of words ending with a period, question mark, or exclamation point.

2. In the 30 selected sentences count every word of three or more syllables. Any string of letters or numerals beginning and ending with a space or punctuation mark should be counted if you can distinguish at least three syllables when you read it aloud in context. If a polysyllabic word is repeated, count each repetition.

3. Estimate the square root of the number of polysyllabic words counted. This is done by taking the square root of the nearest perfect square. For example, if the count is 95, the nearest perfect square is 100, which yields a square root of 10. If the count lies roughly between two perfect squares, choose the lower number. For instance, if the count is 110, take the square root of 100 rather than that of 121.

4. Add 3 to the approximate square root. This gives the SMOG Grade, which is the reading grade that a person must have reached if he or she is to understand fully the text assessed.

SMOG Score and Interpretation

Grade Level (Score)	Level of Style	Typical Magazine Example
6–7	Very Easy	Comics
8	Easy	Pulp fiction
9–10	Average	*Reader's Digest*
11–13	Fairly Difficult	*Atlantic Monthly*
14–16	Difficult	Academic magazines; *Psychoanalytic Review, Child Welfare*
17+	Very Difficult	Scientific, professional magazines; *Music Educator Journal*

Source: Directions for SMOG grading are reprinted with permission from *Journal of Reading* (May 1969:639), Copyright © 1969, International Reading Association Inc.

Sample Self-Management Training Record

Signature and Initials: _____

Diabetes Education Materials Given: _____

Referrals: PT/Exercise: ___ Social Work: ___ Psychologist: ___ Child Life: ___
                  Discharge Planning: ___

Barriers To Learning: _____

Key: o = does not know/do
       / = needs improvement
       + = competence
       NA = not applicable

Topics Instructed	Assess	Teach	Review/ Verbalize	Return Demo	Class
General Information					
Identifies own type of DM and characteristics	____	____	____	____	____
Lists factors that affect blood glucose control	____	____	____	____	____
States rationale for diabetes management	____	____	____	____	____
Discusses incorporating DM management into ADL	____	____	____	____	____
Nutrition					
States meal plan/time schedule	____	____	____	____	____
Selects foods according to meal plan	____	____	____	____	____
States relation between food, weight, and diabetes	____	____	____	____	____
Demonstrates food selection ( )	____	____	____	____	____
Monitoring					
Demonstrates monitoring	____	____	____	____	____
States target blood glucose levels	____	____	____	____	____
States monitoring schedule (times/frequency)	____	____	____	____	____
Knows methods and rationale for ketone testing	____	____	____	____	____
Records results of blood and urine tests in log book	____	____	____	____	____
Understands purpose of HbA$_{1c}$ lab test to monitor control	____	____	____	____	____

Source: Courtesy of Joslin Diabetes Center, Boston, Massachusetts.

Medication

States rationale for diabetes medication

States action, onset, peak, duration, side effects of meds

Knows schedule for administration

Demonstrates insulin technique ( ) self; ( ) _____

Describes rotation/site selection schedule

Knows rules for insulin storage

Disposes syringes appropriately

Complications

Knows sx, cause, prevention, tx—Hypoglycemia

S.O. demonstrates glucagon administration

Knows sx, cause, prevention, tx—Hyperglycemia

States sick-day rules/risks of DKA

Identifies chronic complications and prevention

Exercise

States plan for exercise/play

Knows benefits of exercise

Knows adjustment in food/meals for exercise

Daily Living Concerns/Home Management

States recommendations for drugs/alcohol/dating

Demonstrates foot care; personal hygiene

Wears/carries identification

Identifies support person and community resources

Instructs other caregivers (school nurse, daycare)

Chapter 10

Counseling Skills for Improved Behavioral Change

Michael J. Powers

COUNSELING PROCESS

The process of counseling usually begins when a client or patient seeks help in solving a problem, making a decision, or making a change in behavior. In nutritional counseling for the person with diabetes, the process is more likely to begin when a patient is referred for help in developing and complying with a nutritional and medical treatment plan that will result in diabetes control. There are many similarities between education and counseling, but with counseling, the primary emphasis is on implementation of a plan, rather than teaching new information. The goal of counseling then is to help patients identify some desired state and to help them move in stages from their present state to that desired state.[1,2] To understand the present state, the counselor gathers information about the patient's personality, problems he or she is experiencing, and his or her strengths. Desired state refers to what the person's life would be like if he or she succeeds in making changes.

The counseling process is conducted in five stages: (1) developing a cooperative alliance (establishing rapport), (2) gathering information (understanding the present state), (3) setting goals (constructing a realistic desired state), (4) intervening to attain goals (using techniques that lead to the desired state), and (5) maintaining change. These stages are not as separate as the sequential numbering of them might imply. There can be considerable cycling through these various stages, both within one session and over the whole process of counseling.

STAGE 1: DEVELOPING A COOPERATIVE ALLIANCE

Empowering Assumptions

A patient empowerment approach to managing diabetes advocates that the diabetes counselors/educators adopt a positive set of assumptions about their patients.[3] Success as a nutritional counselor will be enhanced if you meet the patient with certain positive assumptions in mind. Patients respond well to evidence that the counselor believes they can and will succeed.[4] The following five assumptions will facilitate the development of a cooperative alliance and patient empowerment.

1. *Each patient already has all the resources he or she needs to succeed.*[4] A major part of successful counseling requires the counselor to become skillful in helping patients mobilize their own internal resources. Resources are the strengths and abilities to learn or do whatever is needed to attain the desired state. The onset of a major illness, such as diabetes, often debilitates patients and they lose touch with how resourceful they can be.

2. *Each patient is making the best choice he or she can make at any given moment.*[4] No matter how self-defeating or irrational a patient's behavior appears, it is important to give the patient the benefit of the doubt. Assume that if the patient is making poor

choices, something is blocking his or her motivation to make better ones. Holding this assumption will reduce the tendency to judge patients out of frustration as "weak-willed," "lazy," "unmotivated," "immature," or "wanting to be sick."

3. *It is better to have choice than no choice.*[4] Choice, especially informed choice, is the central theme in the patient empowerment approach. It is essential to approach patients with the attitude of helping them find more adaptive behaviors rather than restricting their choices. Patients may be sent to a dietitian after being told that they "must" lose weight or begin insulin. This kind of message may create resistance, because it is given as an order with an attached threat. Threats can be motivating for some patients but not for most. The counselor's first task then is to relieve some of the client's pressure by turning the order into a choice. This can be done by engaging the patient in an empathetic discussion about how it is in the patient's interest to lose weight and realistically what might happen if the weight is not lost. Choice is also involved in deciding how much weight, how quickly, and by what method it will be lost.

4. *Resistance is only a form of feedback.*[5] We often see resistance as the opposite of compliance. The patient empowerment model offers an alternative to a compliance-based approach to diabetes management.[3] Resistance, or noncompliance, can be thought of as feedback that tells us that our current approach is not working and it is time to try something else.[5] Holding this assumption will keep us flexible and willing to vary our approach or timing with different patients. This assumption can prevent much of the familiar frustration that counselors feel when they "know" what the patient "should" do to resolve the problem, but are unable to get the patient to cooperate. This stance of "expert" does not promote patient empowerment and with some patients may actually spark resistance.

5. An assumption that closely follows the previous one is that *there is no such thing as failure as long as you are willing to try something new.*[5] You only fail when you stop trying. The more flexible you are in your willingness to try new and creative approaches, the more likely you are to meet the needs of a variety of patients with differing needs. Failures come quickly when we become wedded to one "right" approach and administer it to everyone.

Establishing Rapport through Pacing

Two fundamental processes in all communication are *pacing* and *leading*.[4–6] Pacing is the process of accepting the patient as he or she is, whereas leading (discussed later) is the process of influencing the patient. Rapport is established and maintained through pacing. It is the counselor's responsibility to initiate the building of rapport. There is usually a social phase at the beginning of each session during which the counselor can make the patient feel welcome and comfortable. It need only last a few minutes and is basically a polite convention that many people need to "break the ice." During and after the social phase, the counselor can use verbal and nonverbal pacing skills to establish a helping relationship. Pacing refers to the counselor's ability to "stay with" the patient. As we see later, patients come to nutrition counseling in different stages of readiness to change. Pushing when they are not quite ready will be a mismatch that decreases rapport. There are two kinds of pacing—verbal and nonverbal—both of which are essential to the building of rapport.

Verbal Pacing

Verbal pacing is the type most frequently described in counseling literature. It is developed through the counselor's careful attention, validation, and acceptance of the feelings and beliefs that the patient verbalizes. The following listening skills adapted from Ivey and Authier can be used to pace patients as they express themselves.[7]

- Open-ended questions—usually beginning with "what," "how," "why," or "could"; allow the patient more of a chance to open up
- Attentive silence—can be a further invitation to talk
- Reflection of feeling—feedback that focuses on the patient's emotions more than on content
- Paraphrasing—feeds back to the patient the essential content of previous statement
- Nonverbal encouraging to talk—head nods and "um hmms"
- Summarizing—similar to paraphrasing or reflection of feeling but used after a longer period of time

These are verbal pacing techniques because they make it easy for the patient to open up and talk. They demonstrate your interest and attention to them in a personal way. Verbal pacing is experienced emotionally by the patient as acceptance, empathy, trust, and understanding.

Nonverbal Pacing

Nonverbal pacing can be observed as a synchronized rhythm of movement, tone of voice, tempo of speech, body posture, and many other physical similarities between the counselor and client.[5,6,8] In most communication, nonverbal pacing is manifested naturally without conscious awareness. It can be observed in most social situations, such as in restaurants or around the water cooler. However, it goes largely unnoticed because we are usually absorbed in verbal content much more than its nonverbal accompaniment. It is, nevertheless, an essential ingredient in making communication feel comfortable. Establishing a counseling relationship frequently requires patients to reveal personal details of their lives to a stranger, whom they cannot even be sure likes them or can understand their problems and fears. They may be of a different gender, race, culture, socioeconomic sta-

tus, or geographic region. This relationship is often begun under very stressful circumstances for the patient. The patient may have just been diagnosed as having diabetes, or he or she may be hospitalized for complications. The patient may be feeling overwhelmed, apprehensive, or angry, and there are many other possible responses to the situation. The dietitian is responsible for beginning a helping relationship under these difficult conditions. The nutritional counselor also may be working under the stress of a too-busy schedule or other constraints. Rapport is possible only if these adverse conditions can be managed and any patient–counselor differences can be bridged. Verbal pacing takes time to use because it is dependent on the patient's verbal self-expression. Nonverbal pacing, however, can begin as soon as you meet the patient.

Mirroring

One useful way to think about nonverbal rapport is as the harmony of movement that is created when two or more individuals are in rhythm with one another. With a couple dancing, there is a noticeable synchrony of movement that indicates that they are in step with one another and are moving together. Similarly, persons in rapport exhibit many movements that mirror one another. These physical manifestations are representative of a harmony on other levels. The studies of how we naturally match one another's movements have not only been useful in defining nonverbal rapport but also in teaching the use of mirroring to establish rapport quickly and intentionally under adverse circumstances and with those persons with whom we normally would not expect to "click."[5,6,8] The technique of mirroring gives us a set of steps in our own repertoire that we can use to bring about rapport, especially under those circumstances in which we might have in the past felt defensive, scared, or unsure of how to proceed with a particular patient. Mirroring involves imitating the posture, movements, rhythms, and other nonverbal qualities of people's behavior. The following are some of the nonverbal behaviors that can be mirrored.[5,6,8]

---

1. PHYSICAL POSITIONS TO MIRROR

Body posture—Sitting or standing

Arm positions—Arms at the side, crossed, or supporting the head

Leg positions—Crossed or uncrossed

Head tilt—Persons often have a characteristic head tilt, especially when listening or reflecting

2. MOVEMENTS TO MIRROR

Repetitive gestures—Touching the face, smoothing the clothing, using the hands to emphasize a point, nodding the head

Breathing rate—A most subtle of mirroring choices that requires careful observation and practice, but is quite effective

3. VOICE QUALITIES TO MIRROR

Vocal qualities—Vocal qualities are considered nonverbal because they concern "how" words are spoken, rather than "what" is said

Voice tempo—The rate of speech

Voice volume—How loudly or quietly the patient speaks

Voice tone—Harsh or soft

These are only a few of many subtle behaviors we may notice during our interactions with patients. And these provide a starting point to train your critical observation skills. By mirroring these aspects of the person's behavior, we enter their present physical state. We match them in a profound way that forms a bond of contact and trust. Once practiced, it is not unusual to find that you can establish effective rapport with persons with whom you might previously have predicted having a poor relationship. One of the reasons rapport can be achieved is that, while you are pacing the patient, you will discover that you have turned off your critical judging process, which often prevents the kind of empathic openness necessary for solid rapport. Being in nonverbal rapport makes it easier to listen attentively and to use verbal pacing skills for establishing deeper rapport.

To develop mirroring skills, first begin by noticing how naturally it occurs as you observe others interact. After you are satisfied that it occurs quite naturally in normal conversation, begin to practice mirroring your patients for very brief (1 minute) periods at the beginning of each counseling session. As with any new skill, it will feel awkward at first. With practice, however, it will become second nature and a valuable skill to be able to count on for working with difficult and hard-to-reach patients.

Mirroring should be used as unobtrusively as possible. It operates at the nonverbal and even unconscious level, and it is best left unmentioned to patients. If brought to their attention, it will only serve to make them self-conscious. They may even think they are being mocked and may respond suspiciously or angrily. In addition to being a concrete behavioral technique to use to establish rapport quickly, mirroring also provides an easy way to test whether you are still in rapport at any stage of the counseling process. By simply observing whether you and the patient are mirroring one another, you can tell if you are in rapport. If you are not, you can return to mirroring until it is established. Frequent "rapport checks" will provide the nutritional counselor with ongoing feedback on the state of the relationship.

STAGE 2: INFORMATION GATHERING

Information gathering is the process of learning about the patient's *present state* from patient self-report and from careful observation. Research shows that individualizing the delivery of nutrition information to a patient based on their stage of readiness for change improves outcomes in changing dietary behavior. Therefore, it is important to collect information about your patient that will assist you in planning effective interventions. The information-gathering process can be used to involve patients so they feel better about themselves. A main goal in this respect is to gather information about patients' strengths, beliefs, and readiness for change that will serve as leverage later in motivating them to make changes. Most of the skills for gathering information were summarized above in the section on verbal pacing. These listening skills are basic and should be a part of every counselor's training.

Observational Skills

Another set of valuable skills that should be developed are observational skills. The accuracy of the assessment of the patient's present state depends on the dietitian's skill in what Mayerson calls "critical observation."[9] Critical observation is being able to "read between the lines." It involves noticing whether nonverbal messages are congruent with verbal messages and being able to recognize how a person looks, acts, and sounds in his or her present state so that changes from that state can be recognized. It is important to observe how patients do or do not express emotion, how carefully they listen, and other potentially significant behaviors they display.

Competency-Focused Interviewing

It has been estimated that the person with diabetes usually provides 95% or more of his or her daily care. Successful management of diabetes depends ultimately on patients' motivation and competence in setting and achieving goals. Therefore, it is vital to help them attain a sense of empowerment so they will succeed.[10] Their self-esteem is based largely on their feelings of competence at the tasks of daily living and self-management.

It is important to remember that gathering information requires asking many questions and that these questions themselves can offend or carry hidden implications. For example, notice the implications in the question, "How many times have you tried to lose weight before?" This seemingly harmless question implies the patient has tried before and has failed and perhaps failed repeatedly. It can leave one focused on past failures and the debilitating feelings of failure. They may not be in a resourceful state for the counselor to motivate them to succeed. A more competency-focused approach would be to establish an expectation of success before asking about previous failures. For example, "To help you be successful in losing weight, it is important that I know of any previous experiences with losing weight." The positive side to hidden implications is that they can also be used to facilitate goal attainment. As long as we know patients do respond emotionally to hidden implications, why not ask questions that imply that they are competent, such as

- "What will be the key difference this time that *will enable you* to lose those 10 lb?"
- "How will your life be different *when you reach* your goal?"
- "What is the biggest obstacle *you will overcome* this week?"
- "What is the most important thing that *you were able to learn*?"
- "*Which change* would you like to *start* with?"

Using competency-focused and success-oriented questions is a skill that can be acquired by first observing the differing effects that certain questions and phrasings can have on patients and then gradually practicing ways to ask questions containing positive implications.

Keep in mind that the principle of pacing and leading still applies to competency-focused interviewing. Sometimes the patient begins very negatively, and you will need to pace that negativity before leading him or her into a more positive frame of mind with a positive question. If the person begins by saying, "I really screwed up my diet this week. I just couldn't seem to stick with it," you can pace by saying, "Yes, according to the food record here, you really did screw up last week (pacing). And if you had the week to do over again what would you do differently (leading)?"

Competency-focused interviewing is meant to help persons regain access to their own inner resources and strengths that they have exhibited at some time in their lives. It can be approached directly by asking persons to name the resource they need to be successful now. Then ask them to remember a time when they demonstrated that they had the resource. For example, "Can you tell me a time when you were successfully able to make a difficult personal change?" They might recall that they gave up smoking several years ago, and they will recall the satisfaction and strength in knowing that they accomplished something difficult.

What other kinds of information should a good assessment cover? You cannot expect to have the time to do a full in-depth assessment of every factor, so it is important to learn to look for what Gregory Bateson called "the difference that makes a difference."[11] Not every variable is vitally important as an impact point for your interventions. The art of counseling is much like that of the sculptor, who must know the stone intimately to know exactly where to place the chisel.

Incongruent Communication

One of the most commonly encountered phenomena in counseling is the patient who is incongruent about change. *Incongruence* occurs when persons experience an internal conflict in which part of them wants to change but another part does not. Both parts can be representing valid concerns of the patient. Sometimes incongruence is expressed as a split between rationality and emotions; for example, when someone says, "I know I should do it (rationality), but I am afraid to try (emotions)." It may be a conflict between what they stand to gain and what they will lose in making the change. There are two types of incongruence that patients typically display: simultaneous and sequential.[2]

Simultaneous Incongruence

Simultaneous incongruence occurs when a person sends two contradictory messages within the same communication.[1,2,11] The contradiction can occur between the verbal and nonverbal parts of the communication. A common example that frequently goes unnoticed is when a person verbally says "yes" to something while nonverbally shaking his or her head "no." The contradiction can also occur between the words and the tone of voice. This is often caricatured comically when a person yells, "I am not angry," in an angry tone of voice. Another common form of simultaneous incongruence occurs when both parts of the conflicting message are in the verbal message, as when qualifiers are used to weaken the impact of a message. How many times have you heard patients say, "I *guess* I'll try to follow the diet?" Other popular qualifiers include "maybe," "sort of," "I hope," "might," and "if I have time." There are myriad ways that patients can be incongruent, and if this ambivalence is observed and responded to effectively, then precious time is not wasted.

Responding to incongruent messages requires skill because the person is typically unaware of one part of the internal conflict. One response is to first bring it to the patient's awareness so that it can be discussed. For example, "I notice that while you are saying 'Yes, I know I must lose weight,' your voice sounds rather flat, and you don't seem to have much energy about really losing weight." Such a statement often evokes a response that gives you more information about the conflict.

A way to test for simultaneous incongruence is to ask direct questions.

- "Do you believe your condition is serious?"
- "Do you believe you can test more often?"
- "Will you follow through this week on x, y, and z?"
- "Are you willing to make changes in your life style to adjust to your diabetic condition?"

Pay careful attention to "how" the patient answers, as well as "what" he or she answers. If you detect a hesitancy or distinct lack of energy in the voice tone, a negative shake of the head, the use of qualifiers, a sigh, or a rapid change in rate or volume of speech, it would be wise to find out if the person is aware of an internal conflict.

Sequential Incongruence

Sequential incongruence is harder to detect, because instead of one communication carrying two contradictory messages, there are two different communications at separate times that contradict one another. The patient is not in conflict when he or she commits (even enthusiastically) to follow the meal plan. The conflicting part only emerges after the session. When the patient returns the next week, it is clear that there was no follow-through. Sequential incongruence can only be detected and responded to by systematic follow-up that compares what is promised with what is accomplished.

Sequential incongruence may be a signal that some situational cue at home overrides patients' best intentions and efforts. They may be fully congruent at the time that they agree to cut down on unhealthy snacks. Then later at home when they see potato chips, they lose control and forget their commitment. This can be a signal that they need family cooperation or need special attention to coping skills in the face of temptation.

Patient Readiness for Change

An area that has received much attention lately is the research of Prochaska and colleagues on how individuals go through predictable stages in the process of changing behaviors. The stages outlined by Prochaska and associates are closely aligned with the stages of the counseling process.[12,13] During the information-gathering stage of counseling, it is essential to use the observation skills, pacing and leading communication skills, and competency-focused interviewing skills covered above to assess the patient's stage of readiness to change nutrition behaviors.

Prochaska et al[13] lists five distinct stages in the process of changing a specific behavior:

1. *Precontemplation*—represents the period when the patient is not considering change and does not even consciously recognize there is a real need to change

2. *Contemplation*—the patient is aware of a desire or need to change but is only considering it

3. *Preparation*—the patient has decided to change and is actively planning how to accomplish the change

4. *Action*—the patient begins implementing the plan he or she chose

5. *Maintenance*—if successful, the patient will continue the new behaviors and work to prevent relapse

Exhibit 10-1 shows the characteristics to be aware of as the agent of support and change for your patients. The stages of the counseling process will naturally align with the stages of the patient's readiness to change if the counselor is pacing and leading appropriately. Mismatching stages will break rapport and may lead patients to avoid further sessions. Mismatching stages can take several forms.[13] It may result from pushing for action too early before a patient is congruently committed, or it could also mean talking too long *about* change with a patient who is ready to "just do it!" It will generally be a waste of the counselor's time to begin skills training on how to use a glucose meter when the patient has not congruently agreed to incorporate this into his or her daily life. As a rule of thumb, the early stages in the process of change (precontemplation, contemplation, preparation) require more cognitive work, whereas the later stages (preparation, action, maintenance) will require more skills training and action orientation. Prochaska et al[13] predicts considerable recycling and spiraling through these stages rather than a simple linear progression. Exhibit 10-1 summarizes the stages of readiness to change and the characteristics the counselor can observe in the patient. It also relates these stages of readiness to the overall stages of the counseling process.

Family Involvement

Family involvement is a highly relevant aspect of assessment of the present state of the pa-

Exhibit 10-1 Stages of Readiness for Change

Stage of Readiness to Change	Characteristics	Focus of Counseling
Precontemplation	Patient has no plan to change in near future; unaware or denying there is a problem; may initiate half-hearted changes just to "get others off his or her back"	Develop cooperative alliance through verbal and nonverbal pacing; listen and use gentle information-gathering methods; if there is rapport, you may use mild confrontation; avoid goal setting and action-oriented focus
Contemplation	Patient is aware of a problem and "thinking about" overcoming it, but no decision or commitment yet; may verbalize that he or she is "not quite ready yet"; watch for incongruent communication—"yeah, I guess maybe I should do something about my weight"	Continue rapport and build on relationship by exploring the idea of change without actively making plans; continue information gathering; use listening skills to explore pros and cons of change; pace both parts of the incongruence—"On the one hand, you'd feel better, but on the other hand, it's an effort to go for daily walks." Lead toward a commitment
Preparation	Patient is planning action within the next month or so or has already begun small efforts toward change May also be a patient bouncing back from a relapse	Continue rapport and lead patient into goal-setting stage; use information you have gathered about motivation, life style, and personal strengths to set realistic goals and plan steps and methods for achieving them
Action	Patient acts on plan; begins to follow meal plan, performs self-monitoring, or other behaviors that lead toward the goal	Use your rapport and influence to encourage, support, and reinforce any steps, no matter how small, toward success; use the interventions in your bag of tricks to promote observable behavioral change
Maintenance	Patients often experience a relapse after successfully making changes. They will still need to work at maintaining and consolidating accomplishments they have achieved	Continue to support and encourage; help them deal with temptation to relapse; build self-esteem by keeping them aware of their internal resources

Note: Although Prochaska later added a sixth stage called termination, this stage is omitted here in recognition that managing diabetes requires life-long commitment and health care.

Source: Adapted with permission from Curry SJ, Kristal AR, Bowen DJ. An application of the stage model of behavior change to dietary fat reduction. *Health Education Research.* 1992;7:1. Copyright © 1992, Oxford University Press.

tient. There is no question of the powerful impact that a family can have on an individual member. For many persons, the family is the main or even the sole source of emotional support. Or, in the case of a patient from a dysfunctional family, the family system could disrupt any progress you attempt to encourage. Family systems theory is an integral part of understanding and intervening in families with medical problems. Some references that can present family systems ideas are listed in the Suggested Reading section at the end of this chapter.

STAGE 3: REALISTIC GOAL SETTING

Zifferblatt and Wilbur[14] show the dangers of unrealistic expectations that may be held by the referring physician, the dietitian, or the patient in nutritional counseling. Realistic goals allow for a reasonable amount of time to make the change; are accomplished in graduated stages; and do not exaggerate the counselor's responsibility and power to influence the patient. Goals can be usefully divided between the long-term goals that describe where the patients will end up and short-term goals that describe the milestones they will accomplish as they make day-to-day changes.

Long-Term Goals

Long-term goals describe the *desired state*. They should be significant and relevant enough to the patient to be motivational. Long-term goals should be well defined so that both patient and counselor will clearly know when the goal has been achieved.

Short-Term Goals

Short-term goals describe the behavioral process that patients will follow to attain the desired outcome. They keep long-term goals realistic by breaking them down to smaller, more manageable actions. They specify the healthy eating habits that the patients will adopt on a daily basis (ideally for a lifetime) to reach the desired state. An example of a long-term goal might be to lose 20 pounds. The corresponding short-term goals might be to reduce daily caloric intake by substituting lower-calorie foods such as fish for red meat, eating more slowly, using a sugar substitute, and taking a walk in the afternoon instead of snacking. Short-term goals should be defined according to these guidelines:

- They should be a statement of what to do rather than what not to do. Telling a patient not to snack without offering a replacement behavior is negative, limits choice, and may trigger resistance.

- They should be under the individual's control. Suggesting modifications in a patient's diet will have little effect if he or she is not the one who does the shopping and cooking.

- They should be developed with as much patient participation as possible.

- They should be specific enough to be measured and evaluated. Avoid vague phases such as "cut down on." This will reduce the chance of uncertainty or denial as excuses.

- They should describe *when* and *where* the behavior is to take place.

STAGE 4: INTERVENTION

Interventions are intended to *lead* more than *pace*. Leading is the type of communication that influences the patient to *move toward* established goals.[5,6] Interventions can range in degree of power from mild suggestions to strong directives.

Most of the interventions presented here deal with cognitive changes that lead to behavioral changes. Such interventions as skills acquisition (weighing food accurately or reading food labels) or informational learning, such as understanding food exchanges, are better covered under the topic of patient education. Many of the tried-and-true methods of increasing adherence through the behavioral techniques of baseline frequency counts, stimulus control, positive reinforcement, successive approximation, and modeling have been covered extensively in other publications.[15–17] The techniques mentioned here are meant to complement and supplement these more widely known behavioral techniques.

Steps in Intervention

1. Check Rapport

The first step in intervention is always to check rapport. Because an intervention is a "lead," it is more effective when it follows appropriate "pacing" of the patient's behavioral and cognitive state. The principle of "pacing and leading" continues to apply throughout the counseling relationship. Janis[18] presents a nicely developed schema that shows the phases and key variables that help determine the amount of "referent power" that counselors can develop as agents of change. He defines referent power as the power of persuasion patients ascribe to the counselor, making the counselor a powerful source of support and approval for the patients. Nutritional counselors can be most effective when they are comfortable with this role and use this power for the benefit of the patient. Never underestimate the power that others may give over to you, and never forget that it can quickly vanish if it is under- or overused. An intervention should also be parsimonious in requiring the least amount of change necessary to make the important difference in the patient's nutritional adjustment. The intervention should therefore be well thought out and individualized to the patient.

2. Secure Congruent Commitment

When rapport is already sufficient or is re-established, the next step is to secure a congruent commitment from the patient to the outcome of the intervention. If the goal is to decrease caloric intake and to increase exercise, then it is important to ask directly if the patient agrees to do it. Doing so gives you the chance to observe direct feedback in the patient's facial expression, voice tone, body posture, and gestures. This feedback can signal to you there is some other consideration, objection, or fear to be dealt with first before the patient will commit to a change. Making this congruency check can save both the dietitian and patient a lot of time and frustration over poor adherence. This verbal commitment also provides a reasonable basis for confronting any later failure to follow-through.

3. Fit Suggestions to the Person

The next step of intervention is to propose the intervention to the patient in a way that will increase his or her acceptance of it. You must be able to use much of what you have learned about the patient's attitudes, beliefs, and interests in a way that makes the suggested intervention fit with the patient's life style and belief system. Once the person's motivational key is found, you can propose the needed changes so that they are congruent with the person's motivation. A person who needs to exercise but has already declared plainly that he or she detests it should obviously not be told that exercise is fun. It would be better to accept their statement and find another avenue of approach. If the patient is the kind of person who is very dutiful, then exercise can be proposed as distasteful but as an obligation for good control.

4. Follow-Up

Interventions lose power if follow-up is neglected. They need to be reinforced when successful and modified when unsuccessful. Zifferblatt and Wilbur[14] correctly point out that if a patient is asked to keep a food record, it should then be used in the sessions or the patient gets the message that it is not very important and will stop. Many patients and referring physicians do not have realistic ideas of the need for follow-up contacts with the nutritional counselor. They may believe that one or two sessions are enough to effect lasting changes. Therefore, the expectation of follow-up should be built into the commitment or contract as early as possible in the counseling relationship.

Intervention Techniques

Confrontation

Confrontation is a technique that can be used to challenge a patient's incongruent behavior, misinformation, counselor–patient misunderstandings, irrational fears and beliefs, denial of problems, disowning of responsibility, ignoring of consequences, or manipulation and game playing.[19–21] Leslie et al[22] suggest confrontation as a key skill in dealing with a patient's reluctance to accept the use of insulin in managing diabetes.

Hauenstein et al[20] report that, although 85.6% of surveyed dietitians counseling individuals with non–insulin-dependent diabetes mellitus perceive confrontation as "very important/helpful," a smaller number (70.1%) felt "very adequately prepared to use the techniques." Part of the preparation for using confrontation should include how to distinguish among levels of intensity in confrontation and how to use it effectively. The term confrontation for many nutritional counselors may be associated with anger or verbal assault on the patient. However, at the milder levels a confrontation can be as gentle as, "I notice you have not been monitoring your blood glucose levels regularly. I wonder what's going on?" Or it can be a request that encourages the patient to confront his or her own behavior: "Have you considered the consequences of adding those extra drinks when you go out to dinner?" The more skilled a dietitian becomes at using low-intensity confrontation, the less likely it becomes that stronger ones will be needed. However, for those difficult patients in whom more intense confrontation is necessary, the following guidelines apply:

- Solid rapport is a necessary precondition for using confrontation. Rapport can ensure that the confrontation is intended to be in the patient's best interest rather than done out of the frustration of the nutritional counselor.

- It is most effective when the confrontation is expressed in concrete terms about specific behaviors rather than in general terms about the person.[21] Doing so keeps the focus on observable behaviors rather than subjective judgments that might create defensiveness.

- Using "I-messages" when confronting will reduce patient defensiveness.[23] "Two weeks ago I heard you commit to keeping a food record, and now I see that this is the second week in a row that you haven't followed through." This is confrontative based on the counselor's observation without being judgmental or accusatory.

- Confrontation is more powerful when it is competency focused. Confrontation can express confidence in the patient's strengths while at the same time pointing out discrepancies between goals and behavior.[9] "I hear you saying that you don't have the willpower to cut down on evening snacks, and yet look how well you did during the first month you started."

Visualization

The use of mental imagery in counseling has been increasing in the past several decades.[5,20,24,25] Visualization can be used to set and clarify long-term goals and to rehearse the behaviors involved in achieving short-term goals. A patient can visualize a long-term goal by imagining what things will be like when the goal is attained. If the goal is to lose 20 pounds, then patients could visualize in detail how they will look, how they will dress differently, how they will act differently, how they will feel differently, and how others will respond to them differently. This visualization helps patients begin to prepare for change, just by imagining it. It can also help in anticipating unsuspected problems that could arise as a consequence of even a positive change.

Visualizing a short-term goal might mean having the patient imagine the specific behaviors he or she must adopt to attain the desired state. For the same goal of losing 20 pounds, it would mean visualizing acting on the diet suggestions designed to result in weight loss. This technique works best when the instruction is to visualize positive behaviors. If patients currently snack on too many high-calorie foods, the choices would either be to visualize themselves snacking on alternative low-calorie foods or doing something else instead of snacking, such as taking a walk.

Visualization can be used effectively for having patients "re-view" positive memories that help them reconnect with inner strengths that would help solve present problems. Simple instructions to remember a time when they exhibited the "determination" (or other resource) to overcome a difficulty, or adjust to a change, or solve a problem can help them reach the key emotion they need to face a present problem. It can put them into a more positive frame of mind and be the basis for a feeling of confidence that they can succeed.

Evocative imagery can also be a powerful means of creating a compelling goal that can be used as a motivator. It can also make goals feel more concrete and achievable to patients. It is self-reinforcing for many patients to regularly revisualize a goal and the progress they are making toward it. Mental images by their very nature are personal ones and can increase the patient's ownership of the nutritional goals. Some guidelines for using visualization are presented below:

- Help patients create an image by describing experiences that involve as many of the senses as possible.

- Use general wording that will not interfere with specific details that patients will spontaneously generate.

- If they are uncomfortable at first, begin with some relaxing directions (close your eyes and get comfortable) and imagery (imagine that you are in your favorite relaxing place).

- If a disturbing image emerges, have them change it, so that they realize they have control over their own images.

Reframing

Reframing is a technique used to help give patients a different (usually positive) way of understanding a problem they are having.[5,11,26,27] Recasting the problem so that they have a new way of viewing it often frees them to find a new solution to an old problem. Reframing produces an impact by changing the meaning attached to a problem or a situation. A positive reframing was effectively used by a family therapist in treating a 19-year-old woman with diabetes who had been hospitalized many times due to keto-

acidosis.[28] The counseling goal was to improve her adherence to her prescribed diet. In interviewing her, the therapist found that she had a strong need to be different and that she had been defiant with all the other medical professionals. She had adopted an "I don't care" attitude and was clearly ready for a power struggle over who was going to "get me to change." The therapist paced her defiant side by carefully listening to her complaints and then reframed them as "justifiable anger," rather than resistance. This pacing and reframing made her feel understood for the first time, allowing her to open up further. He continued to pace her by reiterating her complaints of how difficult it must be to live with her diabetes and how angry it must make her. First he labeled her defiance as being "stubborn." Then he positively reframed her stubbornness as "strength of character," because she would not do something (adherence) she did not believe in, even if it meant ending up in the hospital. Finally, the therapist used his fragile alliance to discuss gently how he "wouldn't dream of challenging her, even though he would 'like' to see her eat ... and be happier." At that point, she asked if he could help her to be happy. He avoided accepting this shift of goal and responsibility by responding vaguely, "Perhaps more happy than you are, or less dissatisfied, but that's all I can tell you." He ended the session by realistically settling with her agreement to return the next week to talk about whether she wanted to change. There was eventually a positive outcome with this patient, because for the first time she was listened to, instead of being pushed to change. The usual power struggle was averted, and she no longer needed to defy her diet to maintain her own integrity and sense of self.

Clearly, reframing is not a technique to be used lightly, or it can appear to be mere flattery. Yet, it can be very effective in handling cases in which you may feel stuck by a patient's defensiveness or negativity. If searched for, there is usually some aspect of a person's behavior or situation that can be positively reframed.

There are many ways of using reframing. Some steps to follow are

- Identify the defensive part of the patient's language or behavior. In the previous example, it would be the woman's non-adherent behavior and "I don't care" attitude.

- Pace this defensive part by responding as if this is exactly what you would expect under the circumstances. Accept and try to understand how the patient is viewing the situation.

- Think of another way that this same set of behaviors or attitudes could be explained positively. Defiance becomes stubbornness and stubbornness becomes strength of character. This redefinition deflects the trap of entering a power struggle and allows an alliance to be established.

- Finally, keep expectations realistic and negotiate a goal that the patient can accept as being in his or her best interest.

Reframing is the technique of choice when it seems that there is not enough of a relationship established to tolerate a direct confrontation. It is particularly effective with patients whom counselors usually label "resistant." Instead of "resistant," they are viewed as self-protective. The assumption, discussed earlier, that "resistance is only a form of feedback" is a reframing of resistance that is meant to help the counselor avoid feeling stuck.

STAGE 5: MAINTAINING CHANGE

In the final stage of the nutritional counseling process, it is the counselor's responsibility to help the patient ensure that positive changes made during counseling will be maintained and incorporated into the patient's daily life style. This stage is often left to chance, perhaps, because it is thought that only through later follow-up can we know if the counseling interventions led to adherence to the meal plan. However, we can increase the lasting success of interventions if the following steps are taken.

When a specific suggestion has been made and agreed to, spend a few minutes using visual-ization to rehearse mentally how the patient will implement the change at home. For example, if a newly diagnosed insulin-dependent diabetes mellitus patient's goal is to learn to feel more comfortable doing a fingerstick blood test when dining out, this behavior can be practiced right in the office with mental rehearsal through the use of visualization. The nutritional counselor can ask the patient to close his or her eyes and imagine in detail (where are you, what room are you in, who is with you) the next time that he or she will encounter this situation. Then you can lead the patient through a mental rehearsal of how he or she achieves the desired outcome.

This kind of preparation tends to remove the element of surprise when the patient later must really perform in that situation. It builds in the associations that will cue the appropriate feelings or behavior. It also provides a fail-safe opportunity to anticipate any questions or difficulties that might arise later when you are not available to support the patient.

The patient's success in maintaining the change would normally signal the end of the counseling process. However, there is no cure yet for diabetes and physical as well as life-style changes may require additional adjustments in management. It can be reassuring for persons with diabetes to know that you will be available in the future should they need further counseling.

REFERENCES

1. Ivey AE, Matthews WJ. A meta-model for structuring the clinical interview. *J Am Assoc Counsel Dev.* 1984;63:237.

2. Grinder J, Bandler R. *The Structure of Magic 11.* Palo Alto, Calif: Science and Behavior Books; 1976.

3. Feste C. A practical look at patient empowerment. *Diabetes Care.* 1992;15:922.

4. Lankton S, Lankton C. *The Answer Within: A Clinical Framework of Ericksonian Hypnotherapy.* New York, NY: Brunner/Mazel; 1983.

5. Bandler R, Grinder J. *Frogs into Princes.* Moab, Utah: Real People Press; 1979.

6. Gordon D, Meyers-Anderson M. *Phoenix: Therapeutic Patterns of Milton H. Erickson.* Cupertino, Calif: Meta Publications; 1981.

7. Ivey AE, Authier J. *Microcounseling.* Springfield, Ill: Charles C Thomas; 1978.

8. Campbell MK, DeVellis BM, Strecher VJ, Ammerman AS, DeVellis RF, Sandler RS. Improving dietary behavior: the effectiveness of tailored messages in primary care settings. *Am J Public Health.* 1994;84:5.

9. Mayerson EW. *Putting the Ill at Ease.* Hagerstown, Md: Harper & Row; 1976.

10. Anderson RR, Funnell MM, Butler PM, Arnold MS, Fitzgerald JT, Feste CC. Patient empowerment: results of a randomized controlled trial. *Diabetes Care.* 1995;18:943.

11. Watzlawick P, Weakland J, Fisch R. *Change: Principles of Problem Formation and Problem Resolution.* New York, NY: WW Norton; 1974.

12. Curry SJ, Kristal AR, Bowen DJ. An application of the stage model of behavior change to dietary fat reduction. *Health Educ Res.* 1992;7:1.

13. Prochaska JO, DiClemente CC, Norcross JC. In search of how people change: applications to addictive behaviors. *Am Psychol.* 1992;47:9.

14. Zifferblatt SM, Wilbur CS. Dietary counseling: some realistic expectations and guidelines. *J Am Diet Assoc.* 1977;70:591.

15. Ferguson J. Dietitians as behavior-change agents. *J Am Diet Assoc.* 1978;73:231.

16. Dunbar JM, Stunkard AJ. Adherence to diet and drug regimen. In: Levy R, Rifkind B, Dennis B, Emest N, eds. *Nutrition, Lipids, and Coronary Heart Disease.* New York, NY: Raven; 1979.

17. Meichenbaum D, Turk D. *Facilitating Treatment Adherence: A Practitioner's Guidebook.* New York, NY: Plenum Press; 1987.

18. Janis IL. The role of social support in adherence to stressful decisions. *Am Psychol.* 1983;38:143.

19. Hammond DC, Hepworth DH, Smith VG. *Improving Therapeutic Communication.* San Francisco, Calif: Jossey-Bass; 1977.

20. Hauenstein DJ, Schiller MR, Hurley R. Motivational techniques of dietitians counseling individuals with type II diabetes. *J Am Diet Assoc.* 1987;87:37.

21. Engen HB, Iasiello-Vailas L, Smith KL. Confrontation: a new dimension in nutrition counseling. *J Am Diet Assoc.* 1983;83:34.

22. Leslie CA, Satin-Rapaport W, Matheson D, Stone R, Enfield G. Psychological insulin resistance: a missed diagnosis? *Diabetes Spectrum.* 1994;7:54.

23. Eisenberg S, Delaney DJ. *The Counseling Process.* Chicago, Ill: Rand McNally; 1977.

24. Sommer R. *The Mind's Eye: Imagery in Everyday Life.* New York, NY: Delta Books; 1978.

25. Kosslyn SM. *Ghosts in the Mind's Machine.* New York, NY: WW Norton; 1983.

26. Minuchin S, Fishman HC. *Family Therapy Techniques.* Cambridge, Mass: Harvard University Press; 1981.

27. Watzlawick P. *The Language of Change.* New York, NY: Basic Books; 1978.

28. Hoffman L. I don't want to be a fool. *Family Process.* 1983;22:133.

SUGGESTED READING

Arnold MS, Butler PM, Anderson RM, Funnell MM, Feste C. Guidelines for facilitating a patient empowerment program. *Diabetes Educ.* 1995;21:310–311.

Feste C. *The Physician Within: Taking Charge of Your Well-Being.* Minneapolis, Minn: Diabetes Centers, Inc; 1987.

Hertzler AA, Owen C. Culture, families, and the change process—a systems approach. *J Am Diet Assoc.* 1984;84:535.

Miller SR, Winstead-Fry P. *Family Systems Theory in Nursing Practice.* Reston, Va: Reston Press; 1982.

Minuchin S. *Families and Family Therapy.* Cambridge, Mass: Harvard University Press; 1974.

Minuchin S, Rosman BL, Baker L. *Psychosomatic Families: Anorexia Nervosa in Context.* Cambridge, Mass: Harvard University Press; 1978.

Prochaska JO, Norcross JC, DiClemente CC. *Changing for Good: The Revolutionary Program that Explains the Six Stages of Change and Teaches You How To Free Yourself from Bad Habits.* New York, NY: William Morrow Company; 1994.

Ruggerio L, Prochaska JO. Readiness for change: application of the transtheoretical model to diabetes. *Diabetes Spectrum.* 1993;6:22–60.

Snetselaar LG. *Nutrition Counseling Skills: Assessment, Treatment, and Evaluation: Second Edition.* Gaithersburg, Md: Aspen Publishers; 1989.

Part III

Selecting a Nutrition Education Approach

Chapter 11

Expanding Meal-Planning Approaches

Joyce Green Pastors

There is substantial agreement among both health care professionals and persons with diabetes that "diet" constitutes the biggest problem in diabetes care.[1] We, the medical community, typically blame the person with diabetes. Comments such as "he is noncompliant with his diet" or "she is just not motivated" are routine among health care professionals. A primary reason for "diet failure" and noncompliance is simply lack of nutrition self-management training. Most people with diabetes, especially those diagnosed with non–insulin-dependent diabetes mellitus (NIDDM), received limited or no diabetes nutrition education and are not referred to registered dietitians for nutrition education and counseling.[2,3] Instead, they may experience one of the following scenarios:

1. They are given a "diet sheet" that provides only very basic information about food exchanges, a meal plan, and a sample menu.
2. They are given a list of "good" and "bad" foods.
3. They are told to avoid sugar and/or to lose weight.
4. They are given an exchange list booklet with a prescribed calorie level just before hospital discharge.

This is particularly unfortunate for people with NIDDM, for whom some nutrition/weight control, exercise, and motivational counseling at the time of diagnosis may be all they need to achieve normoglycemia, improve hyperlipidemia and hypertension, or prevent or delay the need for medications and the complications of diabetes. This is evidenced in a recent study conducted to assess the impact of medical nutrition therapy provided by dietitians on medical and clinical outcomes for people with NIDDM. The study also compared basic nutrition care (single visit with a dietitian) to practice guidelines nutrition care (initial visit with a dietitian followed by two follow-up visits during the first six weeks). Medical nutrition therapy by dietitians resulted in significant improvements in medical and clinical outcomes in both the basic care and practice guidelines care groups and is beneficial to people with NIDDM.[4]

FALSE PREMISES

There appear to be some standard premises or beliefs and accepted practices for the treatment of diabetes. In the specific area of nutritional management, a few of these premises are presented below with specific rationale for why they are false.

- *People with diabetes need a highly structured meal plan.* A *meal plan* should not be considered a "diet" but rather a "guide to healthy eating." Diabetes is a *chronic* disease. Nutrition recommendations should be those that can be incorporated on a long-term basis.

  The American Diabetes Association 1994 nutrition recommendations state, "There is no ONE diabetic or ADA diet. Medical nutrition therapy for persons with diabetes should be individualized, with consideration given to usual eating habits and other lifestyle factors" (p. 522).[5]

Not everyone needs structure to make healthy food choices; for some, too much structure may lead to noncompliance. Given that most people with NIDDM are overweight and older than the age of 40, they are a population group who have long-established habits and patterns of eating. An individualized meal plan means more than making adjustments for food preferences and distributing the calories based on usual eating patterns. Selecting an appropriate meal-planning approach based on a person's educational and nutritional needs and willing- ness to control diabetes are the keys to individualizing the meal plan. When the person understands how to plan his or her meals, the nutritional needs can be more easily attained and the diabetes better managed.

- *The exchange system is the only meal-planning approach for people with diabetes.* For some people, food exchange lists may be an antiquated or inappropriate meal-planning approach. In the 1950s when the exchange lists were developed, people ate more simply, they rarely ate mixed dishes, they rarely ate out, and convenience foods were just being introduced and not a necessary part of meal planning. A meal-planning approach simply means the "educational resource" used by the diabetes educator to teach the person with diabetes how to plan his or her meals. A variety of meal-planning approaches are available for the diabetes educator to educate effectively. The type of meal-planning approach used should take into consideration the following points:

1. the person's ability and/or willingness to learn

2. the person's level of motivation to make the needed changes in his or her eating habits

3. clinical goals (eg, target blood glucose and lipid goals)

4. nutrition therapy goals established by the person with diabetes, the registered dietitian, and other members of the diabetes care team (eg, decrease saturated fat and calories, increase physical activity)

5. type and amount of insulin or oral hypoglycemic agent used (if any)

6. the person's activity level

7. the person's life style (job/school schedule; current eating habits; "favorite foods"; religious/ethnic food beliefs; social and economic factors)

PROCESS OF SELF-MANAGEMENT TRAINING

More important than deciding which meal-planning approach to select is that the process of nutrition self-management training be implemented. It is important to differentiate between content and process in diabetes nutrition education. We must consider not only providing information (content) about diabetes and nutrition but also how this information can most effectively be presented (process).

The purpose of self-management training is to assist in acquiring and maintaining the knowledge, skills, attitudes, behaviors, and commitment needed to successfully meet the challenges of daily diabetes management. This is not accomplished by one therapy session but rather by a process of staged teaching over a longer period of time.

Nutritional therapy for the person with diabetes should be approached in a logically organized and consistent manner that is designed to ensure the highest quality of care. A logical sequence for the process of nutrition education includes (1) rapport establishment; (2) assessment; (3) goal setting; (4) intervention; and (5) evaluation and follow-up. The focus of this chapter is on nutrition intervention (ie, meal planning).

SELECTING AN APPROACH

Ideally, nutrition intervention should be conducted in stages. In spite of terminology used to describe these stages, the standard that should be applied to all nutrition intervention is that it is based on a comprehensive nutrition assessment. For the purposes of this chapter, the wording chosen to describe the stages of nutrition intervention is "initial" and "in-depth" intervention.

1. *Initial intervention*—providing basic information about nutrition and nutrient requirements, discussing the diabetes nutrition management guidelines, providing guidance in making initial changes in selection of food choices, and introducing other "beginning" information that may be important specific to the type of diabetes. The educational resources that can be used to teach basic nutrition and diabetes nutrition guidelines can be referred to as *guideline approaches.*

2. *In-depth intervention*—selecting a more structured meal planning approach for achieving individually determined goals and providing continuity of care. It is in the in-depth intervention stage that more emphasis is placed on meal planning, and often a more structured plan for what to eat is developed. Developing an individualized plan of eating can be accomplished through the use of a variety of options including use of menus, food exchanges, or counting of calories, points, or grams of carbohydrate or fat and, as such, can be referred to as *meal-planning approaches.*

A more comprehensive discussion of initial and nutrition intervention, more specific to clinical application of meal-planning approaches, can be found in a recent publication of the American Dietetic Association, *Meal Planning Approaches for Diabetes Management.*[6]

GUIDELINE APPROACHES

The diabetes educator needs to conduct a comprehensive nutrition assessment to make the best decision about how to introduce nutrition and meal planning. Guideline approaches can be used to provide the foundation of basic nutrition information and can also be used as an assessment tool to determine nutrient adequacy. In some cases, they may provide the necessary information for some persons with diabetes to change eating behaviors. Whether or not they are used as stand-alone resources for diabetes nutrition education, they are a good choice for "starting" the education process!

Using guideline approaches will allow the diabetes educator to individualize the education based on the client's knowledge, interest, and ability to make changes in current eating patterns. Specific ideas for improvements in meal planning can be made without having to provide large amounts of detailed information. However, because of the lack of more structured information about meal planning, they may be less effective in achieving the degree of glucose control desired, especially for persons interested in "fine-tuning" their glucose control (ie, giving particular attention to nutrient and caloric intake) and for persons who need to lose weight and would benefit from a structured eating plan with an emphasis on calories and decreased fat intake.

Guideline approaches are intended to provide some consistency in food intake, but the primary emphasis is on making healthier food choices without weighing and measuring foods, using exchanges, or counting points, calories, fat, or carbohydrate.

Basic nutrition guidelines provide an understanding of the basic principles of nutrition and guidance in selecting an adequately balanced eating plan for optimal health. Educational resources (see Appendix 11-A) that can be used to teach basic nutrition guidelines include

- National Dairy Council's *Guide to Good Eating*

- USDA-HHS's *Dietary Guidelines for Americans*

- USDA's *Food Guide Pyramid*

Diabetes nutrition guidelines provide the person with diabetes an understanding of the connection between nutrition and diabetes. They give the person direction in making appropriate food choices for managing their diabetes. Educational resources that can be used to teach diabetes nutrition guidelines from the American Dietetic and the American Diabetes Association include

- *Healthy Food Choices*
- *The First Step in Diabetes Meal Planning*
- *Facilitating Lifestyle Change: A Resource Manual*
- 21 single-topic diabetes resources

Guide to Good Eating

The National Dairy Council's *Guide to Good Eating* categorizes foods according to their major nutrient composition. Each of the food groups (milk, meat, vegetable, fruit, and grain) are characterized by certain leader nutrients; for example, the leader nutrients for each of the five food groups are calcium, iron, vitamins A and C, and fiber, respectively. Foods of low nutrient density, those containing calories primarily from sugar or fat, are placed in the "others" category. Serving sizes of various foods within a food group are approximately equivalent in leader nutrients but not necessarily equivalent in caloric value. A minimum number of daily servings from each group is recommended for each age group to achieve approximately 80% of the daily requirement of nine leader nutrients. It is assumed that if a variety of foods is chosen from each of the food groups, the daily requirement for all nutrients will be met. The intent of the *Guide to Good Eating* is to give guidance in choosing nutritionally adequate daily food intakes. The emphasis is on providing an approach that is simple and easy to understand.

The basic four food groups were developed in 1954 by the USDA, replacing the earlier basic seven, and were intended to translate the quantitative nutrient-based recommended dietary allowance (RDA) information into practical terms

for the average person. The basic four food guide had been the most widely used food grouping system in the United States and one adapted by several organizations. The *Guide to Good Eating* has been adapted several times to reflect the recommendations of the USDA and changes in the RDA and newer knowledge about the nutrient content of foods. In 1993, a revised version was released as a tool to complement the *Food Guide Pyramid,* introduced by the USDA in 1992.

The *Guide to Good Eating* places emphasis on nutritionally sound eating rather than promoting the concept of a "diet" or a modified eating plan. It can also be used as a tool for assessing a person's current food choices, enabling the diabetes educator to check easily for nutrient adequacy. For many persons with diabetes, the guidelines presented in the *Guide to Good Eating* may be all that is required for making changes in their eating habits. For other persons who need more structure or for those who have not obtained the desired blood glucose control, progression to an individualized meal-planning approach may be necessary.

Dietary Guidelines for Americans

Dietary Guidelines for Americans is a basic nutrition guide aimed at all Americans for the purpose of health promotion and the prevention of chronic diseases. The recommended nutrition guidelines are: eat a variety of foods; maintain healthy weight; choose a diet low in fat, saturated fat, and cholesterol; choose a diet with plenty of vegetables, fruits, and grain products; use sugars only in moderation; use salt and sodium in moderation; and if you drink alcoholic beverages, do so in moderation. The current 1990 edition, which is the third edition, of the guidelines was developed and is distributed by the United States Department of Agriculture and the Department of Health and Human Services. The guidelines were adapted from *Dietary Goals for the U.S.*, developed as a result of hearings of the U.S. Senate Select Committee on Nutrition and Human Needs in 1977. The first and second editions of the guidelines were released in 1980 and 1985, respectively. The intent of *Dietary Guidelines for Americans* is to give healthy people guidance in choosing a more nutritionally balanced diet. The emphasis is on providing an approach that is simple, easy to understand, and adaptable to the person's needs.

Food Guide Pyramid

The *Food Guide Pyramid* is an illustration of the eating guidelines presented in the *Dietary Guidelines for Americans*. It is a general guide for persons to choose a well-balanced diet by recommending a variety of foods to obtain the necessary nutrients. It also provides a guide to obtaining the needed calories to maintain a healthy weight.

The *Food Guide Pyramid* is built on using more complex carbohydrates, which form the base (grains, fruits, vegetables). As the pyramid ascends to the peak, lesser emphasis is placed on foods higher in fat and sugar (meats, dairy products). This educational resource provides an excellent visual of the dietary guidelines and the concept of food grouping.

Healthy Food Choices

Healthy Food Choices is a pamphlet that promotes healthy eating. It is divided into two sections: (1) guidelines for making "healthy food choices," and (2) simplified exchange lists to be used as an introduction to the exchange system. Specific guidelines are included for those who want to decrease fat, salt, and sugar intake and increase fiber intake.

Healthy Food Choices was initially developed by the committee that coordinated the revision of the exchange lists in 1986. It was updated again in 1995 to be consistent with the 1995 revision of the *Exchange Lists for Meal Planning*. It is a joint publication of the American Dietetic Association and the American Diabetes Association. The goal in designing this piece and concurrently publishing it along with the revised exchange lists was to enhance the concept that not

all clients need to use the exchange lists for meal planning. It was intended to provide an introduction to diabetes meal planning with an emphasis on healthy eating. The person who desires to advance to the exchange system could use the simplified lists as the initial step. Two approaches to meal planning, diabetes nutrition guidelines and simplified exchanges, are presented in the pamphlet.

Healthy Food Choices is primarily useful for the "initial stage" of education in diabetes meal planning. It must be remembered that many persons with diabetes may remain at the initial level of education for quite some time or may never advance to the "in-depth" education stage. The diabetes educator should not try to progress through it too quickly, rather provide encouragement and guidance while relying on the person's questions and progress as indicators of readiness for advancement. Supplemental reading materials on the various points addressed (fat, sodium, fiber, food preparation, etc) may be provided to take the pamphlet toward the in-depth stage.

Healthy Food Choices is appropriate for most persons with diabetes because it offers an overview of diabetes nutritional management within the framework of basic eating guidelines and the simplified exchange system. Because it introduces two approaches to nutrition education, diabetes nutrition guidelines and a simplified exchange list, there is concern for potential misuse in that both approaches might be introduced at the same time when it is only appropriate to teach a singular approach.

First Step in Diabetes Meal Planning

The First Step in Diabetes Meal Planning is a modified food guide pyramid that teaches basic diabetes meal-planning goals. The primary purpose of this tool is to help persons newly diagnosed with diabetes to choose healthy foods and plan healthy meals until they can see a dietitian. It can serve as a "stand-alone" educational resource without the aid of a dietitian or a diabetes educator. It is intended for persons who may not have immediate access to meal-planning instruction from a dietitian; for example, a person leaving a physician's office or clinic or a person who has called the American Dietetic Association or the American Diabetes Association for information about meal planning.

The pamphlet presents a few concepts very simply, with the literacy level being approximately 5th to 7th grade. Like *Healthy Food Choices*, it is divided into two sections. The first section provides information about the why, how, and how to for beginning diabetes meal planning. The second section is a food pyramid (Figure 11-1) with six different categories (ie, grains/beans/starchy vegetables that form the base of the pyramid; vegetables and fruits represent the next level of the pyramid; milks and meats the third level of the pyramid; and fats, sweets, and alcohol form the apex of the pyramid). Each category is color-coded, provides food examples, lists number of servings per day, and includes a "tips" section.

The First Step in Diabetes Meal Planning was developed by a work group of the American Dietetic Association and the American Diabetes Association Nutrition Education Resources Steering Committee and was made available for publication in March 1995.

Facilitating Lifestyle Change: A Resource Manual

Facilitating Lifestyle Change is a resource manual designed for dietitians and other diabetes educators to assist clients in monitoring to promote changes toward a more healthy life style, specifically with the aspects of healthier eating and increasing physical activity. It is intended for all persons with diabetes, as well as for people who are overweight or for those who are interested in making life-style changes. The manual contains copy-ready reproducible masters of monitoring forms for assessment, goal setting, intervention, and evaluation.

The assessment resources include a *Lifestyle Questionnaire* (contains sections on Nutrition History with a Typical Food Intake Form,

Weight History, Physical Activity History, Record-Keeping History, and Expectations) and an *Eating Behavior Diary*, which is an assessment tool to provide clients with experience in monitoring eating behaviors to become more aware of how they influence eating.

The *Lifestyle Change Plan* is a tool to assist in setting goals to improve problem life-style behaviors. The categories on this form include sections on choosing a goal, developing an action plan, choosing a reward, and evaluating what worked.

The resources developed to self-monitor lifestyle behaviors include a daily record for keeping track and problem solving (*Diabetes Self-Care: Daily Record and Personal Lifestyle Record*), as well as weekly and monthly records to be used for evaluating progress (*Diabetes Self-Care: Blood Glucose-at-a-Glance, Diabetes Self-Care: Month-at-a-Glance,* and *Personal Lifestyle-at-a-Glance*).

In addition to the monitoring forms, this resource manual provides the dietitian/diabetes educator with a guide for how to use each of the resources, including sample cases, and appendixes of additional professional education resources that can be used in working with clients interested in making behavioral/life-style changes.

Single-Topic Diabetes Resources

Each of these 21 diabetes nutrition-related topics is available as a double-sided reproducible master and is interactive, emphasizing goal setting and problem solving (Exhibit 11-2). The 21 topics fit into the three categories of nutrition and food, general diabetes, and diabetes and life style. Examples of the topics include "what about sugars," "understanding fats," "when you cannot eat," "hypoglycemia," "supermarket smarts," and "older persons with diabetes."

A professional guide will accompany the single-topic diabetes resources that will contain general information about how to integrate the use of each piece in the educational process.

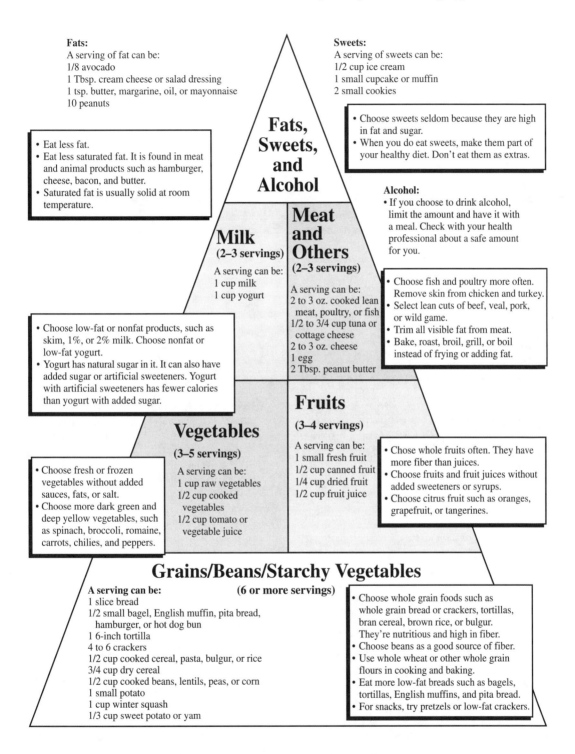

Fats:
A serving of fat can be:
1/8 avocado
1 Tbsp. cream cheese or salad dressing
1 tsp. butter, margarine, oil, or mayonnaise
10 peanuts

Sweets:
A serving of sweets can be:
1/2 cup ice cream
1 small cupcake or muffin
2 small cookies

- Choose sweets seldom because they are high in fat and sugar.
- When you do eat sweets, make them part of your healthy diet. Don't eat them as extras.

- Eat less fat.
- Eat less saturated fat. It is found in meat and animal products such as hamburger, cheese, bacon, and butter.
- Saturated fat is usually solid at room temperature.

Fats, Sweets, and Alcohol

Alcohol:
- If you choose to drink alcohol, limit the amount and have it with a meal. Check with your health professional about a safe amount for you.

Milk
(2–3 servings)

A serving can be:
1 cup milk
1 cup yogurt

Meat and Others
(2–3 servings)

A serving can be:
2 to 3 oz. cooked lean meat, poultry, or fish
1/2 to 3/4 cup tuna or cottage cheese
2 to 3 oz. cheese
1 egg
2 Tbsp. peanut butter

- Choose fish and poultry more often. Remove skin from chicken and turkey.
- Select lean cuts of beef, veal, pork, or wild game.
- Trim all visible fat from meat.
- Bake, roast, broil, grill, or boil instead of frying or adding fat.

- Choose low-fat or nonfat products, such as skim, 1%, or 2% milk. Choose nonfat or low-fat yogurt.
- Yogurt has natural sugar in it. It can also have added sugar or artificial sweeteners. Yogurt with artificial sweeteners has fewer calories than yogurt with added sugar.

Vegetables
(3–5 servings)

A serving can be:
1 cup raw vegetables
1/2 cup cooked vegetables
1/2 cup tomato or vegetable juice

Fruits
(3–4 servings)

A serving can be:
1 small fresh fruit
1/2 cup canned fruit
1/4 cup dried fruit
1/2 cup fruit juice

- Chose whole fruits often. They have more fiber than juices.
- Choose fruits and fruit juices without added sweeteners or syrups.
- Choose citrus fruit such as oranges, grapefruit, or tangerines.

- Choose fresh or frozen vegetables without added sauces, fats, or salt.
- Choose more dark green and deep yellow vegetables, such as spinach, broccoli, romaine, carrots, chilies, and peppers.

Grains/Beans/Starchy Vegetables
(6 or more servings)

A serving can be:
1 slice bread
1/2 small bagel, English muffin, pita bread, hamburger, or hot dog bun
1 6-inch tortilla
4 to 6 crackers
1/2 cup cooked cereal, pasta, bulgur, or rice
3/4 cup dry cereal
1/2 cup cooked beans, lentils, peas, or corn
1 small potato
1 cup winter squash
1/3 cup sweet potato or yam

- Choose whole grain foods such as whole grain bread or crackers, tortillas, bran cereal, brown rice, or bulgur. They're nutritious and high in fiber.
- Choose beans as a good source of fiber.
- Use whole wheat or other whole grain flours in cooking and baking.
- Eat more low-fat breads such as bagels, tortillas, English muffins, and pita bread.
- For snacks, try pretzels or low-fat crackers.

Figure 11-1 Food Pyramid *Source:* Reprinted from *The First Steps in Diabetes Meal Planning* with permission of the American Diabetes Association and the American Dietetic Association, © 1995.

Exhibit 11-2 An Example of a Single-Topic Diabetes Resource

DIABETES: SUGARS AND SWEETS

 What about you?

- Have you ever been told to avoid sugar and sweets?
- What are your favorite sweet foods and sweet drinks?

_____

- How often do you have sweet foods or sweet drinks? _____ times per day _____ times per week
- Do you feel deprived if you try to cut down on sweet foods? yes/no
- Do you read food labels to find out how much sugar is in foods? yes/no

? Why learn about sugars?

- You do not have to give up sugars and sweets when you have diabetes.
- There are many different types of sugars and sweets.
- You can enjoy sweet foods and stay in control of your diabetes if you know how to eat small amounts and how to count sweets in your meal plan.

What will you learn?

- What sugars are and how they affect blood glucose.
- Which foods contain different types of sugar.
- How to fit sugars into your food plan.
- How to use food labels to count sweet and high-sugar foods in your food plan.

From simple to complex

- There are two main types of carbohydrate: sugars (simple carbohydrate), such as jelly beans or hard candy, and starches (complex carbohydrate), such as pasta, bread, or rice.
- Sugars and starches both make your blood glucose go up. They make blood glucose go up about the same amount and about the same speed.

This handout gives general guidelines for everyone with diabetes. Your educator can help you learn more and decide what will work for you.

- Sugars are found naturally in some foods, such as fruit (glucose and fructose) and milk (lactose). Other foods and drinks have sugars added to them, such as high-fructose corn syrup in fruit drinks. Both natural and added sugars have the same effect on your blood glucose.
- Sugars and starches both have 4 calories per gram.
- Sugar alcohols, such as sorbitol, xylitol, and mannitol, have fewer calories than sugars and starches—2–3 calories per gram. They may be found in sugar-free chewing gum, candy, or cookies.

Choosing carbohydrates

- Sugars have the same amount of carbohydrate as starches. But starchy foods also have vitamins, mineals, and fiber.
- If you eat a lot of sugary foods as part of your meal plan, you may miss out on important nutrients.
- Starchy foods are more bulky than sugary foods. You can eat more and you will feel more full if you choose complex carbohydrates, rather than simple carbohydrates.
- These foods all have 15 grams (g) carbohydrate:

Complex carbohydrate	_Simple carbohydrate_
1 6-inch tortilla	1 tablespoon maple syrup
3 cups popcorn	1/4 cup sherbert
1 1/2 cups broccoli	1/24th angel food cake

Note how much more food the same amount of carbohydrate is if the food is complex, rather than simple.
- Foods made with a lot of sugars are often also high in fat. If you choose to eat these foods, you will need to count the fat in your meal plan, too. For example:

　2 small sandwich cookies with creme filling = 15 g carbohydrate and 5 g fat
　1 glazed doughnut = 30 grams carbohydrate and 10 g fat
　1/2 cup ice cream = 15 g carbohydrate and 10 g fat

(Note: If you use exchanges, 15 g carbohydrate = 1 carbohydrate exchange, 5 g fat = 1 fat exchange.)

Courtesy of

Reading food labels

- Read the ingredient list. There are many forms of sugar, such as:

corn syrup	dextrose
fruit juice concentrate	fructose
high-fructose corn syrup	glucose
honey	lactose
maple syrup	maltose
molasses	sucrose
raw sugar	

- The Nutrition Facts panel shows you the total amount of carbohydrate in one serving of the food. It also shows how much of the total carbohydrate is sugars. The amount of sugars includes the natural sugar in milk, fruit, and some vegetables, as well as any added sugars.

- Check the serving size. Is this the amount you normally eat? Your educator can show you how to use the numbers on food labels to fit sweet foods into your food plan.

- By law:
  - -Sugar-free foods have less than 1/2 gram sugars per serving.
  - -Reduced-sugar foods have at least 25% less sugar than regular foods.
  - -Foods with no added sugars do not have any form of sugar added during processing or packaging, do not contain high-sugar ingredients, and can be used instead of a high-sugar food.

- Sugar-free foods are not necessarily low in calories. Check the Nutrition Facts panel.

Eating sugars and sweets

- It's OK to have high-sugar foods or sweet drinks for part of the carbohydrate in your food plan once in a while. Think about which carbohydrate foods you will trade for high-sugar foods.

- Eat small amounts of high-sugar foods. Split a dessert with a friend or order a small scoop in an ice cream shop.

- Check your blood glucose before and after eating high-sugar foods to learn how your body responds to sugars.

- Take advantage of foods or drinks made with low-calorie sweeteners rather than sugars for a sweet taste without the calories.

Set your sights

1. I will have _____(amount) of _____(high-sugar food) instead of _____(carbohydrate food) at _____(meal or time of day)_____times per week

2. _____
   _____
   _____
   _____
   _____

Keep track

Food item: _____

Amount eaten: _____

Blood glucose levels:

   Before eating_____mg/dL

   1 hour after eating_____mg/dL

   2 hours after eating_____mg/dL

Here's the challenge: What's your solution?

1. You and others at work take turns bringing treats on Fridays. Most people bring in cookies, brownies, or doughnuts. You want to enjoy the sweets. How will you fit them into your food plan?

   _____

2. Your food plan has four carbohydrate selections or a total of 60 grams of carbohydrate at dinner. A restaurant meal comes with baked potato, rice, or steamed vegetables as well as homemade dinner rolls. The dessert menu includes fresh fruit and layer cake. What will you choose to eat?

   _____

3. _____
   _____
   _____
   _____
   _____
   _____
   _____
   _____

Source: Developed by Karen M. Bolderman Sporney, RD, CDE. Reprinted with permission from *Single Topic Resources—Diabetes: Sugars and Sweets*, Copyright © 1995, American Diabetes Association and The American Dietetic Association.

MEAL-PLANNING APPROACHES

The in-depth stage of the nutrition intervention process provides more information about meal planning. In-depth nutrition education, specifically, is information that provides more structure to the process of meal planning and/or provides specific nutrient (ie, fat, carbohydrate) or calorie information to assist with meal planning.

As with many other aspects of health care, decisions need to be made about nutrition education that often require using your best clinical judgment. A few of these often-faced decisions are addressed below.

1. *Do I need to advance everyone from the basic to the in-depth stage of education?* Many people do well with guideline information and do not need more structured information about meal planning. This decision is based on more than intellect or literacy level. Many well-educated people may only need or want basic information. They may not have time to use a more in-depth system of meal planning or they do not need it to adopt a healthy eating plan and meet their diabetes-nutrition therapy goals. Conversely, those who are not able to comprehend a more in-depth approach to meal planning (exchanges or a system of counting) may need to remain at the basic stage of nutrition education indefinitely. This does not mean that they only need one education session or that any follow-up sessions should be just a review of information. The challenge is to present new information using techniques that are individualized to their particular needs. The information should empower them to make gradual changes in their life style and eating behaviors that are permanent.

2. *What nutrition education materials should I use?* It is important to choose from a variety of materials rather than always disseminating the same standardized educational material. We all work with persons whose backgrounds, life styles, needs, interests, and diabetes management goals are vastly different, and as a result, their educational needs will differ considerably. Our goal should be to individualize the education and counseling sessions for each person with diabetes rather than to use the same procedure for everyone.

3. *Do I need to provide educational materials to every person with diabetes?* It is okay to decide that the educational material you usually use and that is available to you may not be appropriate. Instead, you may want to develop your own materials or choose not to give any printed material. Another strategy may be to start by establishing short-term eating behavior goals with the person, writing them out on a piece of paper, and simply giving that as your educational resource.

4. *What are the in-depth meal-planning approaches?* For purposes of simplification, the in-depth meal planning approaches that are discussed have been placed into subcategories based on their similarities. The three subcategories and meal planning approaches include (1) Menu approaches to meal planning (individualized menus and *Month of Meals-1 to 5*), (2) exchange list approaches (*Exchange Lists for Meal Planning*), and (3) counting approaches to meal planning (calorie counting, fat counting, fat/calorie counting, carbohydrate counting).

Menu Approaches

The menu is the basis of all meal-planning approaches. It is the written description of what actually can and should be eaten. Ideally, the dietitian will incorporate some degree of menu planning into whatever nutrition counseling approach is chosen. In fact, the dietitian should write out at least one sample menu to illustrate how meals can be designed to fit the person's individual nutrition care plan.

Exhibit 11-3 Individualized Menus

Breakfast **Time: 8:00 A.M.**	**Breakfast** **Time: 8:00 A.M.**

Breakfast　　　　**Time: 8:00 A.M.**
- Hot cereal (1/2 cup oatmeal, cream of wheat, or grits)
- Margarine (1 tsp)
- 2% milk (1 cup)
- Fresh orange (1 small) **or** grapefruit half
- Coffee

Lunch　　　　**Time: 12:30 P.M.**
- Sandwich:
  –Bread (2 slices) or hamburger roll (1)
  –Meat (2 oz roast beef, ham, turkey, chicken, or tuna)
  –Mayonnaise or margarine (1 tsp)
- Sliced fresh carrots and/or celery (1/2 cup)
- Diet iced tea

Dinner　　　　**Time: 6:30 P.M.**
- Meat/fish/poultry (select 3 oz of one of the following: baked or broiled ground beef patty, chicken breast, fish, or pork chop)
- Collards, broccoli, **or** green beans
- Whole wheat bread (1 slice) with margarine (1 tsp)
- Applesauce (1/2 cup unsweetened) **or** 1 small apple
- Diet drink

Snack　　　　**Time: 10:00 P.M.**
- Reduced calorie hot chocolate (1 pkt.)
- 2 graham cracker squares

Breakfast　　　　**Time: 8:00 A.M.**
- Sliced banana (1/2) **or** drained crushed pineapple (1/2 cup) mixed with
- Nonfat plain yogurt (1 cup)
- Bagel (half) **or** English muffin (half)
- Margarine (1 tsp) **or** cream cheese (1 Tbsp)
- Coffee

Lunch　　　　**Time: 12:30 P.M.**
- Hot soup (1 cup broth-based, eg, chicken rice, beef vegetable)
- Ritz crackers (7)
- Cheese (2 oz mozzarella, Velveeta, **or** Casino)
- Tomato (1 fresh **or** 1/2 cup tomato juice)
- Diet lemonade

Dinner　　　　**Time: 6:30 P.M.**
- Sandwich
  –Bread (2 slices) or hamburger roll (1)
  –Meat (3 oz ground beef, roast beef, turkey, chicken, tuna)
  –Mayonnaise or margarine (1 tsp)
- Salad, tossed
- Reduced calorie dressing (1 Tbsp)
- Diet drink

Snack　　　　**Time: 10:00 P.M.**
- Bran flakes or wheat chex (1/2 cup)
- 2% milk (1/2 cup)

This section describes three types of menu planning that may be useful in nutrition counseling. The first, individualized menus, shows how menus can be written with the person to meet his or her individualized nutrition therapy goals. The second is menu planning based on the set of publications, *Month of Meals,* by the American Diabetes Association.

The use of preprinted menus, another menu-planning approach, is traditionally discouraged by dietitians on the basis that they are not individualized. There may be situations, however, in which preprinted menus could be developed specifically for a certain population (and therefore be more individualized to the eating style of that group). They can be useful for the dietitian when counseling time is very limited and there will be an opportunity at a later time to follow-up with a more customized approach.

The term *individualized menus* is defined as a method of meal planning whereby the dietitian works with the person to prepare menus that specify the foods (and appropriate quantities) that should be eaten over a period of days. The written menus reflect the individualized nutrition goals established between the person with diabetes and the dietitian (Exhibit 11-3). The menus can be very specific or involve some choices. The person is not expected to follow the menus forever but will gradually be learning, with the help of the dietitian, how to select foods and appropriate portion sizes.

The simplicity of this approach is its major advantage. Persons who have fairly routine eating habits and who eat at consistent times and in consistent places are likely to do better than those who have no routine. However, this method is also good for persons who follow no routine because it forces some structure and discipline while allowing freedom of choice regarding menu selection. The primary disadvantage with this approach is that, because of the structure, individualized menus may be too restrictive or monotonous in regard to food choices.

Month of Meals-1, Month of Meals-2, Month of Meals-3, Month of Meals-4, and *Month of Meals-5* are five separate books that teach the menu-planning approach for persons with diabetes. Each book contains 28 days of complete menus for breakfast, lunch, dinner, and snacks to provide a balanced healthy diet. Menus are written for a basic meal plan of 1500 calories daily, including three meals, plus two 60-calorie snacks or one 125-calorie snack. Lists of 125- and 170-calorie snacks are also provided to be used in the 1800-calorie diet pattern. Instructions are provided for how to adjust the calorie level upward or downward, with sample patterns for 1800 or 1200 calories.

Menus are designed to follow guidelines for good nutrition and/or the six food exchange groups. Menus provide 45 to 50% of calories from carbohydrate, 20% from protein, and about 30% from fat. Because each breakfast, lunch, and dinner contain approximately the same number of calories (350, 450, and 550, respectively), the person is encouraged to mix-and-match meals (which can be done as the pages are cut into thirds) to suit his or her own tastes. Whenever a special recipe is described, the actual recipe ingredients and preparation directions are included in a back section. Many menus incorporate recipes reprinted from American Diabetes Association cookbooks or *Diabetes Forecast*, whereas others are originals or from other sources provided by contributing authors of *Month of Meals.*

While certain elements are consistent in all five volumes, each volume has unique features.

Thus, the five volumes can be used individually or as a set. All five volumes include a review of diabetes nutrition guidelines, as well as the six food groups in *The Exchange Lists for Meal Planning*; "how-to" features are available in each volume. *Month of Meals-1* includes a special occasions section. *Month of Meals-2* adds in more ethnic foods and quick-to-fix items and meals, with a special chapter on dining out. *Month of Meals-3* continues the emphasis on time-saving meals, incorporating convenience foods and microwave recipes. Special sections cover food labeling lingo, fast foods, fiber, meal planning during illness, and picnics and barbecues. *Month of Meals-4* contains menus emphasizing old-time family favorites such as pot roast and meal loaf. Recipes for one or two people are featured, as well as hints for turning family-size meals into healthy left-overs. *Month of Meals-5* has a special focus on vegetarian meals.

Month of Meals-1 to 5 were developed by committees of the Council on Nutritional Science and Metabolism of the American Diabetes Association and staff members of the ADA National Service Center in 1989, 1990, 1991, 1992, and 1994, respectively. The publications were developed in response to frequent requests for menus to the ADA National Service Center from persons with diabetes and their families.

As with individualized menus, the simplicity of this approach is the major advantage. Persons with diabetes who have fairly routine eating habits and who eat at consistent times and in consistent places are likely to do better than the person who has no routine. Another advantage would be that the person with diabetes does not require any prior knowledge or experience with any meal-planning approach and would be able to follow the menus easily. Also, this option provides structure with food choices and amounts. The primary disadvantage with this approach is that because of the structure, some persons may find individualized menus too restrictive or monotonous in regard to food choices. If this is the case, the dietitian can modify the recipes to include additional foods and/or increased amounts of food.

Exchange List Approaches

Exchange Lists for Meal Planning originally grouped foods into six lists called, appropriately enough, exchange lists. Each list was a group of measured foods of approximately the same nutritional value; therefore, foods on each list could be substituted or "exchanged" with other foods in the same list. The six exchange lists were starch/bread, meat and meat substitutes, vegetables, fruit, milk, and fat. Within each food group, one exchange or choice was approximately equal to another in calories and in the amount of carbohydrate, protein, and fat it contains.

In 1995, a work group of the American Dietetic Association and the American Diabetes Association Nutrition Education Resources Steering Committee revised the *Exchange Lists for Meal Planning*. The exchange lists have been divided into three food groups:

1. Carbohydrate Group—this includes the Starch List, Fruit List, Milk List, Other Carbohydrate List, and the Vegetable List.

2. Meat and Meat Substitutes Group—this group contains four meat categories and represents the major source of protein in the exchange lists.

3. Fat Group—this group contains three fat categories.

See Chapter 12 for further information about the 1995 revisions of the *Exchange Lists for Meal Planning*.

Exchange Lists for Meal Planning also alerts consumers to foods that are good sources of dietary fiber and foods that contribute significant amounts of sodium. Foods on the fruit, vegetable, and whole-grain bread and cracker lists contribute an average of about 2 g of dietary fiber per exchange serving; however, a fiber symbol is next to foods that have 3 g or more fiber per serving. A sodium symbol is next to foods that contain 400 mg or more sodium per exchange serving; however, another symbol is next to foods that will also contribute 400 mg or more sodium per serving when two or more exchanges are eaten in 1 day.

The concept of "exchange" or "substitution" of different foods acceptable for use by clients was developed by the American Dietetic Association and the American Diabetes Association in 1950. Before their development, meal-planning approaches in the United States were chaotic, with no agreement on educational and meal-planning approaches among the major organizations involved with diabetes and nutrition. The goal was to develop an educational tool that would provide uniformity in meal planning and allow a wider variety of foods to be included.

Exchange Lists for Meal Planning can be used for persons with insulin-dependent diabetes mellitus (IDDM) or NIDDM. For persons with IDDM, these lists can be used to emphasize the need for consistency in the timing of food intake and to identify the amount of food to be eaten at meals and snacks while providing for needed variety and flexibility. For persons with NIDDM, they can be used to teach the caloric and fat values of foods.

When used with appropriate clients, the *Exchange Lists for Meal Planning* offers the following advantages: first, it provides a framework for grouping foods that takes into account the calorie, carbohydrate, protein, and fat content of foods; second, it emphasizes important nutritional management concepts such as calorie control, fat modifications, fiber content, and an awareness of high-sodium foods. *Exchange Lists for Meal Planning* can be used to teach persons with diabetes and health professionals the amount of carbohydrate, protein, fat, and calories contributed by foods. With an understanding of the basis of the exchange lists, clients and professionals can use nutrient values from food labels and can incorporate a wider variety of foods into the meal plan. *Exchange Lists for Meal Planning* is not appropriate for use if the person with diabetes and/or family members cannot understand the concept of "exchanging" foods or if they are unable to measure food portions accurately.

Counting Approaches

Calorie Counting

Calorie counting is a meal-planning approach that places major emphasis on the caloric density of food. This structured approach provides a specific calorie limit to the person with diabetes to achieve a weight loss, usually of 0.5 to 2 lb/wk. A calorie reference book is provided to the client to look up calorie values of food, and completed food diaries and calorie calculations are expected.

A major advantage of the calorie-counting approach is the expanded choice of foods and the flexibility in meal planning. Also, this approach promotes the concept of preplanning, through the technique of "banking" calories. Persons with diabetes can develop skills to make choices through the accounting/budget calorie process. For example, a special occasion dinner may cost 800 calories. The person could limit the day's calories or "bank" extra calories for several days to "spend" on the special occasion. The "banking" technique is most appropriate for persons who are not on insulin or oral hypoglycemic agents (OHA), for whom spacing of meals and calories is not as much of a concern. For persons on insulin or OHAs, glucose monitoring would be essential, and adjustment of medication may be necessary when planning a special occasion when a disproportionate amount of calories are being consumed.

A disadvantage of calorie counting is the amount of time involved in record keeping and calculation. Calorie counting may also be more difficult to follow than other less structured alternative approaches because it involves a restriction of calories. Calorie counting, by itself, does not produce a "nutritionally balanced" diet; combined with a guidelines approach, it does.

Fat Counting

Fat counting offers an alternative method of meal planning for overweight persons who are willing to keep food records. It is a simple self-monitoring approach that allows persons to have a considerable amount of flexibility and control over their food choices. A daily fat allowance is established, and the person with diabetes counts the grams of fat he or she eats at each meal and snack. When explaining the concept, it is useful to compare the daily fat allowance to a bank account. Instead of money, a limited number of fat grams is deposited into the person's account each day. These fat grams can be "spent" as desired until the account is empty. The daily fat allowance is calculated in three steps:

1. Estimate daily calorie requirements.
2. Multiply daily calorie requirement by 30% (or the percentage individually determined as appropriate) to determine how many calories per day should come from fat.
3. To convert daily calories from fat into daily grams of fat, divide calories from fat by nine (1 g fat = 9 calories).

Counting grams of fat evolved during the 1980s as a self-monitoring tool for persons following low-fat diets to reduce risk for cancer. The system has been successfully used in several cancer prevention trials, in which clients learned to reduce fat intake to 15 to 25% of total calories. In developing the nutrition components of these trials, researchers realized the difficulties of establishing dietary guidelines based on percentage of calories from fat. Counting grams of fat was simpler, and the concept was easier for people to grasp, because most Americans are familiar with counting calories or carbohydrates.

Gradually, the concept has become more widely used in two other areas—cardiovascular disease and weight management. The system helps people learn how to reduce calorie intake by making low-fat food choices while still maintaining a sense of control over what they eat. They tend to react more positively, because they do not feel restricted or externally controlled.[4]

The fat-counting approach is useful as a weight reduction tool for both IDDM and NIDDM, particularly those who have become frustrated by previous unsuccessful attempts to lose weight. It is also appropriate for people with elevated blood lipids and for those who have had difficulty with meal-planning approaches and would benefit from a new approach.

Fat/Calorie Counting

As consumers continue to increase their awareness about total fat consumption and its relationship to overall health, *fat/calorie counting* is an alternative to calorie counting as the preferred method of monitoring total calorie consumption.

Fat/calorie counting is a structured meal-planning approach that emphasizes caloric density of food and the percentage of calories from fat. Specific guidelines regarding total number of calories and percentage of calories from fat designed to facilitate weight loss of 0.5 to 1 lb/wk can be identified by the dietitian. The person with diabetes is provided with calorie/fat reference books to use in making food choices. A food diary booklet is also provided to record both the daily total calorie and fat calorie intake. The person is instructed how to calculate the total daily calories, the calories from fat, and the resultant percentage of calories from fat, as well as how to evaluate the results and set goals for future counseling sessions.

To facilitate change to a low-fat eating style, persons are taught to keep daily food diaries and evaluate their food choices using a fat and calorie counting guide called *Health Counts.*[7] The guide is designed to show the relationship between the fat content of commonly eaten foods and their corresponding caloric density.

Fat/calorie counting is most appropriate for the overweight persons with NIDDM who have been unsuccessful with previous weight loss attempts. This approach provides more flexibility and a broader range of food choices beyond what is provided by other structured approaches. It provides greater accuracy and specificity in calorie content of foods for the user.

This approach places emphasis on calories and fat, which are the major culprits for which to target change, especially for persons who are overweight. Fat/calorie counting is more visual or direct in its appeal toward helping the person understand the high calorie and fat contribution of some of his or her favorite foods. It may be a revelation for them to discover that their favorite snack food contains less than 50% of its calories from fat!

Carbohydrate Counting

Counting approaches to meal planning provide varying levels of structure and flexibility for persons with IDDM or NIDDM. The number of counting approaches has increased over the past years as advances in diabetes management, technology (blood glucose meters, insulin, and insulin delivery systems), and patient empowerment have increased demand. With the increased use of intensive insulin therapy, specifically multiple daily injections (MDI), and continuous subcutaneous insulin infusion (CSII), greater flexibility in meal planning and food portion sizes is possible.

A meal plan can be developed based on grams of carbohydrate to be consumed at each meal and snack. The meal-planning objective is to coordinate food intake (primarily carbohydrate), exercise, and insulin, by matching the peak activity of insulin with the peak levels of glucose resulting from the digestion and absorption of food. Some clinicians and persons with diabetes take this method a step farther and devise insulin-to-carbohydrate ratios. The most often used beginning ratio is 1 U of insulin to 10 to 15 g of carbohydrate.[8–10] The insulin doses should then be "fine-tuned" based on achieving target 2-hour postprandial and premeal blood glucose levels.

Carbohydrate counting can be used by both persons with IDDM and NIDDM, primarily those on insulin. It is most appropriate for persons with IDDM, who use intensive insulin therapy for diabetes management. The main advantage of using carbohydrate counting is increased flexibility with meal timing, food choices, and portion sizes. Persons with diabetes who travel frequently or who have irregular work or school schedules find this method very

Table 11-1 Summarizing the Meal-Planning Approaches[a]

	Degree of Emphasis on Weight Loss	Degree of Emphasis on Metabolic Control	Degree of Literacy Required	Degree of Structure	Degree of Complexity
Guideline Approaches					
Guide to Good Eating	low-moderate	low	low	low	low
Dietary Guidelines for Americans	low-moderate	low	low	low	low
Food Guide Pyramid	low-moderate	low	low	low	low
Healthy Food Choices (guideline section)	moderate	low	low	low	low
The First Step in Diabetes Meal Planning	moderate	low	low	low	low
Meal-Planning Approaches					
Individualized menus	moderate-high	moderate-high	low	moderate	low
Month of Meals-1 to 5	moderate	moderate	low	moderate	low
Exchange Lists for Meal Planning	moderate	moderate-high	moderate-high	moderate-high	moderate-high
Healthy Food Choices (poster section)	moderate	moderate	moderate	moderate	moderate
Calorie counting	high	low	moderate	moderate-high	moderate
Fat counting	high	low	moderate	moderate-high	moderate
Fat/calorie counting	high	low	moderate	moderate-high	moderate
Carbohydrate Counting: Getting Started	low	high	high	high	high
Carbohydrate Counting: Moving On	low	high	high	high	high
Carbohydrate Counting: CHO/Insulin Ratios	low	high	high	high	high
Lifestyle Change Approaches					
Facilitating Lifestyle Change: A Resource Manual	high	moderate-high	moderate	high	moderate

[a] This table represents the author's judgment and experience with meal-planning approaches. The readers are encouraged to modify the table based on their own experiences.

Source: Adapted with permission from Green JA. *The Diabetes Educator* (1987;13:146), Copyright © 1987, The American Association of Diabetes Educators.

Table 11-2 Selection of Meal-Planning Approaches According to Type of Diabetes[a]

Category	Type	IDDM	NIDDM Nonobese	NIDDM Obese
Guideline Approaches				
Basic nutrition	*Guide to Good Eating*	X	X	X
	Dietary Guidelines for Americans	X	X	X
	Food Guide Pyramid	X	X	X
Diabetes nutrition guidelines	*Healthy Food Choices* (guideline section)	X	X	X
	The First Step in Diabetes Meal Planning	X	X	X
	Single Topic Diabetes Resources[b]	X	X	X
Meal-Planning Approaches				
Menus	Individualized menus		X	X
	Month of Meals-1 to 5		X	X
Exchanges	*Exchange Lists for Meal Planning*	X	X	X
	Healthy Food Choices (poster section)	X	X	X
Counting	Calorie counting			X
	Fat counting			X
	Fat/calorie counting			X
	Carbohydrate Counting: Getting Started	X	X	X
	Carbohydrate Counting: Moving On	X	X	X
	Carbohydrate Counting: CHO/Insulin Ratios	X		
Life Style Change Approaches				
	Facilitating Lifestyle Change: A Resource Manual	X	X	X

[a] This table represents the author's judgment and experience with meal-planning approaches. The readers are encouraged to modify the table based on their own experiences.

[b] There are 21 individualized topics in the Single-Topic Series ranging from topics such as "Sugars and Sweets" and Understanding Fats" to "Exercise and Diabetes" and "Hypoglycemia and Diabetes."

useful. Improved glycemic control is possible as insulin doses can be adjusted up or down according to food intake, and injections (with MDI) or boluses (with CSII) can be taken early or delayed. Persons using this approach need to be aware of the tendency to gain weight and the need to monitor portion sizes and caloric intake.

In 1995, a work group of the American Dietetic Association and the American Diabetes Association Nutrition Education Resources Steering Committee developed three new educational resources for people with diabetes interested in carbohydrate counting. Three levels of carbohydrate counting were identified, based on progressing levels of complexity and requiring increasing knowledge and skills. Patient and professional education publications were developed for the following three levels:

- *Carbohydrate Counting: Getting Started* (Level 1)
- *Carbohydrate Counting: Moving On* (Level 2)
- *Carbohydrate Counting: Carbohydrate/ Insulin Ratios* (Level 3)

Getting Started, the basic level booklet, is designed to encourage consistent amounts of carbohydrate at meals and snacks to allow some predictability of postmeal glucose excursions. *Moving On*, the intermediate level booklet, is aimed at learning to interpret more complex relationships between food, medication, activity, and blood glucose, and assist the client to see patterns. *Carbohydrate/Insulin Ratios*, the advanced level booklet, is designed to help the client learn how to adjust insulin changes in food or activity, using the ratio of carbohydrate intake to insulin dosage. Individualized nutrition assessment will determine which level is appropriate for each particular client.

CONCLUSION

Table 11-1 provides a summary of the meal-planning approaches that have been discussed with regard to the degree of emphasis on weight loss, glucose control, healthy eating, literacy required, structure, and complexity. Table 11-2 provides a recommendation on which meal-planning approaches would be best suited to each type of diabetes.

There is no one "right" or "wrong" method for meal planning. Certainly, not everyone needs a complex system of meal planning. Any method, technique, or teaching tool that supports the nutrition management goals of achieving or maintaining desirable body weight, and appropriate serum glucose and lipid levels, promotes good nutrition, and is realistic and workable for the person with diabetes should be considered acceptable as an approach to diabetes nutrition management.

When providing nutrition education, the educator should be flexible and creative. Boredom can set in with any regimen and also lead to noncompliance. It is the responsibility of the dietitian educator to promote continuity of learning by introducing new ideas and concepts and altering the learning environment.

As educators, we also need to remember that we cannot force our values and knowledge on clients and assume that they will make changes in their eating behaviors because we think they should. Rather, we need to try and diminish the distance between "where they are" and "what

we know." We can help them to discover new choices and make them aware of new possibilities. Taking the time to listen to people and hear what they are telling us and providing them with new possibilities will promote more permanent behavior changes than giving them a standardized or structured tool for meal planning.

Many educational resources are available to teach meal planning. The important issue is not only to individualize the resource to the person but also to use an effective method of education and counseling that will promote positive changes in eating behavior. Gradual change is often the key to incorporating changes into life-long eating habits. Education and counseling about meal planning and eating behaviors is a continual process!

REFERENCES

1. Lockwood D, Fey ML, Gladish NA, et al. The biggest problem in diabetes. *Diabetes Educ.* 1986;12:30–33.
2. Arnold MS, Stephien CJ, Jess GE, Hiss RG. Guidelines vs practice in the delivery of diabetes nutrition care. *J Am Diet Assoc.* 1993;93:34–39.
3. Anderson RM, Stephien CJ, Fitzgerald JT. The diabetes patient education experience of randomly selected patients under the care of community physicians. *Diabetes.* 1993;42(suppl 1):150A.
4. Monk A, Barry B, McClain K, et al. Practice guidelines for medical nutrition therapy provided by dieticians for persons with non–insulin dependent diabetes mellitus (NIDDM). *J Am Diet Assoc.* 1995; in press.
5. American Diabetes Association. Nutrition recommendations and principles for people with diabetes mellitus. *Diabetes Care.* 1994;17:519–522.
6. Green Pastors J, Holler H. *Meal Planning Approaches for Diabetes Management.* Chicago, Ill: American Dietetic Association; 1994.
7. Stevens VL, Rossner J, Greenlic M, Stevens N, Frankel HM, Craddick S. Freedom from fat: a contemporary multicomponent weight loss program for the general population of obese adults. *J Am Diet Assoc.* 1989;89:1255–1258.
8. Muchmore DB, Miller M. Making carbohydrate count. *Diabetes Forecast.* 1989;42:25–30.
9. Brackenridge BP. Carbohydrate gram counting: a key to accurate mealtime boluses in intensive diabetes therapy. *Pract Diabetol.* 1992;22–28.
10. Weinrauch S, Kulkarni K, Tomky D, et al. External insulin pump. *On the Cutting Edge.* 1992;13:24.

Resource Materials for Diabetes Nutrition Education

BASIC NUTRITION AND DIABETES NUTRITION GUIDELINES

- **Guide to Good Eating**—For information about the *Guide to Good Eating*, 1992 edition, contact your local Dairy and Food Nutrition Council Office or the National Dairy Council, 6300 North River Road, Rosemont, IL 60018-4233, Tel:(718) 696-1860, ext. 220.

- **Daily Food Guide Pyramid**—For information about the *Daily Food Guide Pyramid,* 1994 edition, contact your local Dairy and Food Nutrition Council Office or the National Dairy Council, 6300 North River Road, Rosemont, IL 60018-4233, Tel: (718) 696-1860, ext. 220.

- **Dietary Guidelines for Americans** (1990 edition)—Single copies are available free from the Consumer Information Center, Department 514-X, Pueblo, CO 81009. For information about the printing of bulk orders, contact the Superintendent of Documents, US Government Printing Office, Washington, DC 20401, Tel: (202) 783-3238.

- **Food Guide Pyramid**—To order a copy of the *Food Guide Pyramid* booklet, send a $1.00 check or money order made out to the Superintendent of Document to: Consumer Information Center, Department 159-Y, Pueblo, CO 81009. For information about the printing of bulk orders, contact the Superintendent of Documents, US Government Printing Office, Washington, DC 20401, Tel: (202) 783-3238.

- **The First Step in Diabetes Meal Planning**—Order from The American Dietetic Association, 216 West Jackson Boulevard, Chicago, IL 60606-6995, Tel: 1-800-877-1600 or the American Diabetes Association, Inc., Diabetes Information Service Center, 1600 Duke Street, Alexandria, VA 22314, Tel: 1-800-ADA-DISC.

- **Healthy Food Choices**—Order from The American Dietetic Association, 216 West Jackson Boulevard, Chicago, IL 60606-6995, Tel: 1-800-877-1600 or the American Diabetes Association, Inc., Diabetes Information Service Center, 1600 Duke Street, Alexandria, VA 22314, Tel: 1-800-ADA-DISC.

MENU APPROACHES

- **Month of Meals-1, -2, -3, -4, and -5**—Copies of *Months of Meals-1 to 5* are available from the American Diabetes Association, Inc., Diabetes Information Service Center, 1600 Duke Street, Alexandria, VA 22314. Tel: 1-800-ADA-DISC.

EXCHANGE APPROACHES

- **Exchange Lists for Meal Planning** (1995 revision)—Order from The American Dietetic Association, 216 West Jackson Boulevard, Chicago, IL 60606-6995, Tel: 1-800-877-1600 or the American Diabetes Association, Inc., Diabetes Information Service Center, 1600 Duke Street, Alexandria, VA 22314, Tel: 1-800-ADA-DISC.

COUNTING APPROACHES

- **Calorie Counting**
- —Kraus, B. *Carbohydrate and Calorie Guide.* New York: New American Library, 1992.

—Netzer, C. *The Complete Book of Food Counts*, Third Edition. New York: Dell Publishing, 1994.

• **Fat Counting**

—Bellerson, KJ. *The Complete and Up-To-Date Fat Book*. Garden City Park, NY: Avery Publishing, 1993.

—Netzer, C. *The Complete Book of Food Counts*, Third Edition. New York: Dell Publishing, 1994.

• **Fat/Calorie Counting**

—Kaiser Permanente. *Health Counts, A Fat and Calorie Guide*. New York: John Wiley and Sons, Inc., 1991.

—Kaiser Permanente. Pocket Food Diaries. Available through the Department of Health Education and Health Promotion, 7201 N. Interstate Avenue, Portland, OR 97217, Tel: (503) 286-6880.

—Bellerson, KJ. *The Complete and Up-To-Date Fat Book*. Garden City Park, NY: Avery Publishing, 1993.

• **Carbohydrate Counting**

Carbohydrate Counting: Adding Flexibility to Your Food Choices. International Diabetes Center. Distributed by Chronimed Publishing Company, PO Box 59032, Minneapolis, MN 55459-9686, Tel: 1-800-848-2793.

• **Food Composition Tables:** Pennington, J. *Food Values of Portions Commonly Used*. Philadelphia: J.B. Lippincott Company, 1993.

• **Reference Books for Grams of Carbohydrate:**

—Kraus, B. *Carbohydrate Guide to Brand Names and Basic Foods*. New York: The New American Library, 1992.

—Kraus, B. *Carbohydrate and Calorie Guide*. New York: New American Library, 1992.

• **Guides for Exchange Values:**

—*Convenience Food Facts*, *Exchanges for All Occasions*, and *Fast Food Facts*. Inter-

national Diabetes Center. Distributed by Chronimed Publishing Company, PO Box 59032, Minneapolis, MN 55459-9686, Tel: 1-800-848-2793.

—In October 1995, the American Dietetic Association and the American Diabetes Association will have 3 new publications on carbohydrate counting:

  –*Carbohydrate Counting: Getting Started* (Level 1)

  –*Carbohydrate Counting: Moving On* (Level 2)

  –*Carbohydrate Counting: Using Carbohydrate/Insulin Ratios* (Level 3)

Contact the Publications Departments of both associations for information on availability and pricing: The American Dietetic Association, Tel: 1-800-877-1600; American Diabetes Association, Tel: 1-800-ADA-DISC.

LIFE STYLE CHANGE RESOURCES

In October 1995, the American Dietetic Association and the American Diabetes Association will have available the new publication entitled *Facilitating Lifestyle Change: A Resource Manual*.

Contact the Publications Departments of both associations for information on availability and pricing: The American Dietetic Association, Tel: 1-800-877-1600; American Diabetes Association, Tel: 1-800-ADA-DISC.

SINGLE-TOPIC DIABETES RESOURCES

In October 1995, the American Dietetic Association and the American Diabetes Association will have available 21 nutrition-related topics to be sold as 1-page double-sided reproducible masters.

Examples of topics include "When You Can't Eat," "Hypoglycemia," "Supermarket Smarts," and "Older Persons with Diabetes."

Contact the Publications Departments of both associations for information on availability and pricing: The American Dietetic Association, Tel: 1-800-877-1600; American Diabetes Association, Tel: 1-800-ADA-DISC.

Chapter 12

The Exchange System: A Comprehensive Review

Harold Holler

Medical nutrition therapy for diabetes mellitus relies heavily on a complete nutrition assessment, establishment of goals, nutrition intervention, and evaluation. The nutrition intervention involves developing a meal plan that will take into account the individual's eating pattern, life style, ability to learn, and willingness to change eating habits. The exchange system is one of the most commonly used and oldest meal-planning approach.

The basic structure developed in 1950 of food groups based on calories, carbohydrates (CHO), proteins (PRO), and fat continues to be used today. The purposes of the exchange system are to provide:

1. a framework to group foods with similar calorie, CHO, PRO, and fat content

2. a universal system for nutritional management of diabetes (as clients move from one location to another, it is beneficial to all involved to have a uniform system for meal planning)

3. a system that allows clients to be accountable for what they eat

4. a wide variety of food choices and flexibility in planning meals

5. a tool to plan nutritionally adequate meals[1]

HISTORY OF THE EXCHANGE SYSTEM

In its early recorded history, diabetes was treated by a diet of fat, meat (even rancid meat), boiled vegetables (boiled to eliminate excess carbohydrate), and even bran.[2] Overall, the diet that predominated until the advent of insulin was a high-fat, low-carbohydrate regimen because carbohydrate was associated with glucose spilling into the urine. The advent of insulin in 1921 allowed clinicians to be more flexible with allowed food intakes. This flexibility, however, meant long and tedious calculation because there was no standardization of portion sizes or food interchange tables. Variations in menus had to be individually developed. The diet system proved to be difficult for the patient to follow as it was different from the rest of the family's meals and took great efforts to follow consistently, due to its limited range.

To solve the problems inherent in the diet, The American Dietetic Association, American Diabetes Association, and U.S. Public Health Service in 1950 issued a food exchange system for use with diabetes diet calculations.[3] The goal was to allow for more rapid calculations and greater variations in food choices while staying within the boundaries of a modified meal plan. The system was structured by grouping foods with similar distributions of CHO, PRO, and fat so foods within a group could be interchanged or exchanged. The six original groups were milk, meat, vegetable A and B, fat, fruit, and bread.

The exchange system was seen as a tool that would solve adherence problems by providing a tremendous range of food choices. It was perceived as an orderly method of diet instruction after years of individually calculating diets. To simplify its use even further, tear-off precalculated diet sheets were developed. These diet

Table 12-1 1976 and 1986 Revisions in the 1950 Exchange System

Food Group	1950 Edition	1976 Edition	1986 Edition
Milk	Whole milk used as the basis for calculations	Skim milk used as the basis for calculations ***Reason for change:*** increased emphasis on low-fat, low-cholesterol meal plans	The milk group is divided into 3 subgroups depending on the amount of fat in the choice ***Reason for change:*** allows for individualization of milk choice and eliminates the concept of omitting fat exchanges
Vegetables	Two groups of vegetables used—A & B—with the divisions based on carbohy-drate content. Group A were allowed as free foods if less than 1 cup was consumed. B group included some starchy vegetables.	One group of vegetables with a list of low-calorie vegetables to be eaten "free." Starchy veg-etables moved to the bread list ***Reason for change:*** having fewer groups would be easier to understand	No major change
Bread	Included several typical desserts	Simple sugar choices, such as ice cream and angel food cake, omitted ***Reason for change:*** emphasis on decreasing fat and avoidance of all simple sugars	The name is changed to starch/bread list. The protein content increased from 2 g to 3 g. The fat content is noted to be a trace. For calculation purposes, 0.5–1 g can be used ***Reason for change:*** name change describes the food group more accurately. The nutrient data base clearly indicated a need to change the protein and fat content
Fruit	—	—	The fruit list is now 15 g of CHO and 60 calories per serving ***Reason for change:*** the change more accurately reflects the food values for choices within the group

continues

Table 12-1 continued

Food Group	1950 Edition	1976 Edition	1986 Edition
Meat	1 oz of meat used as the basis for calculations	Meats divided into three groups based on fat content. Low-fat meat used as basis for calculations ***Reason for change:*** greater adaptability of the diet to a low-fat, low-cholesterol regimen; clear guidelines for the user	The three meat subgroups are still used—low, medium, and high fat. Recommended calculations are based on the usual type of meat consumed
Fat	One teaspoon of butter used as the basis of exchange	Fats high in polyunsaturates highlighted ***Reason for change:*** to increase the emphasis on low-cholesterol and high-polyunsaturated fat choices	No major change
			Other changes: 1. Two additional categories were added: combination foods and foods for occasional use. 2. The order in which the exchange lists are listed is changed to reflect the emphasis on a high-CHO, low-fat diet. The starch group is listed first, and fat is listed last. 3. Foods containing more than 3 g of dietary fiber or 400 mg sodium are noted by symbols to assist in tailoring the diet to a high-fiber or low-sodium meal plan. 4. Omitting fat to allow certain food choices is not needed; rather the food is listed at its correct value. This is done to make diet calculations clearer.

Exhibit 12-1 The 1995 ADA/ADA Exchange System Grouping of Food

---

Carbohydrate Group: Name of food group that represents food sources of carbohydrate. Foods from the starch list, fruit list, milk list, and the other carbohydrates list can be interchanged in the meal plan. Each list represents foods with 15 g of carbohydrate. The vegetable list is included in this group.

- Starch list: name changed from starch/bread list to starch list
- Fruit list: no major changes
- Milk list: no major changes
- Other carbohydrates list: new list of foods. Each food item is equivalent to 15 g CHO and can be exchanged for one starch or fruit or milk exchange
- Vegetable list: no major change to list. The calories and CHO content are not counted for in the meal plan unless the client is counting calories or CHO. The client is encouraged to eat 1–2 exchanges per meal

Meat and Meat Substitute Group: Name of food group that represents food sources of protein and fat. The group is divided into 4 lists: very lean, lean, medium-fat, and high-fat meats and meat substitutes. Emphasis of this group is to reduce total fat, especially saturated fats.

Fat Group: Name of food group that represents food sources of fat. The group is divided into 3 lists: monounsaturated, polyunsaturated, and saturated fats. Emphasis of this group is to reduce saturated fats.

---

sheets were an enormous time-saver but eliminated the individualization.

The basic structure developed in 1950 is still in effect today, having been modified in 1976, 1986, and 1995. Each revision updated the system to reflect the latest concepts in medical nutrition therapy. The 1976 revision emphasized decreasing fat and cholesterol intake. The 1986 version also stressed the modification of fat intake, as well as decreasing sodium intake and increasing fiber consumption. The 1995 revision provides for expanded food lists (the inclusion of fat-modified food items, vegetarian foods, and fast-food items) and revised food lists (the addition of three fat list categories; addition of a very lean meat category; renaming the starch/bread list to the starch list). The 1994 American Diabetes Nutrition Recommendations[4] served as the basis for the revisions to the 1995 exchange lists. Table 12-1 outlines the changes between the 1950, 1976, and 1986 versions. Exhibit 12-1 identifies the changes from the 1995 revision.

DEFINITIONS

The term *exchange* has been criticized by both clients and practitioners as being confusing. The use of this term encompasses the idea of "a choice, a trade-off and a portion size."[5] The designers of this system searched for terminology that would connote the "exchange" idea. The term remains in use today because of the many diabetes-related publications that contain the terminology. Some practitioners prefer to use such words as *list, serving,* or *choice.* To avoid confusion, the dietetic professionals should thoroughly discuss the concept of an exchange with the client. If the term cannot be understood, then the exchange system may not be the appropriate meal-planning approach to use.

All foods are divided into three main groups—carbohydrate group, meat and meat substitute group, and fat group. The carbohydrate group is divided into five exchange lists: starch list, fruit list, milk list, other carbohydrates list, and vegetable list. The meat and meat substitute group is divided into very lean, lean, medium-fat, and high-fat meat and meat substitutes lists. The fat group is divided into monounsaturated fat list, polyunsaturated fat list, and saturated fat list. Each exchange list reflects an average value for calories, CHO, PRO, and fat based on the foods in each list. A data base serves as the resource for average values of each list (a new data base for the 1995 exchange lists for meal planning will be published in early

Table 12-2 Summary of the 1995 Exchange Lists

List	CHO (g)	PRO (g)	Fat (g)	Calories
Carbohydrates				
Starch	15	3	1 or less	80
Fruit	15	—	—	60
Milk				
Skim	12	8	0–3	90
Low-fat	12	8	5	120
Whole	12	8	8	150
Other carbohydrates	15	Varies	Varies	Varies
Vegetables	5	2	—	25
Meat/meat substitutes:				
Very lean	—	7	1	35
Lean	—	7	3	55
Medium fat	—	7	5	75
High fat	—	7	8	100
Fat	—	—	5	45

Source: Exchange Lists for Meal Planning. The American Dietetic Association and American Diabetes Association, Copyright © 1995, Chicago, Illinois.

1996).[6,7] Table 12-2 provides a summary of the nutrient composition of the exchange lists.

USE OF THE EXCHANGE LISTS

The use of the exchange lists requires the development of a meal plan. A meal plan is a guide that aids clients to make appropriate food choices based on their predetermined diabetes nutrition goals. It provides them with specific information on the amount of food to be used from each exchange list at a meal or snack.

Some individuals need the structure provided by an exchange list meal plan. The following situations give the practitioner an idea of when to use an exchange list meal plan[1]:

1. Client has inconsistent patterns of eating.
   - Skips meals and snacks
   - Varies caloric intake significantly from meal to meal and day to day
   - Is totally unaware of eating pattern
2. Client has a poorly balanced food intake (ie, has no concept of normal nutrition needs).
3. Client needs specific directions to make food choices.

- Is unable to select appropriate food choices at meals/snacks
- Is unaware of appropriate food portions

4. Client desires more information about nutrition (eg, desires knowledge of the specific nutrient content of foods).
5. Client's established diabetes goals are not being accomplished, such as
   - Blood glucose levels are unresponsive to changes in food choices
   - Weight management is not obtained
   - Fat intake is too high

ESTABLISHING A MEAL PLAN USING EXCHANGE LISTS

These steps are followed to establish a meal plan using the exchange list:

1. Compare current body weight with reasonable body weight (RBW), to establish RBW (refer to Chapter 19). When establishing a RBW for a client, realize that it may not be a realistic weight for the individual to achieve. It is more important to

Exhibit 12-2 Evaluation of Usual Food Intake Based on Food Records or a 24-Hour Food Recall

Diet History

Breakfast
1 cup orange juice
1 slice toast
3/4 cup cereal
1/2 cup milk (2%)
2 tsp butter

Evening Snack
3 cups popcorn
4 tsp butter

Lunch
sandwich
   2 slices bread
   1/2 cup tuna
   3 tsp mayonnaise
1 cup cream soup
12 crackers
1 cup milk (2%)

Dinner
6 oz roast beef
1 cup mashed potatoes
3 tsp butter
1/2 cup peas
1/2 cup carrots
1 slice bread
2 tsp butter
1 cup milk (2%)
coffee, black

Food Group	Breakfast	Snack	Lunch	Snack	Dinner	Snack	Total Servings/ day	CHO (g)	Protein (g)	Fat[a] (g)	Calories
Starch	2		5		4	1	12	15	3	1	80
Vegetables	0		0		1		1	5	2		25
Fruits	2		0		0		2	15			60
Milk 2%[b]	1/2		1		1		2 1/2	12	8	5	90
Meats/substitutes	0		2		6		8		7	5	75
Fats	2		3		5	4	1 4			5	45

Meal/Snack/Time (header above columns)

	CHO	Protein	Fat	Calories
Total				
Calories	× 4 =	× 4 =	× 9 =	Total =
Percent Calories				

[a] Calculations are based on medium-fat meats and skim/very low-fat milk. If diet consists predominantly of lean meats, use the factor 3 g instead of 5 g fat; if predominantly high-fat meats, use 8 g fat. If low-fat (2%) milk is used, use 5 g fat; if whole milk is used, use 8 g fat.

[b] This example has been adjusted to use 2% milk.

Source: The Exchange Lists are the basis of a meal-planning system designed by a committee of The American Diabetes Association and The American Dietetic Association. While designed primarily for people with diabetes and others who must follow special diets, the Exchange Lists are based on principles of good nutrition that apply to everyone. © 1995 American Diabetes Association, Inc., American Dietetic Association.

assist the client in identifying a weight that he or she can reach.

2. Assess the client's calorie needs (refer to Chapter 19, Exhibit 19-2). Evaluating the current calorie intake and comparing it with the recommended calorie needs may prove helpful in determining the actual calorie needs of the client. Consider the example in which the calorie needs are 1200 calories and the client's actual calorie intake is 2600 calories per day. A reduction

Exhibit 12-3 Calculating the CHO, PRO, Fat, and Calorie Intake of Each Exchange List

Food Group	Meal/Snack/Time						Total Servings/day	CHO (g)	Protein (g)	Fat[a] (g)	Calories
	Breakfast	Snack	Lunch	Snack	Dinner	Snack					
Starch	2		5		4	1	12	180 ^15	36 ^3	12 ^1	960 ^80
Vegetables	0		0		1		1	5 ^5	2 ^2	0	25 ^25
Fruits	2		0		0		2	30 ^15	0	0	120 ^60
Milk 2%[b]	1/2		1		1		2 1/2	30 ^12	20 ^8	12.5 ^5	300 ^90
Meats/substitutes	0		2		6		8	0	56 ^7	40 ^5	600 ^75
Fats	2		3		5	4	14	0	0	70 ^5	630 ^45
						Total					
						Calories		× 4 =	× 4 =	× 9 =	Total =
						Percent Calories					

[a] Calculations are based on medium-fat meats and skim/very low-fat milk. If diet consists predominantly of lean meats, use the factor 3 g instead of 5 g fat; if predominantly high-fat meats, use 8 g fat. If low-fat (2%) milk is used, use 5 g fat; if whole milk is used, use 8 g fat.

[b] This example has been adjusted to use 2% milk.

Source: The Exchange Lists are the basis of a meal-planning system designed by a committee of the American Diabetes Association and The American Dietetic Association. While designed primarily for people with diabetes and others who must follow special diets, the Exchange Lists are based on principles of good nutrition that apply to everyone. © 1995 American Diabetes Association, Inc., American Dietetic Association.

of 500 to 1000 calories from the current intake would result in a calorie level of 1600 to 2100, which may prove to be a more appropriate starting point when attempting to establish a realistic calorie level.

3. Assess the client's current food intake and schedule demands. To determine calorie and nutrient needs, frequency of meals/snacks, and food quantity, the practitioner needs to understand the client's current eating pattern. These baseline data will serve as the basis for developing a meal plan that will meet the client's life style and schedule.

• Determine the number of exchanges from each meal and snack based on food records or a 24-hour recall (Exhibit 12-2). There are no current scientific data to support the precise distribution of nutrients between meals/snacks. The number of exchanges for each meal/snack is based on current eating patterns, insulin/oral hypoglycemic agents, and the results of blood glucose monitoring.

• Determine the usual intake in grams of CHO, PRO, and fat and calories according to the total number of exchanges per day by using the chart in Exhibit 12-3. To determine the total grams of CHO, PRO, and fat and total calories for each exchange list, multiply the total servings per day by the grams of CHO, PRO, and fat and calories.

• Total the daily intake in grams of CHO,

Exhibit 12-4 Calculating the Total CHO, PRO, Fat, and Calories from the Usual Food Intake

Food Group	Meal/Snack/Time						Total Servings/ day	CHO (g)	Protein (g)	Fat[a] (g)	Calories
	Breakfast	Snack	Lunch	Snack	Dinner	Snack					
Starch	2		5		4	1	12	180 ^{15}	36 ^{3}	12 ^{1}	960 ^{80}
Vegetables	0		0		1		1	5 ^{5}	2 ^{2}	0	25 ^{25}
Fruits	2		0		0		2	30 ^{15}	0	0	120 ^{60}
Milk 2%[b]	1/2		1		1		2 1/2	30 ^{12}	20 ^{8}	12.5 ^{5}	300 ^{90}
Meats/substitutes	0		2		6		8	0	56 ^{7}	40 ^{5}	600 ^{75}
Fats	2		3		5	4	14	0	0	70 ^{5}	630 ^{45}
Total								245	114	134.5	
Calories								× 4 = 980	× 4 = 456	× 9 = 1210.5	Total = 2647
Percent Calories											

[a] Calculations are based on medium-fat meats and skim/very low-fat milk. If diet consists predominantly of lean meats, use the factor 3 g instead of 5 g fat; if predominantly high-fat meats, use 8 g fat. If low-fat (2%) milk is used, use 5 g fat; if whole milk is used, use 8 g fat.

[b] This example has been adjusted to use 2% milk.

Source: The Exchange Lists are the basis of a meal-planning system designed by a committee of the American Diabetes Association and The American Dietetic Association. While designed primarily for people with diabetes and others who must follow special diets, the Exchange Lists are based on principles of good nutrition that apply to everyone. © 1995 American Diabetes Association, Inc., American Dietetic Association.

PRO, and fat and calories per day (Exhibit 12-4).

- Calculate the percentages of CHO, PRO, and fat in the diet using the formula shown in Exhibit 12-5.
- Assess the usual food intake using the following questions:
  - Is the usual calorie intake similar to the estimated calorie needs (within 100 to 200 calories)?
  - Is the usual fat intake within the recommended percentages of calories for management of blood lipids?
  - Are the meals/snacks eaten at a consistent time?
  - Is the action time of insulin or oral hypoglycemic agents matched with the distribution of calories? Insulin and oral hypoglycemic agents can be adjusted, with physician approval, to maintain the client's usual eating pattern.
  - Is the diet adequate in nutrient composition?
  - Is consideration given to a routine exercise pattern?

4. Develop the meal plan using the exchange lists. If the usual eating pattern meets all the criteria noted above, then no further adjustments need be made. If changes are needed, use the diet history to guide the development of a meal plan. The client must be actively involved in the development of the meal plan for it to be realistic and livable. Exhibit 12-6 demonstrates the devel-

Exhibit 12-5 Calculating Percentages of Calories from Carbohydrate, Protein, and Fat

1. To determine percentage of calories from CHO:

$$\frac{\text{g CHO x 4 cal/g}}{\text{Total calories}}$$

2. To determine percentage of calories from PRO:

$$\frac{\text{g PRO x 4 cal/g}}{\text{Total calories}}$$

3. To determine percentage of calories from fat:

$$\frac{\text{g fat x 9 cal/g}}{\text{Total calories}}$$

Sample Calculation

Percentage of calories from CHO:

$$\frac{245 \text{ g CHO x 4}}{2647} = \frac{980}{2647} = 37\%$$

Percentage of calories from PRO:

$$\frac{114 \text{ g PRO x 4}}{2647} = \frac{456}{2647} = 17\%$$

Percentage of calories from Fat:

$$\frac{135 \text{ g fat x 9}}{2647} = \frac{1215}{2647} = 46\%$$

Source: Powers MA, Barr P, Franz M, Holler H, Wheeler M, Wylie-Rosett J. *Nutrition Guide for Professionals: Diabetes Education and Meal Planning.* Chicago, Ill: American Diabetes Association/The American Dietetic Association; 1988.

opment of the meal plan using the pattern obtained from a sample diet history. This meal plan has retained the client's daily pattern of eating three meals and a bedtime snack. The number of exchanges at each meal were reduced to help control total calorie intake. Also, the type of milk used was changed, and fruits and vegetables were increased. The changes would be discussed and agreed on by the client and practitioner. The new meal plan provides a more balanced eating pattern that is lower in calories and fat. The initial meal plan may not meet all the recommendations for diabetes nutrition management, but any change(s) to the current eating pattern may have a positive effect on metabolic control.

SELF-MANAGEMENT TRAINING

After assessing the client's knowledge of nutrition and diabetes, the practitioner can individualize the education. The first step should include information about basic nutrition and how it relates to diabetes. This will help the client understand why and how the exchange lists work to plan meals. A first encounter with a client should not necessarily result in giving a meal plan using exchanges. However, once the client understands basics of nutrition and diabetes, he or she may be a candidate for using the exchange lists.

If the client is taught to use the exchange lists for meal planning, blood glucose monitoring will be helpful for evaluating the effect of changed eating behaviors. During follow-up visits, the dietitian and client will be able to assess the appropriateness of the meal plan, make adjustments to it, and if necessary, make recommendations to the physician for a change in insulin or oral hypoglycemic agents.

APPLICATION

Case Study 1

Carol, a 30-year-old woman with newly diagnosed type I diabetes, is seen in the outpatient diabetes clinic for initial control and education. She does not have any family history of diabetes and has never been on any type of diet. Carol lives alone, infrequently eats away from home, and works as a computer programmer. Her weight is within normal limits. During the initial nutrition screening, it is apparent that Carol has very limited knowledge about nutrition. She expresses interest in learning about nutrition and meal planning. During the initial counseling session, information about nutrients in foods and food grouping is discussed. The second counseling session revolves around the importance of the timing of meals and the need to be consistent with food portions. On the third counseling ses-

Exhibit 12-6 Meal Plan for 1700 Calories

Diet History

Breakfast
1 cup orange juice
1 slice toast
3/4 cup cereal
1/2 cup milk (2%)
2 tsp butter

Evening Snack
3 cups popcorn
4 tsp butter

Lunch
sandwich
  2 slices bread
  1/2 cup tuna
  3 tsp mayonnaise
1 cup cream soup
12 crackers
1 cup milk (2%)

Dinner
6 oz roast beef
1 cup mashed potatoes
3 tsp butter
1/2 cup peas
1/2 cup carrots
1 slice bread
2 tsp butter
1 cup milk (2%)
coffee, black

Meal/Snack/Time

Food Group	Breakfast	Snack	Lunch	Snack	Dinner	Snack	Total Servings/ day	CHO (g)	Protein (gg)	Fat[a] (g)	Calories
Starch	2		3		2	1	8	120^{15}	24^{3}	8^{1}	640^{80}
Vegetables	0		1		1–2		2–3	15^{5}	6^{2}	0	75^{25}
Fruits	1		1		1		3	45^{15}	0	0	180^{60}
Milk, skim[b]	1		0		1		2	24^{12}	16^{8}	2^{5}	180^{90}
Meats/substitutes	0		2		3		5	0	35^{7}	25^{5}	375^{75}
Fats	1		2		2		5	0	0	25^{5}	225^{45}
Total								204	81	60	
Calories								× 4 = 816	× 4 = 324	× 9 = 540	Total = 1680
Percent Calories								49	19	32	

[a]Calculations are based on medium-fat meats and skim/very low-fat milk. If diet consists predominantly of lean meats, use the factor 3 g instead of 5 g fat; if predominantly high-fat meats, use 8 g fat. If low-fat (2%) milk is used, use 5 g fat; if whole milk is used, use 8 g fat.

Source: The Exchange Lists are the basis of a meal-planning system designed by a committee of the American Diabetes Association and The American Dietetic Association. While designed primarily for people with diabetes and others who must follow special diets, the Exchange Lists are based on principles of good nutrition that apply to everyone. © 1995 American Diabetes Association, Inc., American Dietetic Association.

sion, the dietitian introduces the nutrition resource *First Step in Diabetes Meal Planning* and individualizes the number of servings from each of the food groups. Carol and the dietitian plan several menus using some of her favorite foods. During the next follow-up appointment, Carol has many questions about foods she would like to use in her meals, but she is unsure of the portion sizes. The dietitian introduces the concept of food exchanges using the resource *Healthy Food Choices* and together they establish a meal plan. After several weeks, Carol returns for a follow-up visit and again has many questions about foods not found in the *Healthy Food*

Choices brochure. At this time, the dietitian introduces the *Exchange Lists for Meal Planning*, and the client and dietitian establish a meal plan and review a sample menu. Over the course of time, Carol did very well with using the exchange lists and did gradually learn to count carbohydrates.

Case Study 2

Mike, a 45-year-old accountant with a strong family history of diabetes, is diagnosed with type II diabetes. The client is 25 lb overweight and does some of the food preparation at home. Mike's physician would like to implement nutrition therapy only for control of the diabetes for 6 months, and Mike is very motivated because he does not want to take any medications or insulin. During the first nutrition counseling session, Mike and his wife demonstrate some knowledge of using food exchanges but have very little information about general nutrition. The dietitian reviews the basic nutrients and their food sources and asks Mike to keep a food record. On his return visit, the dietitian observes that Mike has kept very detailed food records. The dietitian shows Mike that the number of calories consumed is over the recommended amount and that he does not always select foods from all the food groups. The dietitian provides Mike with some suggestions for changing some of his food choices and stresses the need to continue keeping food records. On the next visit, Mike asks the dietitian to give him a plan to identify what to eat at each meal and how much to eat. The dietitian introduces the *Exchange Lists for Meal Planning* and helps Mike and his wife plan menus. After 2 months, Mike has lost 12 lb, and his blood glucose levels have improved. Mike and his wife feel comfortable with using the exchange lists.

CONCLUSION

The booklet *Exchange Lists for Meal Planning* (Appendix 12-A) should be used for clients who understand the concept of "exchange" and who would like more detail for meal planning. The booklet provides a greater variety of food choices and has many features such as a list of foods with added fats and sugars (other carbohydrates list), combination foods (includes some fast-food items), and free foods.

The exchange lists are one system of meal planning that can provide the client and practitioner with a tool to manage diabetes. Appendix 12-B has ethnic food exchanges and other educational resources are found in Appendix 12-C. If the client and practitioner select the exchange list, the meal plan developed must include the client's suggestions and should be based on previous nutrition and diabetes education provided. The exchange lists can provide variety, flexibility, nutrition adequacy, and a system that helps a client successfully change eating behaviors to improve diabetes management.[1]

REFERENCES

1. Holler HJ. Understanding the use of the exchange lists for meal planning in diabetes management. *Diabetes Educ*. 1992;17(6):474–482.

2. Wood FC, Bierman EL. New concepts: diabetic dietetics. *Nutr Today*. 1972;7:4.

3. American Diabetes Association. *The American Dietetic Association Exchange Lists for Meal Planning, 1950*. Chicago, Ill: American Diabetes Association; 1950.

4. American Diabetes Association. Nutrition recommendations and principles for people with diabetes mellitus. *J Am Diet Assoc*. 1994;94:504–509.

5. Wyse BW. Nutritional analysis exchange lists for meal planning. *J Am Diet Assoc*. 1979;75:238.

6. Powers MA, Barr P, Franz M, Holler HJ, Wheeler M, Wylie-Rosett J. *Nutrition Guide for Professionals—Diabetes Education and Meal Planning*. Alexandria, Va: American Diabetes Association and American Dietetic Association; 1988.

7. Holler HJ, Pastors JG, eds. *Diabetes Medical Nutrition Therapy: A Guide for Professionals*. Chicago, Ill: The American Dietetic Association and American Diabetes Association; in press.

Exchange Lists for Meal Planning

STARCH LIST

Cereals, grains, pasta, breads, crackers, snacks, starchy vegetables, and cooked dried beans, peas, and lentils are starches. In general, one starch is:

- 1/2 cup of cereal, grain, pasta, or starchy vegetable,
- 1 ounce of a bread product, such as 1 slice of bread,
- 3/4 to 1 ounce of most snack foods. (Some snack foods may also have added fat.)

Nutrition Tips

1. Most starch choices are good sources of B vitamins.
2. Foods made from whole grains are good sources of fiber.
3. Dried beans and peas are a good source of protein and fiber.

Selection Tips

1. Choose starches made with little fat as often as you can.
2. Starchy vegetables prepared with fat count as one starch and one fat.
3. Bagels or muffins can be 2, 3, or 4 ounces in size, and can, therefore, count as 2, 3, or 4 starch choices. Check the size you eat.
4. Dried beans, peas, and lentils are also found on the Meat and Meat Substitutes list.
5. Regular potato chips and tortilla chips are found on the Other Carbohydrates list.
6. Most of the serving sizes are measured after cooking.
7. Always check Nutrition Facts on the food label.

**One starch exchange equals
15 grams carbohydrate,
3 grams protein,
0–1 grams fat, and
80 calories.**

Bread

Bagel	1/2 (1 oz)
Bread, reduced-calorie	2 slices (1 1/2 oz)
Bread, white, whole-wheat, pumpernickel, rye	1 slice (1 oz)
Bread sticks, crisp, 4 in. long x 1/2 in.	2 (2/3 oz)
English muffin	1/2
Hot dog or hamburger bun	1/2 (1 oz)
Pita, 6 in. across	1/2
Roll, plain, small	1 (1 oz)
Raisin bread, unfrosted	1 slice (1 oz)
Tortilla, corn, 6 in. across	1
Tortilla, flour, 7–8 in. across	1
Waffle, 4 1/2 in. square, reduced-fat	1

Cereals and Grains

Bran cereals	1/2 cup
Bulgur	1/2 cup
Cereals	1/2 cup
Cereals, unsweetened, ready-to-eat	3/4 cup
Cornmeal (dry)	3 Tbsp
Couscous	1/3 cup
Flour (dry)	3 Tbsp
Granola, low-fat	1/4 cup
Grape-Nuts	1/4 cup
Grits	1/2 cup
Kasha	1/2 cup
Millet	1/4 cup
Muesli	1/4 cup
Oats	1/2 cup

Starch List continued

Pasta	1/2 cup
Puffed cereal	1 1/2 cups
Rice milk	1/2 cup
Rice, white or brown	1/3 cup
Shredded Wheat	1/2 cup
Sugar-frosted cereal	1/2 cup
Wheat germ	3 Tbsp

Starchy Vegetables

Baked beans	1/3 cup
Corn	1/2 cup
Corn on cob, medium	1 (5 oz)
Mixed vegetables with corn, peas, or pasta	1 cup
Peas, green	1/2 cup
Plantain	1/2 cup
Potato, baked or boiled	1 small (3 oz)
Potato, mashed	1/2 cup
Squash winter (acorn, butternut)	1 cup
Yam, sweet potato, plain	1/2 cup

Crackers and Snacks

Animal crackers	8
Graham crackers, 2 1/2 in. square	3
Matzoh	3/4 oz
Melba toast	4 slices
Oyster crackers	24
Popcorn (popped, no fat added or low-fat microwave)	3 cups
Pretzels	3/4 oz
Rice cakes, 4 in. across	2
Saltine-type crackers	6
Snack chips, fat-free (tortilla, potato)	15–20 (3/4 oz)
Whole-wheat crackers, no fat added	2–5 (3/4 oz)

Dried Beans, Peas, and Lentils
(Count as 1 starch exchange, plus 1 very lean meat exchange.)

Beans and peas (garbanzo, pinto, kidney, white, split, black-eyed)	1/2 cup
Lima beans	2/3 cup
Lentils	1/2 cup
Miso*	3 Tbsp

---

*400 mg or more sodium per exchange.

Starchy Foods Prepared with Fat
(Count as 1 starch exchange, plus 1 fat exchange.)

Biscuit, 2 1/2 in. across	1
Chow mein noodles	1/2 cup
Corn bread, 2 in. cube	1 (2 oz)
Crackers, round butter type	6
Croutons	1 cup
French-fried potatoes	16–25 (3 oz)
Granola	1/4 cup
Muffin, small	1 (1 1/2 oz)
Pancake, 4 in. across	2
Popcorn, microwave	3 cups
Sandwich crackers, cheese or peanut butter filling	3
Stuffing, bread (prepared)	1/3 cup
Taco shell, 6 in. across	2
Waffle, 4 1/2 in. square	1
Whole-wheat crackers, fat added	4–6 (1 oz)

Some food you buy uncooked will weigh less after you cook it. Starches will often swell in cooking, so a small amount of uncooked starch will become a much larger amount of cooked food. The following table shows some of the changes.

Food (Starch Group)	Uncooked	Cooked
Oatmeal	3 Tbsp	1/2 cup
Cream of Wheat	2 Tbsp	1/2 cup
Grits	3 Tbsp	1/2 cup
Rice	2 Tbsp	1/3 cup
Spaghetti	1/4 cup	1/2 cup
Noodles	1/3 cup	1/2 cup
Macaroni	1/4 cup	1/2 cup
Dried beans	1/4 cup	1/2 cup
Dried peas	1/4 cup	1/2 cup
Lentils	3 Tbsp	1/2 cup

Common Measurements

3 tsp = 1 Tbsp	4 ounces = 1/2 cup
4 Tbsp = 1/4 cup	8 ounces = 1 cup
5 1/3 Tbsp = 1/3 cup	1 cup = 1/2 pint

FRUIT LIST

Fresh, frozen, canned, and dried fruits and fruit juices are on this list. In general, one fruit exchange is:

- 1 small to medium fresh fruit,
- 1/2 cup of canned or fresh fruit or fruit juice,
- 1/4 cup dried fruit.

Nutrition Tips

1. Fresh, frozen, and dried fruits have about 2 grams of fiber per choice. Fruit juices contain very little fiber.

2. Citrus fruits, berries, and melons are good sources of vitamin C.

Selection Tips

1. Count 1/2 cup cranberries or rhubarb sweetened with sugar substitutes as free foods.

2. Read the Nutrition Facts on the food label. If one serving has more than 15 grams of carbohydrate, you will need to adjust the size of the serving you eat or drink.

3. Portion sizes for canned fruits are for the fruit and a small amount of juice.

4. Whole fruit is more filling than fruit juice and may be a better choice.

5. Food labels for fruits may contain the words "no sugar added" or "unsweetened." This means that no sucrose (table sugar) has been added.

6. Generally, fruit canned in extra light syrup has the same amount of carbohydrate per serving as the "no sugar added" or the juice pack. All canned fruits on the fruit list are based on one of these three types of pack.

**One fruit exchange equals
15 grams carbohydrate and 60 calories.
The weight includes skin, core,
seeds, and rind.**

Fruit

Apple, unpeeled, small	1 (4 oz)
Applesauce, unsweetened	1/2 cup
Apples, dried	4 rings
Apricots, fresh	4 whole (5 1/2 oz)
Apricots, dried	8 halves
Apricots, canned	1/2 cup
Banana, small	1 (4 oz)
Blackberries	3/4 cup
Blueberries	3/4 cup
Cantaloupe, small	1/3 melon (11 oz) or 1 cup cubes
Cherries, sweet, fresh	12 (3 oz)
Cherries, sweet, canned	1/2 cup
Dates	3
Figs, fresh	1 1/2 large or 2 medium (3 1/2 oz)
Figs, dried	1 1/2
Fruit cocktail	1/2 cup
Grapefruit, large	1/2 (11 oz)
Grapefruit sections, canned	3/4 cup
Grapes, small	17 (3 oz)
Honeydew melon	1 slice (10 oz) or 1 cup cubes
Kiwi	1 (3 1/2 oz)
Mandarin oranges, canned	3/4 cup
Mango, small	1/2 fruit (5 1/2 oz) or 1/2 cup
Nectarine, small	1 (5 oz)
Orange, small	1 (6 1/2 oz)
Papaya	1/2 fruit (8 oz) or 1 cup cubes
Peach, medium, fresh	1 (6 oz)
Peaches, canned	1/2 cup
Pear, large, fresh	1/2 (4 oz)
Pears, canned	1/2 cup
Pineapple, fresh	3/4 cup
Pineapple, canned	1/2 cup
Plums, small	2 (5 oz)
Plums, canned	1/2 cup
Prunes, dried	3
Raisins	2 Tbsp
Raspberries	1 cup

Fruit List continued
Strawberries .... 1 1/4 cup whole berries
Tangerines, small .... 2 (8 oz)
Watermelon .... 1 slice (13 1/2 oz)
 or 1 1/4 cup cubes

Fruit Juice
Apple juice/cider .... 1/2 cup
Cranberry juice cocktail .... 1/3 cup

Cranberry juice cocktail,
 reduced-calorie .... 1 cup
Fruit juice blends, 100% juice .... 1/3 cup
Grape juice .... 1/3 cup
Grapefruit juice .... 1/2 cup
Orange juice .... 1/2 cup
Pineapple juice .... 1/2 cup
Prune juice .... 1/3 cup

MILK LIST

Different types of milk and milk products are on this list. Cheeses are on the Meat list and cream and other dairy fats are on the Fat list. Based on the amount of fat they contain, milks are divided into skim/very low-fat milk, low-fat milk, and whole milk. One choice of these includes:

	Carbohydrate (g)	Protein (g)	Fat (g)	Calories
Skim/very low-fat	12	8	0–3	90
Low-fat	12	8	5	120
Whole	12	8	8	150

Nutrition Tips

1. Milk and yogurt are good sources of calcium and protein. Check the food label.

2. The higher the fat content of milk and yogurt, the greater the amount of saturated fat and cholesterol. Choose lower-fat varieties.

3. For those who are lactose intolerant, look for lactose-reduced or lactose-free varieties of milk.

Selection Tips

1. One cup equals 8 fluid ounces or 1/2 pint.

2. Look for chocolate milk, frozen yogurt, and ice cream on the Other Carbohydrates list.

3. Nondairy creamers are on the Free Foods list.

4. Look for rice milk on the Starch list.

5. Look for soy milk on the Medium-Fat Meat list.

**One milk exchange equals
12 grams carbohydrate and
8 grams protein.**

Skim and Very Low-Fat Milk
(0–3 grams fat per serving)

Skim milk .... 1 cup
1/2% milk .... 1 cup
1% milk .... 1 cup
Nonfat or low-fat buttermilk .... 1 cup
Evaporated skim milk .... 1/2 milk
Nonfat dry milk .... 1/3 cup dry
Plain nonfat yogurt .... 3/4 cup
Nonfat or low-fat fruit-flavored yogurt
 sweetened with aspartame or
 with nonnutritive sweetener .... 1 cup

Low-Fat
(5 grams fat per serving)

2% milk .... 1 cup
Plain low-fat yogurt .... 3/4 cup
Sweet acidophilus milk .... 1 cup

Whole Milk
(8 grams fat per serving)

Whole milk .... 1 cup
Evaporated whole milk .... 1/2 cup
Goat's milk .... 1 cup
Kefir .... 1 cup

OTHER CARBOHYDRATES LIST

You can substitute food choices from this list for a starch, fruit, or milk choice on your meal plan. Some choices will also count as one or more fat choices.

Selection Tips

1. Because many of these foods are concentrated sources of carbohydrate and fat, the portion sizes are often very small.
2. Always check Nutrition Facts on the label. It will be your most accurate source of information.
3. Many fat-free or reduced-fat products made with fat replacers contain carbohydrate. When eaten in large amounts, they may need to be counted. Talk with your dietitian to determine how to count these in your meal plan.
4. Look for fat-free salad dressings in smaller amounts on the Free Foods list.

Nutrition Tips

1. These foods can be substituted in your meal plan, even though they contain added sugars or fat. However, they do not contain as many important vitamins and minerals as the choices on the Starch, Fruit, or Milk list.
2. When planning to include these foods in your meal, be sure to include foods from all the lists to eat a balanced meal.

One exchange equals 15 grams carbohydrate, or 1 starch, or 1 fruit, or 1 milk.

Food	Serving Size	Exchanges per Serving
Angel food cake, unfrosted	1/12th cake	2 carbohydrates
Brownie, small unfrosted	2 in. square	1 carbohydrate, 1 fat
Cake, unfrosted	2 in square	1 carbohydrate, 1 fat
Cake frosted	2 in. square	2 carbohydrates, 1 fat
Cookie, fat-free	2 small	1 carbohydrate
Cookie or sandwich cookie with creme filling	2 small	1 carbohydrate, 1 fat
Cupcake, frosted	1 small	2 carbohydrates, 1 fat
Cranberry sauce, jellied	1/4 cup	2 carbohydrates
Doughnut, plain cake	1 medium (1 1/2 oz)	1 1/2 carbohydrates, 2 fats
Doughnut, glazed	3 3/4 in. across (2 oz)	2 carbohydrates, 2 fats
Fruit juice bars, frozen, 100% juice	1 bar (3 oz)	1 carbohydrate
Fruit snacks, chewy (pureed fruit concentrate)	1 roll (3/4 oz)	1 carbohydrate
Fruit spreads, 100% fruit	1 Tbsp	1 carbohydrate
Gelatin, regular	1/2 cup	1 carbohydrate
Gingersnaps	3	1 carbohydrate
Granola bar	1 bar	1 carbohydrate, 1 fat
Granola bar, fat-free	1 bar	2 carbohydrates
Hummus	1/3 cup	1 carbohydrate, 1 fat
Ice cream	1/2 cup	1 carbohydrate, 2 fats
Ice cream, light	1/2 cup	1 carbohydrate, 1 fat
Ice cream, fat-free, no sugar added	1/2 cup	1 carbohydrate
Jam or jelly, regular	1 Tbsp	1 carbohydrate
Milk, chocolate, whole	1 cup	2 carbohydrates, 1 fat

Other Carbohydrate List continued

Pie, fruit, 2 crusts	1/6 pie	3 carbohydrate, 2 fats
Pie, pumpkin or custard	1/8 pie	1 carbohydrate, 2 fats
Potato chips	12–18 (1 oz)	1 carbohydrate, 2 fats
Pudding, regular (made with low-fat milk)	1/2 cup	2 carbohydrates
Pudding, sugar-free (made with low-fat milk)	1/2 cup	1 carbohydrate
Salad dressing, fat-free*	1/4 cup	1 carbohydrate
Sherbet, sorbet	1/2 cup	2 carbohydrates
Spaghetti or pasta sauce, canned*	1/2 cup	1 carbohydrate, 1 fat
Sweet roll or danish	1 (2 1/2 oz)	2 1/2 carbohydrates, 2 fats
Syrup, light	2 Tbsp	1 carbohydrate
Syrup, regular	1 Tbsp	1 carbohydrate
Syrup, regular	1/4 cup	4 carbohydrates
Tortilla chips	6–12 (1 oz)	1 carbohydrate, 2 fats
Yogurt, frozen, low-fat, fat-free	1/3 cup	1 carbohydrate, 0–1 fat
Yogurt, frozen, fat-free, no sugar added	1/2 cup	1 carbohydrate
Yogurt, low-fat with fruit	1 cup	3 carbohydrates, 0–1 fat
Vanilla wafers	5	1 carbohydrate, 1 fat

VEGETABLE LIST

Vegetables that contain small amounts of carbohydrates and calories are on this list. Vegetables contain important nutrients. Try to eat at least 2 or 3 vegetable choices each day. In general, one vegetable exchange is:

- 1/2 cup of cooked vegetables or vegetable juice,
- 1 cup of raw vegetables.

If you eat 1 to 2 vegetables choices at a meal or snack, you do not have to count the calories or carbohydrates because they contain small amounts of these nutrients.

Nutrition Tips

1. Fresh and frozen vegetables have less added salt than canned vegetables. Drain and rinse canned vegetables if you want to remove some salt.
2. Choose more dark green and dark yellow vegetables, such as spinach, broccoli, romaine, carrots, chilies, and peppers.
3. Broccoli, brussels sprouts, cauliflower, greens, pepper, spinach, and tomatoes are good sources of vitamin C.
4. Vegetables contain 1 to 4 grams of fiber per serving.

Selection Tips

1. A 1-cup portion of broccoli is a portion about the size of a light bulb.
2. Tomato sauce is different from spaghetti sauce, which is on the Other Carbohydrates list.
3. Canned vegetables and juices are available without added salt.
4. If you eat more than 4 cups of raw vegetables or 2 cups of cooked vegetables at one meal, count them as 1 carbohydrate choice.
5. Starchy vegetables such as corn, peas, winter squash, and potatoes that contain larger amounts of calories and carbohydrates are on the Starch list.

---

*400 mg or more sodium per exchange.

Vegetable List continued

**One vegetable exchange equals
5 grams carbohydrate,
2 grams protein,
0 grams fat, and
25 calories.**

Artichoke
Artichoke hearts
Asparagus
Beans (green, wax, Italian)
Bean sprouts
Beets
Broccoli
Brussels sprouts
Cabbage
Carrots
Cauliflower
Celery
Cucumber
Eggplant
Green onions or scallions
Greens (collard, kale, mustard, turnip)

Kohlrabi
Leeks
Mixed vegetables (without corn, peas,
   or pasta)
Mushrooms
Okra
Onions
Pea pods
Peppers (all varieties)
Radishes
Salad greens (endive, escarole, lettuce,
   romaine, spinach)
Sauerkraut*
Spinach
Summer squash
Tomato
Tomatoes, canned
Tomato sauce*
Tomato/vegetable juice*
Turnips
Water chestnuts
Watercress
Zucchini

MEAT AND MEAT SUBSTITUTES LIST

Meat and meat substitutes that contain both protein and fat are on this list. In general, one meat exchange is:

- 1 oz meat, fish, poultry, or cheese,
- 1/2 cup dried beans.

Based on the amount of fat they contain, meats are divided into very lean, lean, medium-fat, and high-fat lists. This is done so you can see which ones contain the least amount of fat. One ounce (one exchange) of each of these includes:

	Carbohydrate (g)	Protein (g)	Fat (g)	Calories
Very Lean	0	7	0–1	35
Lean	0	7	3	55
Medium-fat	0	7	5	75
High-fat	0	7	8	100

Nutrition Tips

1. Choose very lean and lean meat choices whenever possible. Items from the high-fat group are high in saturated fat, cholesterol, and calories and can raise blood cholesterol levels.

2. Meats do not have any fiber.

3. Dried beans, peas, and lentils are good sources of fiber.

4. Some processed meats, seafood, and soy products may contain carbohydrate when consumed in large amounts. Check the Nutrition Facts on the label to see if the amount is close to 15 grams. If so, count it as a carbohydrate choice as well as a meat choice.

*400 mg or more sodium per exchange.

Meat List continued

Selection Tips

1. Weigh meat after cooking and removing bones and fat. Four ounces of raw meat is equal to 3 ounces of cooked meat. Some examples of meat portions are:
   - 1 ounce cheese = 1 meat choice and is about the size of a 1-inch cube
   - 2 ounces meat = 2 meat choices, such as
     – 1 small chicken leg or thigh
     – 1/2 cup cottage cheese or tuna
   - 3 ounces meat = 3 meat choices and is about the size of a deck of cards, such as
     – 1 medium pork chop
     – 1 small hamburger
     – 1/2 of a whole chicken breast
     – 1 unbreaded fish fillet
2. Limit your choices from the high-fat group to three times per week or less.
3. Most grocery stores stock Select and Choice grades of meat. Select grades of meat are the leanest meats. Choice grades contain a moderate amount of fat, and Prime cuts of meat have the highest amount of fat. Restaurants usually serve Prime cuts of meat.
4. "Hamburger" may contain added seasoning and fat, but ground beef does not.
5. Read labels to find products that are low in fat and cholesterol (5 grams or less of fat per serving).
6. Dried beans, peas, and lentils are also found on the Starch list.
7. Peanut butter, in smaller amounts, is also found on the Fat list.
8. Bacon, in smaller amounts, is also found on the Fat list.

Meal Planning Tips

1. Bake, roast, broil, grill, poach, steam, or boil these foods rather than frying.
2. Place meat on a rack so the fat will drain off during cooking.
3. Use a nonstick spray and a nonstick pan to brown or fry foods.
4. Trim off visible fat before or after cooking.
5. If you add flour, bread crumbs, coating mixes, fat, or marinades when cooking, ask your dietitian how to count it in your meal plan.

Very Lean Meat and Substitutes List

**One exchange equals
0 grams carbohydrate,
7 grams protein,
0–1 grams fat, and
35 calories.**

One very lean meat exchange is equal to one of the following items.

Poultry: Chicken or turkey (white meat, no skin), Cornish hen (no skin) .... 1 oz
Fish: Fresh or frozen cod, flounder, haddock, halibut, trout; tuna fresh or canned in water .... 1 oz
Shellfish: Clams, crab, lobster, scallops, shrimp, imitation shellfish .... 1 oz
Game: Duck or pheasant (no skin), venison, buffalo, ostrich .... 1 oz
Cheese with 1 gram or less of fat per ounce:
Nonfat or low-fat cottage cheese .... 1/4 cup
Fat-free cheese .... 1 oz
Other: Processed sandwich meats with 1 gram or less fat per ounce, such as deli thin, shaved meats, chipped beef,* turkey ham .... 1 oz
Egg whites 2
Egg substitutes, plain .... 1/4 cup
Hot dogs with 1 gram or less fat per ounce* .... 1 oz
Kidney (high in cholesterol) .... 1 oz
Sausage with 1 gram or less fat per ounce .... 1 oz

Count as one very lean meat and one starch exchange.

Dried beans, peas, lentils (cooked) .... 1/2 cup

---

*400 mg or more sodium per exchange.

Lean Meat and Substitutes List

**One exchange equals
0 grams carbohydrate,
7 grams protein,
3 grams fat, and
55 calories.**

One lean meat exchange is equal to any one of the following items.

Beef: USDA Select or Choice grades of lean beef trimmed of fat, such as round, sirloin, and flank steak; tenderloin; roast (rib, chuck, rump); steak (T-bone, porterhouse, cubed), ground round .... 1 oz
Pork: Lean pork, such as fresh ham; canned, cured, or boiled ham; Canadian bacon*; tenderloin, center loin chop .... 1 oz
Lamb: Roast, chop, leg .... 1 oz
Veal: Lean chop, roast .... 1 oz
Poultry: Chicken, turkey (dark meat, no skin), chicken white meat (with skin), domestic duck or goose (well-drained of fat, no skin) .... 1 oz
Fish:
  Herring (uncreamed or smoked) .... 1 oz
  Oysters .... 6 medium
  Salmon (fresh or canned), catfish............. 1 oz
  Sardines (canned) .... 2 medium
  Tuna (canned in oil, drained) .... 1 oz
Game: Goose (no skin), rabbit................... 1 oz
Cheese:
  4.5%-fat cottage cheese...................... 1/4 cup
  Grated Parmesan .... 2 Tbsp
  Cheeses with 3 grams or less
  fat per ounce .... 1 oz
Other:
  Hot dogs with 3 grams or less
  fat per ounce* .... 1 1/2 oz
  Processed sandwich meat with
  3 grams or less fat per ounce,
  such as turkey pastrami or kielbasa.......... 1 oz
  Liver, heart (high in cholesterol).............. 1 oz

Medium-Fat Meat and Substitutes List

**One exchange equals
0 grams carbohydrate,
7 grams protein,
5 grams fat, and
75 calories.**

One medium-fat meat exchange is equal to any one of the following items.

Beef: Most beef products fall into this category (ground beef, meatloaf, corned beef, short ribs, Prime grades of meat trimmed of fat, such as prime rib) .... 1 oz
Pork: Top loin, chop, Boston butt, cutlet .... 1 oz
Lamb: Rib roast, ground .... 1 oz
Veal: Cutlet (ground or cubed, unbreaded) .... 1 oz
Poultry: Chicken dark meat (with skin), ground turkey or ground chicken, fried chicken (with skin) .... 1 oz
Fish: Any fried fish product .... 1 oz
Cheese with 5 grams or less fat per ounce:
  Feta .... 1 oz
  Mozzarella .... 1 oz
  Ricotta .... 1/4 cup (2 oz)
Other:
  Egg (high in cholesterol,
  limit to 3 per week) 1
  Sausage with 5 grams or
  less fat per ounce .... 1 oz
  Soy milk .... 1 cup
  Tempeh.. 1/4 cup
  Tofu .... 4 oz or 1/2 cup

High-Fat Meat and Substitutes List

**One exchange equals
0 grams carbohydrate,
7 grams protein,
8 grams fat, and
100 calories.**

Remember these items are high in saturated fat, cholesterol, and calories and may raise blood

---

*400 mg or more sodium per exchange.

cholesterol levels if eaten on a regular basis. One high-fat meat exchange is equal to any one of the following items.

Pork: Spareribs, ground pork,
pork sausage .... 1 oz
Cheese: All regular cheeses,
such as American,* cheddar,
Monterey Jack, Swiss .... 1 oz
Other: Processed sandwich meats
with 8 grams or less fat per ounce,
such as bologna, pimento loaf, salami ..... 1 oz

Sausage, such as bratwurst, Italian,
knockwurst, Polish, smoked .... 1 oz
Hot dog (turkey or chicken)* 1 (10/lb)
Bacon .... 3 slices (20 slices/lb)

Count as one high-fat meat plus one fat exchange.

Hot dog (beef, pork, or
combination)* 1 (10/lb)
Peanut butter
(contains unsaturated fat) .... 2 Tbsp

FAT LIST

Fats are divided into three groups, based on the main type of fat they contain: monounsaturated, polyunsaturated, and saturated. Small amounts of monounsaturated and polyunsaturated fats in the foods we eat are linked with good health benefits. Saturated fats are linked with heart disease and cancer. In general, one fat exchange is:

- 1 teaspoon of regular margarine or vegetable oil,
- 1 tablespoon of regular salad dressings.

Nutrition Tips

1. All fats are high in calories. Limit serving sizes for good nutrition and health.
2. Nuts and seeds contain small amounts of fiber, protein, and magnesium.
3. If blood pressure is a concern, choose fats in the unsalted form to help lower sodium intake, such as unsalted peanuts.

Selection Tips

1. Check the Nutrition Facts on food labels for serving sizes. One fat exchange is based on a serving size containing 5 grams of fat.
2. When selecting regular margarine, choose those with liquid vegetable oil as the first

ingredient. Soft margarines are not as saturated as stick margarines. Soft margarines are healthier choices. Avoid those listing hydrogenated or partially hydrogenated fat as the first ingredient.

3. When selecting low-fat margarines, look for liquid vegetable oil as the second ingredient. Water is usually the first ingredient.
4. When used in smaller amounts, bacon and peanut butter are counted as fat choices. When used in larger amounts, they are counted as high-fat meat choices.
5. Fat-free salad dressings are on the Other Carbohydrates list and the Free Foods list.
6. See the Free Foods list for nondairy coffee creamers, whipped topping, and fat-free products, such as margarines, salad dressings, mayonnaise, sour cream, cream cheese, and nonstick cooking spray.

Monounsaturated Fats List

**One fat exchange equals
5 grams fat and 45 calories.**

Avocado, medium .... 1/8 (1 oz)
Oil (canola, olive, peanut) .... 1 tsp
Olives: ripe (black) .... 8 large
　　　 green, stuffed* .... 10 large

---

*400 mg or more sodium per exchange.

Fat List continued

Nuts:

almonds, cashews	6 nuts
mixed (50% peanuts)	6 nuts
peanuts	10 nuts
pecans	4 halves
Peanut butter, smooth or crunchy	2 tsp
Sesame seeds	1 Tbsp
Tahini paste	2 tsp

Polyunsaturated Fats List

One fat exchange equals
5 grams fat and 45 calories.

Margarine: stick, tub, or squeeze	1 tsp
lower-fat (30% to 50% vegetable oil)	1 Tbsp
Mayonnaise: regular	1 tsp
reduced-fat	1 Tbsp
Nuts: walnuts, English	4 halves
Oil (corn, safflower, soybean)	1 tsp
Salad dressing: regular*	1 Tbsp

reduced-fat	2 Tbsp
Miracle Whip Salad Dressing®: regular	2 tsp
reduced-fat	1 Tbsp
Seeds: pumpkin, sunflower	1 Tbsp

Saturated Fats List**

One fat exchange equals
5 grams fat and 45 calories.

Bacon, cooked	1 slice (20 slices/lb)
Bacon, grease	1 tsp
Butter: stick	1 tsp
whipped	1 tsp
reduced-fat	1 Tbsp
Chitterlings, boiled	2 Tbsp (1/2 oz)
Coconut, sweetened, shredded	2 Tbsp
Cream, half and half	2 Tbsp
Cream cheese: regular	1 Tbsp (1/2 oz)
reduced-fat	2 Tbsp (1 oz)
Fatback or salt pork, see below †	
Shortening or lard	1 tsp
Sour cream: regular	2 Tbsp
reduced-fat	3 Tbsp

FREE FOODS LIST

A free food is any food or drink that contains less than 20 calories or less than 5 grams of carbohydrate per serving. Foods with a serving size listed should be limited to three servings per day. Be sure to spread them out throughout the day. If you eat all three servings at one time, it could affect your blood glucose level. Foods listed without a serving size can be eaten as often as you like.

Fat-Free or Reduced-Fat Foods

Cream cheese, fat-free	1 Tbsp
Creamers, nondairy, liquid	1 Tbsp
Creamers, nondairy, powdered	2 tsp
Mayonnaise, fat-free	1 Tbsp
Mayonnaise, reduced-fat	1 tsp

Margarine, fat-free	4 Tbsp
Margarine, reduced-fat	1 tsp
Miracle Whip®, nonfat	1 Tbsp
Miracle Whip®, reduced-fat	1 tsp
Nonstick cooking spray	
Salad dressing, fat-free	1 Tbsp
Salad dressing, fat-free, Italian	2 Tbsp
Salsa	1/4 cup
Sour cream, fat-free, reduced-fat	1 Tbsp
Whipped topping, regular or light	2 Tbsp

Sugar-Free or Low-Sugar Foods

Candy, hard, sugar-free	1 candy
Gelatin dessert, sugar-free	
Gelatin, unflavored	
Gum, sugar-free	

---

*400 mg or more sodium per exchange.

**Saturated fats can raise blood cholesterol levels.

†Use a piece 1 in. x 1 in. x 1/4 in. if you plan to eat fatback cooked with vegetables. Use a piece 2 in. x 1 in. x 1/2 in. when eating only the vegetables with the fatback removed.

Free Foods List continued

Jam or jelly, low-sugar or light .... 2 tsp
Sugar substitutes†
Syrup, sugar-free .... 2 Tbsp

Drinks

Bouillon, broth, consommé*
Bouillon or broth, low-sodium
Carbonated or mineral water
Cocoa powder, unsweetened .... 1 Tbsp
Coffee
Club soda
Diet soft drinks, sugar-free
Drink mixes, sugar-free
Tea
Tonic water, sugar-free

Condiments

Catsup .... 1 Tbsp
Horseradish

Lemon juice
Lime juice
Mustard
Pickles, dill* .... 1 1/2 large
Soy sauce, regular or light*
Taco sauce .... 1 Tbsp
Vinegar

Seasonings

Be careful with seasonings that contain sodium or are salts, such as garlic or celery salt, and lemon pepper.

Flavoring extracts
Garlic
Herbs, fresh or dried
Pimento
Spices
Tabasco® or hot pepper sauce
Wine, used in cooking
Worcestershire sauce

COMBINATION FOODS LIST

Many of the foods we eat are mixed together in various combinations. These combination foods do not fit into any one exchange list. Often it is hard to tell what is in a casserole dish or prepared food item. This is a list of exchanges for some typical combination foods. This list will help you fit these foods into your meal plan. Ask your dietitian for information about any other combination foods you would like to eat.

Food Entrees	Serving Size	Exchange per Serving
Tuna noodle casserole, lasagna, spaghetti with meatballs, chili with beans, macaroni and cheese**	1 cup (8 oz)	2 carbohydrates, 2 medium-fat meats
Chow mein (without noodles or rice)	2 cups (16 oz)	1 carbohydrate, 2 lean meats
Pizza, cheese, thin crust**	1/4 of 10 in. (5 oz)	2 carbohydrates, 2 medium-fat meats, 1 fat
Pizza, meat topping, thin crust**	1/4 of 10 in. (5 oz)	2 carbohydrates, 2 medium-fat meats, 2 fats
Pot pie*	1 (7 oz)	2 carbohydrates, 1 medium-fat meat, 4 fats
Frozen Entrees		
Salisbury steak with gravy, mashed potato*	1 (11 oz)	2 carbohydrates, 3 medium-fat meats, 3–4 fats
Turkey with gravy, mashed potato, dressing**	1 (11 oz)	2 carbohydrates, 2 medium-fat meats, 2 fats

---

* 400 mg or more sodium per choice.

** 400 mg or more sodium per exchange.

† Sugar substitutes, alternatives, or replacements that are approved by the Food and Drug Administration (FDA) are safe to use. Common brand names include: Equal® (aspartame); Sprinkle® (saccharin); Sweet One® (acesulfame K); Sweet-10® (saccharin); Sugar Twin® (saccharin); Sweet 'n Low® (saccharin)

Combination Foods List continued

Entree with less than
  300 calories* .... 1 (8 oz) .... 2 carbohydrates, 3 lean meats

Soups

Bean* .... 1 cup .... 1 carbohydrate, 1 very lean meat
Cream (made with water)* .... 1 cup (8 oz) .... 1 carbohydrate, 1 fat
Split pea (made with water)* .... 1/2 cup (4 oz) .... 1 carbohydrate
Tomato (made with water)* .... 1 cup (8 oz) .... 1 carbohydrate
Vegetable beef, chicken noodle,
  or other broth-type* .... 1 cup (8 oz) .... 1 carbohydrate

---

FAST FOODS LIST

Food	Serving Size	Exchange per Serving
Burritos with beef**	2	4 carbohydrates, 2 medium-fat meats, 2 fats
Chicken nuggets**	6	1 carbohydrate, 2 medium-fat meats, 1 fat
Chicken breast and wing, breaded and fried**	1 each	1 carbohydrate, 4 medium-fat meats, 2 fats
Fish sandwich/tartar sauce**	1	3 carbohydrates, 1 medium-fat meat, 3 fats
French fries, thin	20–25	2 carbohydrates, 2 fats
Hamburger, regular	1	2 carbohydrates, 2 medium-fat meats
Hamburger, large**	1	2 carbohydrates, 3 medium-fat meats, 1 fat
Hot dog with bun**	1	1 carbohydrate, 1 high-fat meat, 1 fat
Individual pan pizza**	1	5 carbohydrates, 3 medium-fat meats, 3 fats
Soft-serve cone	1 medium	2 carbohydrates, 1 fat
Submarine sandwich**	1 sub (6 in.)	3 carbohydrates, 1 vegetable, 2 medium-fat meats, 1 fat
Taco, hard shell*	1 (6 oz)	2 carbohydrates, 2 medium-fat meats, 2 fats
Taco, soft shell*	1 (3 oz)	1 carbohydrate, 1 medium-fat meat, 1 fat

---

*400 mg or more sodium per exchange.
** 400 mg or more of sodium per serving.

Note: Ask your fast-food restaurant for nutrition information about your favorite fast foods.

Ethnic Food Exchanges

Food	Serving	Food Exchange
Mexican Foods		
Burrito, bean	1 small	2 starch
	1 large	1 medium-fat meat, 3 starch, 2 fat
Burrito, meat (beef)	1 small	1 starch, 1 medium-fat meat
	1 large	2 1/2 starch, 3 medium-fat meat, 1 fat
Chili	1 cup	2 starch, 2 medium-fat meat, 1 fat
Chili sauce	2 tsp	1/3 fruit
Corn chips	1 oz (1 cup)	1 starch, 2 fat
Enchilada: meat or cheese	1 small (6" tortilla)	1 medium-fat meat
Refried beans	1/2 cup	1 starch, 1 medium-fat meat
Spanish rice	1 cup	2 starch, 1 fat
Spanish sauce	1/2 cup	1/3 fruit, 1 fat
Tamale with sauce	1	1 starch, 1 medium-fat meat
Tortilla/taco shell	6" diameter	1 starch
Taco (meat, cheese, lettuce, tomato)	1	1 starch, 2 medium-fat meat
Tostada		
with refried beans	1 small	2 starch
with meat	1 small	1 starch, 1 high-fat meat
Chinese Foods		
Egg flower, soup	1 cup	1/2 medium-fat meat
Fried rice (rice, meat, eggs, onions)	1 cup	1 1/2 starch, 1/2 medium-fat meat
Fortune cookies	1	1/2 starch or 1/2 fruit
Egg roll	1	1/2 starch, 1 vegetable
Chow mein	1 cup	1 starch, 1 medium-fat meat, 1 vegetable
Sukiyaki	1 cup	3 medium-fat meat, 1 fat
Tofu	2 oz	1/2 medium-fat meat
Chop suey	1 cup	2 medium-fat meat, 1 vegetable
Pepper steak	1 cup	1 starch, 3 medium-fat meat, 1 vegetable
Chow mein noodles	1/2 cup	1 starch, 1 fat
Egg foo young	1	1 vegetable, 2 medium-fat meat, 2 fat
East Indian Foods		
Alu Mattar (curried potatoes and peas)	1 cup	1 vegetable, 1 1/2 starch, 3 fat
Alu Paratha	6" diameter	2 1/2 starch, 6 fat
(flat whole wheat bread with spiced potato filling)		
Chana Dal (curried chick peas)	1/2 cup	2 medium-fat meat
Kheema do Pyaza	1 cup	2 vegetable, 3 lean meat, 3 fat
(curried ground lamb with onions)		
Kofta	3 balls	3 high-fat meat, 4 fat
	(approx. 1 1/2" diameter)	

Source: McCance and Widdowson's The Composition of Foods by AA Paul and DA Southgate, Elsevier Science Publishing Company Inc, © 1985; *Food Values of Portions Commonly Used* by JAT Pennington and HN Church, Harper & Row Publishers, © 1980.

Food	Serving	Food Exchange
Machli aur tomatar (curried halibut)	3 oz fish	1/2 vegetable, 3 lean meat, 1 1/2 fat
Masala dosai (crepe-like pancake with spiced potato filling)	1	2 starch, 4 fat
Chicken curry	3 oz chicken	1/2 vegetable, 3 lean meat, 2 fat
Samosas (deep-fried filled pastries)	1 large or 3 small (potato filling)	1 starch, 2 fat
	1 large or 3 small (lamb filling)	1 starch, 1/2 lean meat, 2 1/2 fat
Italian Foods		
Vermicelli soup	1 cup	1 starch
Minestrone soup	1 cup	1 starch, 1 fat
Pasta, cooked	1/2 cup	1 medium-fat meat
Italian ham (Prosciutto)	1 oz	1 medium-fat meat
Meatballs	1 oz	1 medium-fat meat
Chicken cacciatore	3 oz chicken with sauce	3 lean meat, 1 vegetable, 1 fat
Eggplant parmesan	1 cup	2 medium-fat meat, 2 vegetable, 1 starch, 1 1/2 fat
Veal parmesan	1 cutlet (4 oz)	1 starch, 4 medium-fat meat, 1 vegetable, 1 fat
Italian spaghetti	1 cup	2 starch, 2 vegetable, 2 medium-fat meat
Lasagna	1 (3" x 4") serving	1 starch, 1 vegetable, 2 1/2 medium-fat meat
Manicotti	1 shell	1 1/2 starch, 1 vegetable, 3 medium-fat meat, 2 fat
Pizza with cheese, sausage, pepperoni	1/4 of 16 oz pizza	2 starch, 1 vegetable, 2 medium-fat meat, 1 fat
Ravioli		2 starch, 1 vegetable, 1 medium-fat meat, 1 fat
with cheese	1 cup	
with beef	1 cup	2 starch, 1 vegetable, 1 medium-fat meat, 1 fat
Jewish Foods		
Bagel	1/2	1 starch
Bialy	1	1 starch
Challah	1 slice	1 starch
Matzo, 6" diameter	1	1 starch
Matzo, crackers	7 (1 1/2" square each)	1 starch
Potato latkes (calculate the fat used in cooking)	1/2 cup	1 starch
Kippered herring	1 oz	1 lean meat
Pickled herring	1 oz	1 lean meat
Smoked salmon (lox)	1 oz	1 lean meat
Corned beef	1 oz	1 high-fat meat
Chopped liver	1 oz	1 high-fat meat

Resource List

EXCHANGE LIST EDUCATION RESOURCES

1. *Healthy Food Choices*

This pamphlet presents general nutritional guidelines. It opens into a mini-poster in which foods are grouped by exchange groups. Blank lines are provided for writing a personalized meal plan. Available in Spanish.

Available from The American Dietetic Association, Tel: 1-800-877-1600, Ext. 5000 and American Diabetes Association, Tel: 1-800-232-3472, Ext. 5000).

2. *The Exchange Lists for Meal Planning*

Available from The American Dietetic Association and the American Diabetes Association.

3. *HCF Exchanges: A Sensible Plan for Healthy Eating*

The focus of the HCF Exchanges is high-fiber nutrition with an emphasis on soluble fiber to lower insulin needs and blood lipid levels. Because of this emphasis, the HCF Exchanges categorize foods into the following groups: cereal, starches, beans, garden vegetables, fruit, milk, protein, and fat.

Available from J.W. Anderson, MD, HCF Diabetes Foundation, 1987, PO Box 22124, Lexington, KY 40522. Tel: 1-800-727-4423.

4. *HCF Guide Book*

This guide book offers practical advice for incorporating the HCF nutrition plan into daily eating habits. It outlines specifics of the nutrition plan, different kinds of fiber, importance of exercise, and information on how smoking and stress affect health. Practical suggestions are made on cooking, eating out, and shopping.

Available from JW Anderson, MD, HCF Diabetes Foundation, 1987, PO Box 22124, Lexington, KY 40522. Tel: 1-800-727-4423.

5. *Exchange It: An Aid to Diet Control in Diabetes*

The kit consists of a folder with two sets of six pockets, labeled for each meal and snack. A clock face is pictured on each pocket, showing the average meal time for the person with diabetes. Several *Exchange It* tickets labeled with food group choices and a picture symbol to correspond with a particular food group are included. On the back of each ticket are listed several foods and allowed portions. Also included are tickets for diabetes medications.

Available from F. Charles Hospital, R. Clark, LPN, Exchange It Program, 2600 Navarre Avenue, Oregon, OH 43616. Tel: (419) 691-2225.

6. *Better Meals for You*

This booklet uses the ADA/ADA Exchange Lists to teach the basics of meal planning. Exchanges for combination foods, as well as information on fiber, fat, cholesterol, and sodium and guidelines for weighing and measuring, are included.

Available from Diabetes Association of Greater Cleveland, 2022 Lee Road, Cleveland, OH 44118. Tel: (216) 591-0800.

7. *Menu Planning—Simple!*

It offers advice on how to understand, use, and individualize meal plans. Exchange lists, non-nutritive sweeteners, and fast-food information are also featured. It has a helpful question/answer format.

Available from Joslin Diabetes Center, One Joslin Place, Boston, MA 02215. Tel: (617) 732-2695.

RENAL DIET EXCHANGE LIST RESOURCES

1. *National Renal Diet*

This was developed by renal dietitians from the ADA Renal Dietetic Practice Group and National Kidney Foundation Council on Renal Nutrition. Professional guide and client education booklets offer standardized guidelines for nutrition intervention and client education in renal disease.

Available from The American Dietetic Association, Tel; 1-800-877-1600, Ext. 5000

2. *Eating Right ... The Diabetic Low Protein Way*

This nutrition education booklet uses a system of exchange lists to control protein, carbohydrate, phosphorus, and sodium intake while maintaining palatable nutrition with a variety of food choices. It includes sources of low-protein products and directions for using nutrition labeling to select appropriate foods, along with several days of sample menus.

Available from Dialyrn, 914 South Eighth Street, D-4, Minneapolis, MN 55404. Tel: (612) 347-5949.

ADDITIONAL EXCHANGE LIST RESOURCES

1. *Convenience Food Facts* by A. Monk

This book includes nutrition information and exchanges for thousands of convenience foods found in any grocery store. Listings are given for more than 1500 popular brand names.

Available from Chronimed Publishing, 13911 Ridgedale Drive, Minnetonka, MN 55305. Tel: 1-800-848-2793.

2. *Exchanges for All Occasions* by M.J. Franz

This book can help anyone to effectively use the diabetes exchange system for meal planning. This book includes exchanges for Italian, Oriental, and Jewish foods, sample meal plans, and planning suggestions for just about any occasion.

Available from Chronimed Publishing, 13911 Ridgedale Drive, Minnetonka, MN 55305. Tel: 1-800-848-2793.

3. *The Exchange Game* by M. Canterbury

This game is a hands-on teaching tool designed to teach the concepts of nutrition and diabetes specifically with the exchange system, using audio, visual, and kinesthetic techniques. The materials are appropriate for use in educating a variety of age groups and literacy levels and can be used with individuals and groups.

Available from Health Partners, Center for Health Promotion, 8100 34th Avenue, PO Box 1309, Minneapolis, MN 55440. Tel: (612) 883-6724.

4. *The Art of Cooking for the Diabetic, Third Edition* by M. Abbott Hess

This is an excellent example of cookbooks available for people with diabetes. It provides diabetes nutrition information in the front of the book followed by 375 recipes. Exchanges are given for each recipe as well as calories, carbohydrate, protein, total fat, saturated fat, cholesterol, fiber, and sodium.

Available from Contemporary Books, 2 Prudential Plaza, Suite 1200, Chicago, IL 60601. Tel: (312) 540-4500.

5. *Cookbooks for People with Diabetes; Diet and Nutrition: Guides, Manuals, Fact Sheets and Cookbooks for People with Diabetes*

This publication is an annotated bibliography providing information on cookbooks and diabetes nutrition resources.

Available from National Diabetes Information Clearinghouse, Box NDIC, 9000 Rockville Pike, Bethesda, MD 20892. Tel: (301) 654-3327.

6. *Ethnic and Regional Food Practices Series: Food Practices, Customs, Holidays*

This series of booklets details food-related traditions and customs of various ethnic groups living in the United States. Supplementary exchange lists and recipes are included.

Available from American Dietetic Association, Tel: 1-800-877-1600, Ext. 5000; also available from American Diabetes Association, Tel: 1-800-232-6733.

Chapter 13

Carbohydrate Counting for Diabetes Nutrition Therapy

Betty Brackenridge

Several distinct meal-planning systems are used in diabetes therapy. Each one stresses a different factor important to dietary management: calories, portion control, food choices, fat or carbohydrate content, and so on. The relative importance of these factors for a given patient is related to characteristics such as diagnosis, clinical goals, and the patient's preferences, knowledge, and learning ability. The appropriateness of the various approaches for diabetes patients with specific personal and clinical characteristics has been evaluated[1,2] and is discussed in Chapter 11. This chapter examines the rationale for and implementation of one such system, carbohydrate counting. Relatively little hard data regarding carbohydrate counting appears in the diabetes literature. It is an empirical approach based on a simplistic understanding of the glucose effects of major food fuels. Much of its power comes from frequent and proactive use of blood glucose monitoring, from its simplicity, and from its attractiveness to persons with diabetes.

Carbohydrate counting is specifically focused on techniques to optimize blood glucose control. In type I diabetes, it is used to match premeal insulin doses to the demand created by food. Doses are adjusted up or down on the basis of actual intake. However, for persons with type II diabetes for whom caloric restriction is a goal, adjustment of the insulin dose for greater-than-normal food intake is not encouraged. Rather, carbohydrate counting may be more useful in such cases to ferret out the cause of unexplained glucose excursions, to accommodate the use of favorite high-carbohydrate foods, or as an alternative to more complicated meal-planning approaches for managing consistent daily food intake.

When carbohydrate counting is used, other aspects of the nutritional plan such as nutritional adequacy, quality and quantity of fat eaten, protein intake, fiber intake, and so forth, must be addressed separately, as needed by the individual client.

RATIONALE FOR INTENSIVE INSULIN THERAPY

Diabetes destroys the body's elegant, precise, and fully automatic system for maintaining glucose homeostasis. Patients and health care providers seek to compensate for that defect with an external system that includes sampling blood glucose levels and manipulating diet, medication, and exercise in response to the findings. One of the primary goals of implementing such an externally imposed system is to match the timing and the quantity of available insulin, whether from endogenous or exogenous sources, to the demands created by the ingestion of food and by the energy consumption of physiologic processes.

The non–insulin-using person with type II diabetes controls blood glucose by balancing food intake with the endogenous insulin supply, with or without the added assistance of oral agents, and physical activity. In such persons there is a discreet limit on the amount of insulin action that can be achieved and so food intake must be calibrated against that limit. Therefore, when postprandial glucose excursions are excessive, limitation of food intake—either through reduction of total intake or through its redistribution in the day—is needed.

In insulin-treated patients, insulin doses may be static or variable, depending on a variety of clinical and personal factors. Static insulin regimens require that the patient maintain static nutritional intake in order to achieve reasonable glucose control. In contrast, protocols by which the patient can vary insulin doses in response to changing circumstances facilitate greater flexibility in food choices and portions. In short, the greater the extent to which external insulin replacement mimics physiologic insulin delivery, the more likely it is that the desirable goals of stable glucose control and life-style flexibility can be achieved. Of all forms of insulin therapy currently in use, delivery of insulin by continuous subcutaneous insulin infusion (CSII) allows the closest approximation of physiologic insulin action. A more physiologic insulin profile can also be approximated through various regimens of multiple daily injections (MDI). CSII and, to a somewhat lesser degree, MDI facilitate the delivery of precise amounts of insulin at discreet points in time. However, capitalizing on these more physiologic insulin delivery schemes requires significant skill in determining the specific insulin rates and doses required to meet changing needs.

For example, in CSII, accurate calibration of the basal rate(s) allows for total freedom in the timing of meals. A given meal can be delayed or even eliminated if patient preference or life circumstances dictate it. Bolus doses of regular insulin are then used to match meal-related insulin demand when food is actually eaten. Precise calibration of these boluses is critical in achieving excellent diabetes control. This need for precise calibration of premeal bolus doses to meal-related insulin demand is also true of MDI regimens. In conventional (ie, one, two, and three injection) insulin regimens, insulin adjustments are more likely to be based on several days of blood glucose patterns than on

meal-to-meal variations in blood glucose levels and food selection.

RATIONALE FOR CARBOHYDRATE COUNTING

Dietary carbohydrate is the main determinant of meal-related insulin demand. Although the absolute glucose excursion and rate of glucose appearance differ among individual carbohydrate foods,[3] it is estimated that 90 to 100% of digestible dietary carbohydrate enters the bloodstream as glucose in the first few hours after a meal.[4] Although a portion of dietary protein and fat are metabolized to glucose, overall these nutrients yield much less glucose than does an equal quantity of carbohydrate.[4] Also, the glucose released by the metabolism of fat and protein does not appear in the bloodstream in the immediate postprandial period. For these reasons, protein and fat are assumed to contribute relatively little to meal-related insulin demand. When fat and protein intake is relatively consistent from day to day, the basal or intermediate-acting insulin present between meals is adjusted to handle the glucose released by their metabolism.

A quite precise estimate of the insulin demand created by a particular meal or snack can, therefore, be derived by simply counting the grams of carbohydrate it contains. For certain patients, this simple approach can be more precise, more easily taught, and less limiting than more complex systems. Carbohydrate counting can make excellent glucose control possible at a very acceptable cost in terms of both effort and life-style restraint for many diabetes patients. It is uniquely suited for those following intensive modes of therapy that utilize flexible insulin regimens.

Alcohol, even though it yields calories, is not considered here because its metabolism does not release glucose to the bloodstream. However, in addition to their alcohol content, sweet wines and mixed drinks made with caloric mixers contain carbohydrate that may need to be included in the carbohydrate count for a meal.

DERIVING THE CARBOHYDRATE COUNTING MEAL PLAN

The basic meal plan for a patient who uses carbohydrate counting is composed of gram totals of carbohydrate to be consumed at each planned meal and snack. There are two ways to develop such a plan. The preferred method for patients with type I diabetes is to base the plan on the patient's current eating habits. An average or usual meal pattern can be identified using several days of food records provided by the patient. This pattern can then be translated into the carbohydrate gram equivalent that is consumed at each meal or snack. This approach can also be used for patients with type II diabetes, with adjustments to the usual intake negotiated to better match intake with available insulin (endogenous or exogenous) or reduce caloric intake as needed. Any desirable changes to improve overall nutritional intake or to address specific risk factors are negotiated on an incremental basis as education progresses.

Alternatively, a carbohydrate plan can be derived from an estimated or calculated calorie prescription by multiplying the desired caloric intake by the desired proportion of carbohydrate and dividing the resulting value by 4. For example, a patient is estimated to require 2000 calories for weight maintenance and the goal is for him to consume 50% of calories as carbohydrate. Multiply 2000 kcal by 0.5 and divide the resulting value (1000) by 4 kcal/g of carbohydrate. The total daily carbohydrate allowance would be 250 g. This total allowance is then distributed among the day's meals and snacks with attention to the patient's preferences for meal size and composition, and subsequently fine-tuned on the basis of blood glucose results.

When the meal plan is developed in this fashion, the calculated carbohydrate allowance must be compared with the patient's current intake. Care should be taken to minimize dramatic differences between the calculated carbohydrate allowance and the actual intake in insulin-using patients because current insulin doses were undoubtedly derived in association with the customary carbohydrate intake. Insulin doses may need to be altered to prevent loss of glucose control if large changes are made in the calorigenic composition of the diet.

The basic meal plan should be followed fairly closely as the patient learns the carbohydrate counting system and stabilizes diabetes control. A stable food intake makes it much easier to correctly adjust the basic insulin doses and, later, to accurately derive the patient's insulin-to-carbohydrate ratio, if insulin adjustments for varied food intake will be used. When this ratio is known, the patient can match insulin doses to actual food intake to accommodate variations in appetite, food availability, personal or work circumstances, and other factors.

CALCULATING PREMEAL DOSES OF REGULAR INSULIN USING THE INSULIN-TO-CARBOHYDRATE RATIO

For each individual with diabetes, there is an identifiable ratio between grams of carbohydrate eaten and the number of units of insulin required to use them. This ratio can be used to calculate the appropriate premeal dose of insulin (bolus) for any meal or snack of known carbohydrate content. The ratio varies significantly from patient to patient: from as little as 5 g of carbohydrate per unit of insulin up to as many as 20 g. Observation suggests that lower ratios might be expected in insulin-resistant individuals with type II diabetes and higher ratios in thin, fit persons with type I diabetes. For example, in my practice I counsel a 154-lb male marathon runner who requires only 1 U of insulin for each 22 g of carbohydrate. However, I have found that most of my patients with type I diabetes require 1 U of premeal bolus regular insulin for each 10 to 15 g of dietary carbohydrate. In general, the lower the total daily insulin dose, the greater the number of grams of carbohydrate covered by a single unit of insulin.

However, because such estimates and generalizations are not adequate to optimize control, the precise ratio for each person should be individually determined. This determination must be made when the diabetes is in good control and meals of known carbohydrate composition are being eaten. Attempting to derive the ratio when glucose control is poor or when an extremely variable diet is being consumed may produce a false value.

Establishing control requires maintaining a stable meal plan while performing frequent blood glucose tests. The basic meal plan can be expressed as grams of carbohydrate to be eaten at each meal and snack or as food exchanges. The basic insulin doses should then be adjusted on the basis of blood glucose values until control stabilizes within the patient's target blood glucose range. As a guideline, most of the patient's fasting and premeal blood glucose tests should be less than 180 mg/dL before attempting to derive the insulin-to-carbohydrate ratio. The premeal reading before any actual meal tested should be between 80 and 150 mg/dL. At this level, we can be confident that the premeal bolus dose will actually be used to cover the food eaten at the meal. If the blood glucose is high, on the other hand, some unpredictable portion of the bolus insulin will be used by the body to meet basal needs.

A rough estimate of the insulin-to-carbohydrate ratio acts as the starting point for identifying the correct ratio. One basis for choosing a starting estimate, based on the patient's weight, is shown in Table 13-1.

Another approach to selecting an initial insulin-to-carbohydrate ratio is to review food and insulin dose records, calculating the patient's average ratio of insulin to carbohydrate on a meal-by-meal basis. A final option is to simply select a ratio in the most common range (1 unit per 10 to 15 g) as the starting point. All of the methods are used successfully by various clinicians. The estimate is then fine-tuned using the results of pre- and postmeal blood glucose determinations. The appropriate ratio has been identified when postprandial blood glucose levels return to the desired range 1 to 5 hours after the meal, depending on how glucose goals are expressed. If the postprandial glucose is higher

Table 13-1 *Estimated* Insulin-to-Carbohydrate Ratio Based on Patient Weight (Grams of Dietary Carbohydrate Covered by 1 U of Regular Insulin Given as a Premeal Bolus)

Weight (lb)	Units:Carbohydrate (g)
100 – 109	1:16
110 – 129	1:15
130 – 139	1:14
140 – 149	1:13
150 – 169	1:12
170 – 179	1:11
180 – 189	1:10
190 – 199	1:9
200 – 219	1:8
220 – 239	1:7
240+	1:6

Source: Adapted from Walsh J, Roberts R. *Pumping Insulin* (p 66) with permission of Torrey Pines Press, ©1994.

than the target value, then a lower insulin-to-carbohydrate ratio should be tried at the next meal or snack. For example, if the patient shown in Exhibit 13-1 found a 2-hour postprandial blood glucose of 220 mg/dL, she might try using 1 U of insulin for each 13 or 14 g of carbohydrate at the next meal.

The process of deriving the insulin-to-carbohdyrate ratio and of monitoring ongoing control in those using carbohydrate counting can be greatly enhanced by using record-keeping forms specifically suited to this meal-planning approach. Two examples are shown in Exhibits 13-2 and 13-3. Exhibit 13-2 is most appropriate for persons just learning carbohydrate counting because it incorporates a food record with space to write in carbohydrate counts for specific foods. The person with diabetes can accumulate information about carbohydrate counts and their respective effects on blood glucose until they have become adept at estimating carbohydrate counts. Exhibit 13-3 may be more appropriate for established users of carbohydrate counting. It allows meal carbohydrate totals, insulin doses, and resulting blood glucose values to be graphed in relation to each other.

Exhibit 13-1 Sample Bolus Calculation by Different Methods

Patient:	37-year-old woman, 112 lb
Estimated Ratio:	15 g carbohydrate (CHO) per unit insulin **or** 1 interchange per unit of insulin

	Method of Carbohydrate Counting			
Sample Meal	**Gram Counting**	**Interchanges**	**Exchanges**	**TAG**
1 ham sandwich	36 g CHO	2 interchanges	2 Starch = 30 g	36 g CHO + 12.6 g CHO (21 g protein x 0.6)
4 oz cup bean soup	11 g CHO	1/2 interchange	1/2 Starch = 8 g	11 g CHO + 1.8 g CHO (3 g protein x 0.6)
Green salad	5 g CHO	Free	Free	5 g CHO
8 oz low-fat milk	12 g CHO	1 interchange	1 Milk = 12 g	12 g CHO + 4.8 g CHO (8 g protein x 0.6)
3 fresh apricots	12 g CHO	1 interchange	1 Fruit = 15 g	12 g CHO
Total carbohydrate	**76 g**	**4 1/2 interchanges**	**65 g**	**95.2 g**
Calculated premeal dose of short-acting insulin or bolus	5.1 U[a]	4.5 U[a]	4.3 U[a]	6.3 U[a,b]

[a] Doses containing fractional units can be given by pump; for injections with syringe or pen, round dose to nearest whole unit.

[b] In patients using systems such as total available glucose (TAG) that account for dietary protein in the bolus insulin dose calculation, total daily insulin doses will not be different, as compared with the same patient using simply carbohydrate counting. However, different basal insulin rates or insulin-to-carbohydrate ratios may be derived under the TAG approach because of the different way in which premeal doses are being determined.

HOW MANY BOLUSES?

One of the most common uses of carbohydrate counting is to identify the bolus dose of regular insulin needed to cover the glucose peak produced by each meal and snack. The more gradual release of glucose between meals, whether from dietary fat and protein or from endogenous sources such as hepatic glucose release, is covered by the basal insulin rate of insulin pumps or the intermediate-acting or long-acting insulin present between meals. Does that mean that anytime a patient eats carbohydrate,

another bolus dose of regular insulin is required? Not necessarily. The correct answer for each patient must be developed on the basis of experience and blood glucose testing.

The peaks produced by the regular insulin currently available are much broader than the peaks of endogenous insulin. As a result, regular insulin injected at meal time will be present in the bloodstream for 3 to 5 hours after the meal. This broad peak makes it wise to be cautious about taking doses of regular insulin too close together. Peaks may overlap, producing unwanted glucose-lowering effects. Small unplanned snacks, containing

Exhibit 13-2 Example #1 of Record-Keeping Form

Day/Date _____ **Insulin-to-CHO Ratio** _____ **High BG Supplement:** ± 1 unit R/ _____ mg/dL from goal

Note: To make it easier for you to see the results of your meals and insulin doses, blood glucose values are graphed directly above the CHO counts and bolus doses that are related to that reading.

Glucose Graph

	Fasting BG	2 h after bkfst	Before lunch	2 h after lunch	Predinner	2 h after dinner	Bedtime	3 AM
320								
280								
240								
200								
180								
160								
140								
120								
100								
70								
50								

Food Record

Breakfast Time ___	g CHO ___	Snack Time ___	g CHO ___	Lunch Time ___	g CHO ___	Snack Time ___	g CHO ___	Dinner Time ___	g CHO ___	Snack Time ___	g CHO ___
Total		Total		Total		Total		Total		Total	

Insulin

Type	Time	U	Time	U	Time	U	Time	U	Time	U	Time	U
CHO BOLUS												
HIGH BG BOLUS												
BASAL RATE												
U, NPH, L												

Exhibit 13-3 Example #2 of Record-Keeping Form

Day	FBS	pc Bfst	ac Lunch	pc Lunch	ac Dinner	pc Dinner	HS	3 AM	FBS	pc Bfst	ac Lunch	pc Lunch	ac Dinner	pc Dinner	HS	3 AM	Exercise, illness, new/unusual foods
Glucose																	
320																	
280																	
240																	
200																	
180																	
160																	
140																	
100																	
70																	
50																	
G Carbohydrate	Bkfst	Snack	Lunch	Snack	Dinner	Snack			Bkfst	Snack	Lunch	Snack	Dinner	Snack			
105																	
90																	
75																	
60																	
45																	
30																	
15																	
Insulin	CHO Bolus	CHO Bolus	CHO Bolus	CHO Bolus	CHO Bolus	CHO Bolus		CHO Bolus	CHO Bolus	CHO Bolus	CHO Bolus	CHO Bolus	CHO Bolus	CHO Bolus		CHO Bolus	
9																	
8																	
7																	
6																	
5																	
4																	
3																	
2																	
1																	
BG Suppl.																	
Basal Rate/ NPH Dose																	

Source: Copyright © 1993. Learning Prescriptions, Phoenix, Arizona.

Exhibit 13-4 Isocarbohydrate Meals

	Item	CHO (g)	Fat (g)	Fiber (g)
Meal 1:	8 oz orange juice	27	0	<1
	2 slices white bread	26	2	2
	2 oz part-skim cheese	2	8	<1
	1 oz puffed rice cereal	13	0	<1
	4 oz skim milk	6	0	<1
	Black coffee	0	0	0
	Total	**74**	**10**	**~4**
Meal 2:	1 apple (3/lb)	18	1	3
	2 slices bran bread	26	4	6
	2 tsp soft margarine	1	10	<1
	1/2 cup 100% Bran	23	2	13
	4 oz low-fat milk	6	3	<1
	Total	**74**	**~20**	**~22**

15 g of carbohydrate or less, do not usually require an additional bolus, especially if the glucose level is near the lower end of the desired range before eating. Larger snacks may require a bolus, especially if blood glucose is already at the higher end of the desired range before eating. There are no hard and fast rules about this. The most effective strategy must be identified by each person with diabetes through personal experimentation and will be greatly affected by the specific insulin regimen being used.

FACTORS AFFECTING GLUCOSE RESPONSE

Although counting carbohydrates is an effective meal-planning approach, it is far from exact. The glucose responses created by meals of the same total carbohydrate content can differ significantly. For example, in a study involving eight patients with well-controlled type I diabetes, Ahern and colleagues[5] observed a significantly higher glucose response after a pizza meal, as compared with an isocaloric and isocarbohydrate control meal. The exaggerated glucose rise occurred between 4 and 9 hours after the pizza meal, even though the insulin regimen was held constant and the other test meal included high glycemic index foods. Among the factors thought to play a role in such departures from a predictable carbohydrate response are fat and fiber content of the meal, food form (particle size and cooked versus raw), protein content, time of day, and between-subject variation. Responses may also vary according to the glycemic index of specific foods chosen, to the premeal blood glucose status, and to the timing of the meal-related insulin dose. Some postprandial blood glucose results, such as the previously described "pizza effect," can be difficult to explain. Documenting food intake, activity, insulin doses, and blood glucose results will build an individualized history that reveals each clients' particular responses to specific foods. This eventually makes it possible to precisely calibrate insulin doses and timing for many circumstances to achieve the best possible glycemic control.

Fat and Fiber Intake

Carbohydrate foods, when eaten alone, have fairly predictable rates of digestion and absorption, which translate into predictable glucose release and insulin demand. However, foods are most often eaten in combination (eg, not potatoes alone but potatoes with meat, gravy, margarine, vegetables, and wine). Some food combinations alter rates of carbohydrate digestion and absorption, modifying the pattern of glucose rise after the meal. When this occurs, although the total amount of glucose released into the bloodstream may remain unchanged, the postprandial glucose excursion can be delayed or blunted, changing the interaction between insulin demand and availability.

Therefore, the two isocarbohydrate meals shown in Exhibit 13-4 may produce significantly different 2-hour postprandial glucose levels. Postmeal glucose testing should be used to determine the optimal size and timing of the premeal insulin bolus for specific meals.

Food Form

Glucose response can also be impacted by food form. Form refers to the physical characteristics of a food such as its relative particle size and whether it is cooked or raw. When cooked, some foods elicit a more abrupt glucose rise than they do when raw, presumably because of enhanced digestibility and absorption of the carbohydrate they contain. This effect may be less noticeable when the food is eaten as part of a mixed meal containing foods of various forms.

High Protein Intake

The exact proportion of protein metabolized to glucose varies, depending on factors such as availability of other fuels and metabolic state. Any glucose yielded by dietary protein does not appear in the bloodstream immediately after the meal but is released slowly over several hours. When protein intake falls within the general guidelines of the diabetes diet (eg, 15 to 20% of calories or 0.8 g/kg), the impact on postprandial blood glucose levels is negligible. However, meals that include considerably more protein than the usual intake may be followed by significant delayed rise in serum glucose. It is not known whether this response is due to the effect of protein per se or to the effect of associated fats on the rate of absorption of the carbohydrates contained in the meal.

Various sources suggest that 50 to 70% of dietary protein can be converted to glucose under certain conditions,[6,7] but there have been no definitive studies of this effect in diabetic persons. Clinically, providers and patients alike observe blood glucose elevations that appear to be related to protein ingestion and, therefore, some clinicians prefer to account for the presence of dietary protein in determining meal-related insulin doses. If glucose goals are not being met by counting carbohydrate alone or if an apparent effect of protein is observed, the approach described below can be used to incorporate protein into the calculation of meal-related insulin doses. Using this approach does not typically affect the total daily insulin dose. Rather, non–meal-related insulin doses (intermediate- and long-acting insulins or basal insulin rates in pump users) get adjusted accordingly.

If we begin with the assumption that approximately 60% of dietary protein can be metabolized to glucose, then each ounce of protein—which contains 7 g of protein—should yield about 4 g of glucose. For example, Joe eats 12 oz of his mom's delicious pot roast at Sunday dinner, instead of his usual 3 oz protein portion. This would be expected to release approximately 38 extra g of glucose, as compared with his usual meal (9 extra oz of meat × 7 g protein per ounce × 0.6 = 38 g glucose). Depending on the patient's insulin-to-carbohydrate ratio, this would change the optimal premeal dose of short-acting insulin by between 2 and 4 U. In addition to increasing the amount of the premeal dose for excess protein intake, the client may also need to delay the injection or split it into premeal and postmeal segments to better match the anticipated appearance of serum glucose when a very high-protein meal is eaten.

The glucose effect of protein is consistently accounted for in calculating premeal insulin doses in the total available glucose (TAG) system.[7] This is done by multiplying the grams of protein consumed by 0.6, as shown in the example above, and then adding the resulting value to the number of grams of carbohydrate in the meal. The additional mathematics required may detract from the simplicity of carbohydrate counting for some patients. However, if glucose targets are not achieved using simple carbohydrate counting, this additional step may enhance control.

Time of Day

Many persons with diabetes find that they require relatively more insulin to handle a given amount of carbohydrate at breakfast than if it were eaten later in the day. This is assumed to be related to secretion of higher levels of counterregulatory hormones (CRHs), especially growth hormone, in the early morning hours, the so-called dawn effect. The CRHs are insulin antagonists. Their presence in the bloodstream reduces the effectiveness of insulin.

Some patients attempt to compensate for this fact by minimizing carbohydrate at the morning meal. This can prove difficult in application because so many traditional breakfast foods are composed largely or completely of carbohydrate: fruits and fruit juices, cereals, toast, bagels, and so on. Also, many breakfast food choices of lower-carbohydrate content such as bacon and eggs are undesirable as a steady diet because of their high saturated fat content.

Possible strategies for dealing with this problem include increasing the basic prebreakfast insulin dose, altering the insulin-to-carbohydrate ratio used for the breakfast bolus calculation, choosing lower glycemic index carbohydrates, or modifying the availability of basal insulin during early morning hours to overcome the transient insulin resistance. For example, a person whose usual insulin-to-carbohydrate ratio is 1:12 might use a ratio of 1:10 at breakfast and limit fruit and fruit juice at that meal. Alternatively, if using MDI, the individual might increase the bedtime dose of intermediate-acting insulin to compensate for the changing early-morning insulin requirement. If using an insulin pump, this person could program a higher basal rate during early morning hours. The individual on oral agents or nonpharmacologic treatment alone has fewer options. The amount of breakfast carbohydrate would need to be limited to what could be effectively handled by the endogenous insulin supply.

Individual Variation

Finally, there are significant individual differences in the glycemic response to specific foods. Blood glucose monitoring allows each person with diabetes and his or her caregivers to identify the optimal bolus for any dietary "wild cards" that exist. The effort required to find individual quirks in glycemic response can produce rewards in at least two ways. First, it may uncover the cause of previously puzzling episodes of poor glucose control. Also, testing to identify optimal boluses sometimes uncovers uncharacteristically flat glucose responses to foods wrongly assumed to be destructive to diabetes control. Such discoveries allow the patient a greater degree of freedom and flexibility in food choices while maintaining good glucose control.

IMPLEMENTING CARBOHYDRATE COUNTING

Sources of Information

Food labels state the grams of carbohydrate contained in a serving of the packaged food. Pocket size and larger reference books on the composition of foods are widely available in locations such as bookstores and even supermarket check-out counters. Exchange food lists reveal the carbohydrate content and corresponding portion sizes for many foods. However, because exchange carbohydrate values are averages, using this source of information will result in some loss of precision when counting carbohydrates.

Teaching Carbohydrate Counting

There are several ways that patients can be taught the inherently straightforward process of determining carbohydrate counts. Four possible approaches to carbohydrate counting are described in Table 13-2. These approaches vary in both simplicity and accuracy. In general, the simpler the method, the less precise or accurate the result. The specific approach chosen should

Table 13-2 Ways To Count Carbohydrate

Method	Description	Ease vs Accuracy	Premeal or Bolus Dose Calculation*
1. Counting carbohydrate exchanges ("interchanges")	Count each serving of starch, fruit, and milk as one carbohydrate exchange and consider them all to be equal in carbohydrate value	Easiest method but also the least accurate. Requires the least math skill	Calculate premeal dose as units/exchange
2. Counting food exchanges	Add the carbohydrate values of all exchanges that contain carbohydrate (including vegetables) to obtain the carbohydrate total for a meal	Easy and fairly accurate	Calculate premeal dose as units/exchange, counting vegetables as 1/3 exchange **OR** Calculate the bolus by dividing the total grams of carbohydrate in the meal by the insulin-to-carbohydrate ratio
3. Carbohydrate gram counting	Add carbohydrate gram values for all foods eaten to obtain carbohydrate total for meal	More time-consuming than methods 1 and 2 but also quite accurate. Requires more math skill to add and divide 2- and 3- digit numbers, because calculations are often done mentally	Calculate the premeal dose by dividing the total grams of carbohydrate in the meal by the insulin-to-carbohydrate ratio
4. Calculating available glucose	Count grams of carbohydrate for all foods eaten. Then calculate the glucose available from protein and add this value to the carbohydrate grams to obtain the meal total	Most difficult. Requires the most math skill of all the methods	Multiply grams of protein in meal by 0.6 to obtain available glucose, add to grams of carbohydrate. Calculate the dose by dividing this total by the insulin-to-carbohydrate ratio

* Short-acting insulin administered before meals to control the meal-related glucose rise. The calibration of insulin to food intake is a recommended strategy for individuals with type I diabetes, especially those following intensified diabetes regimens.

take into account the patient's abilities and motivation as well as the blood glucose results. Some patients achieve excellent glucose control when only estimating the carbohydrate values of meals. Others require much more precision, including the weighing and measuring of foods, to achieve the same results.

Interchanges

The simplest (and least precise) approach to carbohydrate counting uses carbohydrate "interchanges." All the exchange groups that are rich sources of carbohydrate contain similar quantities of carbohydrate per exchange-size serving: one starch or fruit exchange is estimated to contain 15 g carbohydrate and one milk exchange 12 g carbohydrate. Therefore, these groups can be "interchanged"; that is, an 8-oz glass of milk can be assumed to require about the same amount of insulin as a slice of bread or a small piece of fruit. With this approach, the insulin-to-carbohydrate ratio is expressed as "units per exchange." The patient is instructed to count only starch, fruit, and milk in calculating mealtime boluses. This approach may work for certain patients with relatively stable diabetes. It is also a good first step in teaching more precise methods of carbohydrate counting. If glucose goals are not achieved with this method, progressively more precise strategies should be used.

Exchanges

Additional precision is gained when exact exchange carbohydrate values are used and when *all* foods that contribute carbohydrate, including vegetables, are counted.

There are two important benefits to be gained from teaching carbohydrate counting on the basis of the exchange system. The first advantage is that building on existing knowledge limits the amount of new material that the patient must learn. The second is that counting exchanges or interchanges greatly reduces the potential for math errors. The numbers involved will all tend to be less than 10. The patient who counts actual grams of carbohydrate may have to deal with single meal totals greater than 100. This makes the addition and division of two- and three-digit numbers—something generally done mentally—a potential source of error for some people.

Carbohydrate Gram Counting

Despite the greater ease of using exchanges to quantify carbohydrate intake, many clinicians prefer that their patients count all sources of carbohydrate, using exact values from food labels or reliable food tables and references. This is the most precise approach to carbohydrate counting.

Whether patients are taught to count grams per se or to estimate them via exchanges, close attention to portion size is still important. This attention is necessary to obtain the full value of carbohydrate gram counting by *accurately quantifying* carbohydrate intake. Being able to calculate and deliver a bolus down to a fraction of a unit of insulin is of little practical use if the food portion estimate is not accurate.

Measuring Equipment

Precision is enhanced when the patient uses appropriate measuring equipment: liquid measures for liquids, dry measures for items quantified by volume, and gram scales for items quantified by weight. Computerized food scales programmed with food composition data are a convenience but may be too expensive for some patients. Using good measuring tools and technique helps ensure that the portion eaten actually provides the amount of carbohydrate shown on the food label or other listing.

In everyday circumstances, people usually eat more or less than a standard portion of a given food. Therefore, patients must eventually learn to calculate or estimate carbohydrate gram values for servings larger or smaller than standard portions shown on food labels and in reference books. The simplest approach is to use multiples (eg, I'm eating two small apples so I multiply the gram value of a single apple by two) or simple fractions (eg, I'm eating half a carton of yogurt so I multiply the grams of carbohydrate shown on the label by 0.5) of stated portions. Patients with good math skills and motivation can, of course, do more precise calculations based on accurate portion weights if they so choose. Also, those who count carbohydrates using exchanges must be aware that the serving sizes shown on food labels or in reference books may *not* be exchange-size servings. When this occurs, they could either calculate the exchange equivalent portion or simply eat the stated portion and add its carbohydrate gram count to the total for the rest of the meal that was estimated using exchanges. In practice, many patients use a combination of exchange values and actual carbohydrate counts from labels or reference books in deriving the carbohydrate counts for meals.

CONCLUSION

Carbohydrate counting is effective, easy to teach and to use, and supports a less restrictive life style for the patient. It is an excellent meal-planning approach for patients with type I diabetes, especially those using intensive insulin therapy. It is also useful as an adjunct to other meal-planning approaches in type II diabetes to help fine-tune postprandial blood glucose control. Optimal use of carbohydrate counting in type I diabetes requires that the insulin-to-carbohydrate ratio be individually derived for each patient. This is done by starting with an estimated ratio—in the range of 1 U of insulin for each 10 to 15 g of carbohydrate—and then fine-tuning that estimate on the basis of postprandial blood glucose values. The appropriate ratio has been identified when the serum glucose returns to the target range 1 to 5 hours after the meal.

The insulin-to-carbohydrate ratio can be used to calculate the appropriate premeal insulin dose for any meal or snack of known carbohydrate content. Food labels, books of food composition, and food exchange lists are accessible sources of information regarding the carbohydrate content of foods. Accurate determination of portion sizes is critical to successful use of carbohydrate counting.

REFERENCES

1. Pastors JG. Alternatives to the exchange system for teaching meal planning to people with diabetes. *Diabetes Educ.* 1992;18(1):57–62.

2. Holler HJ, Pastors JG, eds. *Meal Planning Approaches for Diabetes Management,* 2nd ed. Chicago, Ill: American Dietetic Association; 1994.

3. Jenkins DJ, Wolever TM, Taylor RH, et al. Glycemic index of foods: a physiological basis for carbohydrate exchange. *Am J Clin Nutr.* 1981;34:184–190.

4. Choppin J, Jovanovic-Peterson L, Peterson C. Matching food with insulin. *Diabetes Professional.* 1991 (Spring); 1–14.

5. Ahern JA, Gatcomb PM, Held NA, Petit WA, Tamborlane WV. Exaggerated hyperglycemia after a pizza meal in well-controlled diabetes. *Diabetes Care.* 1993;16(4): 578–580.

6. Nuttal FQ, Gannon MC. Plasma glucose and insulin response to macronutrients in nondiabetic and NIDDM subjects. *Diabetes Care.* 1991;14:824–834.

7. Oexmann MJ. *Total Available Glucose, Diabetic Food System.* Charleston, SC: Medical University of South Carolina Printing Service; 1987.

Chapter 14

Using Very Low-Calorie Diets To Achieve Weight Reduction

Anne Daly

Obesity is one of the most common and important medical conditions facing Western societies.[1,2] Because of the association of obesity with a wide variety of medical risk factors and serious health consequences,[3,4] obesity poses not only personal costs in terms of quality and length of life for the individual but also a significant economic burden to the health care system. Of all the leading causes of death in the United States, diabetes is the one most closely linked to obesity.[2] At least 80% of persons with non–insulin-dependent diabetes mellitus (NIDDM) are more than 15% in excess of desirable body weight at the time of diagnosis. Because 90% of diabetes is NIDDM, the type most closely associated with obesity, federal sources say about 45% or more of all diabetes can be considered preventable through control of obesity. It is suggested that new cases could be reduced by nearly half by preventing obesity in middle-aged adults.[2] Also, gestational diabetes mellitus is linked to obesity.

Weight reduction is one of the most effective therapies for obese NIDDM, but the success rate with conventional diets has been disappointing. The development of very low-calorie diets (VLCDs) over the past two decades has provided an alternative approach to the treatment of uncomplicated obesity and is increasingly being used to treat obese NIDDM.[5] Medical nutrition therapy designed to promote weight loss, maintain a reasonable body weight, and achieve target metabolic goals remains the primary treatment of obese NIDDM.[6,7] This requires not only control of hyperglycemia but management of as-

sociated metabolic disorders that have an effect on the complications of NIDDM, particularly obesity, hypertension, hyperinsulinemia, and hyperlipidemia.[4] When adequate metabolic control cannot be achieved with conventional nutrition therapy, VLCDs are now recognized as an effective alternative form of therapy, used either alone or in combination with pharmacological intervention.[5] Although the medical benefits of weight loss in such individuals are indisputable, there has been recurrent controversy over the exact composition, safety, and long-term efficacy of VLCDs.

This chapter reviews the historical development of VLCDs, clinical use of VLCD therapy in obese NIDDM, typical VLCD programs structure, potential benefits, long-term results, and a discussion of the pros and cons of VLCD use.

DEVELOPMENT OF VLCDs

The development of VLCDs in the 1920s arose out of a need to attain larger and more rapid weight loss than was possible with conventional diets but to avoid dangers of total starvation.[8] These diets were originally designed to provide 300 to 400 calories/d of high-quality protein as conventional food or liquid formula, with or without carbohydrate, and supplemented with vitamins and minerals.[5]

During the mid-1970s, VLCD use experienced rapid growth after the introduction of the so-called liquid protein-modified fast popularized in *The Last Chance Diet Book*.[9] Some commercial preparations were made largely from collagen or gelatin hydrolysates and thus contained low biologic value protein. These diets tended to have inadequate micronutrient supplementation and were often consumed without medical supervision. Reports of ventricular dysrhythmias and sudden death during liquid protein diets prompted formal investigation of their use and complications. These reports led to a more conservative use and attempts to improve the quality and balance of nutrients.

CONTENT OF VLCDs

Most VLCDs now provide 45 to 100 g of protein with high biologic value (from dairy or egg sources) per day.[10] Carbohydrates are included in varying amounts, up to 100 g/day. Some products also provide up to 15 g soluble fiber per day. Fats in the form of oils containing essential fatty acids have also been increased in VLCDs, as have vitamin and essential minerals. The most fundamental change in VLCDs in recent years has been a gradual increase in the number of calories from 300 to 600 per day originally to 420 to 800 per day in current products.[10,11] There are basically two types of VLCDs that are defined by their protein and carbohydrate content. One form is protein-sparing modified fast (PSMF), in which high protein intake is provided by natural foods such as lean red meat, fish, or fowl that contains minimal fat and little or no carbohydrate. Because patients on these diets learn to consume restricted amounts of natural foods, it has been proposed they more easily make the subsequent transition to a weight maintenance diet. Although highly effective, PSMF is not commonly used because of its inconvenience and the need for food preparation.

The second and most popular type of VLCD is commercially available mixed-formula diets that contain 100% of the recommended daily allowance (RDA) for amino acid, essential fatty acids, vitamins, minerals, and trace elements. Liquid formulas are usually available as a powder, which is reconstituted to liquid with water. Currently, there is no scientific evidence that

Exhibit 14-1 Desirable Characteristics for VLCD Candidates

- **Clinical Indicators**
  - BMI >30
  - Medical conditions present
  - History of diet "failures"

- **Patient Characteristics**
  - Ready for serious commitment to life-style change
  - Able to manage diabetes, including self-monitoring blood glucose
  - Positive support system, financial resources
  - Emotional, psychological stability

Note: Not all patients will meet all these characteristics. Individualized assessment by a skilled registered dietitian is required.

suggests that any particular VLCD, either in terms of composition or calorie content, has advantages over another in the treatment of obese NIDDM. Various forms of VLCD have been used to achieve weight loss and metabolic benefits in NIDDM subjects, and all have been highly efficacious[5] (see Appendix 14-A).

CLINICAL USE OF VLCD THERAPY IN NIDDM

Although VLCD therapy is not recommended as primary therapy for NIDDM, there is a potential role for VLCD treatment in almost every obese NIDDM patient with otherwise uncomplicated diabetes.[5] The dietitian's expertise is essential to consider different nutrition strategies and determine which approach best meets the individual needs of the client. Factors to be considered include weight, distribution of body fat, morbidity of complications, family history, previous weight loss attempts, age, and patient motivation. Desirable characteristics for VLCD candidates are listed in Exhibit 14-1. Bray[12] proposed an algorithm (Figure 14-1) for determining medical risk according to increasing body mass index (BMI) and accompanying risk factors.

Risk Classification Algorithm

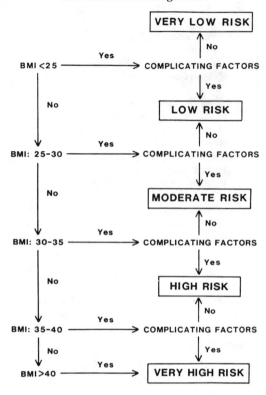

Figure 14-1 Risk Classification Algorithm. *Source:* Copyright © 1988, George A. Bray, MD.

WEIGHT INDICATORS

Some investigations suggest restricting the use of VLCDs to patients more than 50% above ideal body weight, whereas others use VLCDs for patients more than 30% over ideal body weight, especially if there is a history of repeated dietary failure or medical complications of obesity.[11] VLCDs are usually not recommended for patients with BMI of 30 or less. For patients with BMI of 25 to 30, a low-calorie diet (800 to 1200 calories) is usually considered. VLCD is more strongly indicated when fat is located in the upper body or abdomen, because upper body obesity is highly related to heart disease, stroke, diabetes, and death, independent of the degree of obesity.[2,12]

When complications of diabetes and obesity are present, such as hypertension, hyperlipidemia, coronary heart disease, or cardiopulmonary failure, a more aggressive treatment such as a VLCD is warranted. The American Diabetes Association endorses VLCDs for patients with pronounced fasting hyperglycemia to quickly reduce symptoms.[5,13] Strong family history of hyperlipidemia and coronary heart disease also suggest earlier and more aggressive intervention. VLCD therapy has also been used successfully to treat sleep apnea and arthritis and in presurgical management (ie, abdominal, back, hip, knee, and foot surgeries).

BEHAVIORAL INDICATORS

VLCD should only be considered in patients who have tried to lose weight previously and have been unsuccessful in losing weight and/or maintaining weight loss. Behavioral advantages to a VLCD include limited food choices and ease of preparation. The primary advantage, however, is that they do what they were designed to do—produce maximal short-term weight loss. On average, patients on VLCDs lose 20 kg in 12 weeks.[11,14] Men lose more than women, and heavier patients lose more than lighter patients.[14] Patients need to be ready to make a serious commitment to life-style change when they begin a VLCD. Because weekly attendance is required, their personal schedule must be cleared on the day they are scheduled for their medical visit and behavioral education class. Anyone who is not interested in following a behavior modification program *after* weight loss on a VLCD is *not* a candidate to start a VLCD. Discussions about the importance of a long-term maintenance phase should begin with even the first contact with program staff.

CONTRAINDICATIONS—ABSOLUTE AND RELATIVE

Most lists of contraindications to VLCD therapy originated primarily from studies in nondiabetic obese patients. Modification to focus on the risk of VLCD therapy in the NIDDM population is necessary to take into account the increased morbidity and mortality from NIDDM.[5] Contraindications to VLCDs may be absolute or relative[5,8] and are controversial in some instances. A relative contraindication indicates that caution is required, and that treatment may or may not be appropriate, depending on individual circumstances. Exhibit 14-2 is a suggested list of contraindications to VLCD therapy in obese NIDDM patients.[5]

Areas of controversy remain in medical situations in which the balance between risk of VLCD therapy versus benefit to the person with NIDDM may differ compared with the obese nondiabetic patient.

Renal Disease

There is no question that end-stage renal disease is a contraindication to VLCD therapy, but there have been reports of NIDDM patients with renal insufficiency (creatinine >1.5 mg/dL) who were treated with VLCD therapy successfully without further compromise of renal function.[15] In another report, subclinical proteinuria and creatinine clearance improved after VLCD therapy in obese NIDDM patients.[16] Thus, the benefits from VLCD therapy in these specific situations may outweigh the risks.[5]

Cardiovascular Disease

Most cardiovascular diseases are at least relative contraindications for VLCD therapy, yet obesity has significant adverse cardiovascular effects that may be improved by weight loss. Based on reports of successful treatment of patients of coronary artery disease,[17,18] investigators have concluded that VLCD therapy can probably be safely used even in the presence of cardiovascular disease in carefully selected and monitored patients.[5] These patients may experience not only improved glycemic control but management of associated cardiovascular risk factors (ie, hypertension and hyperlipidemia) as well.

Exhibit 14-2 Contraindications to Very Low-Calorie Diet Therapy

- **Absolute contraindications**[a]
  Cardiac disease
    Significant cardiac arrhythmias
    Recent myocardial infarction
    Unstable angina
    Decompensated congestive heart failure
  Major organ system failure
  Cerebrovascular disease—recent stroke
  Protein wasting conditions
  Untreated hypothyroidism
  Active substance abuse

- **Relative contraindications**[a]
  >65 years of age
  <130% ideal body weight
  Nephrolithiasis
  Cholelithiasis
  Gout
  Gilbert's disease
  Psychiatric disorders
  Previous noncompliance or recidivism
  Concurrent medications with known cardiac side effects or sensitive to fluid and electrolyte shifts
  Lactose intolerance[b]

- **Diabetes-related contraindications**
  Insulin-dependent diabetes mellitus
  Non–insulin-dependent diabetes mellitus and obesity due to other endocrinopathies
  Retinopathy?
  Neuropathy?

Note: Modified from reports in nondiabetic obese patients.

? indicates not a well-accepted or established side effect or is controversial.

[a] See text for applicability to non–insulin-dependent diabetes mellitus.

[b] Use formulation without lactose as carbohydrate source.

Source: Reprinted with permission from Henry R, Gumbiner B, Benefits and Limitation of Very Low Calorie Diet Therapy in Obese NIDDM. *Diabetes Care* (1991;14:802–803), Copyright © 1991, American Diabetes Association.

Gallbladder Disease

Gallbladder disease is more prevalent among the obese population, particularly obese females, than the normal weight population. The relative risk of gallbladder disease among moderately obese women (BMI $\geq$32) is six times higher than that of lean women.[19] Between 10 and 25% of obese men and women may develop gallstones within a few months of beginning a VLCD, and perhaps one-third of these will develop symptoms of gallstones. Persons with highest BMI before weight loss and those who lose weight most rapidly appear to be at greatest risk for gallstones. Treatment with urso-deoxycholic acid at the first indication of gall-bladder disease has been effective in dissolving small cholesterol stones, the type most likely to occur in a VLCD-treated population. Although it may appear prudent to exclude persons with pre-existing gallstones from weight loss, no evidence supports this approach.[20] Obese patients contemplating weight loss, particularly a VLCD, should be aware they are at increased risk for developing gallstones. There is a notable lack of literature on the relationship of gallbladder disease and weight loss, and more studies are needed on the effects of low-calorie diets on persons with pre-existing gallstones.

Yo-Yo Dieting

Another controversial contraindication to VLCD therapy is repetitive bouts of dieting. Because many patients regain their weight, some reinstitute dieting, often without medical supervision. This pattern, often referred to as yo-yo dieting, is discussed in greater detail later in this chapter. However, in the case of obese NIDDM, one can argue there are significant metabolic benefits derived from caloric restriction per se.[5,21] Future studies may show it is feasible to evenly restrict caloric intake for short periods as a form of "booster therapy" to improve glycemia, responsiveness to conventional pharmacologic therapy, and control of hypertension and hyperlipidemia.

Insulin-Dependent Diabetes Mellitus

Insulin-dependent diabetes mellitus (IDDM) is usually listed as a relative contraindication to VLCD therapy. Because of the potential for se-

vere ketosis and/or hypoglycemia, VLCDs should be used with caution and close medical monitoring.[8] Patients with IDDM need to have previously received comprehensive diabetes education, and medical monitoring during the VLCD by staff with diabetes expertise (ie, an endocrinologist, certified diabetes educator) is advisable. Other unique contraindications to consider are diabetic complications that may be exacerbated by rapid glycemic control.[5] This has not been adequately studied, but a possibility exists for progression of existing diabetic complications.

Children

In children, weight loss should be carried out under the supervision of a physician, taking into account the child's age, height, and degree of overweight.[8] Caloric intake should be high enough to support normal growth, and protein intakes should be set at higher levels than recommended for adults on VLCDs. Treatment should include behavioral techniques and family involvement. Restrictive diets, such as VLCDs, may be useful in the management of some severely obese children and adolescents[22,23] but should be considered experimental and carried out with careful and experienced medical supervision.[8]

Pregnancy and Lactation

VLCD are contraindicated in pregnant and lactating women due to increased nutritional requirements. If a woman undergoing VLCD therapy becomes pregnant, accelerated refeeding should begin.

Older Persons

Unfortunately, little information exists regarding safety of VLCDs in older individuals. Although weight losses are equivalent to younger persons on VLCDs and improvements in blood pressure and cholesterol are similar, older persons may be at increased risk for negative nitrogen balance because of an already depleted lean body mass and lowered immuno-logic responses.[8] These increased risks must be balanced with the potential benefit of weight loss in older persons.

Clearly, it is important to continue to study the risk-benefit ratio of VLCD therapy in NIDDM patients and revise the list of contraindications accordingly.

PHASES OF COMPREHENSIVE VLCD PROGRAMS

Only comprehensive long-term weight control programs can provide effective treatment for obesity.[24,25] Generally, such a program includes four phases: (1) induction, (2) weight loss, (3) transition or refeeding, and (4) maintenance. An overview of VLCD therapy components is listed in Exhibit 14-3.

Exhibit 14-3 VLCD Therapy Components for Persons with Diabetes

- **Medical Screening and Assessment**

- **Medical Monitoring**
  - Blood Glucose Monitoring
  - Medication Adjustments

- **The VLCD**
  - 400–700 cal/d
  - Protein: $\geq$70 g (1.2–1.5 g/kg desirable body weight)
  - Carbohydrate: up to 100 g
  - Vitamins/Minerals: RDA

- **Intense Behavioral Education**
  - Weight Loss Phase
  - Maintenance Phase

- **Individualized Follow-Up**

Induction Phase

The first step of a comprehensive VLCD behavioral program is an orientation. An orientation is a no-cost, no-obligation information session for prospective patients interested in learning more about the program(s) available. The orientation is an essential first step of the treatment program, not an option that can be missed. Educators begin to lay foundations that will increase patient compliance and success after they have joined, including a program overview, medical issues, side effects and possible risks of the diet, fees, class times, insurance issues, etc, as well as the importance of participation in a comprehensive long-term maintenance program.

The second step of the induction phase, for which there is a fee, is a thorough medical screening and evaluation to determine whether VLCD therapy can be used safely with a given patient. The evaluation should include a nutrition history, a medical history, and physical examination, along with laboratory testing, not only for screening purposes but also as a baseline for monitoring treatment. Tests should include a general chemistry panel (glucose, electrolytes, uric acid, cholesterol, triglyceride, re-nal, and liver tests), complete blood count, urinalysis, thyroid function tests, and a resting electrocardiogram (ECG) with rhythm strip to screen for active cardiac diseases, dysrhythmias, or prolonged QT interval.[5,8]

Weight Loss Phase

Medical supervision and monitoring are imperative for safe VLCD therapy. The over-the-counter preparations that entice individuals to treat themselves with a VLCD should be vigorously discouraged.[26] A physician with specialized training in the use of VLCDs and a supervising physician treating NIDDM should oversee medical therapy throughout the VLCD and during refeeding. Multidisciplinary specialists trained in clinical nutrition and diabetes therapy (ie, registered dietitians, certified diabetes educators, behavioral psychologists) can effectively and safely manage patients with adequate physician support.[5]

Patients with concomitant medical conditions, such as diabetes or hypertension, require close monitoring of medications, usually weekly (Table 14-1). Because oral agents pose the risk of hypoglycemia, many clinicians discontinue them on the first day of the diet and reinstitute them during or after diet therapy if necessary. If a patient is treated with insulin, insulin dose is typically decreased by approximately 50% on VLCD initiation. Close monitoring of self-monitoring blood glucose (SMBG) (two to four times daily) is necessary to prevent hypoglycemia and monitor glucose response to VLCDs. Diuretics are usually discontinued entirely to avoid potentiating electrolyte and fluid shifts associated with VLCD. Antihypertensive medications can be tapered rapidly as well. Continued laboratory monitoring every 2 weeks and periodic ECGs are advisable.

Side effects from VLCD therapy are common during the first 2 weeks of treatment when the rate of weight loss is highest.[17,27] The most common possible side effects that the patient should be informed of are bowel changes, lightheadedness, headaches, and fatigue. Most side effects are easily managed by taking prescribed supplement and fluids.

More frequent contact with NIDDM patients and more intensive monitoring are required for obese NIDDM patients taking insulin. SMBG should begin on the first day of the diet; unlike conventional dieting, the rapid fall in fasting hyperglycemia may immediately reinforce the positive effects of the diet.[5,21] Specific instructions regarding spacing of the supplement and the possible need to use an additional supplement to balance blood glucose levels are necessary. Patterns of supplement intake could vary depending on nutrient composition of the product being used, but taking one serving of a supplement at least every 2.5 to 3 hours during the day is a typical pattern. Individual life style is an important consideration, however, which is the same as with any other medical nutrition therapy regimen.

Daily telephone contact with the health care team to discuss SMBG results and adjust medications may be warranted for the first 1 to 2 weeks. SMBG should continue subsequently at least 3 times per week and more frequently if patients remain on hypoglycemic agents. Urine ketones should be checked during clinic visits

and are useful to monitor supplement compliance and fluid intake. Urine ketones remain negative when the VLCD contains larger amounts of carbohydrate (>50 g/day) and the patient follows the prescribed supplement and fluid regimen. Some NIDDM patients may need basic diabetes education to supplement the behavioral education component of the VLCD program.

The question regarding appropriate duration of treatment has been discussed at length but has never been addressed in a controlled study.[5] Opinion is divided between those who recommend limiting the duration of VLCDs to an arbitrary period of 12 to 16 weeks and those who support open-ended duration of VLCDs until patients reach goal weight or a weight loss plateau. Most clinical investigations have lasted for 12 to 16 weeks,[17,27,28] but others have treated patients safely for longer periods,[5] including myself. The length of time a patient is on a VLCD depends on the judgment of the physician providing medical supervision. The point at which the diet should be terminated is usually obvious to the patient and the health care providers; at less than 130% ideal body weight, VLCDs are generally contraindicated, and conventional dieting should replace the VLCD.[5]

Behavioral Education Intervention

The behavioral education provided the VLCD patients must include the facts and procedures they will need to adopt new life-style behaviors to self-manage their weight over time. Structure of these programs will vary depending on the program site and whether the commercial product being used has developed such a program. A typical format includes a 90-minute behavioral group weekly.[29] The content of the behavioral education is organized into three sequential sections.

The first of these sections extends over the first 12 to 16 weeks and is sometimes referred to as "core." The core behavioral groups are designed to touch basic program content in a relatively structured way and help patients adhere to the VLCD as closely as possible. Content areas include recordkeeping, physical activity, how to balance calories in food with physical activity expenditure, environmental control, nutrition, and failure and avoidance responses.

These sessions are followed by "ongoing" groups for patients who are still on the VLCD beyond 12 to 16 weeks because they have substantial amounts of weight to lose. Ongoing groups allow for expansion and interrelating (weaving) of core information. The educator will individualize the program for patients by demonstrating the problem-solving, learning-based approach to managing issues during the weight loss and maintenance phases. Ongoing sessions offer active "hands-on" learning opportunities (ie, food labs, record-based groups, physical activity sampling, supermarket nutrition, etc). The third section is the maintenance

behavioral education, which is described later in this chapter.

Role of Physical Activity

Physical activity plays a vital role in the management of all persons with diabetes, especially VLCD-treated patients. Physical activity lowers blood glucose both short and long term, as indicated by glycosylated hemoglobin concentrations. Many investigators have demonstrated that regular physical training or activity increases insulin sensitivity, whereas deconditioning and physical inactivity are associated with the development of insulin resistance.[30] Recently, physical activity has been shown to be a critical factor in preventing NIDDM,[31] largely due to its role in preventing or treating obesity. This protective effect is especially pronounced

Table 14-1 Medical Monitoring of NIDDM During Weight Loss Phase

Week	Self-Monitoring Required	Laboratory Tests	Phone Contact Frequency	Medication Changes To Consider
1	Self-monitoring blood glucose (SMBG) bid if on oral agent; SMBG qid if on insulin. Food and fluid records	None	Daily if on insulin; 2–3x/week otherwise	Continue/reduce/stop oral agent Reduce insulin by 50%; continue/ adjust hypertensive/ diuretic
2	Same as above plus physical activity (PA) records	Urinalysis	2–3x/week or more as needed	Reduce oral agent/ insulin per SMBG
3	Same as above plus calculate PA expenditure	Complete blood count Chemistry panel	1–2x/week	Reduce/stop oral agent/insulin per SMBG
4	Reduce SMBG to bid once diabetes medication stopped; continue food, fluid, PA records	Urinalysis	1–2x/week	Same as above plus adjust hypertensive/ diuretic/lipid agents, frequently not needed at this stage
5	Same as above	Chemistry panel	1x/week or more as needed	Continue to monitor
6–12+	Same as above	Alternate blood and urine labs Complete blood count monthly	Same as above	Same as above

in persons at the highest risk for chronic diseases, including NIDDM, hypertension, and hyperlipidemia.[32] The occurrence of NIDDM decreased by 6% for each increment of 500 kcal of weekly physical activity expenditure.[32] Increasing physical activity is the number one predictor of long-term weight maintenance,[7,29] especially in patients who have lost significant amounts of weight, indicating the need for major life-style changes. Patients who increase physical activity are more likely to (1) stay in the program and reach goal weight, (2) join the maintenance program, and (3) keep their weight off long term.

During the weight loss phase, the educator must convince patients that physical activity is important to their success and teach them how to integrate physical activity into their life style. Program content should include physical and psychological benefits of physical activity, how to develop an exercise program, how to keep records of physical activity, and how to calculate caloric expenditure of physical activity. Getting patients to exercise during the weight loss phase helps minimize drop in basal metabolic rate, preserve lean body mass, but more important, help prepare them for the task of weight maintenance. A goal of 2000 calories of physical activity per week by week 6 is recommended for long-term success. This could be accomplished by walking 10 minutes out the door and 10 minutes back three times per day, or a total of 45 minutes to 1 hour of walking per day. Initially, obese persons usually record physical activity by the minute and gradually increase their activity as they lose weight and their tolerance improves. Choosing activities they enjoy encourages frequency. Walking remains the most popular type of physical activity for a variety of reasons; however, sampling new types of physical activity is encouraged. Problem solving about how to get physical activity is a continuous topic in behavioral education content.

Refeeding Phase

The third phase, refeeding, is a transition phase and generally lasts 3 to 6 weeks, during which foods are reintroduced gradually and supplement intake is decreased.[8] Medical monitoring by physician and laboratory assessment continue during this phase, along with behavioral education. The purpose of gradual refeeding is to provide a structured re-entry to eating from full-fasting status. The goals are to minimize medical risk and the magnitude of any water fluctuations and to give patients a greater sense of control and initial success in maintenance. Patients are counseled to expect some of the water weight lost during the first 1 to 2 weeks on the VLCD to be regained during refeed, although individual responses vary. Starting with small amounts of low-fat foods helps minimize side effects and shape behavior change toward healthy eating. Typical refeed instructions are to begin with a limited list of cooked vegetables only (baked potato, green beans, carrots, zucchini), plus their usual amount of supplements for week 1; week 2, some fruits are added, plus a variety of vegetables, decreasing supplement; weeks 3 and 4, vegetables and fruits are increased up to a total of at least five per day, plus low-fat protein foods and limited starches with minimal fat are added (see Exhibit 14-4). In my experience, a calorie-counting approach with emphasis on portion sizes, limiting high-fat foods, and adding in low-fat foods has been more successful in treating post-VLCD patients than the traditional exchange system. Counting carbohydrates can also be used in IDDM patients to achieve euglycemia. Virtually all NIDDM patients who reach goal weight will no longer require medications. SMBG should be continued as indicated by glucose response, usually twice daily at least three to four times per week.

Maintenance Phase

It is crucial that a strong weight maintenance phase be continued after the patient is off the VLCD. Unfortunately, many programs, even some physician-led programs, do not stress this because the profits in the program come from selling the formula.[26] There is little profit during

Exhibit 14-4 Sample Guidelines for Refeeding Phase

Week	Additional Foods and Suggested Amounts Daily	Supplement Prescription	Approximate Total Calories Prescribed
1	Cooked vegetables only; baked potato, green beans, carrots, zucchini Total 300 calories food/day	Continue same as weight loss phase ex: 5 supplements per day	800–1000
2	Add other cooked vegetables, plus some fruits; raw vegetables by end of week as tolerated Total 500 calories food/day	Decrease supplement from week 1 by one ex: 4 supplements per day	900–1000
3	Add 4–6 oz. very lean protein (fish, cottage cheese), plus continue vegetables and fruits, up to at least 5 servings total/day Total 700 calories food/day	Decrease supplement from week 2 by one ex: 3 supplements per day	1000
4	Add lean meat (turkey or chicken breast), low-fat dairy products, and starches in limited portions (100 calories per serving) Total 900-1000 calories food/day	Continue 3 supplements per day	1200–1500

Note: Refeeding instructions vary on an individual basis, depending on client's food intake during weight loss phase, duration of weight loss phase, food tolerances and preferences, life style, etc. Refeed phase can be extended to 6 to 8 weeks for clients who were total fasters for 6 to 12 months or longer. Clients do not complete weight loss phase/medical supervision until supplement intake is ≤3 per day. Upon entering the maintenance phase, medical supervision is transferred back to patient's primary care provider(s).

the maintenance phase, and patients are often not encouraged to continue. This is a great failing of many VLCD programs.

The maintenance phase is the time for "hands on" practice of procedures and skills for long-term successful weight maintenance. Effective behavioral techniques to provide hands-on practice are topic-specific projects, potlucks with themes, supermarket tours, restaurant field trips, and calorie food labs. Successful weight maintenance will involve physical activity on a regular basis, changes in some food choices, and many environmental control procedures. All previously obese patients need time to extinguish old previous behaviors and replace them with new problem-solving, calorie-balancing behaviors. Some patients having successfully completed the weight loss phase of the program may feel overly confident they can maintain their weight loss without the need for the maintenance phase. Virtually all these patients will regain most of their weight. Most patients will gain some weight and will feel discouraged at times. Thus, it is essential to maintain involvement with the program and contact with a health educator. Weekly attendance is a program commitment, not merely a recommendation. Flexible class schedules support long-term group attendance. Length of maintenance programs varies, but a minimum of 18 months is recommended.[29]

EFFECTS OF VLCD

Although obese NIDDM patients treated with conventional therapy lose an average of 1 to 1.5 lb/wk,[7] VLCD-treated patients lose more weight[33] more rapidly, with a weight loss range of 2.5 to 5 lb/wk. Weight loss tends to be greater during the first 1 to 2 weeks of treatment due to fluid diuresis. As VLCD therapy progresses, the contribution of fluid and protein to overall weight loss gradually decreases while fat loss increases.[34]

Many studies have shown that fasting hyperglycemia can be markedly reduced or even normalized with only 10 to 20 lb weight loss.[6,7,17,18,34,35] The fasting plasma glucose level falls rapidly after the initiation of VLCD diet therapy, with most of the reduction occurring within the first 7 to 14 days of treatment.[5] In most cases, the decline in fasting glucose is so dramatic that oral hypoglycemic agents or exogenous insulin must be tapered or discontinued before or within the first few days of the VLCD use. Caloric restriction per se appears to be a significant factor in improving blood glucose and insulin sensitivity.[5,7,18] Urinary glucose excretion rapidly decreases and glycosylated hemoglobin gradually returns to normal nondiabetic levels.[36]

During VLCD, hepatic glucose output uniformly decreases parallel to the decrease in fasting plasma glucose.[37] The exact mechanism of how hypocaloric diet therapy reduces elevated hepatic glucose output in NIDDM is unknown, but increased rates of glucose recycling and increased hepatic insulin extraction have been postulated.[5]

Studies of VLCD therapy on impaired insulin secretion have been conflicting.[5] Although pancreatic ß-cell function is improved by weight loss,[38] insulin secretion remains significantly impaired in these NIDDM patients. Weight loss is well recognized to improve glucose tolerance, and several studies have assessed the contribution of enhanced insulin action to these changes.[5]

The most dramatic and consistent effect of VLCD therapy in obese NIDDM patients is reduced serum triglycerides (TG) levels, which usually range from 40 to 60%.[16,17,34,37] TG levels tend to fall rapidly, often with maximal response by 2 to 4 weeks of therapy. After weight loss, TG

levels also rise significantly by 10 days of weight maintenance refeeding, implying that calorie content and/or diet composition mediate much of this effect.[36] Total cholesterol is reduced by VLCD therapy 20 to 30%, whereas effect on high-density lipoprotein-cholesterol has been inconsistent.[5]

Effect on Blood Pressure

VLCD therapy has beneficial effects on both systolic and diastolic blood pressure in obese NIDDM patients.[5,17,18] Virtually all patients experience some reduction in blood pressure, usually within the first week of VLCD therapy. In many cases, antihypertensive medication can be reduced or discontinued. Diuretics should be discontinued before beginning the diet, due to risks of hypertension and electrolyte abnormalities.[8] More studies are needed to elucidate benefits and mechanisms of weight loss on blood pressure in obese NIDDM.[5]

Long-Term Results

Recidivism is a significant problem after weight reduction, whether achieved by VLCD therapy or conventional dieting. Comprehensive programs combining medically monitored VLCDs with life-style education have shown better long-term weight maintenance[10,39,40] than either treatment alone. In comprehensive VLCD programs, patients maintain an average of 78% of their initial weight loss 1 year after treatment,[41] approximately 56% 2 years after treatment,[10] and approximately 35% 3 to 3.5 years after treatment.[42] The use of medically monitored VLCDs without life-style education usually results in poor weight maintenance.[41] Behavioral education alone produces only modest weight loss.[43] Studies comparing behavioral programs using balanced low-calorie regimens (1000 to 1500 calories/d) versus behavioral programs including VLCDs have shown increased weight losses at 20 weeks using VLCDs (19.3 kg in VLCD plus behavior therapy versus 14.3 kg in behavior therapy with balanced low-calorie regimen).[41,44] No significant differences in weight maintenance between treatments were found at 1-,[40] 3-, or 5- year follow up.[45] Another study of obese NIDDM patients[37] found greater weight regain at 1 year post-VLCD than with behavior therapy.

More studies are urgently needed to compare weight regain of patients on different regimens, yet the number of published studies declines yearly. Unfortunately, research on long-term weight loss is difficult and frustrating, requiring large numbers of study participants. Many researchers find themselves pressured to publish multiple research studies in short periods of time, making this work less enticing to young researchers. Another concern is the tendency of research studies to report group averages, losing sight of individual positive success stories. Recently, an analysis of successful patient stories has been published,[46] illustrating that a variety of weight management strategies can be effective.

Very little is known about psychological factors that may affect the course of treatment with VLCD; however, this seems an important question. Clearly, VLCDs have generally positive effects on depression, anxiety, and hunger.[8,44,47] Compared with moderate weight loss programs, little is known about the effects of VLCD treatment on components of body image. More research is needed in this area.

WEIGHT CYCLING

Many studies have examined potential adverse effects of weight cycling—weight loss followed by weight regain. Key questions have been (1) does weight cycling lead to changes in metabolic rate or body composition, making weight loss more difficult and weight regain easier? and (2) does weight cycling increase risk of mortality, especially cardiovascular mortality?[12] A recent review of literature[48] concluded that most studies show no negative effects of weight cycling on total body fat, body fat distribution, or resting energy expenditure and do not support the hypothesis that weight cycling

makes subsequent efforts at weight loss more difficult. Thus, optimism is warranted concerning patients' ability to lose weight, regardless of severity of an individual's history of weight cycling.[49] By contrast, there is stronger evidence that weight cycling may have adverse effects on cardiovascular mortality. However, many methodology concerns have been raised in this literature.[48] Further research is needed to examine the effects of weight cycling on glycemic control.

BALANCING THE PROS AND CONS

Considerable data now exist on the use of VLCDs containing high-quality protein and macronutrient supplementation for the treatment of obese NIDDM patients. When conventional nutrition therapy fails, VLCDs provide an opportunity to lose clinically significant amounts of weight rapidly and safely and control hyperglycemia, hyperlipidemia, and hypertension, which reduces the excessive risk for premature cardiovascular complications in NIDDM. Measurements of successful VLCD outcomes are listed in Exhibit 14-5. The structure imposed by the VLCD and the simplicity of eating limited food choices and/or liquid formula is an important factor in the success of these diets. Patients report that they like not having to think or make decisions related to food. More important, VLCDs do what they were designed to do—produce large initial weight losses, relatively safely and easily. Another point to remember is that VLCDs were not developed to improve maintenance. As previously discussed, evidence does not indicate VLCDs make maintenance worse than conventional diets. Rather, weight maintenance is a challenge regardless of the weight loss method.

VLCDs require careful supervision and monitoring by a physician and health care team knowledgeable in the principles, methods, and limitation of hypocaloric nutrition therapy and NIDDM. A considerable commitment by staff is required to develop and maintain a successful VLCD program, not unlike intensive insulin therapy. Participation in ongoing staff training is essential to maintain staff morale and develop skills. On completion of the VLCD, patients continue to require ready access to staff and frequent individualized follow-up.

A disadvantage of VLCD therapy is the high cost, estimated at approximately $3000 for a 26-week program, which might produce an average of 60 lb weight loss.[8] However, the cost per kilogram of weight loss on a VLCD program is estimated to be similar to a 26-week behavioral program, when allowances are made for costs of food and medical supervision. Frequently, insurance reimbursement is available, depending on the amount of weight the patient needs to lose and medical conditions present. Individualized letters to insurance companies to explain medical necessity of VLCD therapy are highly effective. One factor patients need to consider is the cost of current medications, which can be decreased or eliminated with weight loss. For example, an obese NIDDM patient taking an oral agent and hypertensive medication may spend $150/month on medication alone. With maintenance of a 40-lb weight loss for 1 year, the patient breaks even, monetarily, not to mention improvements in health status and quality-of-

life factors. However, when no medical conditions are present, the use of VLCD in the treatment of obesity may not be justified, because long-term outcomes of standard behavioral programs are similar to long-term outcome of VLCD.[38] Further research is needed to determine the characteristics of NIDDM clients who will respond to a VLCD.

Long-term maintenance of weight loss with VLCD, as with all obesity treatments currently available, remains disappointing.[8] However, it is important to remember that VLCDs were not developed to improve maintenance.[50] VLCDs do accomplish their goal of producing large weight losses, which is powerful technology.[14] Despite recidivism, VLCD therapy may still be beneficial when one considers the natural history of obese NIDDM may be steady and progressive weight gain. VLCDs may also be superior to alternate forms of diabetes therapy, such as oral hypoglycemic agents or exogenous insulin, as these treatment modalities tend to increase peripheral insulin levels, favor development of atherosclerosis, and promote weight gain.[5]

CONCLUSION

Most experts agree obesity can have serious health consequences. In persons with NIDDM, obesity sets off a cascade of metabolic disorders that can be deadly.[3,4] Despite well-publicized controversies surrounding the use of VLCDs, this treatment modality offers distinct advantages and benefits to most obese NIDDM patients that outweigh its risks.[5] Only comprehensive, long-term weight management programs can provide effective treatment for obesity. Changes in life style and behavior that support maintenance of a reasonable weight require time and experience. Even programs of 6 to 12 months may be too short for persons whose habits have developed over 20 or 30 years.[51]

Although weight loss is desirable in obese NIDDM, the ultimate priority should be achievement of glucose and lipid goals[6,52] and improved quality of life. Interventions that focus on life-style changes, not just on weight loss,

---

Exhibit 14-5 Measurements of Successful VLCD Outcomes

- **Improvement in Medical Indicators**
  - Weight
  - Glucose
  - Glycated Hemoglobin
  - Blood Pressure
  - Lipids

- **Life-Style Changes**
  - Increased Physical Activity
  - Decreased Dietary Fat
  - Calorie Balancing
  - Improved Nutrition
  - New Behaviors/Attitudes

- **Improved Quality of Life**
  - Self-Esteem
  - Psychological Factors
  - Occupational Stability

and those that involve the patient as an integral part of the treatment team have a greater likelihood of long-term success.[51]

Many persons have improved the quality of their lives by losing weight and keeping it off.[46] We must not accept difficulty of treatment and high rates of recidivism as reasons for discontinuing efforts.[51] We do not abandon our patients with diabetes because we cannot cure their diabetes.[53] Similarly, health care professionals must share responsibilities for the treatment of obesity or risk leaving our desperate patients in the hands of profiteers and nutrition quacks. We must critically examine strategies for successful weight management, combine this information with knowledge gained from intervention failures, and tailor future treatments accordingly. For most individuals, obesity is a chronic, lifelong disorder requiring ongoing care. Developing effective treatments for obesity is a challenging, long-term process.

REFERENCES

1. National Institutes of Health, Consensus Development Panel on the Health Implications of Obesity. Health implications of obesity. *Ann Intern Med.* 1985;103(6, pt 2):1073–1077.

2. Berg F. *Special Report: Health Risks of Obesity.* Hettinger, ND: Obesity and Health, Healthy Living Institute; 1993.

3. DeFronzo RA, Ferrannini E. Insulin resistance: a multifaceted syndrome responsible for NIDDM, obesity, hypertension, dyslipidemia and atherosclerotic cardiovascular disease. *Diabetes Care.* 1991;14:173–194.

4. Daly A. Diabesity: the deadly pentad disease. *Diabetes Educ.* 1994;20:156–162.

5. Henry RR, Gumbiner B. Benefits and limitations of very low calorie diet therapy in obese NIDDM. *Diabetes Care.* 1991;14:802–823.

6. American Diabetes Association. Position statement: nutrition recommendations and principles for people with diabetes mellitus. *Diabetes Care.* 1994;17:519–522.

7. Franz MJ, Horton ES, Bantle JP, et al. Technical review: nutrition principles for the management of diabetes and related complications. *Diabetes Care.* 1994;17:490–518.

8. National Task Force on Prevention and Treatment of Obesity. Review: very low calorie diets. *JAMA.* 1993;270:967–974.

9. Linn R, Stuart RL. *The Last Chance Diet Book.* Secausus, NJ: Stuart; 1976.

10. Anderson JW, Hamilton CC, Brinkman-Kaplan V. Benefits and risks of an intensive very low calorie diet program for severe obesity. *Am J Gastroenterol.* 1992;87:6–15.

11. Vinik A, Wing RR. The good, the bad, and the ugly in diabetic diets. *Endocrinol Metab Clin North Am.* 1992;21:237–271.

12. Bray GA. Classification and evaluation of the obesities. *Med Clin North Am.* 1989;73:161–184.

13. Raskin P, ed. *Medical Management of Non-Insulin Dependent (Type II) Diabetes.* Alexandria, Va: American Diabetes Association; 1994.

14. Wing RR. Don't throw out the baby with the bathwater. *Diabetes Care.* 1992;15:293–296.

15. Bauman WA, Schwartz E, Rose HG, Eisenstein HN, Johnson DW. Early and long term effects of acute caloric deprivation in obese diabetic patients. *Am J Med.* 1988;85:38–46.

16. Vasquez B, Flock EV, Savage PJ, et al. Sustained reduction of proteinuria in type II (non–insulin-dependent) diabetes following diet induced reduction of hyperglycemia. *Diabetolgia.* 1984;26:1727–1733.

17. Kirschner MA, Schneider G, Ertel NH, Gorman J. An eight year experience with a very-low-calorie formula diet for control of major obesity. *Int J Obes.* 1988;12:69–80.

18. Uusitupa MIJ, Laasko M, Sarlund H, Majander H, Takala J, Penttila I. Effects of a very low calorie diet on metabolic control and cardiovascular risk factors in the treatment of obese non–insulin-dependent diabetes. *Am J Clin Nutr.* 1990;51:768–773.

19. Maclure KM, Hayes KC, Colditz GA, Stampfer MJ, Spezier FE, Willett WC. Weight, diet, and the risk of symptomatic gallstones in middle-aged women. *N Engl J Med.* 1989;321:563–569.

20. Everhart JA. Contributions of obesity and weight loss to gallstone disease. *Ann Intern Med.* 1993;119:1029–1035.

21. Wing RR, Blair EH, Bononi P, Marcus M, Watanabe R, Bergman R. Calorie restriction per se is a significant factor in improvements in glycemic control and insulin sensitivity during weight loss in obese NIDDM patients. *Diabetes Care.* 1994;14:30–35.

22. Merritt RJ, Bistrian BR, Blackburn GL, Suskind RM. Consequences of modified fasting in obese pediatric adolescent patients. I: protein sparing modified fast. *J Pediatr.* 1980;96:13–19.

23. Zwaiuer K, Schmidinger H, Klicpera M, Mayr H, Widhalem K. 24 hour electrocardiographic monitoring in obese children and adolescents during a 3 week low calorie diet (500 cal). *Int J Obes.* 1989;13(suppl 2):101–105.

24. Council on Scientific Affairs. Treatment of obesity in adults. *JAMA*. 1988;260:2547–2551.

25. Atkinson R, Fuchs A, Pastors JG, Saunders JT. Combination of very low calorie diet and behavior modification in treatment of obesity. *Am J Clin Nutr*. 1992;56:199S–202S.

26. Pi Sunyer X. The role of very low calorie diets in obesity. *Am J Clin Nutr*. 1992;56:240S–243S.

27. Wadden TA, Stunkard AJ, Brownell KD. Very low calorie diets: their efficacy, safety and future. *Ann Intern Med*. 1983;99:675–684.

28. Sikand G, Kondo A, Foreyt JP, Jones PH, Gotto AM Jr. Two year follow up of patients treated with very low calorie diet and exercise training. *J Am Diet Assoc*. 1988;88:487–488.

29. Health Management Resources. *Behavioral Reference for Weight Management*. Boston, Mass: Health Management Resources; 1990.

30. Horton ES. Exercise and physical training: effects on insulin sensitivity and glucose metabolism. *Diabetes Metab Rev*. 1986;2:1–17.

31. Horton ES. Exercise and decreased risk of NIDDM. *N Engl J Med*. 1991;325:196–197.

32. Helmrich SP, Ragland DR, Leung RN, Paffenbarger RS. Physical activity and reduced occurrence of non–insulin-dependent diabetes mellitus. *N Engl J Med*. 1991;325:147–151.

33. Pavlou KN, Krey S, Steffee WP. Exercise as an adjunct to weight loss and maintenance in moderately obese subjects. *Am J Clin Nutr*. 1989;49:1115–1123.

34. Henry RR, Wiest-Kent TA, Scheaffer L, Kolterman OG, Olefsky JM. Metabolic consequences of very low calorie diet therapy in obese non–insulin-dependent diabetic and non-diabetic subjects. *Diabetes*. 1986;35:155–164.

35. Wing RR. Use of very low-calorie diets in the treatment of obese persons with non–insulin-dependent diabetes mellitus. *J Am Diet Assoc*. 1995;95:569–572.

36. Wing RR, Koeske R, Epstein L, Nowalk MP, Gooding W, Becker D. Long-term effects of modest weight loss in type II diabetic patients. *Arch Intern Med*. 1987;147:1749–1753.

37. Henry RR, Scheaffer L, Olefsky JM. Glycemic effects of intensive calorie restriction and isocaloric refeeding in non–insulin-dependent diabetes mellitus. *J Clin Endocrinol Metab*. 1985;61:917–925.

38. Wing RR, Marcus MD, Salata R, Epstein LH, Miaskiewicz S, Blair EH. Effects of very-low-calorie diet on long-term glycemic control in obese type II diabetic subjects. *Arch Intern Med*. 1991;151:1334–1340.

39. Wadden TA, Van Itallie T, Blackburn G. Responsible and irresponsible use of very low calorie diets in the treatment of obesity. *JAMA*. 1990;263:83–85.

40. American Dietetic Association. Position of the American Dietetic Association: very-low-calorie weight loss diets. *J Am Diet Assoc*. 1990;90:722–726.

41. Wadden TA, Stunkard AJ. Controlled trial of very low calorie diet, behavior therapy, and their combination in the treatment of obesity. *J Consult Clin Psychol*. 1986;54:483–488.

42. Anderson JW, Hamilton CC, Crown-Weber E, Riddlemoser M, Gustafson NJ. Safety and effectiveness of multidisciplinary very low calorie diet program for selected obese individuals. *J Am Diet Assoc*. 1991;91:1582–1584.

43. Kramer FM, Jeffrey RW, Forester JL, et al. Long term follow up of behavioral treatment for obesity: patterns of weight regain among men and women. *Int J Obes*. 1989;13:123–136.

44. Miura J, Arai K, Tsukahara S, Ohno J, Ikeda Y. The long term effectiveness of combined therapy, behavior modification and very low calorie diet: 2 years follow up. *Int J Obes*. 1989;13:73–77.

45. Wadden TA, Stunkard AJ, Liebschutz J. Three year follow up of treatment of obesity by very low calorie diet, behavior therapy and their combination. *J Consult Clin Psychol*. 1988;56:925–928.

46. Fletcher A. *Thin for Life*. Sheburne, Vt: Chapters Publishing; 1994.

47. Wing RR, Marcus MD, Clair EH, Burton LR. Psychological responses of obese type II diabetic subjects to very low calorie diet. *Diabetes Care*. 1991:14:596–599.

48. Wing RR. Weight cycling in humans: a review of literature. *Ann Behav Med*. 1992;14:113–119.

49. Wadden TA, Bartlett S, Letizia KA, Foster GD, Stunkard AJ, Conhill A. Relationship of dieting history to resting metabolic rate, body composition, eating behavior, and subsequent weight loss. *Am J Clin Nutr*. 1992;56:203S–208S.

50. Kaplan GD, Stifler LT. Very low calorie diets for obesity (letter). *JAMA*. 1994;271:24–25.

51. Robison JI, Hoerr SL, Strandmark J, Mavis B. Obesity, weight loss and health. *J Am Diet Assoc*. 1993;93:445–449.

52. National Institutes of Health Technology Assessment Conference. Methods for voluntary weight loss and control. *Ann Intern Med*. 1992;116:942–949.

53. Frank A. Futility and avoidance: medical professionals in the treatment of obesity. *JAMA*. 1993;269:2132–2133.

Very Low-Calorie Diet and Low-Calorie Diet Products

	kcal	Protein (g)	Carbohydrate (g)	Fat (g)
			Nutrient Composition	
Health Management Resources				
HMR 500 (5 packets)	520	50	79	1
HMR 70 Plus (Lactose-Free) (5 packets)	520	70	61	3
HMR Chicken Soup (5 packets)	510	50	66	5
HMR 800 (5 packets)	800	80	97	10
HMR 120 (per serving)[a]	120	11	15	2
Sandoz Nutrition				
Optifast 70 (5 servings)	420	70	30	2
Optifast 800 (5 servings)	800	70	100	13
Optitrim (Lactose Free)[a] (3 servings)	700	52	87	16
Ross Laboratories				
New Direction				
Vanilla (3 servings)	600	78	30	18
Chocolate (3 servings)	630	81	33	18

[a] Product used primarily as partial meal replacements in addition to food.

Chapter 15

Cultural Considerations in Diabetes Nutrition Therapy

Kathryn P. Sucher
Pamela Goyan Kittler

Changing demographics and high rates of diabetes among people of color make culturally specific nutrition therapy an increasing necessity. Standard nutrition therapy approaches, including the exchange system and weight loss plans, are most effective when applied with consideration of a client's cultural background. Cultural descriptions are generalizations of long-standing habits and are not meant to be offensive or stereotypic.

Dietitians experience special challenges when counseling clients of ethnic or religious backgrounds different from their own. This chapter discusses demographic trends in the United States, the prevalence of diabetes in ethnic populations, the cultural significance of food, the impact of traditional food habits and worldview on food choices, and the importance of the personal interview in effective culturally specific nutrition therapy.

ETHNIC DIFFERENCES IN DIABETES PREVALENCE

Diversification of the Population

Dramatic changes in the American population have occurred over the past 20 years. The nation is rapidly moving from a majority of whites with a few minority groups to a plurality, in which there are many "minorities" and no single group is a majority. It is predicted that by the year 2050 non-Hispanic whites will become fewer than 50% of the U.S. population. According to the 1990 U.S. census data, pluralities already exist in 186 counties, including those with some of the largest cities in the country, such as New York and Los Angeles.[1]

Although 1990 figures show that the total U.S. population increased by approximately 10% during the past decade, many ethnic groups experienced explosive growth. For example, Vietnamese, Koreans, Chinese, and Asian Indians increased at more than ten times the national average; Mexicans and Guamanians grew at more than five times the overall rate[2] (Figure 15-1).

When compared with U.S. population percentages, it is evident that dietitians as a group do not reflect current trends in diversity. A recent survey of membership characteristics by the American Dietetic Association reported that approximately 90% of dietetic professionals are non-Hispanic whites[3] (Figure 15-2). This demographic mismatch between dietitians and the clients they serve makes cross-cultural nutrition therapy a certainty in many regions.

Rates of Diabetes in Ethnic Groups

The high prevalence of diabetes, especially non–insulin-dependent diabetes (NIDDM), among ethnic groups in the United States further increases the probability that a client will be one of color. Although Africans, Asians, and Hispanics living in their respective countries of origin have prevalence rates lower than those of white Americans, diabetes among these groups living in the United States occurs at reportedly two to three times the prevalence rate among whites.[4] Prevalence among some Native American groups is an astonishing 50% for persons 30 years old and older.[5] Of even greater concern are the data on diabetes-related complications among U.S. ethnic groups. High rates of end-stage renal disease in African Americans,[6] retinopathy in Mexican-Americans,[7] and lower extremity amputations in Pima Indians[8] are a few of the reported risks. Many studies are indicative of higher complication rates in other ethnic groups as well, although comprehensive comparative data are limited.

Excess mortality rates from diabetes are experienced by African Americans, Hispanics, and Native Americans. (Both whites and Asian-Americans have rates lower than the national average: see Table 15-1.[9]) Late detection, poor access to health services, and low socioeconomic status are often cited as causes for the disproportionately high number of deaths. Inadequate diabetes care[10] and ineffective treatments for minorities have also been blamed.[11]

If, indeed, standard approaches to diabetes nutrition therapy are unsuccessful with at least some clients of color, what factors contribute to this failure? Culturally based assumptions about

the food habits of a client can interfere significantly with effective nutrition therapy.[12] Dietitians may misunderstand or underestimate the importance of food within a particular culture. The traditional diet, as well as methods of preparation and consumption, may be unfamiliar to the dietitian. Further, nutritional therapy strategies may not be in accordance with a client's worldview, or outlook on life. Beyond the training and skills of the individual dietitian, the health care system serving these clients may not encourage dietary management of diabetes due to the up-front cost and time required for effective intervention. Successful culturally specific nutrition therapy requires sensitivity to all these factors.

EFFECTIVE CULTURALLY SPECIFIC NUTRITION THERAPY

Role of Food

The nonnutritional significance of food far exceeds its importance as sustenance in most societies.[13] Food habits (ie, what foods are eaten,

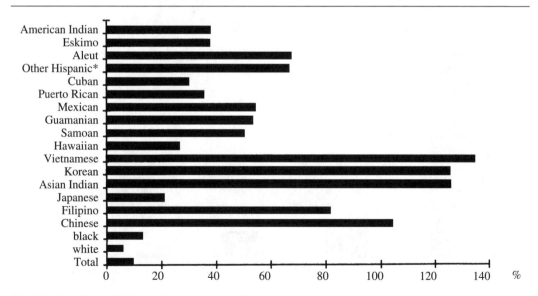

*Includes Brazilians, Chileans, Costa Ricans, El Salvadorans, Jamaicans, Nicaraguans, etc.

Figure 15-1 Percentage Change in U.S. Population Groups from 1980–1990. *Source:* Adapted from CENDATA: Census Bureau Online Service. *1990 US Census Data.* Washington, DC: Division of Population, Bureau of Census; 1994.

how they are eaten, when they are eaten, and by whom they are eaten) are one of the identifying characteristics of a culture. Diet is as much a part of a person's heritage as is language or clothing. Traditional food habits are often the last cultural vestige to change when people immigrate to a new country because they can control their choices in the privacy of their own home.

Food Symbolism

The symbolic use of food can be observed in many ways. It can create cultural cohesiveness and facilitate social interactions. In the United States, some people associate food with certain groups: the poor eat rice and beans; the wealthy consume champagne and caviar; yuppies prefer goat cheese and chardonnay. Women like salads; men want their meat and potatoes. African Americans select soul food, Jews choose deli foods, and Italians pick pizza. Some foods are given prestige in American culture. Filet mignon or lobster is served to special guests, whereas meatloaf and tuna casserole are saved for family meals. A bottle of wine or a box of candy is an appropriate hostess gift; a gallon of milk or a bunch of carrots would be questionable. Health attributes are ascribed to certain foods: chicken soup "cures" the common cold and an apple a day keeps the doctor away. Manners regarding food change according to the occasion. When dining alone, a person might eat a meal straight from the can, without benefit of the good china and candlelight. Eating with fingers is expected at a picnic but not at a black-tie dinner.

Food symbolism and etiquette are unique to each culture. For example, corn is sacred to many Native Americans but is regarded as animal feed in France. Cows are venerated in India, but roast beef is a special occasion food in Britain. Bread is the embodiment of Christ in many Christian religions. Pork is prohibited by both Moslem and Jewish religions. Spicy dogmeat soup is a cold remedy in Korea, and tripe soup alleviates a hangover in Mexico. In Japan, it is considered polite to noisily slurp noodles, and a hostess might receive seaweed (*kombu*) from

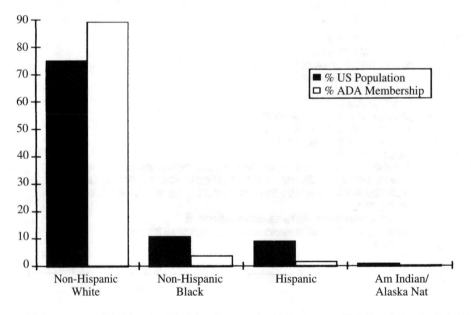

Figure 15-2 Percentage Dietitians by Ethnicity Compared with Percentage U.S. Population by Ethnicity 1990. *Source:* Adapted with permission from Bryk JA, Kornblum TA, Report on the 1991 membership database of the American Dietetic Association. *Journal of the American Dietetic Association.* 1993;93:211–215. Copyright © 1993, The American Dietetic Association.

Table 15-1 Mean Annual Number of Deaths from Diabetes per 100,000 from 1986 to 1988, by Race, Hispanic Origin, and Sex

	Total	Non-Hispanic Whites	Non-Hispanic Blacks	Hispanic	Am Indian/ Alaskan Native	Asian/Pacific Islander
Male	16.1	14.2	25.6	20.8	28.2	12.3
Female	15.7	12.9	31.1	23.7	36.0	10.8

Source: Adapted from Desenclos J, Hahn R. Years of potential life lost before age 65, by race, Hispanic origin, and sex, United States 1986–1988. *Morbidity and Mortality Weekly Report*. 1992;41:13–23.

guests. In most Middle Eastern countries, it is expected that a guest politely refuse food once or twice before accepting it, yet the guest would seriously insult the host if the offered food was completely rejected.

Food habits can be an important aspect of cultural identity for a person. Attempts at nutrition therapy must acknowledge that changes in diet may also inadvertently challenge self-definition. Awareness of the role of food in a client's culture provides context for effective nutrition therapy.

Core Food Habits

Successful nutrition therapy is most likely when recommendations are aligned with the cultural identity of the client. An expanded concept of core foods is a practical application of this concept. As originally described by Passim and Bennett,[14] those foods eaten on a daily or nearly daily basis comprise *core foods* within a culture. Bread and meat in the United States, yams and greens in Nigeria, and tortillas and beans in Mexico are a few examples of such staples. Foods eaten several times each week are classified as *secondary core foods*. Those eaten only occasionally are called *peripheral foods* and are usually the foods that are indicative of individual preference, not cultural group habit. Dietary changes are hypothesized to occur most often with peripheral foods and least often with core foods. It is relatively easy to omit, restrict, or modify foods that are not significant to one's self-definition—it is much more difficult to make adaptations in items integral to one's cultural identity.

Broadening the definition of the core foods model to include food habits can be useful as a nutrition therapy strategy. Identifying those core food habits most associated with the cultural identity of a client and those that are secondary core and peripheral food habits suggest where intervention will be most effective and where compliance may be difficult (Exhibit 15-1).

For many Americans living in the southern United States, pork/chicken/legumes, corn products, greens, fruit beverages, and desserts of all kinds are the core foods. Consideration of core food habits can further guide the management approach: mealtimes are often irregular, heavy snacking is common; frying is the most popular method of preparation, followed by boiling; and healthy persons consume heavy meals; light meals are only appropriate for infants and during illness. Simply recommending increased chicken and legume intake with limited sweetened beverages and desserts may be ineffective nutrition therapy for diabetes without accounting for eating patterns, preparation methods, and the relationship of food and health. It may be difficult to plan for meals when mealtimes are inconsistent. Eating more chicken will be counterproductive if it is fried. Advice to consume smaller meals may be ignored if a client associates hefty portions with well-being.

Impact of Traditional Food Habits

In addition to the core food habits model, another practical approach to culturally specific nutrition therapy is careful preintervention evaluation of traditional food habits. Incorrect

Exhibit 15-1 Core Food Habits Assessment

1. CORE FOOD ASSESSMENT/FREQUENCY			
TYPE OF FOOD	*CORE FOODS* *everyday*	*SECONDARY CORE* *1–3x/week*	*PERIPHERAL* *less than once/wk*
STARCHY FOODS			
wheat/wheat products			
rice/rice products			
corn/corn products			
root vegetables (eg, potatoes, cassava, taro)			
plantains			
other			
PROTEIN FOODS			
red meats			
poultry			
shellfish			
fish			
legumes/legume products (eg, tofu)			
nuts			
other			
DAIRY			
milk			
fresh			
evaporated			
condensed			
other			
fermented dairy			
cheese			
other			

continues

Exhibit 15-1 continued

1. CORE FOOD ASSESSMENT/FREQUENCY			
TYPE OF FOOD	*CORE FOODS* *everyday*	*SECONDARY CORE* *1–3x/week*	*PERIPHERAL* *less than once/wk*
VEGETABLES			
dark green leafy			
nonleafy green/orange			
cruciferous (eg, broccoli, cabbage)			
other			
FRUITS			
high vit. C			
high vit. A			
juices			
canned			
MISC.			
oils			
butter			
lard			
coconut/coconut products			
mayonnaise			
sugar			
honey			
other			
PREPARATION			
deep fat frying			
pan frying			
stir frying			
boiling			

continues

Exhibit 15-1 continued

1. CORE FOOD ASSESSMENT/FREQUENCY

TYPE OF FOOD	CORE FOODS everyday	SECONDARY CORE 1–3x/week	PERIPHERAL less than once/wk
steaming			
roasting			
baking			
barbecuing			
other			

2. MEAL ASSESSMENT

MEALS	TIMING	HOMEMADE OR PURCHASED	TYPE OF FOOD SERVED	PORTION SIZE
#1				
#2				
#3				
#4				
#5				
SNACKS				
#1				
#2				
#3				

3. MEAL CYCLE

a. Are meal patterns the same every day of the week? (Example: Does a Sunday meal pattern differ from a weekday?) If no, how does it differ? _____

b. Are there any special occasions when foods/meals change significantly?_____
   Please identify when and describe food consumed at these times.

       Religious practices _____

       Fasting _____

       Holidays/festivals _____

       Special occasions _____

4. Are there any foods you don't eat because you consider them unhealthy? _____

5. Are there any foods you eat because you believe that they are healthy? _____

6. Do you take any supplements (eg, vitamins/minerals, herbal medicine)? _____

7. Are there any foods you won't eat or dislike? _____

assumptions about food use can occur when the cultural bias of the dietitian interferes with data collection and interpretation. For instance, if a client is fasting, the dietitian may erroneously conclude that this means abstinence from food. In many cultures, fasting is defined as going without certain foods, such as meat and animal products in the Greek Orthodox religion. Fasting may also mean eating specific foods (eg, those cooked in milk in Hinduism). Fasting may be limited in duration, as in the month of Ramadan, when Moslems avoid all food and beverage from sunrise to sunset but can eat and drink in the evening hours. Indeed, a client may eat more on a fast day than on a nonfast day.

The nutritional impact of food habits has been classified by Jellife and Bennett.[15] Modified for use in culturally specific nutrition therapy for diabetes, these categories are

- Food habits that have *positive* consequences on managing the disease and should be encouraged
- Food habits that have *neither positive nor negative* consequences
- Food habits that have *unknown* consequences because culturally specific data is insufficient
- Food habits that have *adverse* consequences on management of the disease and require modification

Cultural variations in a food habit can significantly affect diabetes nutrition therapy. One example is snacking. The French rarely snack. Filipinos prefer fruit snacks and Americans often choose high-fat or high-sugar snacks. The impact of snacking can be beneficial, neutral, or detrimental, depending on the practice. Other food habits are more singular in their dietary effect.

Positive Impact

Many ethnic food practices fit into the positive classification. One example is the emphasis on complex carbohydrates flavored with small amounts of various meats, poultry, fish, and vegetables found in most traditional Asian diets. Also, very few sweets are eaten. In addition, some Asians follow the principles of *yin/yang*, the comprehensive philosophy regarding the harmony of opposing forces in the universe. Applied to diet, it is believed that every meal should include yin (or "cold") foods, such as most vegetables, seaweed, fish, and most herbs, and yang (or "hot") foods, including beef, chicken, fried foods, alcohol, and many spices. Every food falls into one of the categories, although classification varies by region and even by individual. An imbalance of yin/yang in the diet, or in life, can cause disease. In turn, each disease can be cured through consumption of the opposite foods: it has been reported that diabetes is considered a yang disease in China.[16] Vegetables and steamed or boiled foods are advised, and spicy fried foods are to be avoided. (However, dietitians should be aware that, in general, aging is considered to be yin and is balanced by the consumption of more yang foods!) Researchers report that many Asian-Americans (Chinese, Japanese, and Korean), particularly the elderly, maintain many of their traditional food habits.[17] Full or even partial adherence to the typically high-complex carbohydrate–low-sugar diet by some Asian-Americans may explain the low mortality rates compared with higher than average prevalence of diabetes among Asian-Americans in general.

The traditional diets of indigenous cultures throughout the world are another example of food habits with positive consequences. Researchers have found that the starchy staples of the early Native Americans, the Australian aborigines, and Pacific Islanders are high in amylose. It is hypothesized that the unbranched structure of the starch significantly slows carbohydrate digestion. Other researchers suggest that the abundant soluble gums and mucilages in native plants form a biologic slime that physically interfere with carbohydrate breakdown and absorption. In studies, these foods such as acorns, tepary beans, arrowroot, and taro have been shown to decrease insulin production and blood glucose levels. Some indigenous population groups are believed to be genetically predisposed to NIDDM, and that incidence is thought to increase when a diet high in calories from simple carbohydrates and fats is adopted, leading to significant increases in both obesity and insulin levels.[18,19]

Neutral Impact

Food habits that have neither positive nor negative consequences on the diabetes management may still be of importance to a client. Whether a Vietnamese client prefers long-grain rice or a Japanese client selects short-grain rice is of little nutritional significance. Yet the texture of each is closely associated with the respective traditional dishes. Sometimes a food habit with an apparently adverse consequence may be ameliorated through another habit. Puerto Rican women living in New York were reported to consume more calories than those residing in Puerto Rico; however, obesity rates in the United States were lower than those on the island. Although the researchers were unable to explain the discrepancy, their findings also reveal that although the women in Puerto Rico ate more starchy vegetables, such as plantains, breadfruit, or yams, they also consumed more sugar and sweetened foods. The women in New York ate a much wider variety of foods, including meat, fresh fruits, and leafy green vegetables.[20]

Unknown Impact

The consequences of some food habits on diabetes nutrition therapy are unknown due to the paucity of culturally specific research. Two areas of study emerge as inadequate. First, data on nutrient needs of specific populations are limited, although what little information is available suggests that dietary requirements may differ between population groups.[21] Second, nutrient composition data on traditional foods can be difficult to find. Foods may have multiple names, or a single name may be used for several different items. Analysis data, when located, may vary widely from source to source.[22] Grouping foods by plant family or protein source may help in estimating nutrient values and potential impact.

Adverse Impact

Food habits that have adverse consequences on diabetes management include the typical white American eating patterns so widely accepted by immigrants and native populations. Although research suggests that there is no single dietary factor that influences the incidence of diabetes,[23] there is little doubt that many American adaptations of traditional diets are higher in calories and less healthful overall. Among Mexican-Americans, for example, packaged flour tortillas may replace fresh corn tortillas, beans fried in lard may be used more often than simmered pot beans, and consumption of red meat, white bread, sugared cereals, and soft drinks increases compared with Mexicans of the same socioeconomic status living in Mexico.[24]

As noted above, many groups of color do not demonstrate excessive rates of diabetes until they relocate to the United States. This increased prevalence may be associated with increased obesity, a primary risk factor in NIDDM. Mexican-Americans are two to four times more likely than whites to be overweight[25]; research on obesity in other Hispanics is not conclusive. Among blacks, men are only slightly more likely than white men to be overweight. Black women, however, are obese at twice the rate of white women: approximately 50% of black women compared with 22% of white women between the ages of 54 and 65.[26] Indigenous groups of color also show high rates of overweight. One study found two-thirds to three-quarters of some Native American adults to be obese[27]; another reported that overweight is more prevalent in Native American schoolchildren than in any other group of children in the United States, in both sexes and at all ages.[28]

Many reasons for overweight among populations of color have been postulated, including genetic predisposition to weight gain, socioeconomic status, poor diet, and a sedentary life style. Of particular interest to culturally specific nutrition therapy is a different attitude toward body image among some ethnic groups.

Exhibit 15-2 Comparison of Common Values

Anglo American	*Other Ethnocultural Groups*
Mastery over nature	Harmony with nature
Personal control over the environment	Fate
Doing—activity	Being
Time dominates	Personal interaction dominates
Human equality	Hierarchy/rank/status
Individualism/privacy	Group welfare
Youth	Elders
Self-help	Birthright inheritance
Competition	Cooperation
Future orientation	Past or present orientation
Informality	Formality
Directness/openness/honesty	Indirectness/ritual/"face"
Practicality/efficiency	Idealism
Materialism	Spiritualism/detachment

Source: Reprinted from E. Randall-David, *Strategies for Working with Culturally Diverse Communities and Clients*, with permission of the Association for the Care of Children's Health, © 1989.

Historically, overweight has signified affluence in almost all cultures. It has only been in recent times that "one can never be too rich nor too thin" became popular in the United States. In Polynesia, women purposefully fatten-up at adolescence to enhance their beauty. Black women are more comfortable with being overweight than are white women.[29] Among Hispanics, being overweight is associated with well-being for men, women, and children; weight gain for women is expected after marriage as proof that the husband is a good provider.[10] A study of the Dakota people indicates that overweight is associated with health and that weight loss may make a person look ill.[30] The cultural acceptance of overweight combined with the significance of food within daily life makes weight loss especially difficult to achieve in some clients of color.

Encouraging beneficial food habits and sensitive modification of those food habits with adverse consequences can assist in successful culturally specific nutrition therapy. Knowledge of a client's worldview is also advantageous.

Impact of Traditional Worldview

A client's outlook on life is culturally determined. There may be many ways in which the dietitian's viewpoint on health, illness, and treatment differs from that of the client.

Randall-David[31] has identified how the values of the American white majority are in opposition to those of many cultures of color (Exhibit 15-2). These differences result in very practical problems for the dietitian approaching nutrition therapy from the white perspective. A client may be more concerned with helping a family member than with getting to an appointment on time, because personal interactions are more important than time commitments. A client may believe that fate causes diabetes and that little can be done to change the outcome. Similarly, a client may be more interested with what is happening at the moment than what might occur in the future.

Communication

Effective culturally specific nutrition therapy is dependent on sensitive communication strategies.[31,32] A client's worldview can guide verbal and nonverbal approaches. The dietitian should be familiar with cultural norms regarding indirect or direct questioning; formality or informality; eye contact; individual space; and touching.

The Vietnamese, for example, find touching inappropriate. Pointing with the hand or foot (even when the legs are crossed) is disrespectful.

Hispanics consider touching, such as shaking hands, back slapping, and embracing important; sitting closely together is also common. African Americans may be uncomfortable with prolonged eye contact and look away while talking or listening. Native Americans may be insulted by white attempts at directing their lives through intervention. An Asian client might agree with whatever the dietitian says because it would be impolite to question professional expertise. A Mexican-American woman might need her husband's approval before implementing any changes.

Health Beliefs

Cultural health beliefs, especially those regarding the origins of disease, are helpful in determining nutrition therapy approaches. Generally, traditional concepts of well-being and illness reflect the spiritual worldview and the need for harmony in nature. Eliminating the external source of the disease may be of greater concern to a client of color than alleviating the symptoms.

The Navajo believe that illness develops from disharmony and may be caused by loss of the soul, intrusive objects, breach of a taboo, possession by spirits, or witchcraft.[33] Healing occurs when balance is restored. Some Dakota feel that diabetes has afflicted them because their whole lives are out of balance; others believe that diabetes is caused by whites attempting to destroy the Indians through the imposition of disease-transmitting foods.[30] Some blacks attribute illness to the devil's work, as punishment for disobeying God. A few may believe that disease is caused by magic or witchcraft. Some Mexican-Americans subscribe to the idea that illness results from evil supernatural forces; among Caribbean Islanders, especially Haitians, some believe that disease can only be cured by a *voodoo* priest.[31]

As discussed above, the concept of yin/yang is applied to both diet and disease in China. It is also practiced by some Vietnamese. (Yin/yang is rarely used by Japanese, and the Hmong believe most illness is due to conflict in the spirit world.[34]) In rural Mexico, a similar principle of dividing foods into opposing hot-cold categories is also applied to disease. Classification of food varies regionally and is based on the effect of the food on the body, preparation method, or proximity to the sun. Illness can be caused by imbalanced meals and is cured by eating opposing foods. Some Caribbean Islanders also adhere to a hot-cold balance in their diet, as do some Filipinos. Another variation is observed in the Middle East, where some Arabs believe that illness can occur when very hot or very cold foods are eaten, causing extreme temperature shifts in the body.[35]

Traditional healers within a culture usually work in a holistic realm, treating the underlying spiritual causes or natural imbalances of an illness. They can offer important emotional support to a client and relieve anxiety. In most situations, culturally specific nutrition therapy will be most successful when traditional health care is accepted alongside standard treatment. Occasionally, specific folk remedies may compromise therapy. Management of gestational diabetes, for example, could be detrimentally affected by the practice of pica in the rural south[36] or the Chinese belief that smooth skin is maintained by sugar-sweetened broths.[16] But in most cases, folk cures have negligible nutritional consequences and substantial positive psychosomatic results.

The Personal Interview

Thorough knowledge and understanding of a client's cultural background does not ensure successful diabetes nutrition therapy. Such information provides only the foundation for culturally specific nutrition therapy.

Therapy should meet the needs of the individual client, not that of a cultural group. The difficulty with detailing cultural food habits is the impulse to stereotype. Many factors may influence traditional diet and worldview in a client including physical factors (age, gender, health status), socioeconomic factors (income, occupation, education, availability of traditional foods, advertising, community resources), and life-style factors (length of time in the United States, family structure, time constraints, personal preference). An indepth personal interview is necessary to establish acculturative practices and individual preferences.

Lowenberg[37] applied A.H. Maslow's theory of human maturation to food habits. The model describes how a person progresses from eating for existence to eating for self-actualization and provides an overview of how an individual client may use food (Figure 15-3):

1. *Physical needs for survival.* Sufficient nutrients must be regularly available before any other type of food use evolves. This is similar to feeding in animals.

2. *Social needs for security.* After daily needs are met, a society must prepare for future shortages through preservation and storage of foods.

3. *Belongingness.* An individual demonstrates group identity through consuming foods eaten by the group as a whole. Many cultural food habits fall into this category. These foods often represent comfort to a person and may be desired during periods of stress and illness, even if not eaten on a daily basis.

4. *Status.* Social position is defined by what foods are consumed and with whom. Prestige foods in each culture often fall into this category. Eating with a person connotes equality; relationships can be reinforced through dining arrangements, such as when women eat separately from men.

5. *Self-realization.* When all previous stages of food use are satisfied, a person may choose to try foods from different socioeconomic or ethnic groups. Eating for personal satisfaction predominates.

Nutrition therapy is easiest when a client is in the self-realization stage of food use. Higher socioeconomic status is associated with this last stage, as is a willingness to change and adhere to a diet for health purposes. Studies of Mexican-Americans, for instance, have shown that increased affluence and acculturation correspond to decreasing prevalence of diabetes.[38] Successful nutrition therapy becomes more difficult when a client is compelled to maintain cultural identity or social status through food habits. Some clients may be partially at stage 2, where food storage is limited and a nearly hand-to-mouth existence with little dietary planning is common.[39] Effective nutrition therapy is most difficult at this level. Successful intervention with clients in stages 2 and 3 depends on *comprehensive,* culturally specific nutrition therapy that (1) enhances cultural self-definition through increase or adoption of those traditional food habits with positive consequences; (2) emphasizes change in peripheral and secondary core habits; (3) acknowledges the role of food within the culture, building on those practices that are clearly beneficial; (4) incorporates traditional health beliefs into the management approach; and (5) uses appropriate communication techniques. Further, it is important that dietitians ad-

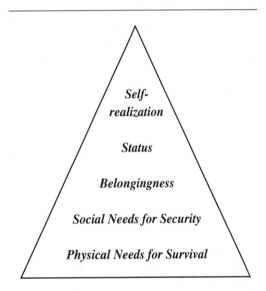

Figure 15-3 Hierarchy of Food Habits Behavior Using Maslow's Theory of Human Maturation. *Source:* Adapted from Lowenberg ME, Socio-cultural basis of food habits. *Food Technology.* 1970;24:27–32. Copyright © 1970, Institute of Food Technologists.

vocate on behalf of their client's need for training: effective therapy approaches take adequate time and resources.

The importance of the indepth interview cannot be overemphasized. Culturally specific nutrition therapy is successful only when it addresses individual needs and effectuates compliance.

RESOURCES

The complexity of culture can make research on ethnic and religious groups frustrating. There is rarely a simple answer to questions about food habits and limited culturally specific diabetes nutrition therapy information is available. Other related resources can be helpful (Appendix 15-A). Dietitians may find that the best cultural sources are their clients, coworkers, a client's family members, and restaurant or market owners in ethnic neighborhoods. This type of fact finding is another form of continuing education for the dietitian, an expansion of the information usually acquired through journals, coursework, and conferences. The knowledge obtained through such nontraditional inquiry increases professional growth and effectiveness. The dietitian who is successful with culturally diverse clients offers far more than technical expertise to the health care team.

More research on the etiology of diabetes in populations of color as well as on effective nutrition therapy approaches is needed. Additional studies on the food habits of ethnic and religious groups would be helpful in all aspects of dietetic practice. In the meantime, communicating cross-cultural experiences and successes with other dietitians can facilitate greater distribution of knowledge and understanding. As the need for culturally specific nutrition therapy increases, an inquisitive mind and an accepting attitude may become a dietitian's most important nutrition therapy tools.

REFERENCES

1. Edmondson B. American diversity. In: *American Diversity*. Ithaca, NY: American Demographics, Inc; 1991: 12–13. Desk Reference Series no. 1.

2. CENDATA (TM): Census Bureau Online Service. *1990 US Census Data*. Washington, DC: Division of Population, Bureau of Census; 1994.

3. Bryk JA, Kornblum TA. Report on the 1991 membership database of the American Dietetic Association. *J Am Diet Assoc*. 1993;93:211–215.

4. Pitts T. Overview of diabetes in ethnic and minority groups. *On the Cutting Edge*. 1991;12:2–3.

5. Sievers ML, Fisher JR. Diabetes in North American Indians. In: Harris MI, Hamman RF, eds. *Diabetes in America*. Washington, DC: U.S. Department of Health and Human Services; 1985. NIH 85-14680.

6. Rostand SG, Kirk RA, Rutsky EA, Pate BA. Racial differences in the incidence of treatment for end-stage renal disease. *N Engl J Med*. 1982;306:1276–1279.

7. Haffner SM, Fong D, Stern MP, et al. Diabetic retinopathy in Mexican American and nonHispanic whites. *Diabetes*. 1988;37:878–884.

8. Gohdes D, Nelson R, Everhart JE, et al. Lower extremity amputations in NIDDM—a 12 year follow-up study in Pima Indians. *Diabetes Care*. 1988;11:8–16.

9. Desenclos J, Hahn R. Years of potential life lost before age 65, by race, Hispanic origin, and sex—United States 1986–1988. *MMWR*. 1992;41:13–23.

10. Davidson, JA. Diabetes in Hispanics. *On the Cutting Edge*. 1991;12:4–5.

11. Kumanyika S. Diabetes, diet and weight control among African Americans. *On the Cutting Edge*. 1991;12:7–10.

12. Kittler PG, Sucher KP. Diet counseling in a multicultural society. *Diabetes Educ*. 1990;16:127–131.

13. Kittler PG, Sucher KP. *Food and Culture in America: A Nutrition Handbook*. New York, NY: Van Nostrand Reinhold; 1989.

14. Passim H, Bennett JW. Social process and dietary change. In: *The Problem of Changing Food Habits*. Washington, DC: National Acadamy of Science; 1943. National Research Council Bulletin 108.

15. Jellife DB, Bennett JW. Cultural and anthropological factors in infant and maternal nutrition. *Fed Proc*. 1961;20:185–188.

16. Ma KM. *Chinese American Food Practices, Customs, and Holidays*. Chicago, Ill: The American Dietetic Association and the American Diabetes Association; 1990. Ethnic and Regional Food Practices: A Series.

17. Kim KK, Yu ES, Liu WT, Kim J, Kohrs MB. Nutritional status of Chinese-, Korean-, and Japanese-American elderly. *J Am Diet Assoc*. 1993;93:1416–1422.

18. Cowen R. Seeds of protection: ancestral menus may hold a message for diabetes-prone descendants. *Sci News*. 1990;137:350–351.

19. Shintani TT, Hughes CK, Beckham S, O'Conner HK. Obesity and cardiovascular risk intervention through the

ad libitum feeding of traditional Hawaiian diet. *Am J Clin Nutr.* 1991;53:1647S–1651S.

20. Immink MDC, Sanjur D, Burgos M. Nutritional consequences of US immigration patterns among Puerto Rican women. *Ecol Food Nutr.* 1983;13:139–148.

21. Kumaniyka S, Helitzer DL. Nutritional status and dietary patterns of racial minorities in the United States. In: *Report of the Secretary's Task Force on Black and Minority Health,* Vol. 2. Washington, DC: U.S. Department of Health and Human Services; 1985:118–130.

22. Ziegler VS, Sucher KP, Downes NJ. Southeast Asian renal exchange list. *J Am Diet Assoc.* 1989;89:85–91.

23. Everhart J, Knowler WC, Bennet PH. Incidence and risk factors for non-insulin dependent diabetes. In: Harris MI, Hamman RF, eds. *Diabetes in America.* Washington, DC: U.S. Department of Health and Human Services; 1985. NIH 85-14680.

24. Wallendorf M, Reilly MD. Ethnic migration, assimilation and consumption. *J Consumer Res.* 1983;10:292–302.

25. Stern MP, Gaskell SP, Hazuda HP, Gardener LI, Haffner SM. Does obesity explain excess prevalence of diabetes among Mexican-Americans? Results of the San Antonio Heart Study. *Diabetologia.* 1983;24:272–277.

26. Lieberman LS. Diabetes and obesity in elderly black Americans. In: Jackson JS, ed. *The Black American Elderly.* New York, NY: Springer Publishing Co; 1988:150–189.

27. Jackson MY. Nutrition in American Indian health: past, present, and future. *J Am Diet Assoc.* 1986;86:1561–1565.

28. Jackson MY. Height, weight, and body mass index of American Indian schoolchildren, 1990–1991. *J AM Diet Assoc.* 1993;93:1136–1140.

29. Kumanyika S, Wilson JF, Guilford-Davenport M. Weigh-related attitudes and behaviors of black women. *J Am Diet Assoc.* 1993;93:416–422.

30. Lang GC. Diabetes and health care in a Sioux community. *Hum Org.* 1985;44:251–260.

31. Randall-David E. *Strategies for Working with Culturally Diverse Communities and Clients.* Bethesda, Md: The Association for the Care of Children's Health; 1989.

32. U.S. Department of Agriculture, U.S. Department of Health and Human Services. *Cross-Cultural Counseling: A Guide for Nutrition and Health Counselors.* Washington, DC: U.S. Department of Agriculture/U.S. Department of Health and Human Services; 1987.

33. Pelican S, Bachman-Carter K. *Navajo Food Practices, Customs, and Holidays.* Chicago, Ill: The American Dietetic Association and the American Diabetes Association; 1991. Ethnic and Regional Food Practices: A Series.

34. Ikeda JP. *Hmong Food Practices, Customs, and Holidays.* Chicago, Ill: The American Dietetic Association and the American Diabetes Association; 1991. Ethnic and Regional Food Practices: A Series.

35. Meleis AI. The Arab American in the health care system. *Am J Nurs.* 1981;81:1180–1183.

36. Hunter JM. Geophagy in Africa and the United States. *Geographical Rev.* 1973;63:170–195.

37. Lowenberg ME. Socio-cultural basis of food habits. *Food Technol.* 1970;24:27–32.

38. Stern MP, Rosenthal M, Haffner SM, Hazuda HP, Franco LJ. Sex differences in the effects of sociocultural status on diabetes and cardiovascular risk factors in Mexican Americans. *Am J Epidemiol.* 1984;120:834–851.

39. Haider M, Wheeler M. Buying and food preparation patterns of ghetto blacks and Hispanics in Brooklyn. *J Am Diet Assoc.* 1979;75:560–563.

Appendix 15-A

Selected Resources

CULTURALLY SPECIFIC NUTRITION AND DIABETES

The American Dietetic Association and the American Diabetes Association. *Ethnic and Regional Food Practices: A Series.* Tel: (800) 877-1600 x5000 or (800) 232-6733.

Algert SJ, Ellison TH, contributors. *Mexican American.* 1989.

Balagopal R. *India and Pakistan.* 1996.

Burke CB, Raia SP. *Soul and Traditional Southern.* 1995.

Claudio VS. *Filipino American Food Practices, Customs, and Holidays.* 1994.

Halderson K. *Alaska Native.* 1993.

Higgins C, Warshaw HS, contributors. *Jewish.* 1989.

Ikeda JP. *Hmong Food Practices, Customs, and Holidays.* 1992.

Leistner CG. *Cajun and Creole.* 1995.

Ma KM. *Chinese Food Practices, Customs, and Holidays.* 1990.

Pelican S, Bachman-Carter K. *Navajo Food Practices, Customs, and Holidays.* 1991.

Woolf N. *Northern Plains Indians.* 1996.

DIABETES AND ETHNICITY

Arnold MS, ed. Selected *Diabetes and Nutrition Education Resources: For the Diabetes Professional.* Chicago, Ill: The American Dietetic Association. 1995.

Bertolli AM, Gallagher A, eds. Diabetes in ethnic and minority groups: a growing challenge. *On the Cutting Edge.* Diabetes Care and Practice Group of the American Dietetic Association. 1991;6:1–24.

Harris MI, Hamman RF, eds. Diabetes in America. U.S. Department of Health and Human Services; 1985. NIH 85-14680.

Stanford Geriatric Education Center Conference. Diabetes in the Elderly: Ethnic Considerations. Conference proceedings. November 2, 1989. Tel: (415) 723-7063.

CULTURALLY SPECIFIC COUNSELING

Kittler PG, Sucher KP. Diet counseling in a multicultural society. *Diabetes Educ.* 1990; 16:127–131.

Randall-David E. *Strategies for Working with Culturally Diverse Communities and Clients.* The Association for the Care of Children's Health. 1989. Tel: (301) 654-6549.

CULTURALLY SPECIFIC FOOD PRACTICES

Kittler PG, Sucher KP. *Food and Culture in America: A Nutrition Handbook*, 2nd ed; in press. West Publishing Company, 610 Opperman Drive, St. Paul, MN 55164-0779.

CULTURALLY SPECIFIC HEALTH BELIEFS

Spector RE. *Cultural Diversity in Health and Illness.* 3rd ed. Norwalk, Conn: Appleton & Lange; 1991.

MINORITY HEALTH

Office of Minority Health Resource Center. Tel: 1-800-444-6472 (professional and consumer information on minority health, risk factors, resources, and programs).

COOKBOOKS

Chantiles VL. *Diabetic Cooking from around the World.* New York, NY: Harper & Row, Publishers; 1989.

Part IV

Macronutrient Influence on Blood Glucose and Health

Chapter 16

Complex and Simple Carbohydrates in Diabetes Therapy

Patti Bazel Geil

The 1994 Nutrition Recommendations and Principles for People with Diabetes Mellitus[1] directs fresh attention to the role of carbohydrate in the diabetes meal plan. Years of traditional thinking have supported the concept that individuals with diabetes mellitus should avoid simple carbohydrate in favor of complex carbohydrate. This belief was based on the assumption that sugars are more rapidly digested and absorbed than starches, resulting in worsening hyperglycemia. New and evolving scientific data have begun to challenge these long-held convictions.

With regard to dietary carbohydrate, the 1994 recommendations emphasize the total amount of carbohydrate rather than type of carbohydrate, liberalize the suggested amount of sucrose, reexamine the function of fructose, and make the same recommendations for dietary fiber for individuals with or without diabetes mellitus. They also address the issue of the recommended distribution of dietary carbohydrate and fat calories, as well as the concept of glycemic response to carbohydrate-containing foods.

The goal of this chapter is to provide registered dietitians with an update of research and practice trends relating to the role of carbohydrate in the diabetes meal plan, with an emphasis on translating scientific information into clinically practical applications. Potential areas of future concern relating to carbohydrate are also reviewed.

HISTORICAL PERSPECTIVE

Diabetes mellitus has traditionally been categorized as a disorder of carbohydrate metabolism, although derangements of fat and protein also result from the disease. Issues surrounding the use of carbohydrate in diabetes meal plans have historically generated controversy.

Early physicians recognized the sweet taste of urine in patients with diabetes, noting the loss of sugar from the body. The earliest diabetes meal plans advocated carbohydrate replacement,[2] based on the theory that dietary carbohydrate should replace the sugar lost in the urine. In 1550 BC, the diabetes diet described in the Ebers Parchment was rich in carbohydrate and consisted of wheat grains, fresh grits, grapes, honey, and sweet beer.[2]

Later, advocates of low-carbohydrate, high-fat diets argued that individuals with diabetes should eat less sugar and carbohydrate to lessen the excess of sugar in the blood and urine. John Rollo, a British Army Surgeon General, recommended a low-carbohydrate, high-fat diet in 1797, noting that even small amounts of bread in the diet enabled "saccharine matter" to return to the urine.[3] He advised complete abstinence from all vegetables, advocating a diet of blood puddings (made of bread and suet) and old meats. This diet met with some success metabolically, but palatability made compliance a problem.

The practice of intermittent fasting and restriction of energy as well as carbohydrate intake characterized the preinsulin era. The famous "Allen starvation treatment," developed in 1910, consisted of a 1000-calorie diet with 10 g of carbohydrate daily.[4] A few clinicians promoted high-carbohydrate, energy-restricted diets before the discovery of insulin, arguing that sugar lost in the urine should be replaced with dietary carbohydrate. "Cures" for diabetes using various carbohydrate sources such as rice, potatoes, and oatmeal were developed.[2]

After insulin was discovered in 1921, low-carbohydrate, high-fat diets were most often used. A common objective of diabetes management was to "desugarize" the patient by temporary elimination or marked reduction of carbohydrate ingestion by use of a low-carbohydrate diet. Later, carbohydrate was added to the diet as the patient's tolerance improved. A minimum of 100 g of carbohydrate daily was advised.[5]

Since the discovery of insulin, the trend has been toward decreasing the amount of fat while increasing the amount of carbohydrate in the diabetes meal plan[6] (Table 3-1, Chapter 3).

Today, the American Diabetes Association recommends that registered dietitians no longer calculate meal plans with strict parameters and percentages of calories from protein, fat, and carbohydrate. Instead, the meal plan is based on a thorough nutrition assessment, and treatment goals are defined, leading to individualized amounts of macronutrients. As a result of these changes, the registered dietitian must be knowledgeable about the chemistry and scientific characteristics of carbohydrate to provide the best medical nutrition therapy for the person with diabetes.

DEFINITIONS

Carbohydrate is the general name for a class of chemical compounds having the empirical form $Cn(H_2O)n$. Digestible dietary carbohydrate has traditionally been classified as "simple" (ie, monosaccharides, disaccharides, and oligosaccharides) or "complex" (ie, polysaccharides) based on its chemical structure. Most foods contain a mixture of both types of carbohydrate.

Monosaccharides are the simplest form of carbohydrate and serve as building blocks of more complex carbohydrates. The three most important monosaccharides in human nutrition are glucose, fructose, and galactose. Glucose and fructose are of particular interest in diabetes.

Glucose is formed from starch digestion; most other sugars are metabolized by the body into glucose. This is the form in which sugar is circulated in the bloodstream and used by the body for energy. *Fructose* is the sweetest of the simple sugars, found primarily in fruits and vegetables. High-fructose corn syrup, which is derived from fructose, is often added to foods (particularly soft drinks) in processing, due to its sweetness. Because fructose produces a smaller rise in blood glucose than isocaloric amounts of sucrose and most starchy carbohydrates,[7] it may be useful as a sweetener for persons with diabetes mellitus. The sugar alcohols, including *sorbitol*, *mannitol*, and *xylitol* are also considered monosaccharides.

Disaccharides are simple sugars made by the linkage of two monosaccharides. Examples are *sucrose* (glucose + fructose), *lactose* (glucose + galactose), and *maltose* (glucose + glucose). Research has shown that substituting small amounts of sucrose for other carbohydrates in the diabetes meal plan does not negatively affect the blood glucose control of persons with diabetes mellitus.[8]

Oligosaccharides are next in complexity, containing between three and ten monosaccharide units. The oligosaccharides *stachyose* and *raffinose* occur in small amounts in legumes such as kidney beans and lentils, and although generally believed to be metabolically inert, they are acted on by bacteria in the lower small intestine and colon, causing increased flatus production in certain individuals.

Polysaccharides are large polymers of glucose, also known as *starch*. Starch consists primarily of amylose (straight chains) and amylopectin (branched chains), both of which yield glucose on digestion.

Indigestible carbohydrate is also known as *dietary fiber*. Dietary fiber refers to all components of food—plant polysaccharides and lignin—that escape digestion because they resist the endogenous enzymes of the human digestive tract. The energy available from indigestible carbohydrate is 50 to 80% of that had glucose been the end-product of starch digestion.[9] Water-

Table 16-1 Summary of Carbohydrate Digestion

Site	Enzyme	Action
Mouth	Salivary amylase: ptyalin	Starch → dextrin → maltose
Stomach	None	Starch hydrolysis continues briefly
Small Intestine	Pancreatic amylase: amylopsin	Starch → dextrin → maltrose
	Intestinal disaccharidases:	
	sucrase	Sucrose → glucose + fructose
	lactase	Lactose → glucose + galactose
	maltase	Maltose → glucose + glucose

soluble fiber, such as that found in oats and legumes, has been shown to reduce the level of serum total cholesterol[10] and may improve glycemic control by delaying nutrient absorption.[11] A more complete discussion of the role of fiber in the diabetes nutrition plan is included in Chapter 21 of this book.

CONSUMPTION TRENDS

Historically, the consumption of carbohydrate in the United States has shown a trend toward more intake of simple sugars and sweeteners and less intake of complex carbohydrate. An increase in the fat content of the diet has simultaneously occurred. Researchers have also noted that the proportion of energy obtained from carbohydrate falls as income rises.[12]

At the turn of the century, 58% of calories in the U.S. diet came from carbohydrate, with the major source being starch. Grains provided almost 56% of carbohydrate calories, whereas sugars and sweeteners provided only 23% of total carbohydrate intake. By 1985, consumption of carbohydrate calories had decreased to 47%. Of these calories, grains were almost 36%, and intake of sugars and sweeteners had risen to almost 40% of total carbohydrate intake.

The form of sugar consumed by Americans has changed from bulk 5- or 10-lb packages used in the home to mostly commercially prepared foods to which sweeteners or sugar has been added in processing.[13]

DIGESTION AND METABOLISM

Digestion of complex carbohydrates begins in the mouth with salivary amylase, which hydrolyzes starch into smaller units. No appreciable additional splitting occurs in the stomach; the bulk of carbohydrate is digested by pancreatic and intestinal digestive enzymes in the upper small intestine.

At this point, complex carbohydrate is reduced to simple carbohydrate, which is absorbed across the plasma membrane into the intestinal mucosa and is transported to the liver via the portal circulation (Table 16-1).

All carbohydrate is eventually metabolized to glucose, which can be used by the body in three ways:

1. to meet immediate energy needs
2. to be stored as glycogen in the liver and muscle for future energy needs. The storage and release of glycogen is controlled by the hormones insulin, glucagon, and epinephrine
3. to be converted to fat and stored as adipose tissue

The digestion and metabolism of carbohydrate is affected by many factors, including the concurrent ingestion of protein, fat, fiber, fluid, and salt, as well as hormonal and neurologic factors. Although the process of carbohydrate digestion and metabolism appears fairly straightforward, the registered dietitian must consider a variety of factors when evaluating the response of a person with diabetes to intake of carbohydrate.

CARBOHYDRATE ISSUES IN DIABETES MANAGEMENT

Type of Carbohydrate

One of the most controversial aspects of the diabetes nutrition plan concerns the type of dietary carbohydrate consumed. As previously noted, dietary carbohydrate has traditionally been classified as either "simple" (sugars, including sucrose, glucose, or fructose) or "complex" (starches) based on their chemical structure. The commonly accepted belief has been that because sugars are smaller molecules, they are more rapidly digested and absorbed than complex carbohydrates. The larger molecules of complex carbohydrate were thought to take longer to be absorbed, resulting in a slower and more moderate rise in blood glucose levels. Patients with diabetes were therefore advised to avoid simple carbohydrate and encouraged to increase their intake of complex carbohydrate.

Researchers began to challenge this dietary dogma, asserting that glycemic changes were not related solely to the molecular structure of the carbohydrate consumed.[14–16] Other factors such as how quickly the food is eaten, how much is eaten, the way in which the food has been processed and cooked, and the combination of foods eaten have a major effect.

Sucrose

Sucrose, also known as table sugar, cane sugar, or beet sugar, is made of one molecule of glucose and one molecule of fructose. It provides 4 calories/g as do other carbohydrates. Sucrose is used extensively in food processing for sweetness and flavor enhancement, and it also occurs naturally in many foods. The average daily per capita consumption of sucrose in the United States is 41 g, which is 9% of total calorie intake.[8] There is no substantial evidence that "sugar causes diabetes"[17]; however, sucrose and other sugars are unquestionably risk factors for the development of dental caries.[18]

Sucrose is primarily absorbed in the small intestine after being hydrolyzed to glucose and fructose by the disaccharidase sucrase, which is located in the brush border. These monosaccharides are then actively absorbed into the portal circulation. Because nearly all sucrose is absorbed as glucose and fructose, its metabolism is essentially that of these two monosaccharides.

Several investigators have conducted research using sucrose in people with diabetes that supports early work indicating that glycemic response is not related solely to the molecular structure of the carbohydrate consumed. Bantle and colleagues[7,19,20] have found that there are no differences in metabolism of glucose between diets containing either predominately starch or simple sugar in patients with either type I or type II diabetes. In one of these studies,[20] 12 persons with type II diabetes consumed, in random order, two isocaloric, 55% carbohydrate study diets for 28 days. In one diet, 19% of energy was derived from sucrose. In the other diet, less than

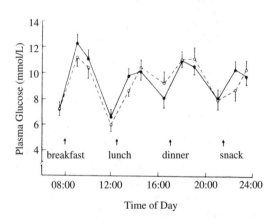

Figure 16-1 Mean ± SE Plasma Glucose Values at Specific Sampling Times on the Final Day (day 28) of the Sucrose (●) and Starch (O) Study Diets. None of the time point differences were significant ($p < .05$) after correction for multiple comparisons. *Source:* Reprinted with permission from Bantle JP, Swanson JE, Thomas W, and Laine DC, Metabolic Effects of dietary sucrose in type II diabetic subjects. *Diabetes Care.* 1993;16:1301–1305. Copyright © 1993, American Diabetes Association.

3% of energy was derived from sucrose; carbohydrate energy came primarily from starch. No significant differences in mean plasma glucose were noted between the study diets at any time point. Figure 16-1 illustrates mean plasma glucose values on the final day of the study. The researchers concluded that a high-sucrose diet did not adversely affect glycemia (or lipemia) in type II diabetic subjects. Additional research has also found no adverse effects of sucrose on glycemia.[21-27] Based on the available data, total restriction of sucrose in the diabetes meal plan to prevent hyperglycemia is not necessary.

Two studies with a small number of subjects[28,29] have concluded that sucrose consumption may have adverse effects on serum triglycerides in persons with type II diabetes; other studies show no such adverse effects.[19,20,23,30-32] It is difficult to make a blanket recommendation based on such limited data; however, Reaven[33] has suggested that there is little evidence to support a negative effect on lipid and carbohydrate metabolism if the intake of refined sucrose is less than 10% of total calories.

Practical Applications. Routine home blood glucose monitoring is the best way to determine an individual's response to the type of carbohydrate consumed. Ultimately, the most important issue is not the type of carbohydrate but the total amount of carbohydrate consumed by the person with diabetes.

On a practical level, if clients want to include *sucrose* in their meal plan, they should be counseled to consume it with a meal, incorporating it in limited amounts as a substitute for other carbohydrate-rich foods. Sucrose-containing foods should not be "added on" to the usual meal plan. Consistency in the meal plan allows for maintaining glycemic control. If sucrose is consumed in higher or lower amounts than usual, changes in the amount of insulin or oral agent may be necessary. For some foods containing sugar, portion sizes will be quite small to keep the carbohydrate intake equal to that of the substituted food.

It may be helpful to point out the nutritional advantages of choosing carbohydrate-rich foods

Table 16-2 Nutrient Content of Whole-Wheat Bread versus Glazed Doughnut

	Whole-Wheat Bread (1 slice)	Glazed Doughnut (1 doughnut)
Calories	60	240
Total fat (g)	1	12
Saturated fat (g)	0	3
% Calories from Fat	17	46
Cholesterol (mg)	0	10
Sodium (mg)	140	160
Total carbohydrate (g)	13	31
Fiber (g)	2	<1
Sugars (g)	2	24
Protein (g)	3	2
% Daily value[a]		
Vitamin A	0	0
Vitamin C	0	0
Calcium	0	0
Iron	4	4

[a] % Daily Value is based on a 2000-calorie diet.

such as whole-wheat bread over the relatively "empty calories" found in another food rich in sucrose. Often, high-sucrose foods also have a high-fat content and a significant number of calories and carbohydrate in small portions. As illustrated in Table 16-2, one glazed doughnut has the same amount of carbohydrate as almost two and one-half slices of whole-wheat bread; yet the bread provides significantly less calories, fat, saturated fat, cholesterol, and sugars. High-sucrose, high-fat foods can be a contributing factor to overweight in patients with type II diabetes.

The 1994 *Nutrition Recommendations and Principles for People with Diabetes Mellitus*[1] gives no specific recommendations for the type of carbohydrate to use in the treatment of hypoglycemia. A general recommendation is 10 to 15 g of carbohydrate to treat mild hypoglycemia and 15 to 30 g for a more severe reaction. Based on the recent findings that the type ("simple" versus "complex") of carbohydrate is not as important as the amount consumed when assessing effect on blood glucose, 15 g of carbohydrate from either 1 tablespoon of table sugar or from six saltine crackers should raise blood glucose in an equal manner. In practice, many registered dietitians recommend that the person with diabetes use the source of carbohydrate that is most convenient and best tolerated during a reaction. Also, a liquid carbohydrate source may raise blood glucose more rapidly because it does not require the time needed to chew and swallow a solid food.

Fructose

Fructose is a monosaccharide that is slightly sweeter than sucrose, provides 4 calories/g and is found naturally in sources such as fruit, honey, and vegetables. It is also available as high-fructose corn syrup and as crystalline fructose. In the United States, the average daily intake of fructose (including fructose occurring naturally in food and the fructose added to food during food processing and preparation with the use of sweeteners) has been reported as 37 g, which represents 8% of energy intake (approximately 148 calories/d).[34]

Fructose undergoes no active absorption in the intestinal mucosa but is slowly and incompletely absorbed by facilitated diffusion. In humans, absorbed fructose is transported to the liver via the portal vein, where it is metabolized. The early stages of fructose metabolism do not require insulin. Under normal conditions, fructose is converted mainly to glucose, glycogen, and lactate and, to a small extent, to triglycerides. Because of its slow absorption, postprandial glucose and insulin response is lower after fructose ingestion than after ingestion of glucose or sucrose.[7] However, in a person with diabetes who is insulin-deficient, fructose stimulates hepatic glucose production, leading to a greater increase in blood glucose concentration.[35] The degree of insulin deficiency required to elicit this effect has not been defined and may vary from person to person.

Fructose may have a potential adverse effect on the serum lipids, particularly triglycerides and low-density lipoprotein-cholesterol (LDL-C), of persons with diabetes. This is of special concern to patients with type II diabetes, most of whom have elevated serum triglycerides and

LDL-C. Several studies have shown increases in serum triglycerides after fructose ingestion[36–39]; other studies note no change.[19,40–42] Additional studies report increased fasting serum total and LDL-C in subjects on a high-fructose diet.[39,41,43,44]

Practical Applications. There is no reason to recommend that persons with diabetes avoid foods in which *fructose* occurs naturally, such as fruits, vegetables, and honey.[8] Persons with diabetes should become aware of sources of added fructose in the diet, such as dietetic foods sweetened with fructose (cookies, puddings, cake mixes, and candy) and regular soft drinks sweetened with high-fructose corn syrup. Fructose may be added to the diet in moderate amounts, although patients with hypertriglyceridemia should avoid consuming more than 20% of their daily calories as fructose. Fructose may have no overall advantage as a sweetening agent in the diabetes meal plan, because large amounts may have potential adverse effects on serum total and LDL-C.[1] Because fructose contains as many calories as sucrose, it should be considered as a source of calories in the meal plan and not viewed as a low-calorie sweetener or free food.

Sugar Alcohols

The sugar alcohols (polyols) are nutritive sweeteners that produce a lower glycemic response than sucrose and other carbohydrates. Mannitol, sorbitol, and xylitol are common sugar alcohols, consisting of monosaccharides that contain alcohol. Isomalt, lactitol, and hydrogenated starch hydrolysates are relatively new nutritive sweeteners that have been used in foods since the 1980s.

Mannitol is derived from mannose, provides 1.6 calories/g, and is approximately 70% as sweet as sucrose. It is found naturally in pineapples, olives, asparagus, sweet potatoes, and carrots and is used as a bulking agent in powdered foods and as a dusting agent for chewing gum.

Sorbitol is derived from glucose, provides 2.6 calories/g and is approximately 60% as sweet as sucrose. It occurs naturally in plums, prunes, berries, pears, apples, and cherries and is used as a sweetener in hard candies, sugarless gum, jams, and jellies. Sorbitol from food sources does not contribute to the sorbitol pathway that leads to neuropathies and retinal changes. Ingested sorbitol is not available once it has been metabolized in the liver; sorbitol found in the nerves and eyes is a result of the reduction of glucose to the sugar alcohol sorbitol by the enzyme aldose reductase.

Xylitol is derived from xylose, provides 2.4 calories/g, and is approximately equally as sweet as sucrose. It occurs naturally in strawberries, raspberries, birchwood chips, and cauliflower. Xylitol has a distinctive sweet, cool taste and is found in gum, mints, and toothpaste in the United States. It is metabolized largely independently of insulin. Xylitol is approved as a direct food additive for use in foods for special dietary uses.

Isomalt is derived from sucrose that has been enzymatically rearranged into equal amounts of two disaccharide alcohols, mannitol and sorbitol. It is 45 to 65% as sweet as sucrose and provides only 2 calories/g. Isomalt is used as both a bulking agent and a sweetener in products such as candies, ice cream, baked goods, and chewing gum. The manufacturers of isomalt cite several research studies showing that isomalt ingestion does not produce sharp increases in blood glucose and insulin levels in individuals with diabetes mellitus. Researchers compared quantities up to 50 g/d (the amount found in approximately 16 pieces of hard candy sweetened with isomalt), which was administered either alone or in addition to the usual diet.[45–50]

Lactitol is a bulk sweetener derived by reducing the glucose portion of the disaccharide lactose. Unlike the metabolism of lactose, this process does not require lactase; lactitol is metabolized by bacteria in the large intestine. It has 40% of the sweetening power of sucrose and provides 2 calories/g. Lactitol is often blended with other low-calorie sweeteners such as acesulfame K, aspartame, and saccharin in foods such as ice cream, candy, baked goods, and

sugar substitutes. Consumption of lactitol does not induce an increase in blood glucose or insulin levels.

Hydrogenated starch hydrolysates (HSH) are formed by the partial hydrolysis (splitting into smaller units by a chemical reaction with water) of corn, wheat, or potato starches and their subsequent hydrogenation (chemical addition of hydrogen to an unsaturated compound) at high temperature under pressure. After hydrogenation, their reducing activity (ability to deoxidize or add hydrogen to another chemical) is eliminated, and they become polyols. Depending on the length of the polymer chains and the parent compound, these polyols may also be known as hydrogenated glucose syrups, maltitol syrups, or sorbitol syrups. HSH serve several roles as food bulking and sweetening agents. They contain no more than 3 calories/g, while providing 40 to 90% of the sweetness of sucrose in products such as candy, baked goods, and dental products.

Polyols are slowly absorbed from the jejunum by passive diffusion and enter the liver independently of insulin, where they are converted to fructose. If a person is properly insulinized, the fructose is then stored as glycogen; if the person is insulin-deficient, the fructose ingestion results in a rise in blood glucose.[35] The caloric values of polyols are difficult to determine and may vary depending on the mode of ingestion and individual factors such as gastrointestinal transit time.[51,52]

Sugar alcohols are often used as substitute sweeteners in food products because of their lower glycemic response, which may assist in blood glucose control. They are also known to prevent tooth decay because they cannot be metabolized by the acid-producing bacteria of the mouth. The main disadvantage of using polyols in a diabetes meal plan is their osmotic diarrhea effect when consumed in large amounts. Abdominal gas, discomfort, and osmotic diarrhea can result when 30 g of sorbitol (the amount found in approximately ten pieces of small hard candy) or more is ingested in a single dose, depending on an individual's gastrointestinal sensitivity; an individual's tolerance level may be as low as 10 g.[53] Because of potential gastrointestinal side effects when ingested in large amounts, the Food and Drug Administration requires the statement, "Excess consumption may have a laxative effect" if reasonable consumption of that particular food may result in a daily ingestion of 50 g.

Practical Applications. There appears to be no significant advantage of sugar alcohols over other nutritive sweeteners in diabetes meal plans, although some polyols are reduced in calories. They assist in the prevention of tooth decay when used in place of a monosaccharide. Sugar alcohols contain calories as do other carbohydrates, but because they are metabolized differently, they produce a lower glycemic response. The potential for osmotic diarrhea if consumed in large amounts is a disadvantage for many individuals with diabetes. It is recommended that foods containing sorbitol be limited to portions containing 20 calories or less (5 g of sorbitol or less).[54] Many individuals with diabetes are under the impression that foods containing sugar alcohols are "free foods." As with any other nutritive sweetener, foods containing sugar alcohols contribute calories and other nutrients and must be accounted for in the meal plan; however, they do provide expanded food choices and can assist in controlling the total carbohydrate content of the diet.

Glycemic Response to Carbohydrate-Containing Foods

There is a wide range of glycemic responses to different carbohydrates. Because the chemical nature of a food (simple versus complex carbohydrate) is not absolutely predictive of its effects on blood glucose, the glycemic index was developed to classify foods based on their impact on blood glucose when compared with a reference food.[55] The glycemic index (GI) is defined as follows:

$$GI = 100 \times F/R$$

in which F and R are the incremental areas under the blood glucose response curve for the test food (F) and reference food (R). Originally, glucose was used as the reference food, but now bread is preferred. The methodology for calculating GI has been described in detail elsewhere.[56]

In theory, the higher the GI value, the higher the blood glucose values would be expected to rise after the ingestion of that food. Results of early GI research proved contrary to previous beliefs about the effect of carbohydrate on blood glucose levels. For example, it was surprising to find that instant potatoes had a higher GI (GI = 120) than ice cream (GI = 69). Knowledge of the glycemic effects of different foods may prove helpful in selecting the types of carbohydrate-containing foods to include in the diabetes meal plan. Table 16-3 shows the approximate GI values of some common foods.

Various factors affect the glycemic response to carbohydrates, including not only the protein and fat content of a meal but also fiber, antinutrients (lectins, phytates, tannins, and amylase inhibitors), food form (pureed versus whole food), rate of ingestion, physiologic effects, methods of processing and cooking, and in the case of fruit, the degree of ripeness.[11]

Simple sugars have been found to be strong determinants of glycemic index. In a study of the dietary GI values of the diet records from 342 patients with non–insulin-dependent diabetes mellitus, the mean diet GI value was 85; an individual's diet GI was inversely associated with intake of simple sugars.[57] Wolever and associates[57] theorize that this is because foods rich in simple sugars such as milk (GI = 46) and fruits (GIs: apple = 52, banana = 84, and orange = 59) tend to have lower GI values than those of common starchy foods such as bread (GI = 100) and potatoes (GI = 70 to 120). The investigators thought that the increased use of simple sugars, which reduces the calculated diet GI, may have a different effect with respect to blood glucose and lipids in diabetic subjects than does reducing dietary GI by the use of low-GI starchy foods.

The GI has not been widely accepted as a useful tool in the nutrition management of diabetes mellitus. Limitations cited include the sugges-

Table 16-3 Glycemic Index of Selected Foods

Food	Glycemic Index	Food	Glycemic Index
Breads		**Legumes**	
White	100	Kidney beans, canned	74
Whole meal	100	Lentils, green, canned	74
Pumpernickel	68	Baked beans, canned	70
		Kidney beans, dried	43
Pasta		Lentils, green, dried	36
Spaghetti, white, boiled 15 min	67	Soybeans, canned	22
Spaghetti, brown, boiled 15 min	61	Soybeans, dried	20
Spaghetti, white, boiled 5 min	45		
		Fruit	
Cereal Grains		Banana	84
Millet	103	Orange juice	71
Rice, brown	81	Orange	59
Rice, instant, boiled 1 min	65	Apple	52
Barley, pearled	36	Apple juice	45
Breakfast Cereals		**Sugars**	
Cornflakes	121	Maltose	152
Puffed wheat	110	Glucose	138
Shredded wheat	97	Sucrose	83
Porridge oats	89	Lactose	57
"All Bran"	74	Fructose	26
Root Vegetables		**Dairy Products**	
Potato, instant	120	Ice cream	69
Potato, mashed	98	Yogurt	52
Potato, new/white, boiled	80	Skim milk	46
Potato, sweet	70	Whole milk	44
Vegetables		**Snack Foods**	
Carrots, cooked	92	Corn chips	99
Peas, frozen	74	Potato chips	77

Source: Data from Wolever TMS. *World Review of Nutrition Dietetics.* 1990;62:120–185, S. Karger AG.

tion that the difference in glycemic effects between foods are clinically insignificant and that the complexities of teaching and applying the GI concept to individual patients makes it impractical. However, it may be necessary to reassess the value of GI in day-to-day meal planning for diabetes.

In clinical trials, improved blood glucose control was seen when diet GI decreased by 12 to 40%; in some cases the low-GI diet reduced serum cholesterol and triglycerides.[57] A meta-analysis of 11 published GI studies[58] summa-

rized results from studies in which the GI of the average diabetic diet was lowered from approximately 66 (bread = 100) to 54 or less and sometimes to 38. This represents an exchange of 50% or more of the carbohydrate from high- to low-GI foods. Over periods ranging from 2 to 12 weeks, on average, low-GI diets reduced glycated hemoglobin by 9% (eg, from 10 to 9.1%), fructosamine by 8%, urinary C peptide by 20%, and daylong blood glucose by 16%. Cholesterol was reduced an average of 6% and triglycerides by 9%. Although these improvements in blood glucose control are only relatively modest, of perhaps greater therapeutic importance is the ability of low-GI diets to induce useful reductions in insulin secretion and blood lipids in patients with hypertriglyceridemia.[55]

Practical Applications. The GI concept is not widely accepted as a method of diabetes meal planning; practical teaching tools have not yet been developed. Until more research has been completed, there are several recommendations that the registered dietitian may make. Persons with diabetes may want to emphasize foods within food groups that demonstrate lower glycemic responses (such as lentils and beans). Raw and unpeeled foods and foods in their whole or minimally cooked form have been associated with lower glycemic responses. However, foods should not be eliminated or included in the meal plan based solely on their glycemic response.

A person with diabetes who is striving for intensive control with near-normal blood glucose levels may be able to determine their own individual GI for certain foods by using self-monitoring of blood glucose. After eating a set meal or snack, blood glucose should be tested in the 1- to 3-hour postprandial period and the results recorded. This procedure should be repeated on different days. Then one food at a time can be changed, repeating the blood glucose monitoring. If a certain food consistently produces a particular response, it is likely to affect blood glucose in a similar manner in the future. The person with diabetes should be cautioned to avoid attributing variations in blood glucose values only to the food that was eaten; it is important to remember that many factors affect blood glucose values.[59,60] When planning meals for the person with diabetes, first priority should still be given to the total amount of carbohydrate consumed rather than its source.

Amount of Carbohydrate

Recommendations for the amount of energy from carbohydrate in the diabetes meal plan have gradually increased over the years, from 20% in 1921 to 60% or less in 1986. However,

the most recent recommendations[1] do not suggest a specific percentage of dietary carbohydrate. Instead, the amount of carbohydrate should be based on the eating habits, clinical condition, and glucose/lipid goals of the individual with diabetes. Because it is recommended that dietary protein contribute 10 to 20% of the total caloric content of the diet, 80 to 90% of caloric intake remains to be divided between dietary fat and carbohydrate. An individual's specific metabolic abnormality will determine the macronutrient content of their meal plan. The percentage of carbohydrate in the diet of an adult with type II diabetes and hypertriglyceridemia may be quite different from that in the diet of a child with type I diabetes.

It has been estimated that up to 50% of persons with diabetes have hyperlipidemia, with the most common lipid abnormality being the hypertriglyceridemia, elevated very low-density lipoprotein-cholesterol (VLDL-C) and decreased high-density lipoprotein-cholesterol (HDL-C) found in individuals with type II diabetes. This lipid profile may be a major factor in the development of coronary heart disease, which is approximately three times higher in the diabetic than nondiabetic population.[61]

People with hypertriglyceridemia or with hyperinsulinemia may be more sensitive to the effects of dietary carbohydrate. Dietary carbohydrates have a major effect on triglycerides, with elevations more likely to occur in older, male, or inactive persons. In some circumstances, sucrose and fructose increase fasting triglycerides more than do starch or glucose.[62]

Early studies showed improved blood lipids and glucose tolerance in persons with diabetes mellitus with the use of a high-carbohydrate diet.[63] More recent research indicates that diets high in carbohydrate increase the serum triglycerides, blood glucose, and insulin levels of persons with poorly controlled type II diabetes.[28,29,64]

Several factors must be considered when determining the carbohydrate content of the diet for diabetes. Including generous amounts of fiber in a high-carbohydrate diet may dampen the rise in blood glucose and triglycerides.[65,66] Improvements in insulin sensitivity have been seen in individuals with impaired glucose tolerance consuming a diet rich in fiber and extremely high in carbohydrate (70% to 80%).[67] The moderate increase in fasting triglycerides and worsening of glycemic control that occurs in the first weeks after beginning a high-carbohydrate diet may be temporary,[62] although this has been challenged.[68]

Another consideration is the increasing evidence that a high-carbohydrate diet plays a role in enhancing weight reduction in persons with diabetes mellitus. High-carbohydrate meals may suppress appetite by increasing the postprandial ratio of the concentration of tryptophan to that of the other large neutral amino acids in plasma. Tryptophan is the precursor of the neurotransmitter serotonin, one of the major regulators of appetite, whose metabolism is abnormal in obese subjects with and without diabetes. Tryptophan has been shown to reduce food intake in healthy subjects and a low plasma tryptophan/large neutral amino acid ratio in diabetics has been shown to be associated with increased perception of hunger.[11]

There are both advantages and disadvantages to using a high-carbohydrate diet in a person with diabetes. The effects of the amount of carbohydrate in the meal plan are related to several factors including both the carbohydrate and fiber content of the diet, the length of time on the diet, and the metabolic status of the patient.

High-Carbohydrate versus High-Monounsaturated Fat Diet

Increasing the carbohydrate content of the meal plan for diabetes was originally intended to lower dietary saturated fat intake, thus decreasing the risk of coronary heart disease. Because of concern about the potential adverse effects of high-carbohydrate diets on lipids and glucose control in some patients, alternative dietary approaches have been developed. One such approach is to replace the dietary saturated fat with monounsaturated fat rather than with carbohydrate.

Several studies have shown that a high-monounsaturated fat diet is metabolically preferable to a high-carbohydrate diet in individuals with type II diabetes. Campbell and associates[69] fed high-monounsaturated fat diets (40% calories as carbohydrate, 38% as fat [21% monounsaturated]) or high-carbohydrate diets (52% calories as carbohydrate, 24% as fat [8% monounsaturated]) to ten men with type II diabetes and found that the high-monounsaturated fat diet resulted in significantly lower 24-hour urinary glucose excretion, fasting triglyceride, and mean profile glucose levels. The fructosamine levels, the fasting total, LDL-C and HDL-C, and the prandial triglyceride concentrations did not differ significantly as a result of the diets.

In a longer-term outpatient study of 42 patients with type II diabetes on oral hypoglycemic agents, Garg and associates[70] found that a high-carbohydrate diet (55% calories as carbohydrate, 30% as fat [10% monounsaturated]) caused persistent deterioration of glycemic control and increased plasma insulin, triglyceride, and VLDL-C levels when compared with a high-monounsaturated fat diet (40% of calories as carbohydrate, 45% as fat [25% monounsaturated]). The results persisted for more than 14 weeks. These studies confirm previous work in the area,[71–77] prompting the suggestion that diets rich in monounsaturated fatty acids should be advised as an alternative to high-carbohydrate diets in both patients with type I and type II diabetes mellitus.[78] A meal plan high in monounsaturated fats can be achieved by including nuts, avocados, olive, and canola oil while carefully avoiding excess calories and *trans*-fatty acids. Guidelines for using this approach to meal planning are outlined in the literature.[69]

Practical Applications

Determining the total amount of carbohydrate to use in the meal plan for the patient with diabetes is challenging; it is not possible to synthesize the research literature into one simple recommendation appropriate for everyone. It seems clear that the amount of carbohydrate in the meal plan must be individualized based on the eating habits, clinical condition, and glucose/lipid goals of the person with diabetes. An adult with type II diabetes, dyslipidemia, and insulin resistance may be more sensitive to carbohydrate and have a decreased capacity to handle a high-carbohydrate diet. Options for a patient such as this include increasing dietary fiber intake if carbohydrate intake is high or using a meal plan rich in monounsaturated fat and low in saturated fat. By contrast, a child with newly diagnosed type I diabetes in good control may be able to include more sucrose and higher levels of carbohydrate in his or her diet if insulin dosage is adjusted to cover carbohydrate intake. Appendix 16-A outlines sample menus and points to consider when incorporating sugar in the diabetes meal plan.

Today, there is no ONE "diabetic" or "ADA" diet.[6] An individualized nutrition assessment conducted by a registered dietitian is crucial, particularly in the determination of the optimal amount of carbohydrate in the meal plan. The collection of clinical data, completion of a nutrition history, and evaluation of food intake are all part of the assessment necessary for successful nutrition care.[79]

FUTURE RESEARCH QUESTIONS

The role of carbohydrate in the diabetes meal plan remains controversial and in urgent need of further research. Unresolved issues include

- What are the effects of the so-called simple versus complex carbohydrates, particularly in the treatment of hypoglycemic reactions? The 1994 Nutrition Recommendations reports that there is little or no scientific evidence to support the traditional belief that sucrose and other sugars are more rapidly digested and absorbed than starches. Will the advice given to persons with diabetes regarding treatment of hypoglycemia change? Are there differences if the source of the 15 g of carbohy-

drate recommended for treatment is glucose tablets versus whole-wheat bread?
- Can specific recommendations be made for the amount of sucrose and fructose to include in the diabetes meal plan? What are the permanent effects of using sucrose and fructose?
- Does increasing dietary carbohydrate adversely affect serum lipids and risk for cardiovascular disease in persons with diabetes?
- What are the long-term effects of high-carbohydrate diets versus high-monounsaturated fat diets on diabetes control and the development of complications?
- Can more practical guidelines be developed for translating potentially useful information such as the GI into user-friendly teaching tools?

Much work in the area of carbohydrate and diabetes mellitus remains. The recommendations we make regarding dietary carbohydrate reflect our present knowledge and may be modified in the future in response to innovative research findings.

REFERENCES

1. American Diabetes Association. Nutrition recommendations and principles for people with diabetes mellitus. *Diabetes Care.* 1994;17:519–522.
2. Wood FC Jr, Bierman EL. New concepts in diabetic dietetics. *Nutr Today.* 1972;7:4–12.
3. Rollo J. *A General View of the History, Nature and Appropriate Treatment of Diabetes Mellitus.* London: T. Gillet for C. Dilly, 1798.
4. Allen FM. Studies concerning glycosuria and diabetes. *JAMA.* 1914;63:639–643.
5. Short JJ. Diabetes mellitus. In: Johnson HJ, ed. *Bridge's Dietetics for the Clinician.* 5th ed. Philadelphia, Pa: Lea & Febiger; 1949:315–346.
6. American Dietetic Association. Nutrition recommendations and principles for people with diabetes mellitus. *J Am Diet Assoc.* 1994;94:504–506.
7. Bantle JP, Laine DC, Castle GW, Thomas JW, Hoogwerf BJ, Goetz FC. Postprandial glucose and insu-

lin responses to meals containing different carbohydrates in normal and diabetic subjects. *N Engl J Med.* 1983; 309:7–12.

8. Franz MJ, Horton ES, Bantle JP, et al. Nutrition principles for the management of diabetes and related complications. *Diabetes Care.* 1994;17:490–518.

9. Macdonald I. Carbohydrates. In: Shils ME, Olson JA, Shike M, eds. *Modern Nutrition in Health and Disease.* 8th ed. Philadelphia, Pa: Lea & Febiger; 1994:36–46.

10. Glore SR, Van Treek D, Knehans AW, Guild M. Soluble fiber and serum lipids: a literature review. *J Am Diet Assoc.* 1994;94:425–436.

11. Wolever TMS, Josse RG. The role of carbohydrate in the diabetes diet. *Med Exerc Nutr Health.* 1993;2:84–99.

12. Perisse J, Sizaret F, Francois P. Carbohydrate consumption patterns. *FAO Newsletter.* 1969;7.

13. Nutrient Content of the US Food Supply. Washington, DC: Human Nutrition Information Service, USDA; 1988. HNIS Adm. Report no. 299-21.

14. Crapo PA, Reaven GM, Olefsky JM. Plasma glucose and insulin responses to orally administered simple and complex carbohydrates. *Diabetes.* 1976;25:741–747.

15. Crapo PA, Reaven GM, Olefsky JM. Postprandial glucose and insulin responses to different complex carbohydrates. *Diabetes.* 1977;26:1178–1183.

16. Crapo PA, Kolterman OG, Waldeck MA, Reaven GM, Olefsky JM. Postprandial hormone responses to different types of complex carbohydrates in individuals with impaired glucose tolerance. *Am J Clin Nutr.* 1980;33:1723–1728.

17. Nuttal FQ, Gannon MC. Sucrose and disease. *Diabetes Care.* 1981;4:305–307.

18. Navia JM. Carbohydrates and dental health. *Am J Clin Nutr.* 1994;59:719S–727S.

19. Bantle JP, Swanson JE, Thomas W, Laine DC. Metabolic effects of dietary fructose and sucrose in types I and II diabetic subjects. *JAMA.* 1986;256:3241–3246.

20. Bantle JP, Swanson JE, Thomas W, Laine DC. Metabolic effects of dietary sucrose in type II diabetic subjects. *Diabetes Care.* 1993;16:1301–1305.

21. Slama G, Haardt MJ, Jean-Joseph P, et al. Sucrose taken during mixed meal has no additional hyperglycemic action over isocaloric amounts of starch in well-controlled diabetics. *Lancet.* 1984;2:122–125.

22. Bornet F, Haarst JB, Costagliola D, Blayo A, Slama G. Sucrose or honey at breakfast have no additional acute hyperglycemic effect over an isoglucidic amount of bread in type II diabetic patients. *Diabetologia.* 1985;28:213–217.

23. Abraira C, Derler J. Large variations of sucrose in constant carbohydrate diets in type II diabetes. *Am J Med.* 1988;84:193–200.

24. Forlani G, Galuppi V, Santacroce G, et al. Hyperglycemic effect of sucrose ingestion in IDDM patients controlled by artificial pancreas. *Diabetes Care.* 1989;12:296–298.

25. Wise JE, Keim KS, Huisinga JL, Willmann PA, Effect of sucrose-containing snacks on blood glucose control. *Diabetes Care.* 1989;12:423–426.

26. Peters AL, Davidson MB, Eisenberg K. Effects of isocaloric substitution of chocolate cake for potato in type I diabetic patients. *Diabetes Care.* 1990;13:888–892.

27. Loghmani E, Rickard K, Washburne L, Vandagriff H, Fineburg N, Golden M. Glycemic response to sucrose-containing mixed meals in diets of children with insulin-dependent diabetes mellitus. *J Pediatr.* 1991;119:531–537.

28. Coulston AM, Hollenbeck CB, Donner CC, Williams R, Chiou YM, Reaven GM. Metabolic effects of added dietary sucrose in individuals with non–insulin-dependent diabetes mellitus (NIDDM). *Metabolism.* 1985;34:962–966.

29. Coulston AM, Hollenbeck CB, Swislocki ALM, Chen YI, Reaven G. Deleterious metabolic effects of high-carbohydrate, sucrose-containing diets in patients with non–insulin-dependent diabetes mellitus. *Am J Med.* 1987;82:213–219.

30. Jellish WS, Emanuele MA, Abraira C. Graded sucrose/carbohydrate diets in overtly hypertriglyceridemic diabetic patients. *Am J Med.* 1984;77:1015–1022.

31. Peterson DB, Lambert J, Gerring S, et al. Sucrose in the diet of diabetic patients—just another carbohydrate? *Diabetologia.* 1986;29:216–220.

32. Colagiuri S, Miller JJ, Edwards RA. Metabolic effects of adding sucrose and aspartame to the diet of subjects with non–insulin-dependent diabetes mellitus. *Am J Clin Nutr.* 1989;50:474–478.

33. Reaven GM. Parma symposium: current controversies in nutrition. *Am J Clin Nutr.* 1988;47:1078–1082.

34. Park YK, Yetley E. Intakes and food sources of fructose in the United States. *Am J Clin Nutr.* 1993;58:737S–747S.

35. Uusitupa MIJ. Fructose in the diabetic diet. *Am J Clin Nutr.* 1994;59:753S–757S.

36. Bohannon NV, Karam JH, Forsham PH. Endocrine responses to sugar ingestion in man. *J Am Diet Assoc.* 1980;76:555–560.

37. Crapo PA, Kolterman OG, Henry RR. Metabolic consequences of two-week fructose feeding in diabetic subjects. *Diabetes Care.* 1986;9:111–119.

38. Nikkila EA, Kekki M. Effects of dietary fructose and sucrose on plasma triglyceride metabolism in patients with endogenous hypertriglyceridemia. *Acta Med Scand Suppl.* 1972;542:221–227.

39. Hallfrisch J, Reiser S, Prather ES. Blood lipid distribution of hyperinsulinemic men consuming three levels of fructose. *Am J Clin Nutr.* 1983;37:740–748.

40. Turner JL, Bierman EL, Brunzell JD, et al. Effect of dietary fructose on triglyceride transport and glucoregulatory hormones in hypertriglyceridemic men. *Am J Clin Nutr.* 1979;32:1043–1047.

41. Bantle JP, Swanson JE, Thomas W, Laine DC. Metabolic effects of dietary fructose in diabetic subjects. *Diabetes Care.* 1992;15:1468–1476.

42. Thorburn AW, Crapo PA, Beltz WF, Wallace P, Witzum JL, Henry RR. Lipid metabolism in non–insulin-dependent diabetes: effects of long-term treatment with fructose-supplemented mixed meals. *Am J Clin Nutr.* 1989;50:1015–1022.

43. Reiser S, Powell AS, Scholfield DC, Panda P, Ellwood KC, Canary JJ. Blood lipids, lipoproteins, apoproteins and uric acid in men fed diets containing fructose or high-amylose cornstarch. *Am J Clin Nutr.* 1989;49:832–839.

44. Swanson JE, Laine DC, Thomas W, Bantle JP. Metabolic effects of dietary fructose in healthy subjects. *Am J Clin Nutr.* 1992;55:851–856.

45. Drost H, Gierlich P, Spengler M, Jahnke K. Blood glucose and serum insulin after oral administration of Palatinit (isomalt) in comparison with glucose in diabetics of the late-onset type. *Verh Dtsch Ges Inn Med.* 1980;86:978–981.

46. Petzold R, Lauer P, Spengler M, Schoffling K. Palatinit (isomalt) in type II diabetics: effects on blood glucose, serum insulin, C-peptides and free fatty acids in comparison with glucose. *Dtsch Med Wochenschr.* 1982;107:1910–1913.

47. Bachmann W, Haslbeck M, Spengler M, Schmitz H, Mehnert H. Investigations of the metabolic effects of acute doses of Palatinit (isomalt). Comparison with fructose and sucrose in type II diabetes. *Aktuel Ernahrung.* 1984;9:65–70.

48. Kaspar L, Spengler M. Effect of oral doses of Palatinit (isomalt) on insulin requirements in type I diabetics. *Aktuel Ernahrung.* 1984;9:60–64.

49. Hutter R, Boswart K, Irsigler K. Consumption by type I diabetics following oral administration of isomalt. *Aktuel Ernahrung Med.* 1993;18:149–154.

50. Pometta D, Trabichet C, Spengler M. Effects of a 12 week administration of isomalt on metabolic control in type II diabetics. *Aktuel Ernahrung.* 1985;10:174–177.

51. Bar A. Factorial calculation model for the estimates of the physiologic caloric value of polyols. In: Caloric Evaluation of Carbohydrates. Proceedings of the International Symposium on Caloric Evaluation of Carbohydrates. January 11–12, 1990. Kyoto, Japan; 1990.

52. Federation of American Societies for Experimental Biology. The Evaluation of the Energy of Certain Sugar Alcohols Used as Food Ingredients. Bethesda, Md; 1994.

53. Jain NK, Rosenberg DB, Wahannan MJ, Glasser MJ, Pitchumoni CS. Sorbitol intolerance in adults. *Am J Gastroenterol.* 1985;80:678–681.

54. American Dietetic Association. Position of the American Dietetic Association: use of nutritive and nonnutritive sweeteners. *J Am Diet Assoc.* 1993;93:816–821.

55. Wolever TMS, Jenkins DJA, Jenkins AL, Josse RG. The glycemic index: methodology and clinical implications. *Am J Clin Nutr.* 1991;54:846–854.

56. Wolever TMS, Jenkins DJA. The use of the glycemic index in predicting the blood glucose response to mixed meals. *Am J Clin Nutr.* 1986;43:167–172.

57. Wolever TM, Nguyen PM, Chiasson JL, et al. Determinants of diet glycemic index calculated retrospectively from diet records of 342 individuals with non–insulin-dependent diabetes mellitus. *Am J Clin Nutr.* 1994;9:1265–1269.

58. Miller JCB. Importance of glycemic index in diabetes. *Am J Clin Nutr.* 1994;59 (suppl):747S–752S.

59. Crapo P. The glycemic response—a new way of looking at starch and sugar. *Clin Diabetes.* 1985;4:12–19.

60. Franz MJ. Evaluating the glycemic response to carbohydrates. *Clin Diabetes.* 1986;4:129–141.

61. Stamler J, Vaccaro O, Neaton JD, Wentworth D for the Multiple Risk Factor Intervention Trial Research Group. Diabetes, other risk factors, and 12-yr cardiovascular mortality for men screened in the Multiple Risk Factor Intervention Trial. *Diabetes Care.* 1993;16:434–444.

62. Truswell AS. Food carbohydrates and plasma lipids—an update. *Am J Clin Nutr.* 1994;59 (suppl):710S–718S.

63. Stone CB, Connor WE. Prolonged effects of a low cholesterol, high carbohydrate diet upon the serum lipids in diabetic patients. *Diabetes.* 1965;12:127–132.

64. Coulston AM, Hollenbeck CB, Swislocki ALM, Reaven GM. Persistence of hypertriglyceridemic effect of low-fat high-carbohydrate diets in NIDDM patients. *Diabetes Care.* 1989;12:94–101.

65. Riccardi G, Rivellese A, Pacioni D, Genovese S, Mastrenzo P, Mancini M. Separate influence of dietary carbohydrate and fibre in the metabolic control in diabetes. *Diabetologia.* 1984;26:116–121.

66. Anderson JW, Ward K. High-carbohydrate, high-fiber diets for insulin-treated men with diabetes mellitus. *Am J Clin Nutr.* 1979;32:2312–2321.

67. Anderson JW. Effect of carbohydrate restriction and high carbohydrate diets on men with chemical diabetes. *Am J Clin Nutr.* 1977;30:402–408.

68. Smith U. Carbohydrates, fat, and insulin action. *Am J Clin Nutr.* 1994;59 (suppl):686S–689S.

69. Campbell LV, Marmot PE, Dyer JA, Borkman M, Storlien LH. The high-monounsaturated fat diet as a practical alternative for NIDDM. *Diabetes Care.* 1994;17:177–182.

70. Garg A, Bantle JP, Henry RR, et al. Effects of varying carbohydrate content in patients with non–insulin-dependent diabetes mellitus. *JAMA.* 1994;271:1421–1428.

71. Grundy SM. Comparison of monounsaturated fatty acids and carbohydrates for lowering plasma cholesterol. *N Engl J Med.* 1986;314:745–748.

72. Garg A, Bonanome A, Grundy SM, Zhang Z, Unger RH. Comparison of high-carbohydrate diet with a high-monounsaturated-fat diet in patients with non–insulin-dependent diabetes mellitus. *N Engl J Med.* 1988; 319:829–834.

73. Rivellese AA, Giacco R, Genovese S, et al. Effects of changing amount of carbohydrate in diet on plasma lipoproteins and apolipoproteins in type II diabetic patients. *Diabetes Care.* 1990;13:446–448.

74. Bonanome A, Visane A, Lusiana L. Carbohydrate and lipid metabolism in patients with non–insulin-dependent diabetes mellitus: effects of a low-fat, high-carbohydrate diet vs a diet high in monounsaturated fatty acids. *Am J Clin Nutr.* 1991;54:586–590.

75. Garg A, Grundy SM, Unger RH. Comparison of effects of high- and low-carbohydrate diets on plasma lipoproteins and insulin sensitivity in patients with mild NIDDM. *Diabetes.* 1992;41:1278–1285.

76. Garg A, Grundy SM, Koffler M. Effect of high carbohydrate intake on hyperglycemia, islet function and plasma lipoproteins in NIDDM. *Diabetes Care.* 1992;15:1572–1580.

77. Parillo M, Rivellese AA, Ciardullo AV, et al. A high-monounsaturated-fat/low-carbohydrate diet improves peripheral insulin sensitivity in non–insulin-dependent diabetic patients. *Metabolism.* 1992;41:1371–1378.

78. Garg A. High-monounsaturated fat diet for diabetic patients. Is it time to change the current dietary recommendations? *Diabetes Care.* 1994;17:242–246.

79. Holler HJ, Pastors JG, eds. *Meal Planning Approaches for Diabetes Management.* 2nd ed. Chicago, Ill: The American Dietetic Association; 1994.

Incorporating Sugar in the Diabetes Meal Plan: Sample Menus and Points To Consider

BASIC 1200-CALORIE MEAL PLAN	1200-CALORIE MEAL PLAN (MODERATE AMOUNT OF ADDED SUGAR)	1200-CALORIE MEAL PLAN (LARGE AMOUNT OF ADDED SUGAR)
Breakfast	*Breakfast*	*Breakfast*
2 slices whole-wheat toast	2 slices whole-wheat toast	2 jelly doughnuts
2 tsp corn oil margarine	2 tsp strawberry jelly	1/2 fresh grapefruit
1/2 fresh grapefruit	1/2 fresh grapefruit	1 packet sugar substitute
1 packet sugar substitute	1 packet sugar substitute	8 oz skim milk
8 oz skim milk	8 oz skim milk	Black coffee
Black coffee	Black coffee	
Lunch	*Lunch*	*Lunch*
Turkey sandwich made with 3 oz sliced turkey breast 2 slices whole-wheat bread 1 tsp regular mayonnaise	Turkey sandwich made with 3 oz sliced turkey breast 2 slices whole-wheat bread 1 tsp regular mayonnaise	Turkey sandwich made with 3 oz sliced turkey breast 2 slices whole-wheat bread 1 tsp regular mayonnaise
Green salad with 1 Tbsp fat-free Italian dressing	Green salad with 1 Tbsp fat-free Italian dressing	Green salad with 1 Tbsp fat-free Italian dressing
1 fresh orange	1 cup frozen yogurt	1 fresh orange
4 oz skim milk	Diet cola	Regular cola
Dinner	*Dinner*	*Dinner*
2 oz broiled fish	2 oz broiled fish	2 oz broiled fish
2/3 cup rice	2/3 cup rice	2/3 cup rice
1/2 cup corn	1/2 cup corn	1/2 cup corn
1 tsp corn oil margarine	1 tsp corn oil margarine	1 tsp corn oil margarine
1 cup broccoli florets	1 cup broccoli florets	1 cup broccoli florets
1 cup cantaloupe cubes	3 gingersnap cookies	1 slice pecan pie
Iced tea	Iced tea	Iced tea
1 packet sugar substitute	1 packet sugar substitute	1 packet sugar substitute

Source: Nutrient analysis performed using Nutritionist IV Software, Version 3.0, 1993, N-Squared Computing, Salem, OR.

BASIC 1200-CALORIE MEAL PLAN

Evening Snack
3 cups air-popped popcorn
Diet cola

Nutrient Profile
Calories 1237
Carbohydrate .... 195 g
Protein .... 58 g
Fat .... 25 g
Sugar .... 57 g

1200-CALORIE MEAL PLAN (MODERATE AMOUNT OF ADDED SUGAR)

Evening Snack
1 slice angel food cake
4 oz skim milk

Nutrient Profile
Calories 1397
Carbohydrate .... 218 g
Protein .... 57 g
Fat .... 33 g
Sugar .... 67 g

Points To Consider
• Overall good nutrition choices are the main consideration when using sugar in the diabetes meal plan. Often, high-sugar foods are high in fat and devoid of other nutrients. In this menu, foods with sugar were carefully *substituted,* not eaten in addition to the usual meal plan.
• Individuals with diabetes should be encouraged to test blood glucose frequently when using sugar in the meal plan to see the effect a specific food may have on them. Adjustment of diabetes medications may be necessary when including sugar in the meal plan.
• An individual with type II diabetes, dyslipidemia, and insulin resistance may be more sensitive to carbohydrate intake and unable to add sugar without resulting in increased blood glucose and lipid levels.

1200-CALORIE MEAL PLAN (LARGE AMOUNT OF ADDED SUGAR)

Evening Snack
1 cup sugared cereal
4 oz skim milk

Nutrient Profile
Calories 2247
Carbohydrate .... 328 g
Protein .... 65 g
Fat .... 75 g
Sugar .... 93 g

Point To Consider
• This menu is an example of the potentially negative effects of *adding* large amounts of sugar to the diabetes meal plan. As this illustrates, foods high in sugar are often high in fat. Making unwise food choices almost doubles the amount of calories originally prescribed. Weight gain and elevated blood glucose and lipid levels may occur if this meal plan is followed over a long period of time.

Chapter 17

Identifying Protein Needs in Persons with Diabetes

Sydne K. Carlson

Historically, dietary recommendations for the treatment of diabetes have been numerous and varied. After it was determined that it was not advisable to feed sugar to persons with diabetes to compensate for glucosuria, prescribed diets often bordered on starvation or were unusually bizarre or distasteful. In the late 1700s, John Rollo, the famous Surgeon General of the Royal Artillery, suggested a diet that consisted of animal products "with an entire abstinence of every kind of vegetable matter." Recommended foods included puddings made only of blood and suet, or fat and old rancid meat.[1] Another approach advocated the yolk of a hen's egg as the only article of food adapted to the needs of the diabetic organism during diabetic acidosis. This was recorded in the book *Fasting and Undernutrition in the Treatment of Diabetes* published in 1916. The "yolk cure" of 10 to 40 egg yolks per day (25 to 100 g protein and 2500 to 10,000 mg cholesterol) was prescribed until the patient showed improvement. After that, eating a yolk once or twice a week was believed to be sufficient.[2]

In contrast to prescribing hypocaloric diets of a distasteful nature, others prescribed high-protein, low-carbohydrate diets consisting of more normal foods. Carbohydrate-containing foods were avoided almost entirely, because they were believed to be directly responsible for glucosuria. Even though the preference of the day may have been to avoid feeding persons with diabetes anything at all, meat and related foods containing protein and fat were eaten liberally as the lesser of two evils.

Moderating the level of protein consumption received more attention after it was discovered that the quantity of nitrogen in the urine decreased with restriction of dietary protein. In 1916, Joslin suggested a safety level of 1 g protein/kg body weight. This was based on the belief that higher amounts stimulated diabetes metabolism and, in severe cases of diabetes, increased the quantity of sugar, as well as nitrogen, in the urine.[3] In the 1930s, it was established that via gluconeogenesis as much as 50 to 58% of the protein from animal products could be metabolized to glucose.[4] In this early work, the glucose yield of casein and egg albumin was found to be about 50% on a weight-for-weight basis, whereas meat resulted in approximately 58% glucose production. This remains the basis for the often-used assumption that an average of 50% of the protein in the diet will be converted to glucose.

From the 1930s until recently, the metabolic response to ingestion of various amounts and types of dietary proteins has received relatively little attention. A high-protein diet has at times been advocated in clinical practice. There has been lack of information to truly substantiate or disclaim the benefit, but rationale for a high level of protein has included the following:

1. Most amino acids are gluconeogenic. Thus, dietary protein was thought to stabilize or "cushion" blood glucose levels by providing a substrate for glucose production when needed.

Table 17-1 Recommended Allowances of Reference Protein and U.S. Dietary Protein

Category	Age (years) or Condition	Weight (kg)	Recommended Dietary Allowance (g/kg)	(g/d)
Babies and children	0–0.5	6	2.2	13
(either sex)	0.5–1	9	1.6	14
	1–3	13	1.2	16
	4–6	20	1.1	24
	7–10	28	1.0	28
Males	11–14	45	1.0	45
	15–18	66	0.9	59
	19–24	72	0.8	58
	25–50	79	0.8	63
	51+	77	0.8	63
Females	11–14	46	1.0	46
	15–18	55	0.8	44
	19–24	58	0.8	46
	25–50	63	0.8	50
	51+	65	0.8	50
Pregnancy	1st trimester		+1.3	+10
	2nd trimester		+6.1	+10
	3rd trimester		+10.7	+10
Lactation	1st 6 months		+14.7	+15
	2nd 6 months		+11.8	+12

Source: Adapted from *Recommended Dietary Allowances,* ed. 10 (p 66), with permission of National Academy Press, © 1989.

2. There are reasons to implicate carbohydrate and fat. However, dietary protein has not previously been considered as important either in regulation of diabetes or as a risk factor for coronary heart disease or cancer.

3. Even before the discovery of insulin, it was known that a high-protein diet caused less of an effect on circulating glucose concentrations.[5] In recent years, a diet containing 40% of calories from protein has been advocated on the basis of improved metabolic control and lower insulin requirements.[6]

Changes in protein intake cannot be viewed in isolation because a simultaneous alteration in the intake of the other macronutrients may have independent consequences. Also, dietary protein studies that are performed are often short term and thus do not necessarily reflect long-term effects. As a consequence, there continue to be many unresolved issues. Questions that remain unanswered include:

1. What is the most appropriate level of protein to ensure adequate nutrition and quality of life?

2. How much of an effect does dietary protein have on metabolic control of diabetes because of altered substrate availability or changes in insulin or counterregulatory hormone secretion?

3. Because a high-protein diet increases glomerular filtration rate,[7] can a low-protein diet delay the progression of diabetic nephropathy? If so, what level of protein is most appropriate?

In summary, there are limited scientific data on which to base firm nutritional recommendations for protein in diabetes. In fact, the protein content of the diet—whether it be high or low, of animal or vegetable origin, etc—has today become one of the more controversial issues in diabetes nutrition therapy.

GENERAL RECOMMENDATIONS FOR PROTEIN INTAKE IN DIABETES

Protein is needed for the provision of energy, but more important, adequate protein is required to ensure normal growth, development, and maintenance of body protein stores. The average protein intake in the United States for all age groups varies from 14 to 18% of total calories.[8] According to the National Health and Nutrition survey data, the percentage of calories from protein for all ages and both sexes is 15.1%.[9] Most persons consume about 1.5 g/kg of protein per day or approximately twice what is needed to meet known nutrient needs. This is true both for persons with or without diabetes.

An expert panel has estimated the average need of adults of high-quality protein is 0.6 g/kg of body weight per day.[10] As half the population should have protein requirements below the average (and half above), public health requirements must be set at a level to cover the needs of those with the highest requirements. To ensure a margin of safety, the current recommended dietary allowance (RDA) for adults for protein is 0.8 g/kg body weight per day.[11] This approximates 10% of the total daily caloric intake and translates to about 63 g/d for a 79-kg (174 lb) man and 50 g/d for a 63-kg (138 lb) woman. In the 1989 revision of the RDAs, the number of grams of protein recommended per day was increased because of the use of observed average body weights for each age and sex rather than the reference weights used previously.

In infants, children, and adolescents, the RDA is increased to support growth and tissue maintenance with progressive decreases toward adulthood. Protein intakes in the range of 12 to 20% of calories (0.9 to 2.2 g/kg per day) are recommended. The RDA for protein during pregnancy is 60 g or an additional allowance of 10 g of reference protein per day throughout pregnancy. The recommended increase for lactation is 12 to 15 g/d. After 6 months of lactation, the volume of milk produced decreases by about 20%, and as a consequence, the RDA increment for protein is decreased by 3 g (Table 17-1).

The current RDAs for protein in the elderly are largely extrapolations from nitrogen-balance studies conducted in healthy young men. Because there are significant changes in body composition, basic metabolic and physiologic processes, and activity and food intake in the elderly, research is being undertaken to make a determination more specific to that age group. Recent findings suggest a safe protein intake for elderly adults of 1.0 to 1.25 g/kg per day of high-quality protein.[12] The higher dietary protein requirement has been found to be necessary despite generally decreased muscle mass suggesting a lower efficiency of protein use.

Protein requirements are based on nitrogen balance studies. Nitrogen balance is the difference between the amount of nitrogen consumed and the amount of nitrogen excreted per day. Provided energy needs are being met, balancing intake with output allows for a state of nitrogen equilibrium.

Positive nitrogen balance (higher intake than output) is necessary for growth or recovery from illness. Merely eating adequate protein does not guarantee a positive balance—the body also needs the right hormonal condition to build tissues. Hormones that stimulate positive protein balance include insulin, growth hormone, and testosterone. Conversely, hormones that encourage negative balance (breakdown of body tissue) include cortisol and thyroid hormone.

There is no longer a traditionally defined "diabetic diet" in terms of percentage of calories. However, for persons with diabetes as well as the general population, the level of protein should fall within the range of 10 to 20% of total calories. There is currently insufficient scientific evidence to support either a higher or lower intake.[8] Protein should be incorporated into the diet considering overall nutrient content and the effect of that level of protein on diabetes control in general.

Amino Acid Requirements

Adult requirements for indispensable amino acids have been established through nitrogen balance studies in much the same way as the total protein requirements have been determined. The difference is that the protein in the basic diet is replaced by a mixture of amino acids so that the quantity of each amino acid can be adjusted separately. Diets containing adequate amounts of all but the amino acid in question with gradually increasing increments of this amino acid are fed to experimental subjects. The intake at which zero nitrogen balance occurs is taken as the requirement for the indispensable amino acid.

In infants and young children, the indispensable amino acid requirements have been established by observing changes in weight after the amount of one amino acid in an otherwise adequate diet is reduced incrementally. As soon as the intake of the amino acid falls below requirement, weight gain will decline. To prevent impairment of growth in these studies, the amount of the limiting amino acid is increased as soon as a change in weight gain is detected.

Amino acid requirements decline much more rapidly with increasing age than protein requirements. The proportion of the total amino acids required as indispensable amino acids is much lower for the adult than for the infant. In other words, a protein may not meet the essential amino acid requirements of a young child when consumed in amounts high enough to meet the total nitrogen requirement. However, this same protein could provide necessary amino acids in excess of the requirements for adults when consumed at a level high enough to meet the adult nitrogen requirement.[13]

PROTEIN DIGESTION

Protein digestion begins in the stomach, where pepsins hydrolyze protein into large peptides. Pancreatic enzymes in the small intestine catalyze the large polypeptides into smaller peptides. They are further hydrolyzed into di- and tripeptides and free amino acids by peptidases on the intestinal brush border. Specific transporters present on the luminal side of the cells then actively transport them into mucosal cells. Once inside these cells, the amino acids diffuse down a concentration gradient into the mucosal capillaries and from there are transported through the portal vein to the liver. The concentration of amino acids in the portal vein increases rather quickly after a high-protein meal. In one study, the peripheral plasma concentration of amino acids was increased 30 minutes after ingestion of a high-protein meal.[14]

In humans, protein digestion may take 6 to 7 hours, but most amino acids in a meal are absorbed within 4 hours.[15] The time required for these processes may be type/dose-dependent as various food proteins have reportedly been digested at different rates.

In the normal person, the peripheral circulating concentration of α-amino-nitrogen (represents total amino acids present) is approximately 3.4 to 6.0 mg/dL. After a high-protein meal, it increases to about 8.7 mg/dL although the increase varies with the amount and type of protein ingested.[15] Fasting results in the release of amino acids (primarily alanine and glutamine, which are major carriers of nitrogen from muscle to liver) equivalent to protein loss of 50 g/d from a 70-kg man.[16] The limited data available in subjects with diabetes suggest that the fasting values as well as the rise after a high-protein meal are similar to those in normal subjects.

PROTEIN AND AMINO ACID METABOLISM

Animal and plant proteins are made up of about 20 common amino acids. The proportion of these amino acids varies as a characteristic of a given protein, but all food proteins (except gelatin) contain some of each. Nine amino acids are not synthesized by mammals and are there-

Table 17-2 Essential and Nonessential Amino Acids

Essential Amino Acids (Indispensable)	Nonessential Amino Acids (Dispensable)	Glucogenic and Ketogenic Amino Acids
Histidine[a]	Alanine	Leucine, lysine (purely ketogenic)
Isoleucine	Arginine	
Leucine	Asparagine	Isoleucine, phenylalanine, tyrosine, tryptophan (both ketogenic and glucogenic)
Lysine	Aspartic acid	
Methionine	Cysteine[b]	
Phenylalanine	Glutamic Acid	Alanine, serine, glycine, cysteine, aspartic acid, asparagine, glutamic acid, glutamine, arginine, histidine, valine, threonine, methionine, proline (purely glucogenic)
Threonine	Glutamine	
Tryptophan	Glycine	
Valine	Proline	
	Serine	
	Tyrosine[b]	

[a] Essential since the rate of synthesis is not adequate to support growth.

[b] Produced from essential amino acids:
phenylalanine → tyrosine
methionine → cysteine.

Source: Data from Brody T, *Nutritional Biochemistry,* Academic Press.

fore essential or indispensable nutrients. The essential amino acids are histadine, isoleucine, leucine, lysine, methionine, phenylalanine, threonine, tryptophan, and valine. Amino nitrogen accounts for approximately 16% of the weight of protein. Both the essential and the nonessential amino acids are listed in Table 17-2. On the average, it takes 6.25 g of dietary protein to yield 1 g of nitrogen, although there is some variability depending on the digestibility of a specific protein.

Amino acids are required for the synthesis of body proteins and nitrogen-containing compounds such as creatine, peptide hormone, and some neurotransmitters. The carbon skeletons of amino acids can also be oxidized to yield energy. Although energy requirements are primarily met by oxidation of carbohydrate and lipids, amino acids are indispensable for protein biosynthesis. Thus, it is important to eat sufficient protein-containing foods of adequate biologic value.

The biologic value (BV) of a protein is a measure of the degree to which its nitrogen can be used for growth or maintenance of total body function. The BV can be determined by measuring the change in nitrogen excretion relative to nitrogen intake. The BV is expressed as

$$BV = \frac{N\ intake - N\ loss\ in\ feces,\ sweat,\ urine}{N\ intake - N\ loss\ in\ feces} \times 100$$

$$= \frac{N\ retained}{N\ absorbed} \times 100$$

The nitrogen in the feces represents the nitrogenous material in the diet that is not digested and absorbed by the body. By contrast, the nitrogen in the sweat and urine arises in large measure from the catabolism of nitrogenous material in the body. Therefore, the BV is a percentage ratio that indicates the extent to which a dietary protein satisfies the amino acid requirement. In general, proteins found in eggs, milk, or

Table 17-3 Examples of High-, Intermediate-, and Low-Quality Proteins[a]

High Quality	Intermediate Quality	Low Quality
Cow milk	Rice	Cassava
Eggs	Potato	Gelatin
Human milk	Oats	Peas
Beef	Soy flour	Cornmeal
Fish		White flour

[a] The protein quality depends on its amino acid composition and digestibility. If a protein contains a disproportionately low amount of one or more amino acids or is not completely digestible, the amount of that protein needed to meet protein requirements will be greater than for a protein that has a well-balanced pattern of amino acids and is easily digested.

Source: Adapted with permission from Harper AE, Yoshimura NN. Protein quality, amino acid balance, utilization, and evaluation of diet containing amino acids as therapeutic agents. *Nutrition*. 1993;9(5):460–469, Copyright © 1993, Nutrition Inc.

meat have a proper proportion of essential amino acids and are considered to be of good protein quality. Vegetable proteins tend to have a lower BV or protein quality because each one has a low level of one or more essential amino acids. Examples of high-, intermediate-, and low-quality proteins are listed in Table 17-3.

Proteins and amino acids are not stored by the body but are being degraded and resynthesized continuously. The amino acid pool should not be thought of as a long-term storage place but rather as a convenient way of representing the sum of the circulating amino acids in the blood and the small amounts present within the cell structures.

Reutilization of amino acids is a major feature of the economy of protein metabolism because several times more protein is turned over daily than is normally consumed. In a 70-kg adult, the amount of protein synthesized daily is 250 to 300 g representing a turnover of protein that is several times the intake of the average diet.[16] Losses of amino acids occur through oxidative catabolism, and as metabolic products—urea, creatinine, and uric acid. Nitrogen is lost in sweat, feces, and other body secretions and is sloughed in skin, hair, and nails. Thus, a continuous supply of dietary amino acids is needed to replace these losses even after growth has ceased. Amino acids consumed in excess of

amounts needed to replace losses are not stored but are degraded. The carbon skeletons left after the removal of the amino groups is either used directly as sources of energy or converted to glucose or fat.

Organs and tissues of the body differ in their ability to use amino acids as energy sources. The liver has the capacity to oxidize most amino acids and, if they are in surplus, oxidizes them in preference to other energy-yielding molecules. Most of the essential amino acids are not oxidized in other tissues. The exception is the branched-chain amino acids—leucine, isoleucine, and valine—which like many nonessential amino acids can be oxidized by most organs and tissues. Some tissues prefer certain amino acids. For example, glutamine and glutamic acid are preferential energy sources of the intestine and lymphocytes.

The Krebs cycle and reactions leading to and from it are the dominant features of the diagram depicting metabolism of the amino acids resulting from the breakdown of proteins (see Figure 17-1). Those portions of amino acids that form Krebs cycle intermediates can be thought of as glucogenic, because oxaloacetate can be converted to phosphoenolpyruvate and then to glucose. Those portions that are ketogenic can give rise to either acetoacetate or acetyl coenzyme A. Some amino acids have the potential to form ei-

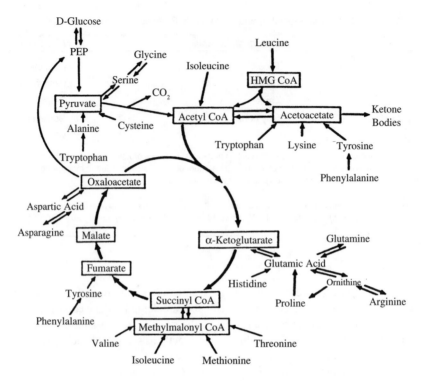

Figure 17-1 Summary of Metabolic Fates of Carbon Skeletons of Amino Acids. *Source:* Adapted from *Biochemistry: A Case Oriented Approach*, ed 4 (p 476) by R Montgomery et al with permission of Mosby-Yearbook, © 1983.

ther glucose or ketone bodies. Although most amino acids are potentially glucogenic, only alanine, serine, threonine, and glycine give rise to significant amounts of glucose. Of these, alanine is the most significant amino acid involved in gluconeogenesis. The only amino acids believed to be ketogenic, but not glucogenic, are leucine and lysine.[17]

INSULIN, GLUCAGON, AND PROTEIN USE

In examining the role of dietary protein in diabetes management, it is necessary to highlight the impact of protein on the secretion of insulin and glucagon. It is widely accepted that the influx of amino acids, as well as glucose, into the peripheral bloodstream stimulates the release of insulin. Insulin enhances muscle amino acid up-

take and stimulates muscle protein synthesis. Certain amino acids—arginine and the branched chains, especially leucine—promote insulin secretion. Other amino acids—asparagine, glycine, serine, cysteine, etc—stimulate secretion of glucagon. In turn, glucagon enhances liver uptake of amino acids and provides for gluconeogenesis and catabolism of the excess amino acids ingested. Normally, the concerted actions of insulin and glucagon serve to reduce plasma amino acid concentrations efficiently.[15]

Gluconeogenesis is the process by which lactate, pyruvate, glycerol, and amino acids are converted to glucose. The liver plays the most significant role in the synthesis of glucose, although under certain conditions, gluconeogenesis does occur in the kidney. Control of the gluconeogenic process within the body can be exerted at three points: (1) the supply of precursors coming from the peripheral tissues, (2) their uptake by the liver, and (3) the subsequent conversion to glucose within the liver.[18] The hormones, insulin and glucagon, are involved in regulation at all three levels. For example, insulin regulates gluconeogenesis by influencing the supply of gluconeogenic precursors entering the liver. Glucagon stimulates gluconeogenesis within the hepatocyte by enhancing the activity of various gluconeogenic enzymes, such as pyruvate carboxylase and fructose diphosphate, and by inhibiting the activity of several glycolytic enzymes. The amount of gluconeogenesis that occurs at specific plasma insulin or glucagon levels remains unknown.

People with diabetes exhibit an absolute or relative lack of insulin along with an absolute or relative excess of glucagon. This alteration in metabolism, as well as the importance of insulin and glucagon in regulating gluconeogenesis, complicates the issue of protein's contribution to achievement of metabolic control. Due to the complexity and the interdependency of hormonal roles, more research is needed to understand fully protein use in diabetes. For now, making appropriate food choices and achieving day-to-day consistency in amounts and distribution of carbohydrates, proteins, and fat to optimize glucose and lipid levels will continue to be major diabetes management goals.

GLUCOSE AND INSULIN RESPONSE TO DIETARY PROTEIN IN PERSONS WITH NON–INSULIN-DEPENDENT DIABETES MELLITUS

Before recommendations for dietary protein can be made, the potential for unique responses to protein ingestion in diabetes needs to be considered. Both forms of diabetes are associated with abnormalities of insulin metabolism—the predominant defect in insulin-dependent diabetes mellitus (IDDM) is insulin deficiency compared with impaired insulin action in non–insulin-dependent diabetes mellitus (NIDDM). Because insulin plays a significant role in pro-

tein metabolism, there is a distinct possibility that variations in protein intake will elicit different responses in the two forms of diabetes.

Enhanced Insulin Secretion

Protein stimulates insulin secretion—an effect that is significantly more pronounced in persons with NIDDM or glucose intolerance, whether obese or not. Arginine, lysine, leucine, and phenylalanine (in descending order) are the most potent amino acid secretagogues. A mixture of indispensable amino acids is more potent than any single amino acid, suggesting a synergistic effect.[19]

Mechanisms by which protein may stimulate insulin secretion are (1) a direct effect of absorbed amino acids on pancreatic ß-cells and (2) an indirect effect mediated through the release of intestinal incretins. Incretins are hormones released from the gastrointestinal tract in response to the ingestion of food, which in turn stimulate, potentiate, or inhibit the secretion of other substances that have metabolic effects. The incretin effect is thought to be significant in enhancing insulin secretion, because ingested amino acids cause a greater insulin response than when amino acids are infused intravenously.[20]

A strong synergistic interaction on insulin secretion can be demonstrated when various sources of protein are ingested with glucose. There is, however, variation in their potency. In one study using several different protein sources, gelatin and cottage cheese were the most potent in enhancing insulin secretion and egg white protein was the least potent.[21]

It is not known whether a lower glycemic response occurs to glucose and protein than to glucose alone in type II diabetes. Increasing the amount of protein in the first of two portions of a breakfast meal separated by a 30-minute interval reduced the glucose and enhanced the insulin response to the second feeding.[22] By contrast, it has been reported that neither the protein nor fat content of a meal affects the glucose response in NIDDM.[23]

In clinical practice, the question becomes— should dietary protein be enhanced to increase insulin secretion with the potential for moderating glucose response? Or conversely, is too much insulin already a large part of the problem? Accelerating levels of insulin could be potentially damaging because epidemiologic data suggest a strong correlation between high circulating insulin concentration, insulin resistance, hypertension, and coronary heart disease.

Increased Gluconeogenesis

Fasting hyperglycemia in poorly controlled NIDDM is largely due to hepatic glucose production, seemingly the result of increased gluconeogenesis. Amino acids (primarily alanine) are substrates for gluconeogenesis. When the liver converts alanine to glucose, the excess amino group is synthesized into urea. A study to assess the relation of urea synthesis to blood alanine levels in NIDDM found that when the diabetes is poorly controlled, an increased conversion of alanine to urea nitrogen occurs at any amino acid concentration. This perturbation was in part normalized by improved metabolic control.[24]

Protein ingestion causes a rise while glucose ingestion causes a lowering of the glucagon concentration in normal persons. Protein is thought to be at least four times more potent in stimulating a rise in glucagon as glucose is in lowering it. In persons with NIDDM, the fasting glucagon concentration is normal or modestly elevated and generally rises in response to a protein meal. Gluconeogenic amino acids arising from protein ingestion (as well as incretins) may stimulate glucagon secretion.[15] In patients with NIDDM, glucagon levels seem to be one reason for increased glucose output despite high insulin levels.[25]

There appear to be many interdependent variables regulating the rate of gluconeogenesis in NIDDM, and protein is only one of them. Due to the paucity of information, adjusting dietary protein to influence gluconeogenesis would only be based on conjecture and theory. Until recommendations can be made based on firm scientific data, the best approach may be to concentrate on helping persons remain adequately nourished while achieving the best metabolic control possible.

Issues of Adequate Protein in NIDDM

As a result of studies implicating a high-protein diet in development of glomerular sclerosis and nephropathy even in the patient with type II diabetes, restriction of dietary protein is being explored. The RDA for protein (0.8 g/kg body weight per day) is recommended for individuals with evidence of microalbuminuria.[26] There are presently not sufficient data to recommend a lower protein diet to delay the onset of nephropathy in persons with type II diabetes. There may actually be more reasons to enhance protein intake.

Although many Americans consume considerably more protein than they need, there are elderly persons with type II diabetes experiencing economic or digestive difficulties who do not. Their potential for malnutrition, as well as recent studies suggesting that older persons require a higher level of protein than previously thought,[12] may be supportive of a higher protein intake overall. Other considerations in support of not restricting protein in type II diabetes include the likelihood of a recommendation for at least a modest reduction in caloric intake compounded by decreased energy needs in general. A minimum guideline of 10% of calories from protein at a caloric level of 1500 is 38 g—an amount that is not adequate. Often a diet containing 20 to 25% calories from protein may be necessary to provide adequate nutrition for these persons.

DIETARY PROTEIN CONSIDERATIONS IN IDDM

Several aspects of the relationship of dietary protein and insulin metabolism in IDDM need to be considered. The first involves the likelihood that protein will be converted to glucose in various diabetic states. More information would allow for adjustments in dietary protein intake and insulin based on anticipated outcomes, resulting in improved diabetes control. Another consideration concerns regulation of protein catabolism during conditions of insulin resistance and deficiency—even intensively treated individuals may experience this at times. During periods of poor control, persons may be prone to accelerated protein turnover with resultant deleterious effects on maintenance of body protein stores. Last, the recent interest in restricting animal protein to decrease glomerular injury and thus delay the progression of renal failure deserves consideration. Questions that evolve from these issues are addressed in the following paragraphs.

- *Because it is known that protein stimulates insulin secretion, can it be assumed that adjustments in insulin are needed to appropriately metabolize various intakes of dietary protein?*

There is convincing evidence that increasing the carbohydrate of a meal increases the glycemic response and therefore the amount of insulin necessary to restore normal glycemia. There are very few studies to substantiate the belief that protein also has a major influence on postprandial glucose response in IDDM. In a recent study of insulin-dependent subjects, Peters and Davidson[27] found the addition of protein energy (200 kcal, 50 g protein) to a meal increased both the postprandial glucose response and the insulin requirement. There was primarily a late (150 to 300 minutes) glucose response, which then also raised the late insulin requirements after the protein-added meal. This finding helps substantiate that extra insulin may be required when large amounts of protein are added to a meal.

As a result of observing studies in the literature indicating dietary protein restriction can reduce insulin requirements, Lariviere et al[28] monitored glucose levels, plasma glucose rate of appearance, and daily insulin requirements of men with uncomplicated tightly controlled IDDM fed a protein-free diet. Twelve similar nondiabetic subjects were also given a maintenance-energy but protein-free diet for 10 days. After adaptation to this protein-free diet, the men with diabetes experienced a 30% decrease in average blood glucose concentrations despite a concurrent 25% decrease in insulin dosages. The short-term protein restriction decreased the postabsorptive glucose and insulin concentrations in the normal men and revealed that the effect of protein restriction is general and not restricted to diabetes. It is not known whether the decreased insulin requirements were a result of increased insulin sensitivity, decreased hepatic output, or both.

As with the study by Peters and Davidson, these results support the contention that higher levels of dietary protein require increased amounts of insulin or, conversely, the lower levels require less insulin. Clinically, it seems logical to conclude that persons with diabetes desiring intensive metabolic control need either to be consistent with the level of protein in their diets, or they need to learn to adjust insulin appropriately for significant changes in dietary protein intake.

- *Can total available glucose be used as a meal-planning system for varying protein intakes?*

It may be clinically relevant for persons on intensive therapy who inject premeal insulin to increase insulin if much more than the usual amount of protein is to be consumed. Patients who do not adjust premeal insulin doses may want to decrease the amount of carbohydrate consumed in a meal if a large amount of protein is eaten to keep the postprandial glucose response roughly equivalent. One meal-planning strategy used to assist patients in making these adjustments is referred to as total available glucose (TAG). The assumption in using TAG is that approximately 58% of animal protein will be converted to glucose. (It must be remembered that this 58% conversion figure is based on a theory promulgated in 1936.) With the TAG system, the TAG values assigned to starch, fruit, and vegetables are the same as carbohydrate grams in the ADA Exchange Diet. To account for additional protein in meat and milk, a 58% conversion factor for protein is used. Because

58% of the protein in one meat exchange is 4 g, the amount of TAG provided by each ounce of meat is 4 g. The TAG for 1 cup of milk is 17 (12 g of carbohydrate plus 5 from 58% of 8 g of protein) (see Exhibit 17-1). The protein from vegetables and starches is ignored both because of the relatively low levels of protein they contain and also as a result of research suggesting that the effects of animal and plant proteins are not the same. Clinically, the TAG system may be of value for the patient who has a good diabetes and nutrition knowledge base, desires intensive control, basically eats a good diet, but who would like the flexibility of significantly varying the amount of meat and milk with some degree

of reliability. TAG is a high-level meal-planning system not appropriate for everyone.

- **Should protein be included as part of a bedtime snack?**

Many experienced practitioners answer this question in the positive, although there have been few data to validate the significance. In the study reported earlier,[27] the greater glucose response to a protein-added meal was primarily due to an increase in the late (150 to 300 minute) postprandial glucose. This can be interpreted as an indication that protein is a good source of long-term energy, which would cause a sustained rise in blood glucose concentration and

---

Exhibit 17-1 Total Available Glucose (TAG) from Diabetic Exchange Groups

Exchange Group	Carbohydrate (g)	Protein (g)	TAG
1 fruit exchange	15	0	15
1 meat exchange	0	7	4
1 milk exchange	12	8	17
1 bread exchange	15	0	15
1 vegetable exchange	5	0	5
1 fat exchange	0	0	0

Sample Menu Using TAG for Goal Level of 90

Food Item	TAG
Grilled chicken breast (4 oz)	16
Baked potato (medium) 2 tbsp sour cream	30
Peas (1/2 cup)	15
Sliced tomatoes	5
Skim milk (12 oz)	25
Total	**91**

Note: The TAG system expands the carbohydrate counting system by assuming that both carbohydrate and animal protein contribute to elevations in blood sugars. TAG is calculated as follows:

TAG = carbohydrate (g) + [animal protein (g) x 0.58]

A meal plan identifies the number of TAG points allowed per meal or snack. Limiting fat intake is also encouraged.

Source: Adapted from Snetselaar LG. *Nutrition Counseling Skills*. 2nd ed. (p 300). Aspen Publishers, Inc.; © 1989.

help prevent nocturnal hypoglycemia. Adding 10 to 20 grams of protein to the bedtime snacks of persons experiencing the nocturnal hypoglycemia is worth a try. Although there is little scientific research to support it, it often seems to help.

- *What is a safe level of dietary protein consumption?*

There has been a great deal of interest in the possibility that a low-protein diet can retard the progression of renal disease, regardless of underlying pathology. A high-protein diet elevates the glomerular filtration rate (GFR) in individuals with or without diabetes, probably by increasing renal blood flow and intraglomerular pressure. Zeller et al[29] and Walker et al[30] showed independently that diets containing 0.6 g/kg ideal body weight and 0.67 g/kg per day, respectively, slowed the decline in GFR in persons with IDDM an average of 75% over a 3-year period. Despite encouraging results such as these, there is also provocative evidence indicating that 0.6 g protein per kilogram ideal body weight is too low for the person with diabetes. Brodsky et al[31] reported that six patients with IDDM experienced decreased muscle strength and increased adiposity with no change in body weight during 3 months of adherence to a protein-restricted diet. Accelerated gluconeogenesis and rates of protein degradation with negative nitrogen balance and muscle wasting occur in patients with diabetes—a process that seems even more pronounced in patients with end-stage renal disease.[32] Thus, low-protein diets should be used with caution.

- *Is vegetable protein safer than animal protein?*

Persuasive data indicate that the clinical course of diabetic nephropathy can be positively influenced by intensive metabolic control, smoking cessation, normalization of blood pressure, certain pharmacologic therapies (captopril and perhaps enalapril), and a possible dietary protein.[26] There are also preliminary findings to suggest that the protein source, whether the protein is animal or vegetable origin, may be important in affecting the progression of renal disease.

Jibani et al[33] studied the effects of a predominantly vegetarian diet in eight insulin-dependent patients with nephropathy. The proportion of vegetable protein was supplemented to maintain a protein intake that approximated the patient's usual diet. The results of the study suggested that it is possible to reduce proteinuria by restricting the animal fraction of the diet while at the same time supplementing the vegetable protein content to maintain a desirable protein intake. Although the authors stated that the patients found the vegetarian diet acceptable, they did not consume as much total protein on the lactovegetarian diet as they did their usual diet. Thus, as in other studies in which the average total protein tends to be lower in the vegan and vegetarian groups,[34] it was not discernible whether the fall in albumin excretion rate was due to a reduction in total protein or from less protein of animal origin. There has been speculation that protein from animal sources is generally more digestible than vegetable protein. The increased availability of amino acids would result in more urea production and a greater workload for the kidneys. More research on vegetable protein versus animal protein is needed to confirm the benefits.

USE OF VEGETARIAN DIETS IN DIABETES

It is the position of the American Dietetic Association that vegetarian diets are healthful and nutritionally adequate when appropriately planned.[35] There are scientific data to suggest a positive relationship between vegetarianism and a reduced risk of many chronic degenerative diseases—not the least of which is diabetes mellitus. The results of a study in which healthy elderly vegetarian women were compared with closely matched nonvegetarian peers showed significantly lower concentrations of serum glucose, low-density lipoprotein-cholesterol, and total cholesterol in the vegetarian group.[36] These vegetarian women (nonconsumers of any flesh

Table 17-4 Comparison of Mean Daily Intakes of the Macronutrients from 7-Day Food Records of Vegetarian and Nonvegetarian Elderly Women

Energy and Nutrients	Vegetarians (no. = 23)	Nonvegetarians (no. = 14)
Energy (kcal)	1452	1363
Protein (g/kg)	0.78	0.88
Protein (% kcal)	12.9	16.2
Carbohydrate (% kcal)	60.0	50.2
Fat (% kcal)	31.7	35.9

Source: Adapted with permission from Nieman DC, Underwood BC, Sherman KM, Arabatzis K, et al. Dietary status of Seventh-Day Adventist vegetarian and non-vegetarian elderly women. *Journal of the American Dietetic Association.* 1989:89(12):1763–1769, Copyright © 1989, American Dietetic Association.

meat) had intakes of the macronutrients (Table 17-4) more in line with guidelines advocated by both the American Heart Association and American Diabetes Association. Both the vegetarian and nonvegetarian groups had a tendency to be low in zinc, vitamin B6, folacin, vitamin B12, calcium, vitamin D, vitamin E, pantothenic acid, copper, and manganese. Based on analysis of the 7-day food records, the nonvegetarians actually had the lower intakes of the two groups with the notable exception of vitamin B12.

For lacto-ovo-vegetarians (who use dairy products and eggs) or lacto-vegetarians (who use dairy products), the RDAs can easily be met depending on the foods and portions of foods consumed. More careful planning may be necessary by the vegan (strict vegetarian who uses neither dairy products or eggs) to attain a nutritionally adequate diet. The nutrients that are most often deficient are calcium, vitamin D, iron, zinc and vitamin B12. Although it is questionable how many people follow a strict vegetarian diet long enough to develop a deficiency of vitamin B12, the risk does exist.

Even though vitamin B12 is found almost exclusively in foods of animal origin, there may be some B12 in the diet on the surface of unwashed plants. Obviously, this makes vegetables an unreliable source of vitamin B12, and vegans need a dependable source of B12 in their diets. Cyanocabalamin, the physiologically active form of the vitamin, is available from vitamin supplements or in fortified foods such as cereals, soy beverages, and some brands of nutritional yeast.

Vitamin B12 is needed by the body in very small amounts. The RDA for vitamin B12 in the adult is 2 µg. Although vitamin B12 is produced by microorganisms present in the gastrointestinal tracts of animals and human beings, it appears to be produced beyond the ileum, which is the site of vitamin B12 absorption.

Calcium deficiency in vegetarians is rare. Calcium from low oxalate vegetable greens such as kale has been shown to be absorbed as well as calcium from milk.[37] Studies have also shown that vegetarians absorb and retain more calcium from foods than do nonvegetarians.[38] If exposure to sunlight is limited, the need for supplementation of vitamin D should be carefully assessed.

The status of iron nutriture is dependent on amount of dietary iron consumed and amount absorbed. In Western diets, there is usually adequate intake of iron from plant products and in the United States from foods fortified with iron to prevent deficiency. Western vegetarians also may consume more ascorbic acid (an enhancer of nonheme iron) than vegetarians in developing countries.[35]

Iron status may be dependent on the type of foods used. In a recent study of young Chinese Buddhist vegetarian and nonvegetarian students, meat was replaced with soy bean products. The researchers concluded that a vegetarian diet rich in soy bean products and limited in bioavailable

Table 17-5 Approximate Amino Acid Content of Different Food Protein Sources

Food Source	Lysine (mg/g protein)	Sulfur Amino Acids (mg/g protein)	Threonine (mg/g protein)	Tryptophan (mg/g protein)
Legumes	64	25	38	12
Cereals	31	37	32	12
Nuts, seeds	45	46	36	17
Fruits	45	27	29	11
Animal foods	85	38	44	12

Source: Adapted with permission from Young VR, Pellet PL. Plant proteins in relation to human protein and amino acid nutrition. *American Journal of Clinical Nutrition.* 1994;59(suppl):1205S, Copyright © 1994, American Society for Clinical Nutrition.

iron was not adequate for maintaining iron balance in either men or women.[39]

Zinc is found in plant sources such as grains, nuts, and legumes—staples of a vegetarian diet. Intakes of zinc are usually adequate when a varied diet and appropriate calories are consumed.

Protein and Amino Acids in Vegetarian Diets

Adequate amounts of essential and nonessential amino acids can be provided by plant food alone as long as the plant proteins come from varied sources and the caloric intake is sufficient to meet energy needs. A common myth that plant proteins are incomplete because they lack specific amino acids is no longer considered accurate. It has been determined that even though specific food proteins may be low in certain amino acids, usual dietary combinations of proteins are complete. For example, soy beans, which are low in sulfur-containing amino acids, can be combined effectively in combination with cereal grains, which are deficient in lysine, to provide a protein quality that is greater than for either protein source alone (Table 17-5).

There has been concern that foods with complementary amino acid patterns be provided within the same meal to achieve maximum benefit. Recent studies in human adults indicate that dietary use is similar whether daily protein intake is distributed among two or three meals. It is of interest that there is a sizable pool of lysine in the intracellular space of free amino acids and that in a diet based predominantly on cereal grains, lysine is likely to be the limiting amino acid. When a protein-rich meal is eaten, 60% of the adult daily requirement for lysine may be deposited into the intracellular pool within 3 hours. If a low lysine meal of corn were ingested some hours later, there would be enough free lysine in the pool to buffer the low lysine content of the amino acid mixture derived from corn. In this case, the overall nutritional quality of the combined meals would be high. In summary, it is not necessary to balance the amino acid profile at each meal, especially under conditions in which the amount of total protein ingested far exceeds minimum physiologic requirements.[40]

COMBINING VEGETARIAN AND DIABETES GUIDELINES

Looking for something they can do to prevent/delay the complications of their disease, persons with diabetes sometimes gravitate toward vegetarianism as a health-supporting dietary alternative. A vegetarian diet in diabetes is entirely workable. In fact, the recommendations made by the American Dietetic Association for planning a vegetarian diet overlap nicely with general nutrition recommendations for persons with diabetes.

The American Dietetic Association guidelines for a well-planned vegetarian diet include

- Choose a wide variety of foods
- Maintain an adequate caloric intake
- Keep nutrient-dense foods (sweets and high-fat foods) to a minimum
- Choose unrefined grain products or fortified or enriched cereals
- If milk products are consumed, use low-fat varieties
- Use a variety of fruits and vegetables, including good sources of vitamin C
- Limit egg yolks to three to four yolks per week

Although the Vegetarian Nutrition Guidelines are similar to the diabetes association nutrition recommendations, persons with diabetes truly interested in adopting a vegetarian life style benefit from a dietitian's assistance. In addition to controlling the quantity and types of foods eaten for metabolic control of diabetes, vegetarianism can add a restrictive dimension. In today's hectic life style, combining the two requires careful planning and forethought. After following a vegetarian diet for several months, one young woman stated she almost cried on entering a fast-food restaurant with friends and realizing the only foods that "really fit" were a dinner salad and a baked potato with a limited amount of margarine.

Planning a vegetarian diet is much like planning any other diabetic diet. When the exchange system is used, the number of servings of vegetables, fruit, starches, fat, milk, or "meat" allowed at each meal is determined. Nuts, nut butters, soy protein, animal product substitutes, tofu, and legumes are common meat alternatives. Because legumes are high in carbohydrate as well as protein, people often require extra help with incorporating them into their meal plan appropriately.

CONCLUSION

The role of clinicians may be to remember that the data are not all in and to assist patients in

moderating rather than severely restricting the level of protein in their diets. It is convenient that the dietary recommendations presently advocated for patients with diabetes do not emphasize protein. Encouraging a high-carbohydrate, low-fat diet usually results in a lowering of dietary protein. It is expected that continued research will provide further insight on the relationship of protein intake to renal complications.

REFERENCES

1. Nuttall FQ. Diet and the diabetic patient. *Diabetes Care.* 1983;6:197–207.
2. Stern H. *Fasting and Undernutrition in the Treatment of Diabetes.* New York, NY: Rebman Company; 1916.
3. Joslin EP. *Treatment of Diabetes Mellitus.* Philadelphia, Pa: Lea & Febiger; 1916.
4. Conn JW, Newburgh LH. The glycemic response to isoglucogenic quantities of protein and carbohydrate. *J Clin Invest.* 1936;15:665–671.
5. Dolger H, Seeman B. *How to Live with Diabetes.* New York, NY: WW Norton & Company, Inc.; 1958.
6. Bernstein RK. *Diabetes. The GlucograF® Method for Normalizing Blood Sugar.* New York, NY: Crown Publishers, Inc.; 1981.
7. Wylie-Rosett J. Evaluation of protein in dietary management of diabetes mellitus. *Diabetes Care.* 1988; 11(2):143–148.
8. Franz MJ, Horton ES, Bantle, JP, et al. Nutrition principles for the management of diabetes and related complications. *Diabetes Care.* 1994;17(5):490–518.
9. McDowell MA, Briefel RR, Alaimo K, et al. *Energy and Macronutrient Intakes of Persons Ages 2 Months and Over in the United States: Third National Health and Nutrition Examinations Survey, Phase 1, 1989–91. Advance Data from Vital and Health Statistics; No 255.* Hyattsville, Md: National Center for Health Statistics, 1994.
10. WHO (World Health Organization). *Energy and Protein Requirements. Report of a Joint FAO/WHO/UNU Expert Consultation.* Geneva: World Health Organization; 1985. Technical Support Series 724.
11. National Research Council. *Recommended Dietary Allowances.* 10th ed. Washington, DC: National Academy Press; 1989.
12. Campbell WW, Crim MC, Dallal GE, et al. Increased protein requirements in elderly people: new data and retrospective reassessments. *Am J Clin Nutr.* 1994;60:501–509.
13. Harper AE, Yoshimura NN. Protein quality, amino acid balance, utilization, and evaluation of diet containing

amino acids as therapeutic agents. *Nutrition.* 1993;9(5): 460–469.

14. Ahmed M, Nuttall FQ, Gannon MC, Lamusga RF. Plasma glucagon and α-amino acid nitrogen response to various diets in normal humans. *Am J Clin Nutr.* 1980;33:1917–1924.

15. Nuttall FQ, Gannon MC. Metabolic response to dietary protein in persons with and without diabetes mellitus. *Diabetes Nutr Metab.* 1991;4:71–88.

16. Shils ME, Olson JA, Shike M, eds. *Modern Nutrition in Health and Disease.* 8th ed. Philadelphia, Pa: Lea & Febiger; 1994.

17. Brody T. *Nutritional Biochemistry.* New York, NY: Academic Press, Inc.; 1994.

18. Brownlee M, ed. *Diabetes Mellitus: Intermediary Metabolism and Its Regulation.* Vol. 3. New York, NY: Garland STPM Press; 1981.

19. Nuttall FQ, Gannon MC. Plasma glucose and insulin response to macronutrients in nondiabetic and NIDDM subjects. *Diabetes Care.* 1991;14:824–838.

20. Henry RR. Protein content of the diabetic diet. *Diabetes Care.* 1994;17(12):1502–1513.

21. Gannon MC, Nuttall FQ, Neil BJ, Westphal SA. The insulin and glucose responses to meals of glucose plus various proteins in type II diabetic subjects. *Metabolism.* 1988;37(11):1081–1088.

22. Seino Y, Ikeda M, Taminato T, et al. Blood glucose and plasma insulin of mild diabetic patients in response to high protein divided meals. *Hum Nutr Appl Nutr.* 1983;37A:222–225.

23. Simpson RW, McDonald J, Wahlqvist ML, et al. Macronutrients have different metabolic effects in non-diabetics and diabetics. *Am J Clin Nutr.* 1985;42:449–453.

24. Almdal TP, Jensen T, Vilstrup H. Control of non–insulin-dependent diabetes mellitus partially normalizes the increase in hepatic efficacy for urea synthesis. *Metabolism.* 1994;43(3):328–332.

25. Wyngaarden JB, Smith LH, Bennett JC. *Cecil Textbook of Medicine.* 19th ed. Philadelphia, Pa: WB Saunders Company; 1988.

26. American Diabetes Association. Consensus development conference on the diagnosis and management of nephropathy in patients with diabetes mellitus. *Diabetes Care.* 1994;17(11):1357–1361.

27. Peters AL, Davidson MB. Protein and fat effects on glucose responses and insulin requirements in subjects with insulin-dependent diabetes mellitus. *Am J Clin Nutr.* 1993;58:555–560.

28. Lariviere F, Chiasson JL, Schiffrin A, et al. Effects of dietary protein restriction on glucose and insulin metabolism in normal and diabetic humans. *Metabolism.* 1994;43(4):462–467.

29. Zeller K, Whittaker E, Sultan L, et al. Effect of restricting dietary proteins on the progression of renal failure in patients with insulin-dependent diabetes mellitus. *N Engl J Med.* 1991;324(2):78–84.

30. Walker JD, Dodds RA, Murrells TJ, et al. Restriction of dietary protein and progression of renal failure in diabetic nephropathy. *Lancet.* 1989;2:1411–1414.

31. Brodsky IG, Robbins DC, Hiser E, et al. Effects of low-protein diets on protein metabolism in insulin-dependent diabetes mellitus patients with early nephropathy. *J Clin Endocrinol Metab.* 1992;75(2): 351–357.

32. Vinik AI, Wing RR. The good, the bad, and the ugly in diabetic diets. *Endocrinol Metab Clin North Am.* 1992; 21(2):237–279.

33. Jibani MM, Bloodworth LL, Foden E, et al. Predominantly vegetarian diet in patients with incipient and early clinical diabetic nephropathy: effects on albumin excretion rate and nutritional status. *Diabetic Med.* 1991;8:949–953.

34. Kontessis P, Jones S, Dodds R, et al. Renal, metabolic and hormonal responses to ingestion of animal and vegetable proteins. *Kidney Int.* 1990;38:136–144.

35. American Dietetic Association. Position of the American Dietetic Association: vegetarian diets. *J Am Diet Assoc.* 1993;93(11):1317–1319.

36. Nieman DC, Underwood BC, Sherman KM, et al. Dietary status of Seventh-Day Adventist vegetarian and non-vegetarian elderly women. *J Am Diet Assoc.* 1989; 89(12):1763–1769.

37. Heaney RP, Weaver CM. Calcium absorption from kale. *Am J Clin Nutr.* 1990;51:656–657.

38. Zemel MB. Calcium utilization: effect of varying level and source of dietary protein. *Am J Clin Nutr.* 1988;48: 880–883.

39. Shaw NS, Chin CJ, Pan WH. A vegetarian diet rich in soybean products compromises iron status in young students. *J Nutr.* 1995;125:212–219.

40. Young VR, Pellett PL. Plant proteins in relation to human protein and amino acid nutrition. *Am J Clin Nutr.* 1994;59(suppl):1203S–1212S.

Chapter 18

Lipid Metabolism and Choices for Persons with Diabetes

Linda V. Van Horn

Dietary fat intake and lipid metabolism are especially important considerations in treating diabetes because of the macrovascular sequelae, including coronary heart disease (CHD), stroke, cardiac failure, and occlusive peripheral artery disease, that are common complications.[1-3] Despite advances in pharmacologic approaches and diagnostic methods for detecting and treating diabetes, the pathogenic mechanisms involved in these relationships remain undefined.[4] Mortality from atherosclerosis is two to three times more common among diabetic compared with nondiabetic individuals, with an expected reduction in lifespan of 5 to 7 years.[5] The major risk factors for this increased cardiovascular mortality include blood lipid/lipoprotein abnormalities, hypertension, and obesity.[5-8] The mechanisms related to this association are not completely known and may be multiple.[4-6] Enhanced low-density lipoprotein (LDL) oxidation, altered cellular function, promotion of thrombogenesis, and increased incidence of hypertension and renal disease are suspected factors. High triglycerides and low high-density lipoprotein-cholesterol (HDL-C) are often present. Non–insulin-dependent diabetes mellitus (NIDDM) is also associated with accumulation of small very low-density lipoprotein (VLDL) particles, intermediate-density lipoprotein (IDL), small dense LDL, and altered composition of HDL.[4,5]

In studies comparing diabetic with non-diabetic control populations, serum total cholesterol levels were consistently found to be higher in the former.[9] Pooled mean cholesterol values from 11 studies were 221 mg/dL in diabetic groups versus 193 mg/dL among the controls. Data from the San Antonio heart study further indicated that combined increase in risk factor levels can predict future diagnosis of clinical diabetes.[10] Increased serum cholesterol may be related to the hypertriglyceridemia common among diabetic individuals. Lack of consistent reporting and measurement of the lipids and lipoproteins in these studies has complicated evaluations regarding qualitative and quantitative differences between diabetic and nondiabetic groups.

In treating diabetes, a comprehensive dietary approach is needed to prevent and/or control these risk factors and regulate glucose metabolism.[3] The diet should be nutrient dense, nonatherogenic, and calorie-controlled, yet practical, palatable, and adaptable to individual tastes and preferences. A skilled dietitian can be invaluable in accomplishing these objectives.

This approach reflects a tremendous change since 1922, when Leonard Thompson, the first diabetic patient in the world to receive insulin, was prescribed a diet that was 70% fat, 20% carbohydrate, and 10% protein.[11] He lived for 13 years on this regimen. He reportedly died from bronchopneumonia, but it seems likely that his high-fat diet would have eventually contributed to hypercholesterolemia and his premature demise through coronary, cancer, or other diseases associated with chronic high-fat, low-fiber intake. The Diet and Health Report of the National Academy of Sciences describes an optimal diet for prevention of disease as nutrition rich in vegetables, fruits, and grains; moderate in low-fat dairy products, fish, poultry, and lean meats; and sparse in salt, alcohol, and refined sugar.[12]

The recommended fat content for patients with insulin-dependent diabetes mellitus (IDDM) has recently been reconsidered due to reports of elevated triglycerides, reduced HDL-C levels in patients following a very low-fat, high-carbohydrate diet, without necessarily reducing LDL-C.[12,13] Nutrition therapy should be consistent with the treatment and control of diabetes, the prevention of macrovascular diseases, and general health and nutritional adequacy. This chapter reviews the role of dietary lipids in lipid metabolism for the prevention and treatment of coronary heart disease and in the overall management and control of diabetes. An update of the scientific background supporting dietary recommendations and practical intervention approaches for achieving them are presented.

BLOOD LIPIDS IN DIABETIC POPULATIONS

With adequate insulin therapy and good control of blood glucose, the plasma lipid levels of patients with IDDM are similar to those of the general population of the same age and sex. Levels of HDL-C may actually be higher than average in some of these patients.[3] In patients with NIDDM, there is a two- to threefold increase in the prevalence of dyslipidemia.[14] Hypertriglyceridemia, increased VLDL-C, and decreased HDL-C are the most frequent lipid abnormalities, and as many as 40% of the patients have high-risk levels (≥160 mg/dL) of LDL-C.[15] Accumulation of small dense LDL particles in plasma, known as phenotype B, is twice as common in patients with NIDDM as in the normal population and is associated with increased risk of cardiovascular disease (CVD).[15] It is suspected that NIDDM and phenotype B are genetically linked and accompany the hyperinsulinemia, insulin resistance and intra-abdominal fat accumulation commonly observed in these patients.[16,17] In the nondiabetic population, elevated plasma triglyceride may or may not contribute to cardiovascular risk,[18] but in persons with diabetes, hypertriglyceridemia and hyperinsulinemia are major CVD risk factors.[19,20]

The American Diabetes Association points out that abnormalities in lipid and carbohydrate metabolism in persons with diabetes may require adjustments in dietary treatment for CVD risk reduction recommended for nondiabetic individuals with elevated LDL-C.[21] The potential risk of further increasing triglycerides with a diet high in carbohydrate must be weighed against the LDL-C lowering benefits of a diet low in total and saturated fat.[3] Quantitative changes in fat (ie, replacing saturated fats with unsaturated fats and reducing cholesterol below 300 mg/d while maintaining total fat intake at about 30% of total kilocalories and carbohydrates at 50 to 55% of kilocalories) offer a strategy for reducing triglycerides and LDL-C without reducing HDL-C.[22] Exercise is also an important intervention strategy. Omega-3 fatty acids have been shown to help reduce CVD risk and triglyceride levels, but in NIDDM, increases in LDL-C and worsening of glucose control have also been reported.[23] Increased fish consumption is generally considered more beneficial than fish oil supplements.

EPIDEMIOLOGIC BACKGROUND

There is overwhelming epidemiologic evidence supporting a direct relationship between level of total fat and LDL-C and rate of CHD. Population studies such as the Pooling Project, as well as the between population studies conducted by Keys et al[24] conclude that CHD is more prevalent in countries where diets high in fat, saturated fat, and cholesterol are consumed.[5] Further evidence from more than 361,000 men screened for the Multiple Risk Factor Intervention Trial (MRFIT) shows that the association between blood cholesterol level and CHD is continuous, across a wide spectrum of cholesterol levels, and graded, (ie, the higher the level, the higher the risk).[25]

Clinical trials have provided additional data showing efficacy of LDL reduction with subsequent improvement in CHD risk.[26] Meta-analyses from primary prevention trials comparing diet and/or drug intervention report that reduced

Exhibit 18-1 National Cholesterol Education Program: Risk Status Based on CHD Risk Factors Other Than LDL-C

Positive Risk Factors (Increased Risk)

- Age:
  Male ≥ 45 years
  Female ≥ 55 years or premature menopause without estrogen replacement therapy
- Family history of premature CHD
- Current cigarette smoker
- Hypertension (≥140/90 mm Hg or on antihypertensive medication)
- Low HDL-C (<35 mg/dL)
- Diabetes mellitus

Negative Risk Factor (Decreased Risk)

- High HDL-C (≥60 mg/dL)

Other Non-Lipid Risk Factors

- Obesity
- Physical inactivity

Source: Expert Panel on Detection, Evaluation, and Treatment of High Blood Cholesterol in Adults. Summary of the second report of the National Cholesterol Education Program (NCEP) expert panel on detection, evaluation, and treatment of high blood cholesterol in adults (Adults Treatment Panel II). *Journal of the American Medical Association.* 1993;269: 3015–3023.

---

total cholesterol levels through either strategy is effective in reducing CHD rates.[27–29] Because of potential serious side effects and economic burden imposed by long-term pharmacologic treatment, dietary intervention, exercise, and weight control without drugs are the preferred strategies whenever adequate lipid lowering can be achieved.

From the mid-1960s, when the CHD mortality rate reached a peak, to the early 1990s, there has been a dramatic decline of about 2% per year. The impact of this decline is reflected in extended life expectancy, with 6.5 million more people older than age 65 in 1985 than there were in 1970 and estimates of double that in the year 2000.[30] Early detection and treatment are credited for much of this improvement, and primary prevention is of paramount importance.[5,13] Despite this decline, CHD remains the leading cause of death in this country, claiming more than 800,000 lives and costing more than $60

billion each year in direct and indirect costs. One-fourth of these deaths occur in people younger than the age of 65, and one in five American men are estimated to develop the disease before age 60.[12] After age 60, one in three men and one in three women will die from CHD.

It is now well accepted that atherosclerosis is a slow, progressive disease that has its roots in the pediatric years but typically becomes symptomatic in middle age during an individual's most productive time of life.[5,8,12] A variety of risk factors are strongly associated with progression of the disease, including hypertension, hypercholesterolemia, smoking, obesity, inactivity, stress, and diabetes mellitus (Exhibit 18-1). Overall risk of developing CHD rises with each additional factor. Nutrition plays an important role in management and control. In treating lipid problems, diet, weight control, and exercise are standard intervention objectives. Evidence from the landmark Lipid Research Clinics Coronary Prevention Trial (LRC-CPT) produced the well-known equation that for every 1% reduction in plasma cholesterol there is an estimated 2 to 3% reduction in incidence of the first major coronary event.[26,27,31]

DEFINITION OF RISK

All individuals, whether diabetic or not, should be evaluated and monitored for risk of CHD on the basis of available genetic, experimental, epidemiologic, and clinical trial evidence on risk status by level of blood cholesterol. The National Cholesterol Education Program (NCEP) was initiated in 1985 and has provided recommendations for dietary treatment, educational programs, research, and greater physician awareness in facilitating lipid lowering on a mass scale.[5] Blood cholesterol values that represent the 75th to the 90th percentiles of the LRC-CPT distribution were used to define the degree of risk.[5,31] The initial classification of risk is based on total cholesterol and HDL-C levels (Exhibit 18-2). Treatment decisions are based on LDL-C level (Exhibit 18-3). Results from more than 350,000 screenees in the

MRFIT indicate that the increased risk of premature CHD associated with increased serum cholesterol is continuous and graded.[25] Risk increased when the serum cholesterol level was more than 180 mg/dL. The serum cholesterol level of more than 80% of the American population is at this level or higher.

Below a certain basal level of plasma cholesterol, obstructive atherosclerotic lesions are seldom seen in humans and are difficult to promote experimentally in animals.[8] These findings suggest that the plasma cholesterol values that are typically accepted as "normal" in the United States and certain other industrialized nations are not ideal. Primary genetic disorders of lipid metabolism occur in only 2 to 3% of the population. Most CHD occurs in so-called normal people with plasma cholesterol levels of 200 to 260 mg/dL.[8] In diabetes, the accompanying disorders of glucose and insulin metabolism may partly account for the excess risk. Not only the concentration but also the actual structure of certain lipoproteins or apoproteins may be altered in diabetes, thereby accelerating the atherogenic process.[4,13]

INSULIN RESISTANCE

In addition to problems of dyslipidemia with high triglycerides and VLDL-C, low HDL-C and high LDL-C, insulin resistance, hyper-insulinemia, glucose intolerance, or NIDDM and hypertension when combined together have been termed *syndrome X*.[32] It is suspected that insulin resistance may be genetically induced and/or may be exacerbated by obesity, particularly central obesity, and inactivity.[32–34] Weight loss and exercise have been shown to enhance insulin sensitivity in peripheral tissues and consequently to decrease insulin resistance.[32]

The prevalence of lipid abnormalities is much higher in NIDDM than in IDDM, further implicating an association with obesity and/or the other risk factors. Insulin plays a key role in lipid

Exhibit 18-2 National Cholesterol Education Program: Classification Based on Total Cholesterol and HDL-C

Total Cholesterol	Classification
<200 mg/dL	Desirable
200–239 mg/dL	Borderline high
≥240 mg/dL	High
HDL-C	
<35 mg/dL	Low

Source: Expert Panel on Detection, Evaluation, and Treatment of High Blood Cholesterol in Adults. Summary of the second report of the National Cholesterol Education Program (NCEP) expert panel on detection, evaluation, and treatment of high blood cholesterol in adults (Adults Treatment Panel II). *Journal of the American Medical Association.* 1993;269: 3015–3023.

Exhibit 18-3 National Cholesterol Education Program: Treatment Decisions Based on LDL-C

Dietary Therapy	Initiation Level (mg/dL)	LDL-Goal (mg/dL)
Without CHD and <2 risk factors	≥160	<160
Without CHD and ≥2 risk factors	≥130	<130
With CHD	>100	≤100
Drug Treatment		
Without CHD and <2 risk factors	≥190	<160
Without CHD and with ≥2 risk factors	≥160	<130
With CHD	≥130	≤100

Source: Expert Panel on Detection, Evaluation, and Treatment of High Blood Cholesterol in Adults. Summary of the second report of the National Cholesterol Education Program (NCEP) expert panel on detection, evaluation, and treatment of high blood cholesterol in adults (Adults Treatment Panel II). *Journal of the American Medical Association.* 1993;269:3015–3023.

metabolism. It promotes fat storage (lipogenesis) and activates the enzyme lipoprotein lipase (LPL) on the outside of the fat cell. LPL promotes the breakdown of triglycerides to fatty acids and glycerol. The fatty acids enter the fat cell, and the glycerol portion goes to the liver. The fatty acid in the fat cell combines with the glycerol portion of α-glycerophosphate to form triglyceride. Triglyceride is then stored in the fat cell. When insulin is deficient, lipolysis or the breakdown of fat occurs, causing increased serum triglyceride levels. Insulin treatment and good control in uncomplicated IDDM usually result in normalized lipid and lipoprotein levels.[3] Weight loss and exercise are essential to improved insulin sensitivity in NIDDM, and this can subsequently lower triglycerides. Dietary intervention is vital in either case.

OVERVIEW OF LIPID METABOLISM

Cholesterol

Cholesterol is one of the fats found in the blood (plasma or serum), along with phospholipids, triglycerides, and fatty acids. In plasma, most of the cholesterol exists as cholesterol esters, with the remainder being unesterified. Although dietary cholesterol found in foods of animal origin contributes to the plasma cholesterol level, endogenous production is believed to account for most of plasma cholesterol. There is no biologic requirement for dietary cholesterol because endogenous cholesterol can be synthesized by the liver, intestinal cells, and in almost all other tissues.[35] Cholesterol is a vital component of the structural membranes of all cells and predominates in nerve and brain cells. Gallstones are also primarily composed of cholesterol. The exact function of cholesterol is not completely understood, but it acts as an intermediate in the biosynthesis of bile acids, adrenocortical hormones, estrogens, androgens, progesterone, and other steroids. Approximately 80% of the metabolized cholesterol is converted to bile acids, which help absorb fats from the intestines. The adrenocortical hormones help control the

sodium-potassium stores of the body and the rates of metabolism of carbohydrate and nitrogen. Cholesterol is also converted by the intestinal mucosa to 7-dehydrocholesterol, the provitamin of cholecalciferol. Cholesterol in the skin along with other lipids helps make the skin resistant to the action of certain chemical agents and restricts water evaporation. When abnormal deposits of cholesterol, called xanthomas, are found in the skin or other tissues, they are typically symptomatic of atherosclerosis.[35,36]

Hydrolysis of cholesterol esters occurs in the intestines, with re-esterification during absorption. Chylomicrons transport cholesterol to the liver via the lymphatic system. The enterohepatic cycle refers to the process of continual reabsorption of cholesterol and bile acids from the intestines back to the liver to be excreted again in the bile. The liver stores and regulates cholesterol synthesis based on the amount present in the body, as well as the amount in the diet (Figure 18-1). It is not clear exactly how much dietary or endogenous cholesterol is absorbed by the body, but investigators agree that it is only partially absorbed, regardless of origin. Triglycerides in the diet facilitate cholesterol absorption by expansion of biliary micelles. A diet high in cholesterol can raise blood cholesterol in most people by 15%, the rest is contributed by endogenous absorption. Plant sterols diminish absorption of dietary cholesterol, probably due to competition with cholesterol for incorporation into micelles and transport across the intestinal mucosa.[36,37] Conversely, on the basis of experimental data, it is further suspected that increased dietary fat intake, saturated or unsaturated, stimulates synthesis of endogenous fatty acids.[37,38]

Lipoproteins

Lipoprotein levels are related to atherogenic risk. Levels of LDL-C, HDL-C, and VLDL-C and their ratios are used to classify hyperlipidemic phenotypes. It is the LDL-C fraction that is atherogenic and comprises most of the atherosclerotic lesions.[39–44] Total cholesterol, LDL-C, and HDL-C distribution based on the

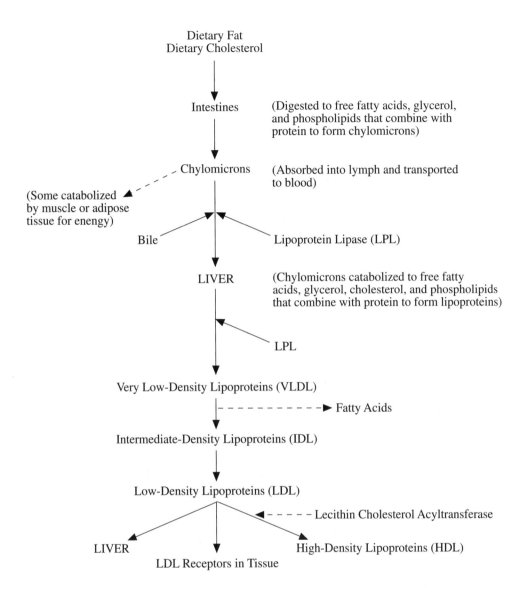

Figure 18-1 Fat Metabolism Simplified

National Health and Nutrition Evaluation Survey (NHANES III) and by age and sex are presented in Appendixes 18A through 18C. The lipoproteins are classified by their densities or by their electrophoretic mobility. The commonly accepted nomenclature is based on their density. Table 18-1 delineates the physical and chemical properties of the lipoproteins.

Chylomicrons

Chylomicrons are synthesized by the small intestines in direct response to the absorption of dietary fat. Once in the systemic circulation, the chylomicron triglycerides are rapidly hydrolyzed by the enzyme LPL. Remnant particles containing apoprotein (apo) E and cholesterol

Table 18-1 Physical Properties and Chemical Constituents of Human Plasma Lipoproteins

	Electrophoretic Mobility	Density (g/mL)	Major Apoproteins[a]	Minor Apoproteins	Major Components	Particle Diameter (A)
Chylomicrons	Origin	<0.95	B C-I C-II C-III	A-I A-II E	90% exogenous triglyceride	750–12,000
VLDL	pre-β	0.95–1.006	B C-I C-II C-III	E	65% endogenous triglyceride	300–800
LDL	β	1.006–1.063	B	E C-I C-II C-III	43% cholesterol 22% phospholipids 25% protein	190–290
HDL₂	α	1.063–1.125	A-I A-II	C-I C-II C-III E	30% phospholipids 18% cholesterol 50% protein	95–115
HDL₃	α	1.125–1.210	A-I A-II	C-I C-II C-III E D	<30% phospholipids 18% cholesterol >50% protein	55–95

[a]Apoproteins comprise the protein component of lipoproteins. At least eight apoproteins have been identified and are metabolically active (ie, apo: C-II acts as a co-factor for lipoprotein lipase in the hydrolysis of triglycerides; apo: A-I activates lecithin cholesterol acyltransferase).

Source: Adapted from *Prevention of Coronary Heart Disease* (p 38) by N Kaplan and J Stamler (Eds) with permission of WB Saunders Company, © 1983.

are formed and are taken up by specific hepatic receptors. With increased hepatic cholesterol content, synthesis of endogenous cholesterol is reduced. In type I hyperlipoproteinemia, LPL is absent, causing increased plasma chylomicrons and triglyceride levels. Table 18-2 lists the five types of hyperlipoproteinemia and their specific lipoprotein abnormalities.

VLDL and Triglyceride

VLDLs are precursors of LDLs and are involved in the transport of endogenous triglycer-ide from the liver to the peripheral tissues. The rate of VLDL secretion from the liver is influenced by many factors, such as the basal diet, insulin level, glucagon, time of day, and the degree of adiposity; therefore, wide variability in these levels is common.[37,40] Wide variation is also caused by differences in laboratory methodology as well. Fasting conditions help reduce the degree of physiologic triglyceride variability. In certain alcohol-sensitive individuals, abstinence from alcohol for 24 hours may also help reduce exaggerated levels. For purposes of dietary counseling, overall progress should be based on

Table 18-2 Five Types of Hyperlipoproteinemia

Type	Lipoprotein Elevated	Elevated Lipid	Probable Metabolic Defect	Possible Secondary Disease (Cause)
I	Chylomicrons	Triglyceride	Lipoprotein lipase deficient	Diabetic acidosis, hypothyroidism, IDDM
IIa	LDL	Cholesterol	Reduced clearance or excess production of LDL-C	Hypothyroidism, nephrosis, dietary excess
IIb	LDL, VLDL	Cholesterol, triglyceride	Excess production or decreased clearance of LDL-C and VLDL-C	
III	IDL	Triglyceride	Familial dysbetalipoproteinemia	Diabetes (rare), hypothyroidism, renal insufficiency
IV	VLDL	Triglyceride (cholesterol)	Overproduction or decreased clearance of VLDL-C	Diabetes, hypothyroidism, liver disease, alcoholism, pancreatitis
V	Chylomicrons: VLDL	Triglyceride	Decreased chylomicron clearance; overproduction or decreased clearance of VLDL-C	Diabetes, hypothyroidism, liver disease, alcoholism, pancreatitis

the mean of at least two fasting values to monitor better the trend over time. This same principle applies to the other lipids and lipoproteins as well. Under normal conditions, VLDL and the apo B component are metabolized to IDL and then to LDL in the presence of apo E. Excessive caloric intake from any source (carbohydrate, protein, alcohol, or fat) causes a high level of unesterified fatty acids in the blood that stimulates increased hepatic synthesis of VLDL.

Whether elevated triglycerides and/or elevated VLDL values are independently and directly atherogenic in nondiabetic individuals remains unclear.[20,21] Serum triglyceride and HDL levels are strongly related to the degree of diabetic control and obesity. Individuals with IDDM who are insulin deficient and ketotic have hypertriglyceridemia and frequently hyperchylomicronemia that subside with insulin treatment. Increased mobilization of free fatty acids and decreased clearance due to reduced LPL ac-

tivity result in elevated levels of triglyceride and VLDL.[4] Insulin regulates both the secretion of VLDL into the plasma from the liver and its removal at the peripheral tissues through its action on endothelial LPL. Improved glycemic control has been associated with reduced VLDL and LDL and increased HDL.[4,39,45–49] In IDDM, qualitative lipoprotein abnormalities may persist including glycosylation and oxidation, increased triglyceride, decreased cholesterol ester in the lipid core, and increased free cholesterol.[4]

In NIDDM,[47,48] disturbances of VLDL, triglycerides, and HDL are even more common and are typically related to obesity. There is general agreement that dietary treatment, including a reduction in total fat and cholesterol, alcohol restriction, and weight loss, results in reduced production of chylomicrons and VLDL, often to within normal ranges. Increased intake of dietary fiber may also be beneficial in moderating carbohydrate impact.[49] HDL often remains lower and serum triglycerides, VLDL, and LDL higher than among the nondiabetic population.[42,43,48]

Low-Density Lipoprotein (LDL)

Each LDL particle contains 45% cholesterol, mostly esterified; 20 to 25% protein, mostly apo B; and the rest as phospholipid (lipids containing phosphorus). The production of LDL is the end-product of intravascular VLDL metabolism. Catabolism of LDL occurs both in the peripheral cells and in the liver, through both receptor- and non–receptor-mediated pathways.[50] LDL serves a major role in transporting cholesterol from the liver to extrahepatic tissues where it is taken up and used primarily by endocrine tissues that produce steroid hormones (see Figure 18-1).

In describing the pathophysiology involved, Brown and Goldstein[50] first reported that LDLs interact with specific high-affinity receptor sites on the surface of fibroblasts that regulate cholesterol synthesis and that these receptor sites are defective among patients with familial hypercholesterolemias. Mahley et al[46] further indicated that certain apoprotein subfractions of LDL and HDL bind to the cell surface receptors and, by suppressing the enzyme 3-hydroxy-3-methylglutaryl-Co-A reductuse (HMG-COA) reductase activity, lead to intracellular cholesterol accumulation. The protein moiety of the lipoprotein determines the specificity for binding. HMG-COA reductase is the rate-limiting factor in cholesterol synthesis by the liver.[51] Chylomicrons seem to be very effective in inhibiting this enzyme. Therefore, when dietary cholesterol intake is high and more chylomicrons are produced, hepatic production of cholesterol is reduced. Increased uptake of cholesterol within the cell inhibits LDL receptor activity. Intracellular esterification of cholesterol increases due to enhanced activity of the enzyme, acyl cholesterol acyltransferase, which is thought to be released when LDL binds to its receptor. Cholesterol can also be incorporated into the cell membrane, thus altering the membrane fluidity and physiologic properties of the cell.[47] In dia-

betic populations the prevalence of hypercholesterolemia (elevated LDL-C) is estimated to range between 20 and 46%. Because abnormalities of cholesterol metabolism are reportedly less common than those of triglyceride metabolism in diabetes, most of the early research concentrated on the latter.

LDL is derived from VLDL, and high triglyceride-VLDL levels in diabetes may accelerate synthesis of LDL. However, because there is also an increased catabolism of LDL in diabetes the plasma levels do not appear abnormally elevated.[52] Studies in both NIDDM and IDDM report that with improved insulin regulation significant serum cholesterol reduction occurs.[3]

The atherogenic lipoprotein phenotype LDL subclass B is associated with increased triglycerides and apo B, VLDL, and IDL and decreased HDL, apo A, and HDL_2. Austin et al[51] reported qualitative associations between small, dense LDL rich in triglycerides and LDL subclass B phenotype. The prevalence of this phenotype in normolipidemic diabetic men is double that of normolipidemic nondiabetic men and even higher in diabetic versus nondiabetic women.[53]

This genetically altered receptor-mediated LDL pathway results in the increased catabolism of LDL via an atherogenic, nonreceptor pathway.[51] Glycosylation and oxidation of LDL may also occur with poor glycemic control, reducing the binding of LDL to its receptors and causing accumulation of cholesterol esters and foam cell formation.[4,15,45,52,54,55] Nutritional status, calorie balance, and glycemic control can help reduce the VLDL synthesis rate.[56]

High-Density Lipoprotein (HDL)

The major production of HDL occurs in the liver. Some additional HDL particles are derived from the metabolism of intestinal chylomicrons. HDL are smallest of the lipoproteins and contain about 26% cholesterol and 49% protein, mostly apoproteins A-I, A-II, E, and C. Two major subfractions of total HDL (HDL-C) are HDL_2 and HDL_3. HDL_2 has a lower density and contains more phospholipids, free cholesterol, and apoprotein A-I than HDL_3. Most of the physiologic variation of HDL-C is accounted for by HDL_3. One of the functions of HDL is the formation of cholesterol esters in plasma catalyzed by the enzyme lecithin acyl cholesterol transferase (LCAT). HDL provides reverse cholesterol transport of membrane-derived cholesterol back to the liver and thus plays a protective role.

An inverse association between HDL and CHD was noted as early as 1951 by Barr et al[55] when low HDL levels were observed among diabetic subjects and individuals who experienced coronaries compared with normal controls.[57] Not until 1966 were these findings repeated when prospective studies again demonstrated the inverse correlation between HDL and cardiovascular mortality.[58] Many studies have since documented this relationship and have further reported that the HDL_2 subfraction has a closer inverse association with atherosclerosis than HDL.[53,59,60] HDL-C and HDL_2 also show an inverse relationship with plasma VLDL and triglyceride levels and are markedly lower among insulin-deficient IDDM patients. Mechanisms underlying low levels of HDL-C and HDL_2 are thought to be multifactorial but relate to the reduced LPL activity because the rate and formation of HDL-C are dependent on the catabolism of chylomicrons and VLDL.[53,61]

Insulin treatment in IDDM restores HDL-C to normal ranges. In NIDDM, HDL-C level is typically normal or reduced. Higher HDL-C concentration is favorably associated with female sex, weight loss, smoking cessation, exercise, and low intake of alcohol.[52] In patients with NIDDM, even glycemic control may not adequately normalize lipids and lipoproteins, especially when these risk factors coexist. Glycosylation and oxidation of HDL further contribute to atherogenesis through impaired HDL-receptor binding and lack of reduction of cholestyl ester content of the macrophage.[4,52,61] Macrophages that become overloaded with oxidated LDL create foam cells that ultimately die and deposit their lipid contents on the walls of arteries. The mechanism whereby HDL is protective involves competition with LDL for binding sites in tissues. By reducing the cellular uptake of LDL, HDL thus retards the atherosclerotic process.[60,62] HDL is instrumental in the removal of cholesterol from the tissues by transporting it to the liver where it is excreted.[62,63] This process involves LCAT, which is HDL-dependent for esterification and is crucial to the removal of cholesterol from the cell. There is also evidence that, through binding to LDL receptor sites and preventing its uptake, HDL may inhibit the proliferation of smooth muscle cells, one of the initial steps in the formation of the atherosclerotic lesion.

Lp(a)

Lipoprotein (a) or Lp(a) looks like LDL but is larger and more dense due to its additional peptide chain and is similar to plasminogen. Lp(a) inhibits plasminogen binding and is thought to contribute to thrombogenesis.[53,60,61] Lp(a) is also prone to oxidation and may be taken up by macrophages that eventually contribute to foam cells. Some studies have reported increased levels of Lp(a) in poorly-controlled diabetes,[53] but others do not.[61,63] The level of this potential association and whether dietary factors influence Lp(a) require further investigation.

RECOMMENDED DIETARY PATTERN

The dietary pattern recommended for prevention and control of hyperlipidemia is nutritionally sound for diabetic and nondiabetic individuals alike. A diet rich in vegetables, fruits, and grains; moderate in protein; and low in total fat, saturated fat, and cholesterol is the basis for good nutrition for all age, sex, and ethnic groups.[12] The dietitian should assess the patient's baseline dietary intake and gradually direct him or her toward behavioral changes that will ultimately accomplish this dietary goal. Such an eating pattern is healthful for the entire family, whose support can help foster better adherence in the individual with diabetes or hyperlipidemia. The NCEP recommends a stepped care approach to dietary change depend-

Exhibit 18-4 National Cholesterol Education Program: Step I and Step II Diets

Factor	Step I	Step II
Total fat	≤30% of total calories (kcal)	
Saturated fat	8–10% kcal	<7% kcal
Polyunsaturated fat	≤10% (kcal)	
Monounsaturated fat	≤15% kcal	
Carbohydrates	≥55% kcal	
Protein	15% kcal	
Cholesterol	<300 mg/d	<200 mg/d
Total calories	To achieve and maintain ideal weight	

Source: National Cholesterol Education Program, National Heart, Lung and Blood Institute, NIH Publication no. 88-2925, January 1988, pg. 30.

Exhibit 18-5 Effect of Changes in Certain Dietary Constituents on the Plasma Lipids and Lipoproteins

Reduction of dietary cholesterol to 100 mg/d

Decreases:
Total plasma cholesterol
LDL
Remnants (IDL)
VLDL (slightly)
HDL (slightly)
LDL/HDL

Reduction of total fat to 20% of total calories and saturated fat to 5% of total calories

Decreases:
Chylomicrons
Total plasma cholesterol
LDL
Remnants
VLDL (slightly)
LDL/HDL

Caloric reduction (if adiposity present)

Decreases:
Plasma triglyceride
VLDL
Remnants
LDL and total cholesterol

Increases:
HDL

Source: Reprinted from *Coronary Heart Disease: Prevention, Complications, and Treatment* (p 61), WE Connor and JD Bristow, eds, with permission of JB Lippincott Company, Copyright © 1985.

ing upon level of risk and dietary adherence.[5] Exhibit 18-4 depicts the NCEP Step I and Step II diets. These guidelines have subsequently been endorsed by the American Heart Association (AHA), the American Dietetic Association, and American Diabetes Association.

Part of the patient's confusion regarding dietary and blood lipids occurs because the same terms are used to describe both. It is important for the dietitian to help the patient differentiate dietary fats from biologic fats, cholesterol, triglycerides, and related issues. Exhibit 18-5 summarizes the impact of dietary changes on plasma lipids and lipoproteins.

Dietary Fat Classification

The role of dietary fat in lipid metabolism has received much research attention. Qualitative and quantitative differences in the fats need careful consideration. Fats can be classified chemically into three types: simple, compound, and derived. Simple fats include fatty acids and glycerides, compound lipids include phospholipids and lipoproteins, and derived lipids include sterols and the fat-soluble vitamins A, D, E, and K. Chemically, fatty acids are comprised of linear chains of carbon atoms with hydrogen atoms attached. There is an acidic carboxyl group at one end and a methyl group at the other. The chain length/number of carbons, ie, C20 and the degree of saturation with hydrogen atoms or the number of double bonds (C20:5 means 5 double bonds for eicosapentaenoic acid) designate each particular fatty acid.

Dietary triglycerides are made up of one glycerol and three fatty acids. They comprise 98 to 99% of most natural fats. Most of these are long-chain triglycerides containing between 12 to 30 carbon atoms, as well as hydrogen and oxygen. The number of double bonds between the carbon atoms determines the degree of hydrogen saturation. Saturated fatty acids (SFA) have no double bonds and are fully hydrogenated. Monounsaturated fatty acids (MUFA) have one double bond, and polyunsaturated fatty acids (PUFA) have several double bonds.

In addition to chain length and the number of double bonds, fatty acids are further identified by the position of the first double bond in relation to the terminal methyl group. The three most common types are n-3 fatty acids, with three carbons between the methyl end and the first double bond; n-6 fatty acids with six carbons between them; and n-9 fatty acids with nine. Common n-3 fatty acids include eicosapentaenoic (C20:5), linolenic (C18:3), and docosahexaenoic acid (C22:6) found in fish and marine oils. The n-6 fatty acids include linoleic (C18:2) and arachidonic acid (C20:4) found in vegetable oils. Oleic acid is the most common n-9 fatty acid (C18:1).

Dietary Cholesterol

Data from carefully controlled metabolic ward studies indicate that dietary cholesterol increases plasma total cholesterol.[64] Approximately 40% of dietary cholesterol is absorbed, and the remainder is excreted.[56] The amount absorbed is added to the cholesterol already synthesized by the body. There is only a partial feedback mechanism for cholesterol synthesis in the human body, because the dietary cholesterol that is not excreted is stored in tissues, including the coronary arteries. Connor and Connor[56] delineate the effects of dietary cholesterol on increased chylomicrons, increased LDL-C, and increased hepatic cell cholesterol. The authors

describe the rapid increase in plasma cholesterol that occurs with increased intake of dietary cholesterol beyond a certain threshold amount of about 100 mg/d. They further suggest a certain ceiling amount of between 300 and 400 mg/d, whereby the rapid rise in plasma cholesterol levels off. Current estimates of the average American intake of dietary cholesterol are about 400 to 500 mg/d. The American Diabetes Association, NCEP, National Academy of Sciences, and AHA recommend less than 300 mg/d. It is estimated that, for every 100 mg/d decrease in dietary cholesterol, plasma cholesterol is reduced by about 7 mg/dL.[56] Because egg yolks provide the single most common source of dietary cholesterol at approximately 211 mg, the NCEP Step I diet advises less than four egg yolks per week.[5] Step II recommends less than two yolks per week. Table 18-3 lists the cholesterol content of various foods and Table 18-4 lists fatty acid contents.

Total Dietary Fat

Reduction in total fat is recommended because the formation and circulation of chylomicrons are directly proportional to the amount of fat consumed and because obesity is a common problem.[58,59] There is no question that weight loss in obese diabetic patients can produce dramatic improvements in plasma glucose concentrations. The typical American intake of 110 g/d of fat produces 110 g of chylomicron triglycerides and can contribute to overweight. The atherogenic remnant production is proportional to the number of chylomicrons synthesized, thereby making total fat intake a major factor in blood lipid level.

There is wide variation in dietary intake within and between individuals, including those with diabetes. Statistical methods have been devised to predict plasma cholesterol response to dietary changes.[57,65,66] The formulas used in predicting plasma cholesterol response to dietary alterations in fat are described in Appendix 18-D. It is recommended that total fat intake should be reduced from the current average of about 34% of total calories to, ideally, less than

Table 18-3 Cholesterol Content of Selected Foods

Food	Amount	Average Cholesterol (mg)
Milk, skim: fluid or reconstituted	1 cup	5
Milk, whole	1 cup	33
Cottage cheese, lowfat (1%)	1/2 cup	10
Cottage cheese, creamed	1/2 cup	17
Cream, light table	1 fl oz	20
Cream, half and half	1 fl oz	12
Ice Cream, regular, approximately 10% fat	1/2 cup	27
Cheese, cheddar	1 oz	30
Butter	1 Tbsp	31
Lard	1 Tbsp	12
Oysters	3 oz	40
Clams	3 oz	55
Salmon	3 oz	74
Shrimp: cooked	3 oz	167
Chicken, turkey, light meat: cooked	3 oz	67
Beef, pork, chicken, turkey, dark meat: cooked	3 oz	75
Lamb, veal: cooked	3 oz	85
Heart, beef: cooked	3 oz	164
Egg	1 yolk or 1 egg	211
Liver (beef, calf, hog, lamb): cooked	3 oz	410
Kidney, cooked	3 oz	329
Brains, raw	3 oz	1700+

Source: Adapted from Hands E. *Food Finder.* ESHA Research, Oregon, 1990.

30%, with the replacement being derived from complex carbohydrate. Table 18-5 presents data on total and saturated fat intake from NHANES III.[67]

Recently, there has been concern regarding high-carbohydrate, very low-fat diets in some diabetic patients due to potential further exacerbation of hypertriglyceridemia and decreased HDL-concentrations.[21,22] The goal in these patients is to reduce saturated and *trans*-fatty acid intake and shift emphasis to monounsaturated fat sources, while maintaining total fat intake around 30% of total calories. It is thought this will minimize hyperinsulinemia and postprandial glucose response to very high-carbohydrate, very low-fat diets.[21]

Saturated Fatty Acids

SFAs are not essential nutrients and are readily synthesized in the body from acetate.

They are known to increase total serum cholesterol by directly increasing chylomicrons and thereby increase the concentration of LDL-C that may promote thrombosis.[5,39]

Except for fish and shellfish, all animal fats are saturated. Animal fats, meats, hydrogenated shortenings (rich in atherogency *trans*-fatty acids), some vegetable oil (palm, coconut, cocoa butter), whole-milk dairy products, and commercial baked goods are major sources of saturated fat in the American diet. The current average SFA intake is about 12% (Table 18-5), and the NCEP recommends not more than 10% of total calories be derived from saturated fat. Dietary adherence to reductions of this type are estimated to reduce plasma cholesterol by about 20 mg/dL within as few as 3 weeks.[56]

Palmitic and myristic fatty acids are hypercholesterolemic, but stearic acid is not. This has caused some confusion in the part of patients who

Table 18-4 Fat Content and Major Fatty Acid Composition of Selected Foods

Food	Total Fat (%)	Saturated [b] (%)	Unsaturated Oleic (%)	Unsaturated Linoleic (%)	P/S [c]
Salad and cooking oils					
Canola	100	6	62	31	5.1/1.0
Safflower	100	10	13	74	7.4/1.0
Sunflower	100	11	14	70	6.4/1.0
Corn	100	13	26	55	4.2/1.0
Cottonseed	100	23	17	54	2.3/1.0
Soybean	100	14	25	50	3.6/1.0
Sesame	100	14	38	42	3.0/1.0
Soybean, special processed	100	11	29	31	2.8/1.0
Peanut	100	18	47	29	1.6/1.0
Olive	100	11	76	7	0.6/1.0
Coconut	100	80	5	1	0.2/1.0
Margarine, first ingredient on label [d]					
Safflower oil (liquid)—tub	80	11	18	48	4.4/1.0
Soybean oil (liquid)—tub	80	15	31	33	2.2/1.0
Butter	81	46	27	2	0.4/1.0
Animal fats					
Poultry	100	30	40	20	0.67/1.0
Beef, lamb, pork	100	45	44	2–6	0.04–0.13/1.0
Fish, raw [e]					
Salmon, sockeye	9	2	2	4	2.0/1.0
Mackerel, Atlantic	13	5	3	4	0.8/1.0
Herring, Pacific	13	4	2	3	0.75/1.0
Tuna, Blue Fin	5	2	1	2	1.0/1.0
Nuts					
Walnuts, black	60	4	21	28	7.0/1
Brazil	67	13	32	17	1.3/1
Peanuts or peanut butter	51	9	25	14	1.6/1
Egg yolk	31	10	13	2	0.2/1
Avocado	16	3	7	2	0.67/1

[a] Total is not expected to equal total fat.

[b] Includes fatty acids with chains containing from 8 to 18 carbon atoms.

[c] P/S = Linoleic acid content/saturated fatty acid content.

[d] Mean values of selected samples, which may vary with brand name and date of manufacture. Includes small amounts of monounsaturated and diunsaturated fatty acids that are not oleic or linoleic.

[e] The amount of ω-3 fatty acids/100 g is salmon, 0.5 g; mackerel, 0.9 g; herring, 1.0 g; tuna 0.4 g (data from USDA Bulletin no. PT-103).

Source: Adapted from *Fats in Food and Diet*, U.S. Department of Agriculture Information Bulletin no. 361.

Table 18-5 Mean Daily Total Food-Energy Intake (TFEI)[a] and Mean Percentage of TFEI from Total Dietary Fat[b] and from Saturated Fat, by Age Group—Third National Health and Nutrition Examination Survey, Phase 1, 1988–91

Age Group (yrs)	Sample Size	Daily TFEI[c]		% TFEI from Total Dietary Fat		% TFEI from Saturated Fat	
		No.	(SE)[c]	%	(SE)	%	(SE)
2–11 mos[d]	871	877	(±10.9)	37.2	(±0.3)	15.8	(±0.1)
1–2[d]	1231	1289	(±21.2)	33.7	(±0.4)	13.9	(±0.2)
3–5	1547	1591	(±20.5)	33.0	(±0.3)	12.6	(±0.1)
6–11	1745	1897	(±25.0)	34.0	(±0.4)	12.8	(±0.2)
12–15	711	2218	(±48.8)	33.4	(±0.6)	12.2	(±0.2)
16–19	765	2533	(±88.2)	34.5	(±0.4)	12.4	(±0.2)
20–29	1682	2484	(±44.4)	34.0	(±0.4)	12.0	(±0.2)
30–39	1526	2372	(±43.4)	34.4	(±0.4)	11.9	(±0.2)
40–49	1228	2146	(±44.5)	34.4	(±0.5)	11.6	(±0.2)
50–59	929	1967	(±30.7)	34.7	(±0.4)	11.6	(±0.2)
60–69	1106	1822	(±39.0)	33.0	(±0.3)	11.2	(±0.2)
70–79	851	1624	(±25.3)	32.9	(±0.5)	11.2	(±0.3)
≥80	609	1484	(±27.4)	32.0	(±0.3)	11.0	(±0.2)
Total	**14,801**	**2095**	**(±20.0)**	**34.0**	**(±0.2)**	**12.0**	**(±0.1)**
≥2	13,314	2123	(±20.4)	33.9	(±0.2)	11.9	(±0.1)

[a] Defined as all nutrients (ie, protein, fat, carbohydrate, and alcohol) derived from consumption of foods and beverages (excluding plain drinking water), measured in kilocalories.

[b] Defined as all fat (ie, saturated and unsaturated) derived from consumption of foods and beverages, measured in grams.

[c] Standard error.

[d] Excludes nursing infants and children.

Source: Reprinted from Daily Dietary Fat and Total Food Energy Intakes; Third National Health and Nutrition Examination Survey Phase 1, 1988-1991, *Morbidity and Mortality Weekly Report.* 1994;43(7):116–117.

might be tempted to eat foods like chocolate or beef that are relatively high in stearic acid. Patients need to be reminded that these foods also contain large amounts of atherogenic palmitic and myristic acid and should limit intake of these foods for these reasons.[37,39]

Monounsaturated Fatty Acids

Monounsaturated fats are predominately derived from oleic acid, an n-9 fatty acid. Major dietary sources include peanut oil and olive oil, but as indicated in Table 18-4, oleic acid is present in all animal and vegetable fats. They are not essential fatty acids (EFA) and are synthesized endogenously. The NCEP recommends that approximately one-third or more of total dietary fat intake be derived from monounsaturated sources. Once thought to have a neutral effect on plasma LDL-C, monounsaturated fats have been shown to help reduce LDL-C without reducing HDL-C.[36,68]

Polyunsaturated Fatty Acids

Polyunsaturated fatty acids (PUFAs) (linoleic, linolenic, and arachidonic acids) cannot be synthesized by the body and are therefore EFAs. Of these, linoleic acid, an n-6 fatty acid, is most commonly found in food.[37] Along with pyridoxine, arachidonic and linolenic acid can be synthesized from linoleic acid by the liver. Current average intake of polyunsaturated fat is approximately 5 to 6% of total calories. PUFAs maintain the function and integrity of cell membranes and are prostaglandin precursors. Prostaglandins are hormone-like compounds that are involved in the regulation of blood pressure, heart rate, lipolysis, and the nervous system.

PUFA of either the n-6 or the n-3 type are known to reduce plasma total cholesterol and LDL-C. The n-3 fatty acids, found in fish or marine oils, have the additional effect of lowering plasma triglyceride levels and especially VLDL-C. Because elevated triglyceride and VLDL-C levels are common in diabetes, this effect has been of particular interest in potential treatment. The normal human requirement for the n-6 structure is about 2 to 3% of total calories supplied as linoleic acid; n-6 and n-3 fatty acids are not interconvertible and seem to have different functions in the body. The n-3 fatty acids are primarily concentrated in the gonads, spermatozoa, retina, phospholipid membranes, and other organs, whereas n-6 fatty acids are found in the phospholipids, cholesterol esters, and other lipids and are involved in lipid transport.[37] Epidemiologic data have reported a protective effect of n-3 fatty acids on the risk of CHD, possibly through this mechanism.[69] Clinical trials on the hypolipidemic effects of fish oil and n-3 fatty acid supplements in NIDDM have reported decreased triglycerides but increased LDL-C and worsened glycemic control.[69–71] This may be due to stimulation of hepatic glucose output and inhibition of insulin secretion. More controlled research is needed to better understand this relationship. Recommendations for increasing fish intake, decreasing red meat consumption, and not resorting to fish oil supplements are widely advocated (see Table 18-6).

Increased intake of PUFA increases the requirement for vitamin E. In the United States, this is not considered to be a problem because most sources of PUFA are also rich in vitamin E.[72] Vitamin E is primarily carried by the lipoproteins, and in normal individuals, there is a high correlation between plasma total lipids and plasma tocopherol concentration.[72] Major sources of PUFA in the U.S. diet are vegetable oils, shortenings, and margarines that are liquid or only partially hydrogenated. The exceptions include palm oil, coconut oil, and cocoa butter that are saturated (fully hydrogenated) despite their vegetable derivation.

Polyunsaturated-to-Saturated Fat Ratio

In regard to the hypo- versus hypercholesterolemic effect, gram for gram, the plasma cholesterol increase from saturated fat is about twice the plasma cholesterol decrease from polyunsaturated fat.[73] The current American diet has an estimated polyunsaturated-to-saturated fat (P/S) ratio of about 0.4, reflecting the greater intake of saturated fat (see Table 18-5). The recommended P/S ratio for reducing plasma cholesterol level is at least 2:1.[56,73] This is impractical for many people who are reluctant to add oils and/or margarine due to their high calorie loads. The dietitian should emphasize reduction of total fat intake to 30% of calories and shift the emphasis from animal sources to vegetable sources. Excessive intake of polyunsaturated fat is not advocated because of potential risk of cholelithiasis, weight gain, altered cell membranes, and cancer.[5,59,74]

Trans-*Fatty Acids*

The process of partial hydrogenation that connects liquid vegetable oils into solid shortenings was developed in the early 1900s and provided the food industry with an economic strategy for extending the shelf life of foods.[75,76] Hydrogenation causes some of the unsaturated bonds to become saturated and others to switch from their natural state in the *cis*-position to the *trans*-position. This creates the more solid state of the fat.

Metabolic research by Mensink and Katan[77] reported increases in LDL-C and Lp(a) and decreases in HDL-C as a result of *trans*-fatty acid intake. Epidemiologic studies have reported positive association between *trans*-fatty acids and CHD.[78,79]

Current food labeling policy does not require listing of *trans*-fatty acid content in foods.[79] The most common sources include solid margarines, salad dressings, and commercial cookies, crackers, baked goods, and other foods made with hydrogenerated shortenings. Patients should be encouraged to use liquid, unsaturated cooking oils, soft (tub) or liquid margarines, and avoid foods whose ingredients include "partially hydrogenated oils."

Current intake of *trans*-fatty acids is approximately 2% of total energy. A recent editorial by Willett and Ascherio[80] estimated that attributable risk of increased total cholesterol to HDL-C ratio is about 7% for the population, potentially resulting in more than 30,000 deaths per year. More research on these associations is needed, and the response of the food industry to these findings will be important to public health.

Intake of Complex Carbohydrates and Fiber

The decrease in total fat intake requires a compensatory increase in some other macronutrient. Because the current intake of dietary protein in this country of about 12 to 20% of total calories is more than adequate, the remaining 50 to 60% of calories should be derived from carbohydrates. Complex carbohydrate sources are nutritionally superior to refined sources and thus should provide most of the calories ingested. These include vegetables, fruits, and grains that are, in addition to their nutrient quality, also major sources of dietary fiber. Dietary fiber had for many years been overlooked as a significant nutritional factor because it does not contain appreciable energy value. Technological improvements in the methods for measuring fiber quantitatively and qualitatively have facilitated the opportunities to study its effects on nutritional status and health (see Chapter 21).

A meta-analysis of intervention studies with oats, rich in soluble fiber, concluded that oat fiber was an effective adjunct to a fat-modified diet in maximizing total and LDL-C reduction without compromising HDL levels.[81] Similarly, studies on soluble-fiber rich foods have reported improved regulation of insulin response among diabetic populations.[82–84] Higher fiber diets in certain populations such as Seventh Day Adventists and South African blacks have also

been associated with lower prevalence of obesity, one of the risk factors for both elevated LDC-C and non–insulin-dependent diabetes.[85,86] Future research is needed on the qualitative as well as quantitative impact of specific forms of dietary fibers as they may modify both lipid and insulin response to certain diets.

NCEP Dietary Guidelines

In 1993, the NCEP Second Report of the Expert Panel on Detection, Evaluation and Treatment of High Blood Cholesterol in Adults (ATPII) issued dietary guidelines (Exhibit 18-4) for prevention and treatment of high blood cholesterol.[5]

This diet is consistent with the dietary guidelines (USDA) food pyramid and provides a sound approach to eating for both healthy and high-risk individuals. It is also recommended that these criteria be phased in gradually, starting with the changes that are easiest for the patient to make. Switching from butter to margarine and using polyunsaturated or monounsaturated oils in cooking are usually easier changes. Increasing intake of fish, skinless poultry, meatless meals, fruits, and vegetables and cutting down portion sizes of meat are more difficult changes. The Step II guidelines offer a more aggressive approach for patients whose serum cholesterol or LDL-C levels have not responded sufficiently with adherence to Step I. Lack of lipid response to this diet will usually require prescription of lipid-lowering drugs by the patient's physician while continued adherence to the diet is recommended. Table 18-6 from the ATPII report provides examples of foods to choose or decrease in adopting the Step I or Step II diets.

Dietary cholesterol intake should not exceed 300 mg/d. Alcohol is not recommended especially for patients with diabetes. For those who drink alcohol, total consumption should not exceed 1.5 oz of pure alcohol per day. This amount equals two mixed drinks, two 4-oz glasses of wine, or two 12-oz glasses of beer. Weight control is emphasized, and regular exercise is advocated. This is especially important for patients

Table 18-6 Examples of Foods To Choose or Decrease for the Step I[a] and Step II Diets

Food Group	Choose	Decrease
Lean Meat, Poultry, and Fish ≤5–6 oz per day	Beef, pork, lamb—lean cuts, well trimmed before cooking	Beef, pork, lamb—regular ground beef, fatty cuts, spare ribs, organ meats
	Poultry without skin	Poultry with skin, fried chicken
	Fish, shellfish	Fried fish, fried shellfish
	Processed meat—prepared from lean meat (eg, lean ham, lean frankfurters, lean meat with soy protein or carrageenan)	Regular luncheon meat (eg, bologna, salami, sausage, frankfurters)
Eggs ≤4 yolks per week, Step I ≤2 yolks per week, Step II	Egg whites (two whites can be substituted for one whole egg in recipes), cholesterol-free egg substitute	Egg yolks (if more than four per week on Step I or if more than two per week on Step II); includes eggs used in cooking and baking
Low-Fat Dairy Products 2–3 servings per day	Milk—skim, 1/2%, or 1% fat (fluid, powdered, evaporated), buttermilk	Whole milk (fluid, evaporated, condensed), 2% fat milk (low-fat milk), imitation milk
	Yogurt—nonfat or low-fat yogurt or yogurt beverages	Whole milk yogurt, whole milk yogurt beverages
	Cheese—low-fat natural or processed cheese	Regular cheeses (American, blue, Brie, cheddar, Colby, Edam, Monterey Jack, whole-milk mozzarella, Parmesan, Swiss), cream cheese, Neufchatel cheese
	Low-fat or nonfat varieties (eg, cottage cheese—low-fat, nonfat, or dry curd [0–2% fat])	Cottage cheese (4% fat)
	Frozen dairy dessert—ice milk, frozen yogurt (low-fat or nonfat)	Ice cream
	Low-fat coffee creamer Low-fat or nonfat sour cream	Cream, half & half, whipping cream, nondairy creamer, whipped topping, sour cream
Fats and Oils ≤6–8 teaspoons per day	Unsaturated oils—safflower, sunflower, corn, soybean, cottonseed, canola, olive, peanut	Coconut oil, palm kernel oil, palm oil
	Margarine—made from unsaturated oils listed above, light or diet margarine, especially soft or liquid forms	Butter, lard, shortening, bacon fat, hard margarine

continues

Table 18-6 continued

Food Group	Choose	Decrease
Fats and Oils ≤6–8 teaspoons per day (continued)	Salad dressings—made with unsaturated oils listed above, low-fat or fat-free	Dressings made with egg yolk, cheese, sour cream, whole milk
	Seeds and nuts—peanut butter, other nut butters	Coconut
	Cocoa powder	Milk chocolate
Breads and Cereals 6 or more servings per day	Breads—whole-grain bread, English muffins, bagels, buns, corn or flour tortilla	Bread in which eggs, fat, and/or butter are a major ingredient; croissants
	Cereals—oat, wheat, corn, multigrain	Most granolas
	Pasta	
	Rice	
	Dry beans and peas	
	Crackers, low-fat—animal-type, graham, soda crackers, breadsticks, melba toast	High-fat crackers
	Homemade baked goods using unsaturated oil, skim or 1% milk, and egg substitute—quick breads, biscuits, cornbread muffins, bran muffins, pancakes, waffles	Commercial baked pastries, muffins, biscuits
Soups	Reduced- or low-fat and reduced-sodium varieties (eg, chicken or beef noodle, minestrone tomato, vegetable, potato, reduced-fat soups made with skim milk)	Soups containing whole milk, cream, meat fat, poultry fat, or poultry skin
Vegetables 3–5 servings per day	Fresh, frozen, or canned, without added fat or sauce	Vegetables fried or prepared with butter, cheese, or cream sauce
Fruits 2–4 servings per day	Fruit—fresh, frozen, canned, or dried Fruit juice—fresh, frozen, or canned	Fried fruit or fruit served with butter or cream sauce
Sweets and Modified Fat Desserts	Beverages—fruit-flavored drinks, lemonade, fruit punch	
	Sweets—sugar, syrup, honey, jam, preserves, candy made without fat (candy corn, gumdrops, hard candy), fruit-flavored gelatin	Candy made with milk chocolate, coconut oil, palm kernel oil, palm oil

Table 18-6 continued

Food Group	Choose	Decrease
Sweets and Modified Fat Desserts (continued)	Frozen desserts—low-fat and nonfat yogurt, ice milk, sherbet, sorbet, fruit ice, popsicles	Ice cream and frozen treats made with ice cream
	Cookies, cake, pie, pudding—prepared with egg whites, egg substitute, skim milk or 1% milk, and unsaturated oil or margarine; ginger snaps; fig and other fruit bar cookies, fat-free cookies; angel food cake	Commercial baked pies, cakes, doughnuts, high-fat cookies, cream pies

[a] Careful selection of processed foods is necessary to stay within the sodium <2,400 mg guideline.

Source: Expert panel on Detection, Evaluation, and Treatment of High Blood Cholesterol in Adults. Summary of the second report of the National Cholesterol Education Program (NCEP) expert panel on detection, evaluation, and treatment of high blood cholesterol in adults (Adults Treatment Panel II). *Journal of the American Medical Association.* 1993;269:3015–3023.

with diabetes since exercise and weight loss can help raise HDL-C and lower VLDC-C. Eating a wide variety of food to achieve optimal intake of all nutrients and fiber is further recommended. Gradual adaptation to these criteria should optimize nonpharmacologic lipid and glucose response.

Pediatric Prevention and Treatment of High Blood Cholesterol

In 1992, the Report of the Expert Panel on Blood Cholesterol Levels in Children and Adolescents was released by the NCEP.[87] This marked the first time that national standards for detection and treatment of high blood cholesterol in children were adopted by the cardiovascular, nutritional, and pediatric communities. Evidence from cross cultural, cross sectional, and prospective epidemiologic studies as well as autopsy data were reviewed from the study of Pathobiological Data on Atherogenesis in the Young.[88] This expert panel concluded that the atherosclerotic process begins in childhood and is affected by high blood cholesterol levels.

The report recommends a two-pronged approach including population and individualized

strategies. For all children older than the age of 2 years, the Step I diet was recommended. Nutritional adequacy should be achieved by eating a wide variety of foods. For certain children considered to be at increased risk due to family history of premature CVD, a more aggressive screening process was recommended but dietary intervention with Step I diet is also the primary

Exhibit 18-6 NCEP Pediatric Lipid/Lipoprotein Classifications

Category	Total Cholesterol (mg/dL)	LDL-C (mg/dL)
Acceptable	<170	<110
Borderline	170–199	110–129
High	≥200	≥130

Source: Expert Panel on Detection, Evaluation, and Treatment of High Blood Cholesterol in Adults. Summary of the second report of the National Cholesterol Education Program (NCEP) expert panel on detection, evaluation, and treatment of high blood cholesterol in adults (Adults Treatment Panel II). *Journal of the American Medical Association.* 1993;269: 3015–3023.

treatment. The Step II diet should be prescribed for children who do not achieve adequate lipid response with the Step I diet. Exhibit 18-6 lists the NCEP cutpoints for classifying pediatric hyperlipidemia. Additional data regarding the efficacy, safety, and acceptability of a fat-modified diet in children with elevated LDL-C are available from the Dietary Intervention Study in Children.[89,90]

UNIFIED APPROACH TO PREVENTION AND TREATMENT: THE OVERALL GOAL

After many years of disagreement about the basic components of a healthful eating pattern, nutrition and health agencies have reached a consensus about basic standards for a healthful eating pattern. Intake of total fat should be less than 30% of total calories, dietary cholesterol should be no more than 300 mg/d, 12 to 20% of calories should be derived from protein, approximately 50 to 60% of calories should come from carbohydrate, and about 40 g of dietary fiber should be ingested each day. The American Diabetes Association, American Dietetic Association, and American Heart Association, as well as the National Cancer Institute, National Heart, Lung and Blood Institute, and numerous local health departments, all advocate such a diet for optimal health and treatment of chronic disease.[53] The 1994 nutritional goals for diabetes management established by the American Diabetes Association list "restoration of normal blood glucose and optimal lipid levels" as a priority.[5] Other goals include promotion of normal growth in children, adequate nutrition for pregnant women, and weight management for the obese. These are ideally accomplished through inculcation of healthy eating habits that optimize nutritional status and reduce risk of chronic disease. Gradual replacement of foods known to increase serum cholesterol with other foods that lower serum cholesterol and do not increase plasma glucose or interfere with insulin regulation is the goal. With time and skillful dietary counseling, such dietary modifications can be successfully adapted to individual needs and taste preferences, regardless of age, sex, or cultural influences.

REFERENCES

1. Kannel WB. Cardiovascular sequelae of diabetes. In: National Heart, Lung and Blood Institute, ed. *Diabetes and Atherosclerosis Connection.* New York, NY: Juvenile Diabetes Foundation; 1981:5–16.

2. Stamler J, Berkson D, Linberg HA. Risk factors: their role in the etiology and pathogenesis of the atherosclerotic diseases. In: Wissler RW, Geer JC, eds. *The Pathogenesis of the Atherosclerotic Diseases.* Baltimore, Md: Williams & Wilkins; 1972:67–69.

3. American Diabetes Association Consensus Statement. Detection and management of lipid disorders in diabetes. *Diabetes Care.* 1993;16 (suppl 2):106–112.

4. Bierman EL. Atherogenesis in diabetes. *Arteriosclerosis Thromb.* 1992;12:647–656.

5. Expert Panel on Detection, Evaluation, and Treatment of High Blood Cholesterol in Adults. Summary of the second report of the National Cholesterol Education Program (NCEP) expert panel on detection, evaluation, and treatment of high blood cholesterol in adults (Adults Treatment Panel II). *JAMA.* 1993;269:3015–3023.

6. Steiner G. Diabetes and atherosclerosis. *Diabetes.* 1981;30 (suppl 2):1.

7. Anderson J. Hyperlipidemia and diabetes: nutrition considerations. In: Jovanovic L, Peterson C, eds. *Nutrition and Diabetes.* New York, NY: Alan R. Liss Inc; 1985:1331–1359.

8. Stamler J, Stamler R. Maturity onset diabetes and asymptomatic hyperglycemia. In: National Heart, Lung and Blood Institute, ed. *Diabetes and Atherosclerosis Connection.* New York, NY: Juvenile Diabetes Foundation; 1981:17–44.

9. Saudek C, Young N. Cholesterol metabolism in diabetes mellitus. The role of diet. *Diabetes.* 1981;20 (suppl 2):76.

10. Haffner SM, Stern MP, Hazuda HP, Mitchell BD, Patterson JK. Cardiovascular risk factors in confirmed prediabetic individuals: does the clock for coronary heart disease start ticking before the onset of clinical diabetes? *JAMA.* 1990;263:2839–2898.

11. Burrow G, Hazlett B, Phillips J. A case of diabetes mellitus. *N Engl J Med.* 1982;306:340–343.

12. National Research Council, Committee on Diet and Health, Food and Nutrition Board Diet and Health. *Implications for Reducing Chronic Disease Risk.* Washington, DC: National Academy Press; 1989.

13. Thom T, Kannel W, Feinleib M. Factors in the decline of coronary heart disease mortality. In: Connor WE, Brinstow JD, eds. *Coronary Heart Disease: Prevention, Complications and Treatment.* Philadelphia, Pa: JB Lippincott; 1985:5–20.

14. Stern MP, Patterson JK, Haffner SM, Hazuda HP, Mitchell BD. Lack of awareness and treatment of hyperlipidemia in type II diabetes in a community survey. *JAMA.* 1989;262:360–364.

15. Feingold KR, Grunfeld C, Pang M, Doerrler W, Krauss RM. LDL subclass phenotypes and triglyceride metabolism in non–insulin-dependent diabetes. *Arteriosclerosis.* 1992;12:1496–1502.

16. Reaven GM. Role of insulin resistance of human disease. *Diabetes.* 1988;37:1595–1607.

17. Reaven GM, Chen Y-DI, Jeppesen J, Maheux P, Krauss RM. Insulin resistance and hyperinsulemia in individuals with small, dense, low density lipoprotein particles. *J Clin Invest.* 1993;92:141–146.

18. Kannel WB, Castelli WP, Gordon T, et al. Serum cholesterol, lipoprotein, and the risk of coronary heart disease. *Ann Intern Med.* 1971;74:1–12.

19. Fontbonne A, Eschwege E, Cambien F, et al. Hypertriglyceridemia as a risk factor of coronary heart disease mortality in subjects with impaired glucose tolerance or diabetes. *Diabetologia.* 1989;32:300–304.

20. Austin MA. Plasma triglyceride as a risk factor for coronary heart disease: the epidemiologic evidence and beyond. *AJ Epidemiol.* 1989;29:249–259.

21. Coulston AM, Hollenbeck CB, Swislocki ALM, Reaven GM. Persistence of hypertriglyceridemic effect of low fat, high carbohydrate diets in NIDDM patients. *Diabetes Care.* 1989;12:94–101.

22. Garg A, Bonanome A, Grundy SM, Zhang AJ, Unger RH. Comparison of a high-carbohydrate diet with high monosaturated-fat diet in patients with non–insulin-dependent diabetes mellitus. *N Engl J Med.* 1988;391:829–834.

23. Malasanos TH, Stacpoole PW. Biological effects of Omega-3 fatty acids in diabetes mellitus. *Diabetes Care.* 1991;41:1160–1179.

24. Keys A. *Seven Countries: A Multivariate Analysis of Death and Coronary Heart Disease.* London: Howard University Press; 1980.

25. Stamler J, Wentworth D, Neaton J. Is relationship between serum cholesterol and risk of premature death from coronary heart disease continuous and graded? *JAMA.* 1986;256:2823–2828.

26. Lipid Research Clinics Program. The Lipid Research Clinics Coronary Primary Prevention Trial results: I. Reduction in incidence of coronary heart disease. *JAMA.* 1984;251:351–364.

27. Holme I. An analysis of randomized trials evaluating the effect of cholesterol-reduction on total mortality and coronary heart disease incidence. *Circulation.* 1990;82:1916–1924.

28. Mann J, Marr J. Coronary heart disease prevention: trials of diets to control hyperlipidemia. In: Miller NE, Lewis B, ed. *Lipoproteins, Atherosclerosis and Coronary Heart Disease.* Amsterdam: Elsevier/North Holland Biomedical Press; 1981:197–210.

29. Roussow J. Clinical trials of lipid lowering drugs. In: Rifkind BM, ed. *Drug Treatment of Hyperlipidemia.* New York, NY: Marcel Dekker Inc; 1991:67–88.

30. U.S. Department of Health and Human Services. *Healthy People 2000.* Boston, Mass: Jones & Bartlett Publishers; 1992.

31. Lipid Research Clinics Program. The Lipid Research Clinics Coronary Primary Prevention Trial results: II. The relationship of reduction in incidence of coronary heart disease to cholesterol lowering. *JAMA.* 1984;251:365–374.

32. Reaven GM. Banting Lecture 1988: Role of insulin resistance in human disease. *Diabetes.* 1988;37:1595–1607.

33. Kaplan NM. The deadly quartet: upper-body obesity; glucose intolerance, hypertriglyceridemia, and hypertension. *Arch Intern Med.* 1989;149:1514–1520.

34. Mykkanen L, Laakso M, Pyörälä K. Association of obesity and distribution of obesity with glucose tolerance and cardiovascular risk factors in the elderly. *Int J Obes.* 1992;16:695–704.

35. Vergroesen AJ, Gottenbos JJ. The role of fats in human nutrition: an introduction. In: Vergroesen AJ, ed. *The Role of Fats in Human Nutrition.* London: Academic Press; 1975:1–41.

36. Grundy SM, Denke MA. Dietary influences on serum lipids and lipoproteins. *J Lipid Res.* 1990;31:1149–1172.

37. Linscheer W, Vergroesen A. Lipids. In: Shils M, Olson J, Shike M, eds. *Modern Nutrition in Health and Disease.* 8th ed. Philadelphia, Pa: Lea & Febiger; 1994;47–88.

38. Howard BV. Lipoprotein metabolism in diabetes mellitus. *J Lipid Res.* 1987;28:613–628.

39. Garg A, Grundy SM. Management of dyslipidemia in NIDDM. *Diabetes Care.* 1990;13:153–169.

40. Brunzell JD, Chait A. Lipoprotein pathophysiology and treatment. In: Rifkin H, Porte D, eds. *Ellenberg and Rifkins's Diabetes Mellitus: Theory and Practice.* 4th ed. New York, NY: Elsevier Science Publishing Co; 1990:756–767.

41. Stern MP, Haffner SM. Dyslipidemia in type II diabetes: implication for therapeutic intervention. *Diabetes Care.* 1991;14:1144–1159.

42. Ginsberg HN. Lipoprotein physiology in nondiabetic and diabetic states: relationship to atherogenesis. *Diabetes Care.* 1991;14:839–855.

43. Taskinen MR. Hyperlipidemia in diabetes. *Ballieres Clin Endocrinol Metab.* 1990;4:743–775.

44. Aberg H, Lithell H, Selinus L, et al. Serum triglycerides are a risk factor for myocardial infarction but not for angina pectoris: results from a ten year follow-up of Uppsala Primary Preventive Study. *Atherosclerosis.* 1985;54:89–97.

45. Lopes-Virella MF, Klein RL, Lyons TJ, Stevenson HC, Witztum JL. Glycosylation of low-density lipoprotein enhances cholesteryl ester synthesis in human monocyte-derived macrophages. *Diabetes.* 1988;37:550–557.

46. Mahley RW. Weisgraber KH, Bersot TP. Effects of cholesterol feeding on human and animal high density lipoproteins. In: Gotto AM, Miller NE, Oliver MF, eds. *High Density Lipoproteins and Atherosclerosis.* New York, NY: Elsevier/North Holland Biomedical Press; 1978.

47. Gotto A. The plasma lipoproteins: metabolism, structure-function relationships and their relevance to atherosclerosis. In: National Heart, Lung and Blood Institute, ed. *Diabetes and Atherosclerosis Connection.* New York, NY: Juvenile Diabetes Foundation; 1981:167–180.

48. Nikkila E. Plasma lipid and lipoprotein abnormalities in diabetes. In: Jarett RJ, ed. *Diabetes and Heart Disease.* New York, NY: Elsevier; 1984:133–167.

49. Anderson J. The role of dietary carbohydrate and fiber in the control of diabetes. *Adv Intern Med.* 1980:26:67–96.

50. Brown MS, Goldstein JL. Receptor mediated control of cholesterol metabolism. *Science.* 1976;191:150.

51. Austin MA, King MC, Vranizan KM, Krauss RM. Atherogenic lipoprotein phenotype: a proposed genetic marker for coronary heart disease risk. *Circulation.* 1990;82:495–506.

52. Klein RL, Wohltmann HJ, Lopes-Virella MF. Influence of glycemic control on interaction of very-low- and low-density lipoproteins isolated from type I diabetic patients with human monocyte-derived macrophages. *Diabetes.* 1992;41:1301–1307.

53. Scanu AM. Lipoprotein(a): a genetic risk factor for premature coronary heart disease. *JAMA.* 1992;267:3326–3329.

54. Margolis JR, Kannel WB, Feinleib M, Dawber TR, McNamara PM. Clinical features of unrecognized myocardial infarction: silent and symptomatic. Eighteen year follow-up: the Framingham Study. *Am J Cardiol.* 1973;32:1–7.

55. Barr DP, Russ EM, Eder HA. Protein-lipid relationships in human plasma in atherosclerosis and related conditions. *Am J Med.* 1951;11:480–493.

56. Connor W, Connor S. The dietary prevention and treatment of coronary heart disease. In: Connor W, Bristow JD, eds. *Coronary Heart Disease: Prevention, Compli-cations and Treatment.* Philadelphia, Pa: JB Lippincott; 1985:44–62.

57. Liu K, Stamler J, Dyer A. Statistical methods to assess and minimize the role of intra-individual variability in obscuring the relationship between dietary lipids and serum cholesterol. *J Chronic Dis.* 1978;31:399–418.

58. Gofman JW, Young W, Tandy R. Ischemic heart disease, atherosclerosis and longevity. *Circulation.* 1966;34:679–697.

59. Ashwel M, ed. *Diet and Heart Disease: A Roundtable of Factors.* London: British Nutrition Foundation; 1993.

60. Duell PB, Oram JF, Bierman EL. Nonenzymatic glycosylation HDL and impaired HDL-receptor-mediated cholesterol afflux. *Diabetes.* 1991;40:377–384.

61. Guillausseau PJ, Peynet J, Chanson P, et al. Lipoprotein (a) in diabetic patients with and without chronic renal failure. *Diabetes Care.* 1992;15:976–979.

62. Carew TE, Koschinsky T, Hayes S, et al. A mechanism by which high density lipoprotein may slow the atherogenic process. *Lancet.* 1976;1:1315–1317.

63. Ritter MM, Richter WO, Lyko K, Schwandt P. Lp(a) serum concentrations and metabolic control [Letter to the Editor]. *Diabetes Care.* 1992;15:1441–1442.

64. Keys A, Anderson J, Grande F. Serum cholesterol response to changes in the diet. *Metabolism.* 1965;14:747–787.

65. Kannel WB, Castelli WP, Gordon T. Cholesterol in the prediction of atherosclerotic disease. *Ann Intern Med.* 1979;90:85–91.

66. Mistry P, Miller N, Laker M. Individual variation in the effects of dietary cholesterol on plasma lipoproteins and cellular homeostasis in man. *J Clin Invest.* 1981;67:493–502.

67. Daily dietary fat and total food energy intakes; Third National Health and Nutrition Examination Survey Phase 1, 1988-1991. *MMWR.* 1994;43(7):123–125.

68. Grundy S. Comparison of monounsaturated fatty acids and carbohydrates for lowering plasma cholesterol. *N Engl J Med.* 1986;314:745–748.

69. Kromhout D, Bosschieter E, Coulander C. The inverse relation between fish consumption and 20 year mortality from coronary heart disease. *N Engl J Med.* 1985;312:1205–1209.

70. Simpoulos A. Omega-3 fatty acids in health and disease and in growth and development. *Am J Clin Nutr.* 1991;54:438–463.

71. Herold P, Kinsella J. Fish oil consumption and decreased risk of cardiovascular disease: a comparison of findings from animal and human feeding trials. *J Clin Nutr.* 1986;43:566–598.

72. National Research Council. *Recommended Dietary Allowances.* 9th ed. Washington, DC: National Academy of Sciences; 1980.

73. Hegsted DM, McGandy RB, Myers ML. Quantitative effects of dietary fat on serum cholesterol in man. *Am J Clin Nutr.* 1965;17:281.

74. Sturdevant R, Pearce M, Dayton S. Increased prevalence of cholelithiasis in men ingesting a serum-cholesterol lowering diet. *N Engl J Med.* 1973;288:24–27.

75. Emken EA. Nutrition and biochemistry of *trans* and positional fatty acid isomers in hydrogenated oils. *Annu Rev Nutr.* 1984;4:339–376.

76. Dupont J, White PJ, Feldman EB. Saturated and hydrogenated fats in food in relation to health. *J Am Coll Nutr.* 1991;10:577–592.

77. Mensink RPM, Katan MB. Effect of dietary *trans* fatty acids on high-density and low-density lipoprotein cholesterol levels in healthy subjects. *N Engl J Med.* 1990;323:439–445.

78. Thomas LH, Winter JA, Scott RG. Concentration of 18:1 and 16:1 transunsaturated fatty acids in the adipose body tissue of decedents dying of ischaemic heart disease compared with controls: analysis by gas liquid chromatography. *J Epidemiol Community Health.* 1983;37:16–21.

79. Willett WC, Stampfer MJ, Manson JE, et al. *Trans*-fatty acid intake in relation to risk of coronary heart disease among women. *Lancet.* 1993;341:581–585.

80. Willett WC, Ascherio A. *Trans* fatty acids: are the effects only marginal? *Am J Publ Health.* 1994;84(5): 722–724.

81. Ripsin CM, Keenan JM, Jacobs DR, et al. Oat products and lipid lowering. A meta-analysis. *JAMA.* 1992;267: 3317–3325.

82. Riccardi G, Rivellese AA. Effects of dietary fiber and carbohydrate on glucose and lipoprotein metabolism in diabetic patients. *Diabetes Care.* 1991;14:1115–1125.

83. Jenkins DJA, Wolever TMS, Taylor RH, et al. Glycemic index of foods: a physiological basis for carbohydrate exchange. *Am J Clin Nutr.* 1981;34:362–366.

84. Ferrannini E, Shieh SM, Fuh MT. Insulin resistance in essential hypertension. *N Engl J Med.* 1987;317:350–357.

85. Barbosa JC, Shultz TD, Filley SJ, Nieman DC. The relationship among adiposity, diet, and hormone concentrations in vegetarian and nonvegetarian postmenopausal women. *Am J Clin Nutr.* 1990;51:798.

86. Walker ARP. Disease patterns in South Africa as related to dietary fiber intake. In: Spiller G, ed. *CRC Handbook of Dietary Fiber in Human Nutrition.* Boca Raton, Fl: CRC Press; 1993:491–495.

87. NCEP. Report of the expert panel on blood cholesterol levels in children and adolescents. *Pediatrics.* 1992;88 (suppl):525–583.

88. PDAY Research Group. Relationship of atherosclerosis in young men to serum lipoprotein cholesterol concentrations and smoking: a preliminary report. *JAMA.* 1990;264:3018–3024.

89. DISC Collaborative Research Group. Dietary Intervention Study in Children (DISC) with elevated LDL-cholesterol: design and baseline characteristics. *Ann Epidemiol.* 1993;3:393–402.

90. DISC Collaborative Research Group. Efficacy and safety of lowering dietary intake of fat and cholesterol in children with elevated low-density lipoprotein cholesterol. *JAMA.* 1995;273(18):1429–1435.

High-Density Lipoprotein Cholesterol in Milligrams per Deciliter for Persons 20 Years of Age and Older by Race/Ethnicity, Sex, and Age: United States, 1988–1991

Race/ethnicity, sex, and age	Number of examined persons	Mean	Selected percentile								
			5th	10th	15th	25th	50th	75th	85th	90th	95th
Men											
20 years and older	3920	46.5	28.0	31.0	34.0	37.0	44.1	53.1	59.1	64.0	73.0
20–34 years	1178	47.1	30.0	34.0	35.1	38.0	46.0	54.0	60.1	64.0	71.0
35–44 years	642	46.3	28.0	30.0	33.0	37.0	44.0	53.0	58.1	63.0	73.1
45–54 years	502	46.6	28.0	30.0	33.0	36.0	43.1	53.0	61.0	66.1	77.1
55–64 years	533	45.6	29.0	31.0	33.0	36.1	43.0	53.0	59.0	62.0	72.0
65–74 years	553	45.3	28.0	31.0	32.0	36.0	43.0	53.0	58.0	62.1	71.0
75 and older	512	47.2	28.0	32.0	34.0	38.0	45.0	54.0	62.0	67.0	75.1
Women											
20 years and older	3855	55.7	34.0	38.0	41.0	44.1	54.0	65.0	71.0	76.1	83.0
20–34 years	1167	55.7	34.0	38.0	41.0	44.1	54.0	64.1	70.1	75.1	83.1
35–44 years	701	54.3	33.0	37.0	40.0	44.0	53.0	64.1	69.1	72.1	79.0
45–54 years	459	56.7	37.0	38.0	41.0	46.0	56.0	65.0	72.1	77.1	84.1
55–64 years	500	56.1	33.0	37.0	40.0	44.0	53.0	66.0	73.0	79.0	87.1
65–74 years	492	55.7	34.0	37.0	40.0	44.1	54.0	65.1	73.0	78.0	83.1
75 and older	536	57.1	33.0	39.0	41.0	44.1	56.0	66.1	73.1	78.1	87.0
Mexican Americans											
Men	1077	46.9	30.0	33.0	34.1	38.0	45.0	54.0	59.0	64.0	69.0
Women	1040	53.3	34.0	37.0	40.0	44.0	52.0	61.0	68.0	72.1	78.0
Non-Hispanic black											
Men	918	53.3	30.0	35.0	38.0	42.0	51.0	62.0	69.1	75.1	86.1
Women	978	57.8	37.0	40.0	43.0	47.0	55.1	67.1	74.0	78.1	86.0
Non-Hispanic white											
Men	1803	45.5	28.0	30.0	33.1	36.1	44.0	52.1	58.0	62.0	71.1
Women	1717	55.7	33.1	37.0	40.0	44.0	54.0	65.1	71.1	77.0	83.1

Source: National Health and Nutrition Examination Survey III, Hyattsville, Md: National Center for Health Statistics, 1993.

Low-Density Lipoprotein Cholesterol in Milligrams per Deciliter for Persons 20 Years of Age and Older by Race/Ethnicity, Sex, and Age: United States, 1988–1991

Race/ethnicity, sex, and age	Number of examined persons	Mean	Selected percentile									
			5th	10th	15th	25th	50th	75th	85th	90th	95th
Men											
20 years and older	1669	131	75	87	95	106	129	154	167	179	194
20–34 years	487	120	67	78	86	97	121	139	152	165	186
35–44 years	274	134	85	92	98	111	131	156	166	176	192
45–54 years	224	138	78	91	100	118	136	163	174	187	195
55–64 years	228	142	78	90	104	117	143	165	175	194	205
65–74 years	259	141	93	104	109	119	134	163	177	185	199
75 and older	197	132	83	88	93	106	130	154	170	186	196
Women											
20 years and older	1673	126	69	81	88	99	122	150	165	175	191
20–34 years	525	110	59	70	75	88	108	129	142	155	173
35–44 years	316	117	67	85	88	97	116	138	146	155	165
45–54 years	214	132	70	87	93	107	130	157	173	182	198
55–64 years	213	145	79	90	101	122	145	170	184	189	209
65–74 years	202	147	92	97	109	119	148	169	185	192	206
75 and older	203	147	90	102	109	121	143	168	189	197	209
Mexican Americans											
Men	448	124	70	77	85	96	120	148	161	172	188
Women	471	122	67	80	86	95	118	144	158	166	189
Non-Hispanic black											
Men	393	126	69	76	82	96	123	146	168	186	206
Women	422	126	67	76	86	100	124	147	162	174	192
Non-Hispanic white											
Men	773	132	76	88	97	108	129	154	168	179	194
Women	729	126	69	82	89	99	122	151	166	176	192

Source: National Health and Nutrition Examination Survey III, Hyattsville, Md: National Center for Health Statistics, 1993.

Total Serum Cholesterol Levels in Milligrams per Deciliter for Persons 20 Years of Age and Older by Race/Ethnicity, Sex, and Age: United States, 1988–1991

Race/ethnicity, sex, and age	Number of examined persons	Mean	Selected percentile									
			5th	10th	15th	25th	50th	75th	85th	90th	95th
Men											
20 years and older	3953	205	143	153	162	176	201	231	247	260	276
20–34 years	1186	189	134	145	151	162	186	211	225	236	260
35–44 years	653	207	144	155	167	182	205	231	245	258	269
45–54 years	508	218	152	170	180	191	215	242	257	268	283
55–64 years	535	221	154	169	180	195	221	245	264	274	285
65–74 years	557	218	157	173	179	190	214	241	256	270	286
75 and older	514	205	145	156	164	175	202	232	248	257	275
Women											
20 years and older	3885	207	143	154	162	175	202	233	252	269	287
20–34 years	1177	185	134	143	150	160	182	204	218	229	254
35–44 years	709	195	142	152	159	170	193	215	232	242	254
45–54 years	464	217	158	165	171	187	212	240	264	279	297
55–64 years	503	237	168	184	191	204	228	264	280	291	323
65–74 years	493	234	168	180	186	205	232	261	278	290	308
75 and older	539	230	163	175	184	198	227	263	279	287	316
Mexican Americans											
Men	1092	202	140	151	159	172	199	225	245	257	277
Women	1046	200	139	149	158	169	195	224	241	258	279
Non-Hispanic black											
Men	922	199	136	149	156	170	195	224	242	252	276
Women	985	203	137	150	159	172	200	227	248	262	286
Non-Hispanic white											
Men	1816	206	144	154	163	177	203	232	247	260	276
Women	1734	208	144	155	163	176	202	234	254	271	288

Source: National Health and Nutrition Examination Survey III, Hyattsville, Md: National Center for Health Statistics, 1993.

Predicting Plasma Cholesterol Response

These formulas, which are based on regression equations, have been developed to predict plasma cholesterol response to manipulations in dietary fat:

Δ Key's Equation:

$$1.26 (2S - P) + 1.5 \ 1000 \ C/E3$$

Hegsted's Equation:

$$2.16 \ \Delta \ S - 1.65 \ \Delta \ P + 6.77C - o \ 53$$

in which S denotes the percentage of calories from saturated fat, P denotes the percentage of calories from polyunsaturated fat, C is dietary cholesterol in milligrams per day, and E is the daily energy intake in kilocalories in Key's equation, and Δ is the change in those values in the second formula.

Some reservations exist regarding the accuracy of these equations. They do not allow for the potential effect of monounsaturated fat, carbohydrate, or fiber. Also, the effect of dietary cholesterol intake is implied to be quantitatively similar, regardless of the mix of neutral fat. Studies have demonstrated both a greater and a lesser effect of dietary cholesterol than that predicted by the formula when saturated fats were increased or decreased relative to polyunsaturated fats. As increasing information is gathered regarding the effect on lipid levels of dietary factors other than fat, a revised formula may be devised. Interindividual variability regarding the bioavailability of dietary cholesterol, as well as other factors related to lipid metabolism, will continue to complicate these efforts, however. Dietary cholesterol, whether it contributes to elevated serum cholesterol or not, may accumulate in already present atherosclerotic lesions. In combination with hypertriglyceridemia and platelet aggregation common in diabetes, this accumulation is likely to accelerate the atherosclerotic process in diabetic individuals. Dietary cholesterol reduction is thus particularly beneficial to these individuals.

Chapter 19

Issues in Prescribing Calories

Monica Joyce

The management goals of diabetes are directly influenced by an adequate and appropriate caloric intake. Attaining and maintaining reasonable body weight often improve glucose tolerance and play a major role in reducing prominent risk factors (obesity, hyperglycemia, hyperlipidemia) associated with atherosclerosis.[1] Nutrition therapy is fundamental to achieving glycemic control in persons with diabetes. The Diabetes Control and Complications Trial (DCCT) showed, however, that achieving near-normal glycemia can result in weight gain.[2] Patients in the intensive therapy group (mean HbA_{1c} of 7.1%) gained an average of 4.6 kg more at 5 years than patients receiving conventional therapy (mean HbA_{1c} of 8.9%). Consequently, the caloric prescription is a critical component of diabetes nutrition therapy and should be carefully selected and monitored.

A calorie level is selected in the same manner for the person with diabetes as the person without diabetes. It should be individualized based on many factors, such as the current caloric intake, food preferences, level of glycemic control, activity level, economics, the environment, genetics, and nutrient requirements. A nutrition assessment is necessary to obtain this information, as is follow-up to evaluate the prescription.

This chapter discusses the various methods available for determining the caloric needs of the person with diabetes at various stages of the life cycle and discusses the principal factors known to affect caloric requirements.

ENERGY REQUIREMENTS

Energy requirements are usually stated in relation to the number of calories a person expends. A calorie is the amount of heat energy required to raise 1 kg of water 1°C (from 15° to 16°C). Daily energy requirements are the result of the sum of the (1) basal metabolism, (2) energy liberated in exercise, and (3) specific dynamic action of food.

Basal Metabolism

Basal metabolic rate (BMR) is the minimum amount of energy needed by the body in a rested and fasted state. It represents the amount of energy needed to sustain such life processes as respiration, cellular metabolism, circulation, glandular activity, and maintenance of body temperature. It is measured in the morning at least 12 hours after a meal and following a normal period of sleep. Resting metabolic rate (RMR) is the energy expenditure under similar conditions but is calculated at any time of the day. Basal metabolism is affected by such factors as surface area, body composition, age, hormones, drug ingestion, nutritional status, physical state, level of physical activity, climate, and specific dynamic action of food.

Basal metabolic needs comprise approximately 50 to 70% of the total daily calorie requirement for most individuals.[3] The standard basal energy requirement for individuals of average height and weight is 1 kcal (4184 KJ)/kg per hour (Exhibit 19-1).[4] A frequently used equation, Harris-Benedict equation (HBE), was derived using adults and has been shown to underestimate caloric needs of children with cystic fibrosis.[5] Although this group of children may have greater energy expenditures than other groups of children, this study points out that formulas should be used cautiously with follow-up evaluation of nutritional status and weight.

Surface Area

The greater the body surface or skin area, the greater the amount of heat loss and, in turn, the greater the need for calories. A tall person has higher basal metabolic needs than a short person, due to more body surface area. Even when the two are the same weight, the tall person will have more surface area.

Body Composition

Adipose tissue requires less oxygen for metabolism; therefore it has a lower BMR than muscle tissue. As a result, the ratio of body muscle to body fat has an important influence on energy requirements. Indeed, body composition partly accounts for why the BMR is 5 to 10% lower in women than men, because men have a greater proportion of lean tissue than women. Exercise training has been shown to increase the ratio of muscle to fat, thereby increasing the metabolic rate.[6] This increase seems to be of particular value to women.

Skinfold calipers have been shown to be as effective as computed tomography (x-rays) in measuring subcutaneous fat in clinical settings.[7] The optimum level of body fat for a particular individual cannot be precisely stated. It has been suggested that, based on data from physically active young adults and competitive athletes, it would be desirable to strive for a body fat content of 15% for men (certainly less than 20%) and about 25% for women (certainly less than 30%).[8] Even with these guidelines, following a series of measurements and assessing the pattern

Exhibit 19-1 Basal Energy Expenditure (BEE)

Basal energy requirement is equal to:

Women:
$655 + (9.6 \times W) + (1.7 \times H) - (4.7 \times A)$

Men:
$66 + (13.7 \times W) + (5 \times H) - (6.8 \times A)$

W = actual weight in kg
   (2.2 lb = 1 kg)
   (1 lb = .45 kg)

H = height in cm
   (1 in = 2.54 cm)

A = age in years

in comparison to caloric intake and activity level is the best determination of what is achievable for a particular individual. For many persons with diabetes, a percentage body fat content measurement is not the most critical measurement to monitor but is a useful indicator to use in those who are undernourished, are striving for a particular level of body fat, or need a different measurement to add "interest" to their health goals.

Age

During the first and second years of life, the BMR reaches its highest point due to rapid tissue growth and development. A lesser rise is experienced during the periods of puberty and adolescence in both males and females. After the age of 21, the BMR begins to decline about 2% during each decade.[9] This decline is attributed to changes in body composition that result in an increase of fat and decrease in muscle, the more metabolically active tissue. There is usually a decrease in activity, also.

Hormones and Drugs

Various hormones—thyroid, growth and sex hormones, insulin, cortisol, and epinephrine—

have been shown to influence metabolic rate. Their degree of influence varies but may be of importance for a few persons with weight problems. Also, several drugs may exert a small, usually insignificant influence on overall energy needs. Hyper- and hypothyroidism have characteristically been noted to cause an increase and decrease, respectively, in BMR. Reduced caloric intake, severe stress, and steroid administration have been shown to influence one of the major thyroid hormones, T3.[10]

Nutritional Status

Starvation or semistarvation results in a lowered BMR, in some cases as much as 50% below normal. The body responds to these adverse conditions by energy conservation; the metabolic rate decreases to conserve energy. Studies show that diets may have this same lowering affect on the metabolic rate.[6,11] Therefore, individuals who are attempting to lose weight by reduced caloric intake may alter their metabolism and thus require fewer calories for weight maintenance.

Physical State

Physical states, such as infection, burns, stress, pregnancy, and lactation, affect energy needs. Fevers or infections increase the BMR approximately 7% for each degree rise in body temperature above 98.6°F or 13% for each degree above 37°C.[3] During pregnancy, the muscle development of the fetus, placenta, and uterus increases the mother's metabolic requirements. Increased respiration and cardiac work also contribute to the elevated BMR in pregnancy. Both pregnancy and lactation require additional calories to meet the energy needs of these demanding periods.

Physical Activity

Physical activity is the dominant factor, second only to basal needs, in influencing one's daily energy requirements. Body size (more energy is expended for heavier persons) and the nature, duration, and intensity of the activity influence total energy requirements.

Additional calories must be added to the BMR based on the activity level of the person: usually 30% more calories are added for a sedentary person, 50% above basal for a moderately active person, and 100% above basal for the very active individual. Energy expenditure for various activities for persons of various weights is given in Table 19-1.

The metabolic rate falls during sleep to about 10 to 15% below awake levels.[4] This decrease is due to muscular relaxation and reduced activity of the sympathetic nervous system.

Climate

People living in the tropics for the most part have a decreased metabolic rate that is 10% less than individuals living in cold climates. In colder climates, people have an increased secretion of thyroxine, which affects metabolic rate. Because most people in the United States are protected against the elements by heating and air conditioning, their BMR is usually not affected by temperature extremes.

Specific Dynamic Action of Food

Metabolic rate increases after a meal because of the specific dynamic action (SDA) of food. This effect causes a 10% increase over basal metabolism for a meal of 1000 kcal.[12] It has been shown in animals that carbohydrate and fat contribute very little to SDA and that the increase is primarily related to protein consumption.

DETERMINING AND INDIVIDUALIZING THE CALORIC PRESCRIPTION

Although weight and height measurements are necessary, other factors that influence energy requirements must also be evaluated in the nutritional assessment. It should include a detailed diet, weight, and family weight history and a review of exercise habits. The daily caloric intake

Table 19-1 Approximate Energy Expenditure during Performance of Various Activities

	Caloric Expenditure (kcal) by Weight and Time					
	120 lb (54.5 kg)		150 lb (68 kg)		220 lb (90.9 kg)	
Activity	Time Needed To Use 250 Calories	Calories Used per Hour of Activity	Time Needed To Use 250 Calories	Calories Used per Hour of Activity	Time Needed To Use 250 Calories	Calories Used per Hour of Activity
Aerobic dancing	27	553	22	691	16	922
Badminton (singles)	47	318	38	396	28	529
Basketball	33	452	27	564	20	753
Bicycling						
6 mph	71	210	57	262	43	349
12 mph	27	553	22	691	16	922
Bowling	100	150	83	180	71	210
Calisthenics	69	216	56	270	42	360
Canoeing (leisure)	104	144	83	180	63	240
Dancing						
Slow	89	167	71	209	54	278
Fast	27	550	22	687	16	916
Football	35	432	28	540	21	720
Golf (walking and carrying bag)	54	278	43	348	32	450
Hockey	42	360	36	420	33	450
Jumping rope	42	360	36	420	33	450
Running or jogging						
5 mph	34	442	27	552	20	736
7.5 mph	24	630	19	792	14	1050
10 mph	18	824	15	1030	11	1375
Sailing	83	180	69	216	57	264
Skating (ice or roller)	61	245	49	307	37	409
Skiing						
Downhill	50	280	40	360	32	450
Cross-country	38	390	31	487	23	649
Soccer	45	330	37	410	29	512
Squash, racquetball	42	357	34	446	25	595
Swimming (fast, freestyle)	36	420	29	522	22	698
Tennis						
Singles	42	357	34	446	25	595
Doubles	71	210	57	262	43	350
Volleyball	93	164	74	205	54	273
Walking						
3 mph	74	206	58	258	44	344
4 mph	49	308	39	385	29	513
Upstairs	32	471	26	589	19	786
Weight training	42	340	34	420	28	520
Wrestling (practice)	23	600	18	800	14	1020

Source: Adapted with permission from PM Kris-Etherton, Nutrition and the exercising female. *Nutrition Today* (1986;21:8), Copyright © 1986, Williams & Wilkins Company.

Exhibit 19-2 Estimating Caloric Intake for Adults

Basal Calories:	10–12 kcal/lb desirable body weight
	20–25 kcal/kg desirable body weight

Add Calories for Activity:	If sedentary—	additional 30% calories
	If moderately active—	50% calories
	If strenuously active—	100% calories

Adjustments:*	*Add* 300 kcal/d during pregnancy
	Add 500 kcal/d during lactation
	Add 500 kcal/d to gain one lb/wk
	Subtract 500 kcal/d to lose one lb/wk

*Adjustments are approximate: weight changes should be monitored and compared to caloric intake.

can be estimated from a 24-hour dietary recall. Formulas such as the HBE can also be used to estimate the required amount of calories (Exhibits 19-1 and 19-2; see Table 25-8 for children). Calories must then be added or subtracted from the diet for the patient to gain or lose weight. Exhibits 19-3 and 19-4 can be used as guides to determine weight goals and degree of obesity.

It is not mandatory that a precise calorie level be selected initially by the practitioner. One can estimate the amount of calories needed and then make the appropriate adjustments during the follow-up period. Doing so enables the patient and dietitian to work together to avoid an underprescription of the actual number of calories required and to make adjustments to the diet if activity or schedule changes occur.

There is a tendency to underestimate the caloric prescription, particularly if the diet is based on the patient's dietary recall. Both lean and obese patients tend to underestimate the actual number of calories they consume as extra foods; alcohol, sweets, sauces, or gravies are sometimes overlooked. Persons who are obese or previously obese may reduce the accuracy of energy expenditure data based on self-reports. Persons who have a prescribed number of calories in the hospital may actually need an increase in calories at the time of discharge, taking into consideration the person's life style, schedule, and activity level changes.

Weight goals must be discussed and clearly defined with the patient. If an inappropriate calorie level is selected, adherence to the food plan will be jeopardized. A gradual steady weight loss of 0.5 to 2 lb/wk or 2 to 8 lb/mo is recommended when weight loss is desired and as a nutrition therapy goal.[1,13,14] Also, patients who are consistently hungry because of too-low calorie levels may consume extra or inappropriate food, such as a snack or larger meals, thereby interfering with optimal blood glucose control. Good clinical judgment, which takes into consideration the person's overall appearance and anthropometric values, is the basis for an accurate and realistic nutritional assessment of caloric needs.

A variety of weight tables are available, as well as formulas, for defining a desirable weight goal. A commonly used one is from the Metropolitan Life Insurance Company (see Exhibit 19-5). The U.S. Department of Agriculture and Health and Human Services issued the one (Exhibit 19-6) in the 1990 Dietary Guidelines for Americans.[14] There are some who feel that an age-adjusted weight chart should be used with persons older than the age of 50 years. The American Diabetes Association states that nutrition therapy should be based on achieving a reasonable weight goal defined as a weight that is achievable and maintainable both short and long term.[1] When this individualized weight goal is

Exhibit 19-3 Estimating Desirable Body Weight in Adults

Frame size	*Women*	*Men*
Medium	100 lb for first 5 ft plus 5 lb for each additional inch	106 lb for first 5 ft plus 6 lb for each additional inch
	or	or
	45 kg for first 150 cm plus 0.9 kg for each additional cm	48 kg for first 150 cm plus 1.1 kg for each additional cm
Small	Subtract 10%	
Large	Add 10%	

Source: U.S. Department of Agriculture and U.S. Department of Health and Human Services, *Nutrition and Your Health: Dietary Guidelines for Americans*, ed. 3, 1990.

set, it should take into account the client's eating habits, activity, musculature, growth and development, and glycemic and lipid goals as well as other health goals. Social and cultural attitudes of the client also need to be considered.[15]

Caloric Prescription for the Person with Insulin-Dependent Diabetes Mellitus

The person with insulin-dependent diabetes mellitus (IDDM) is rarely overweight when diagnosed with diabetes. In fact, one of the clinical symptoms of this type of diabetes is weight loss. The person with IDDM in poor control may excrete up to 100 g/d of glucose (400 kcal); less than 20 g/d is acceptable; less than 10 g/d is preferable.[16] At the time of diagnosis, larger amounts may be excreted due to the untreated diabetes.

A person who lost weight before diagnosis usually gains weight when blood glucose levels are normalized. The prescribed calorie level should be similar to the one the patient was following before diagnosis and onset of symptoms if he or she is not overweight. The dietitian needs to consider that before diagnosis the person with IDDM frequently consumes excess calories due to the uncontrolled diabetes. Therefore, a calorie formula may be most useful when the eating pattern has been abnormal for some time. Calorie levels should not be decreased in

the thin insulin-dependent person in an attempt to improve blood glucose. Lean body mass will be lost if the calorie level is lower than a maintenance level.

If the patient is hospitalized after diagnosis, the calorie level may differ in the hospital than in the outpatient setting. Calories may need to be adjusted at the time of admission and again at discharge. Activity and physical state—diabetes control, stress—are important factors to consider when making this adjustment.

Not only must calories be adequate to ensure normal growth and weight maintenance in the person with IDDM but also the distribution of these calories, in particular carbohydrate, throughout the day is essential to avoid repeated insulin reactions and adjustment of exogenous insulin. In lean patients, satiety, appetite, and hunger are usually reliable guides to caloric requirements; body weight and nutritional status are, of course, the definite long-term guide.[17] Many persons with IDDM are well satisfied initially with prescriptions containing 70 to 80% of their present calorie intake because the ratio of bulk to calories is a little higher in most diabetic diets and because extra calories were previously available in snacks.[18] After a short time, the lean IDDM may need to add necessary calories. The problem with this is that they may be added on an irregular basis leading to a disruption in the

Exhibit 19-4 Body Mass Nomogram

To use this nomograph, place a straightedge across the scales for weight and height. The body mass index (BMI) is the number in the middle scale where the straightedge crosses it.

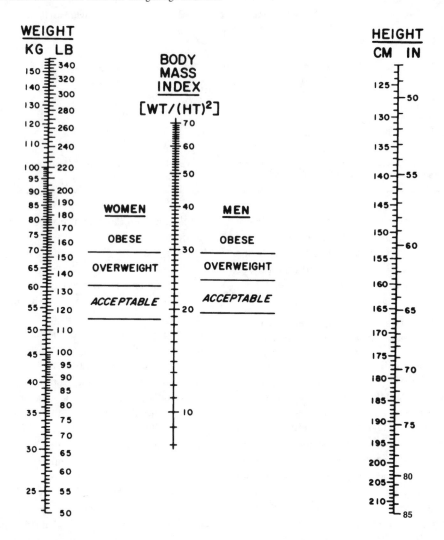

Source: Copyright © George A. Bray, 1978. Used with permission.

Use of BMI to Guide Therapeutic Intervention

BMI

≤23   Normal

>23 to <27   Intervention in the presence of ↑ serum cholesterol or family history of heart disease, diabetes, or hypertension

≥27   Intervention even in the absence of other risk factors

Source: Data from Burton BT, Foster WR, Hirsch J, Van Itallie TB. Health Implications of Obesity: An NIH Consensus Development Conference. *International Journal of Obesity*. 1985;9:155–169, MacMillan Press Ltd.

Exhibit 19-5 Weights Associated with Lowest Mortality for Men and Women, 1983

Height (with Shoes)	Weight (in Indoor Clothing), lb		
	Small Frame	*Medium Frame*	*Large Frame*
Men[a]			
5'2"	128–134	131–141	138–150
5'3"	130–136	133–143	140–153
5'4"	132–138	135–145	142–156
5'5"	134–140	137–148	144–160
5'6"	136–142	139–151	146–164
5'7"	138–145	142–154	149–168
5'8"	140–148	145–157	152–172
5'9"	142–151	148–160	155–176
5'10"	144–154	151–163	158–180
5'11"	146–157	154–166	161–184
6'0"	149–160	157–170	164–188
6'1"	152–164	160–174	168–192
6'2"	155–168	164–178	172–197
6'3"	158–172	167–182	176–202
6'4"	162–176	171–187	181–207
Women[b]			
4'10"	102–111	109–121	118–131
4'11"	103–113	111–123	120–134
5'0"	104–115	113–126	122–137
5'1"	106–118	115–129	125–140
5'2"	108–121	118–132	128–143
5'3"	111–124	121–135	131–147
5'4"	114–127	124–138	132–151
5'5"	117–130	127–141	137–155
5'6"	120–133	130–144	140–159
5'7"	123–136	133–147	143–163
5'8"	126–139	136–150	146–167
5'9"	129–142	139–153	149–170
5'10"	132–145	142–156	152–173
5'11"	135–148	145–159	155–176
6'0"	138–151	148–162	158–179

[a] Weights at ages 25–59 based on lowest mortality. Weight in pounds according to frame (in indoor clothing weighing 5 lb, shoes with 1" heels).

[b] Weights at ages 25–59 based on lowest mortality. Weight in pounds according to frame (in indoor clothing weighing 3 lb, shoes with 1" heels).

Source: Courtesy of Metropolitan Life Insurance Company.

consistency of the meal plan. The dietitian should work closely with the physician regarding the insulin regimen and dosage requirements to promote optimal glycemic levels.

Specific Concerns for Children

The child with diabetes requires vigilant monitoring of growth and development while

Exhibit 19-6 Suggested Weights for Adults

Height[a]	Weight in Pounds[b]	
	19 to 34 years	35 years and over
5'0"	97–128[c]	108–138
5'1"	101–132	111–143
5'2"	104–137	115–148
5'3"	107–141	119–152
5'4"	111–146	122–157
5'5"	114–150	126–162
5'6"	118–155	130–167
5'7"	121–160	134–172
5'8"	125–164	138–178
5'9"	129–169	142–183
5'10"	132–174	146–188
5'11"	136–179	151–194
6'0"	140–184	155–199
6'1"	144–189	159–205
6'2"	148–195	164–210
6'3"	152–200	168–216
6'4"	156–205	173–222
6'5"	160–211	177–228
6'6"	164–216	182–234

[a] Without shoes.

[b] Without clothes.

[c] The higher weights in the ranges generally apply to men, who tend to have more muscle and bone; the lower weights more often apply to women, who have less muscle and bone.

Source: Data from *Diet and Health: Implications for Reducing Chronic Disease Risk.* National Research Council, National Academy of Sciences, 1989.

dietary plan is strongly correlated to blood glucose control,[21] especially in children younger than 16 years of age.[22]

If a rough calorie estimate is necessary before a nutrition consult is possible, the formula of 1000 calories as a base with the addition of 100 calories for each year of life or the recommended dietary allowance (RDA) estimates in Table 25-8 can be used. Energy allowances for children of both sexes decline gradually to about 80 kcal/kg through 10 years of age.[4] After the age of 10, energy allowances decline further to 45 kcal/kg for adolescent boys and 38 kcal/kg for adolescent girls.[9] Formulas should be used only as guidelines because body composition and activity levels can vary considerably in children of the same age. Growth should be monitored frequently using standard growth charts.

The caloric prescription may need to be adjusted several times a year to facilitate normal growth and development and to take into consideration the level of activity, which can change frequently by participation in sports or a change in the school schedule. A review of caloric needs is suggested three to six times a year.[20] This is one of the reasons why the type I Nutrition Practice Guidelines recommend a minimum of quarterly nutrition therapy visits for those beyond initial level nutrition care.[23]

carefully balancing insulin, exercise, and food intake. Frequently, caloric prescriptions are based on a variety of formulas that may or may not reflect the true caloric intake of the child. The latest nutrition recommendations of the American Diabetes Association state that the preferred method of determining a child's caloric needs is through a 24-hour recall or a 2- to 3-day diet history.[19] This method is more time-consuming and may be overlooked when writing the prescription. However, its importance should be stressed as dietary adherence is thought to be compromised by the use of calculated estimates.[20] The calorie review is accomplished as part of the initial nutrition assessment performed by the registered dietitian. This step is necessary as adherence to a

Specific Concerns for Adolescents

Adolescents require guidance and supervision during this time of growth, fluctuations in activity, varying eating patterns, and increased awareness of body image, all of which can affect calorie intake and needs. Weight gain in teenage girls is more prevalent than in males due to metabolic changes at menarche. This is an opportune time to provide sound nutritional guidelines.

The temptation to eat large quantities of food is always present in some adolescents with diabetes. They may know the correct food choices, yet they are apt to choose inappropriate foods to satisfy hunger. The meal plan should be revised frequently, taking into consideration holidays, parties, use of alcohol, and means of dealing effectively with exceptions to the average day.

Hypoglycemia is an ever-present threat to the adolescent with diabetes. To avoid these episodes, the nutrition prescription should allow for necessary snacks (eg, during school hours, before and after exercise, and at bedtime). Yet, the total calorie level must be appropriate to avoid inappropriate weight gain.

Calorie Prescription for the Person with Non–Insulin-Dependent Diabetes Mellitus

Although most persons with non–insulin-dependent diabetes mellitus (NIDDM) are overweight, occasionally the practitioner must prescribe a calorie level for a lean person with NIDDM. Because these patients occasionally attempt to improve hyperglycemia by losing weight, it is important to emphasize that a hypocaloric diet does not improve blood glucose control. These individuals require a diet similar in caloric control to the one followed before the diagnosis of diabetes. Small frequent feedings are often emphasized. For most active patients, weight maintenance requires roughly 30 to 35 kcal/kg.[17]

More than 80% of all persons with NIDDM are obese. In the past, a primary goal in their treatment has been caloric restriction leading to weight reduction.[24] Because traditional dietary strategies have usually not been effective in achieving long-term weight loss, current emphasis is placed on obtaining glucose and lipid goals.[19] This emphasis may destigmatize the ideas of a food plan and actually result in weight loss.

The therapy goal of weight loss should not, however, be overlooked. Weight loss has a definite effect on ß-cell function and insulin sensitivity by increasing the number of insulin receptors and improving intercellular metabolism, which characterizes the insulin resistance of obesity.[16] Mild-to-moderate weight loss (10 to 20 lb; 5 to 10 kg) has been shown to improve diabetes control, even if desirable body weight is not achieved.[19]

In obese persons with type II diabetes, weight reduction has the potential not only of improving glycemic control but even of reversing the disease when it has been present for only a few years.[25] Prescribing an overly restrictive diet with an inappropriate calorie level to achieve weight loss may result in arbitrary food additions that ultimately interfere with the weight management plan. The patient's input is critical in development of the meal plan because it fosters a commitment to the diet and life-style changes necessary to adhere to the nutrition/caloric prescription.

REFERENCES

1. Franz MJ, Horton, HS, Bantle JP, et al. Nutrition principles for the management of diabetes and related complications. *Diabetes Care.* 1994;17(5):490–518.

2. Diabetes Control and Complications Trial Research Group. Weight gain associated with intensive therapy in the Diabetes Control and Complications Trial. *Diabetes Care.* 1988;11:567–573.

3. Guyton AC. Nutrients in food, their digestion, absorption, and metabolism. In: Guyton AC, ed. *Textbook of Medical Physiology.* 5th ed. Philadelphia, Pa: WB Saunders Co; 1976.

4. Harris JA, Benedict FG. *A Biometric Study of Basal Metabolism in Man.* Washington, DC: Carnegie Institute of Washington; 1919. Publication no. 279.

5. Murphy MD, Ireton-Jones CS, Hilman BC, Gorman MA, Liepa GU. Resting energy expenditures measured by indirect calorimetry are higher in preadolescent children with cystic fibrosis than expenditures calculated from prediction equations. *J Am Diet Assoc.* 1995; 95:30–33.

6. Lennon D, Nagle F, Stratman F, Shrago E, Dennis S. Diet and exercise training effects on resting metabolic rate. *J Obes.* 1985;9:39.

7. Orphanidou C, McCargar L, Birmingham L, Mathieson J, Goldner E. Accuracy of subcutaneous fat measurement: comparison of skinfold calipers, ultrasound, and computed tomography. *J Am Diet Assoc.* 1994;94:855–858.

8. Frank I, Katch M, William D, McArdle A. Evaluation of body composition. In: Harris JM, ed. *Intoduction to Nutrition, Exercise, and Health.* 4th ed. Malwern, Pa: Lea & Febiger; 1993.

9. Food and Nutrition Board. *Recommended Dietary Allowances.* 10th ed. Washington, DC: National Academy of Sciences; 1989.

10. Molitch ME, Dahms WT. Endocrinology. In: Schneider HA, Anderson CE, Coursin DB, eds. *Nutritional Support of Medical Practice.* 2nd ed. Philadelphia, Pa: Harper & Row Publishers; 1983:328–351.

11. DeBoer J, VanEs A, Roovrees L, et al. Adaptation of energy metabolism of overweight women to low energy intake studied with whole body calorimeters. *Am J Clin Nutr.* 1986;44:585.

12. Garrow JS. *Energy Balance and Obesity in Man.* Amsterdam: Elsevier/North-Holland Biomedical Press: 1978.

13. American Dietetic Association. *Nurtition Information Series—Losing Weight.* Chicago, Ill: American Dietetic Association; 1986.

14. U.S. Department of Agriculture, U.S. Department of Health and Human Services. *Nutrition and Your Health: Dietary Guidelines for Americans.* 3rd ed. Hyattsville, MD: USDA's Human Nutrition Information Service; 1990.

15. Cassell J. Social anthropology and nutrition: a different look at obesity in America. *J Am Diet Assoc.* 1995;95: 424–427.

16. Marble A, Ferguson D. Diagnosis and classification of diabetes mellitus and non-diabetic meliturias. In: Marble A, Krall LP, Bradley RF, et al, eds. *Joslin's Diabetes Melllitus.* 12th ed. Philadelphia, Pa: Lea & Febiger; 1985:343.

17. West KM. Diabetes mellitus: endocrinology. In: Schneider HA, Anderson CE, Coursin DB, eds. *Nutritional Support of Medical Practice.* 2nd ed. Philadelphia, Pa: Harper & Row Publishers; 1983:302–319.

18. West KM. Diet therapy of diabetes: an analysis of failure. *Ann Intern Med.* 1973;79:425.

19. American Diabetes Association. Position statement: nutrition recommendations and principles for people with diabetes mellitus. *Diabetes Care.* 1994;17:519–522.

20. Connel J, Thomas-Dobersen D. Nutritional management of children and adolescents with insulin-dependent diabetes mellitus: a review by the Diabetes Care and Education Practice Group. *J Am Diet Assoc.* 1991;91: 1556–1564.

21. Delahanty LM, Halford BN. The role of diet behaviors in achieving improved glycemic control in intensively treated patients in the Diabetes Control and Complications Trial, *Diabetes Care.* 1993;16:1453–1458.

22. Burroughs TE, Pontious SL, Santiago J. The relationship among six psychosocial domains, age, health care adherence and metabolic control in adolescents with IDDM. *Diabetes Educ.* 1993;19:396–402.

23. Diabetes Care and Education Practice Group. Nutrition practice group guidelines for type I diabetes mellitus. American Dietetic Association, in preparation.

24. Amercian Diabetes Association. Position statement: nutrition recommendations and principles for individuals with diabetes mellitus. 1986. *Diabetes Care.* 1987;10: 126–132.

25. Arky RA, Wylie-Rosett J, el-Beheri B. Examination of current dietary recommendations for individuals with diabetes mellitus. *Diabetes Care.* 1982;5:62.

Chapter 20

Low-Calorie Sweeteners and Fat Replacers: The Ingredients, Use in Foods, and Diabetes Management

Margaret A. Powers
Hope S. Warshaw

In the past few decades, the number of reduced-calorie, sugar-free, and fat-free foods and beverages has grown tremendously. These foods can be produced because new low-calorie sweeteners and fat-replacer ingredients have been developed and approved for use. Interestingly, low-calorie sweeteners have been available since the 1878 discovery of saccharin, but only in the past several decades have reduced-calorie foods become popular and socially acceptable for many individuals. The emphasis on lowering sugar and fat in the American diet has fostered the development of and desire for these products.

This explosion of new foods has both helped and confused the person with diabetes. Food choices are now more complicated. Consider salad dressing. It used to be just a matter of choosing a flavor. Now, shoppers can choose from regular, reduced-calorie, low-fat, or fat-free as well as deciding on a flavor. The person with diabetes has more palatable sugar-free and fat-free food choices compared with years ago when "special dietary foods" were relegated to the "diet" section of a supermarket aisle. However, persons with diabetes are often left confused about all these foods and may use them inappropriately. Self-management training and education about these choices are needed so that these foods can be appropriately incorporated into an individual's diabetes nutrition therapy plan.

The discussion of low-calorie sweeteners and fat replacers are combined in this chapter because they have many commonalties:

- Both are ingredients used to create nutritionally conscious foods (reduced sugar, fat, and/or calories).

- Low-calorie sweeteners are sometimes combined with fat replacers.

- Manufacturers must follow similar procedures for seeking ingredient approval through the Food and Drug Administration (FDA).

- Educational concepts about their use in diabetes management are similar.

It is important for diabetes nutrition educators to be familiar with the ingredients and resulting foods and know how to advise clients with diabetes about their use.

Questions to be answered are:

1. What obstacles are faced by the food industry to replace sugars and fats in foods?

2. What are low-calorie sweetener and fat-replacer ingredients?

3. Are currently available low-calorie sweeteners and fat replacers safe?

4. What is the FDA regulatory review process for these ingredients?

5. How should these ingredients and resulting foods be used by persons with diabetes?

6. What are the educational concepts to teach about the use of these ingredients and foods in diabetes management?

NUTRITION RECOMMENDATIONS

Americans have been advised to use sugars in moderation and to reduce fat intake to 30% or less of total calories.[1,2] Advice is similar for persons with diabetes, with a few additional twists. Sugar can be part of the total carbohydrate content of the food plan, yet should be consumed within the context of a healthy diet.[3] A specific percentage of total fat is not recommended because the amount of fat intake should be individualized according to food preferences and desired glucose, lipid, and weight goals.[3] Specific advice to individuals with diabetes on fat is to reduce saturated fat intake to less than 10% of total calories and polyunsaturates to no more than 10% with monounsaturated fats contributing the remainder.[3] Meeting these goals may require the use of foods with low-calorie sweeteners or fat replacers.

Neither the American Dietetic Association nor the American Diabetes Association gives specific upper limits for intake in its sweetener or fat-replacer position statements, except for the accepted daily intake values provided by the FDA.[3–6] An assessment of the individual's nutritional, medical, and behavioral needs and habits is the best indicator for specific intake and use recommendations.

The amount of sugar (sucrose), as refined sugar, Americans consume has declined over the past few decades due to cost. However, the consumption of other sugars, high fructose corn syrup (HFCS), corn sweeteners, honey, and syrups, has increased.[7] For example, today regular carbonated soft drinks are sweetened with HFCS, in part because it is less expensive than cane or beet sugar. According to national food consumption data, total fat and saturated fat intake has gradually decreased from 36 and 13%, respectively, in 1978[8] to 34 and 12%, respectively, in 1990.[9] It is conjectured that the availability of reduced-calorie and reduced-fat foods has and will continue to assist Americans in lowering fat intake.[6] However, studies to date indicate that these foods do not assist in girth control.[10,11]

The emphasis on reducing sugar and fat intake has created marketing opportunities for food manufacturers. In fact, food companies were encouraged to develop new foods to help Americans accomplish this goal.[1,12] The critical links in creating sugar-free, low-fat, and fat-free foods are (1) new ingredients to replace sugar and fat, (2) willingness of food manufacturers to produce foods that are lower in sugar, fat, and calories, and (3) consumers' request for and willingness to purchase such foods.

The result has been an exponential growth in the number of foods formulated with low-calorie sweeteners and fat replacers. Estimates are that the sales of low-cholesterol and low-fat foods will climb from $25 billion in 1990 to $33 billion in 1993 and $41.1 billion in 1995.[13] A recent national survey revealed that 86% of all women and 75% of all men consume low-calorie and reduced-fat foods.[14] Although there are no data documenting an increased use of these foods by persons with diabetes, this conjecture is probable. Persons with diabetes are more likely to be searching for products to achieve nutrition therapy goals more easily.

Terminology

In addressing low-calorie sweeteners and fat replacers, a variety of other terms are used. Low-calorie sweeteners are also referred to as intense, noncaloric, nonnutritive, artificial, or alternative sweeteners; sugar substitutes; and sugar replacers. All terms refer to sweeteners that are intensely sweet and contribute minimal calories to a food. Fat replacers are also referred to as fat substitutes and fat replacements. In this chapter, the terms low-calorie sweeteners and fat replacers are used.

CHALLENGES OF FORMULATING NEW FOODS WITH LOW-CALORIE SWEETENERS AND FAT REPLACERS

Food manufacturers who incorporate low-calorie sweeteners and fat replacers into foods are challenged to create products lower in sug-

Exhibit 20-1 Role of Sugars and Fats in Foods

Sugar Provides	*Fat Provides*
Sweetness	Flavor carrier/taste enhancer
Structure and texture (crystalline properties)	Rich and creamy mouth feel
Bulk/volume	Emulsification
Caramelization/browning	Aeration
Lowers freezing point	Heat stability
Moistness and tenderness (humectancy)	Moistness and tenderness (humectancy)
	Aroma precursors

ars, fat, and/or calories while providing consumers with the familiar and desirable taste profile of the "regular" food. Replacing sugars and fats in foods requires total reformulation of the recipe. It is essentially new product development. Both sugars and fats serve a variety of roles in foods and beverages. People are most familiar with the sweetening role sugars provide in foods and beverages and the taste fat adds to foods. Both, however, contribute additional properties and roles (see Exhibit 20-1).

No ideal low-calorie sweetener or fat replacer exists today that has all the necessary functional and taste attributes to allow food manufacturers to replace a regular form of sugar or fat with a low-calorie sweetener or fat replacer. Therefore, when food manufacturers develop or reformulate foods with these ingredients, they use a *multiple ingredient approach*. Several ingredients, each with its unique qualities, are combined to achieve the desired product. For example, the first ingredient on the packets of low-calorie sweeteners is a bulking ingredient such as the carbohydrate-based maltodextrin. The low-calorie sweeteners are so sweet (at least 200 times sweeter than sucrose) that very little is needed. The bulking ingredient is used to provide volume or bulk, not sweetness and calories. These ingredients are less sweet than sucrose and have from 2 to 4 calories/g. Sorbitol and polydextrose are also familiar carbohydrate-bulking ingredients used with high-intensity sweeteners. The multiple ingredient approach is also used when replacing fat. Common combinations of fat replacers are shown in Table 20-1.

Blending Sweeteners

A concept gaining popularity in the low-calorie sweetener marketplace is the blending of several high-intensity sweeteners. Blends of sweeteners are used to take advantage of the benefits of each sweetening ingredient to produce a taste profile not attainable with a single sweetener.[15] For instance, one low-calorie sweetener might produce a quick, briefly sustained sweet taste, and another produces a delayed, longer-perceived taste. A blend of acesulfame K and aspartame resulted in a taste quite similar to that of sucrose when tested in a liquid solution.[16] Blends of two or more sweeteners in varying amounts can be designed to provide a particular food product the best result.

In addition to improved taste profile, blending results in the use of less total sweetener due to sweetener synergy. Sweetener synergy has been defined as a mixture response that is greater than the sweetness of the component sweeteners.[17] Also, using blends can positively affect the heat, liquid, and shelf stability of the food.

The blending of noncaloric sweeteners became popular in the United States from 1960 to 1970. Cyclamate and saccharin were blended until the ban on cyclamate in 1969. Blending has continued with the combination of saccharin and aspartame in the fountain syrup of carbonated soft drinks. Saccharin's benefits are its stable concentrated sweet taste, but its downside is an often reported bitter aftertaste. Some consumers prefer this taste over the taste of other sweeteners. Aspartame's benefits are its clean sweet

Table 20-1 Comparison of Ingredients and Nutrition Information for Regular and Reduced-Fat Foods[a]

Food Product	Fat Replacements Used[b]	Serving Size	Calories	Carbohydrate(g)	Protein (g)	Fat (g)
Salad Dressings						
Hidden Valley Ranch—regular	Maltodextrin, food starch modified, xanthan gum	2 Tbsp	140	1	1	14
Hidden Valley Ranch—light	Modified food starch, tapioca dextrin, xanthan gum	2 Tbsp	80	22	0	7
Hidden Valley Ranch—fat-free	Maltodextrin, modified food starch, xanthan gum	2 Tbsp	45	9	1	0
Kraft Ranch—Fat-Free	Cellulose gel, maltodextrin, food starch-modified, xanthan gum	2 Tbsp	50	11	4	0
Cream Cheese						
Kraft Philadelphia Soft	Stabilizers (xanthan gum, +/or carob bean gum +/or guar gum)	1 oz/2 Tbsp	100	1	2	10
Kraft Philadelphia Light	Stabilizers (xanthan gum, +/or carob bean gum +/or guar gum), carob bean gum	1 oz/2 Tbsp	70	2	3	5
Kraft Philadelphia Fat-Free	Xanthan gum, carrageenan	1 oz/2 Tbsp	35	2	5	0

[a] Note that salad dressing and cream cheese are being used as examples. The products chosen are simply representative products from these food categories. Not all products within the same food product category have the same ingredients or nutrition information.

[b] Listed in order ingredients appear on the ingredient list.

taste, but its downside is loss of sweetness in solution over time. It is predicted that as more sweeteners are approved for use in additional food and beverage categories and more sweeteners approved for use in the United States, more blends will be used. Also, since The NutraSweet Company's U.S. patent on aspartame expired in December 1992, there has been an increase in the blending of aspartame and acesulfame K. This blend has been used internationally for almost a decade.

Sweetener blends are currently seen in chewing gums, instant puddings, dairy shake mixes, and tabletop sweeteners in the United States. Blends in carbonated beverages and fruit drinks are quite popular in Europe and Canada and are expected to be introduced into the United States when more low-calorie sweeteners are approved for use in liquid beverages. Due to the concept of blending, the ideal sweetener blend can now be used rather than searching for the ideal single low-calorie sweetener.[18]

FDA'S REGULATORY REVIEW PROCESS FOR GENERALLY RECOGNIZED AS SAFE SUBSTANCES AND FOOD ADDITIVES

The FDA is responsible for the approval process of fat replacers. Never before have so many potential ingredients been undergoing FDA review. The regulations stipulating the safety review process have been in place for decades. An understanding of the FDA regulatory process and terminology is important to appreciate the FDA regulatory status of low-calorie sweetners and fat replacers.

Low-calorie sweeteners and fat replacers fall into two FDA designated categories, GRAS (generally recognized as safe) and food additive. The approval process for each differs. A detailed review of each process is available elsewhere.[19] Figures 20-1 and 20-2 are flow charts of the GRAS affirmation and food additive petition processes respectively. Briefly, the manufacturer, as well as the FDA, determine the appropriate regulatory process for the product. Saccharin is a GRAS substance, whereas aspartame and acesulfame K are food additives. Most fat replacers available today are GRAS substances.

GRAS approval is granted stipulating the food categories in which the fat replacer can be used. Approvals for food and beverage applications are granted based on those for which the manufacturer applied. An approval does not blanketly approve the use of a substance in any food and beverage. Companies have the option of petitioning for additional product applications after initial approval. The FDA might also require specific food and nutrition labeling guidelines. For example, foods containing a polyol require labeling about their potential laxative effect.

Accepted Daily Intake

A relatively new concept in food additive approvals is the designation of an accepted daily intake (ADI). ADIs have been established for acesulfame K (15 mg/kg body weight) and aspartame (50 mg/kg). In 1977, the National Academy of Sciences recommended limiting saccharin intake to 1 g/d. It is not a food additive and, therefore, does not have an ADI. To date, no fat replacer has been approved as a food additive, although Procter & Gamble has had a petition filed for olestra since 1986. The ADI represents the amount of a food additive that, even if consumed on a daily basis through a person's lifetime, is still considered safe by a 100-fold safety margin. It is not a toxic threshold, and even if an individual occasionally consumed a substance in amounts greater than the ADI, this would pose no health risk.

To calculate an individual's ADI, multiply the assigned ADI for a substance by body weight in kilograms (weight in pounds divided by 2.2). The following is an example using aspartame. One can of diet soda containing 100% aspartame has approximately 200 mg of aspartame. A 60-kg (132 lb) person needs to consume 15 12-oz cans of soda every day to reach the upper limit of the ADI for aspartame. Using packets of aspartame in this example (35 mg aspartame/packet), the person needs to consume 86 packets of the sweetener every day. (One packet of tabletop sweetener sweetened with 100% acesulfame K contains 50 mg of the sweetener; one packet with 100% saccharin contains 40 mg.)

The average amount of aspartame consumed has been monitored by the NutraSweet Company by FDA direction to ensure that safe limits are met. It has been found that the average aspartame consumption by the general population is 2 to 3 mg/kg per day or about 4% of the ADI.[20] It was found that people with diabetes consumed 2 to 4 mg/kg per day.[20]

The World Health Organization's Joint Expert Committee on Food Additives (JECFA) also reviews the safety of food additives and establishes ADIs. Nations that do not have their own FDA-type regulatory agency look to JECFA to sanction the safety of new food ingredients and to provide guidance on their use. Some JECFA and FDA ADIs are similar while others vary.

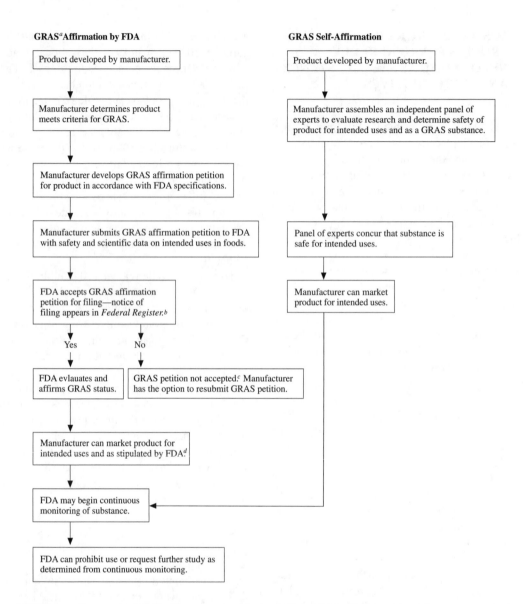

GRAS[a]**Affirmation by FDA**

- Product developed by manufacturer.
- Manufacturer determines product meets criteria for GRAS.
- Manufacturer develops GRAS affirmation petition for product in accordance with FDA specifications.
- Manufacturer submits GRAS affirmation petition to FDA with safety and scientific data on intended uses in foods.
- FDA accepts GRAS affirmation petition for filing—notice of filing appears in *Federal Register.*[b]

    Yes → FDA evlauates and affirms GRAS status.

    No → GRAS petition not accepted.[c] Manufacturer has the option to resubmit GRAS petition.

- Manufacturer can market product for intended uses and as stipulated by FDA.[d]
- FDA may begin continuous monitoring of substance.
- FDA can prohibit use or request further study as determined from continuous monitoring.

GRAS Self-Affirmation

- Product developed by manufacturer.
- Manufacturer assembles an independent panel of experts to evaluate research and determine safety of product for intended uses and as a GRAS substance.
- Panel of experts concur that substance is safe for intended uses.
- Manufacturer can market product for intended uses.

[a] GRAS, generally recognized as safe. There are two methods to achieve GRAS affirmation. Presently, most companies use the FDA route. Some companies choose to use both the FDA and GRAS self-affirmation processes to assure product safety. In addition, FDA can affirm GRAS status of a substance on its own initiative.

[b] Once FDA accepts GRAS Affirmation Petition for filing they have completed an initial evaluation. Unlike with a food additive, the manufacturer can at this point make the decision to market the product for its intended use. However, the manufacturer runs the remote risk of FDA regulatory action.

[c] Manufacturer informed that substance is categorized as food additive and must go through FDA food additive approval.

[d] FDA may stipulate approval conditions. For example, certain labeling requirements.

Figure 20-1 The Process of a GRAS Petition/Review. *Source*: Reprinted with permission from Powers MA, Warshaw HS. Fat Replacers: A Wide Range of Choices. *Diabetes Spectrum*. 1992;5(2):76. Copyright ©1992, American Diabetes Association.

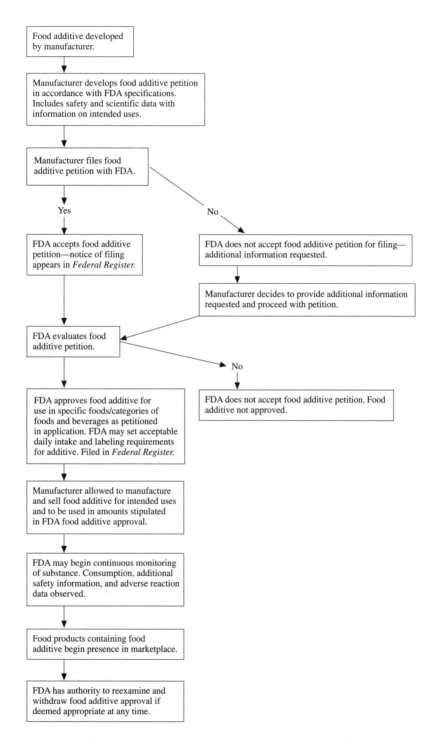

Figure 20-2 The Process of a Food Additive Petition. *Source*: Reprinted with permission from Powers MA, Warshaw HS. Fat Replacers: A Wide Range of Choices. *Diabetes Spectrum.* 1992;5(2):76 Copyright © 1992, American Diabetes Association.

Food Label Requirements

In the approval statement that FDA issues regarding a food additive or a GRAS substance, informational or warning label statements may be mandated. Products containing aspartame must carry the following label "Phenylketonurics: contains phenylalanine." This is necessary for those with phenylketonuria (PKU). Products with saccharin carry a warning label stating "Use of this product may be hazardous to your health. This product contains saccharin, which has been determined to cause cancer in laboratory animals." Saccharin's label must also state the amount of saccharin in the food or beverage. Other labeling requirements, such as what descriptors are used to define a product, health claims, and what must be in the Nutrition Facts box must be followed for products containing low-calorie sweeteners or fat replacers. These are mandated by the 1990 Nutrition Labeling and Education Act (NLEA) implemented in May 1994[21] (see Chapter 22).

The FDA has no special food labeling requirements for products containing fat replacers other than those set forth by the NLEA. Manufacturers are not required to provide any information on the package stating that an ingredient is a fat replacer. Because fat replacers are not designated as such on the ingredient list, most consumers are unaware of what ingredients are fat replacers. Fat replacers might appear as modified corn starch or maltodextrin. By contrast, most consumers know the names of the currently available low-calorie sweeteners and can identify them.

CURRENTLY APPROVED LOW-CALORIE SWEETENERS

The following reviews the current status of the three low-calorie sweeteners currently approved for use in the United States—acesulfame potassium, aspartame, and saccharin—and low-calorie sweeteners with approval or reapproval pending—alitame, cyclamate, and sucralose. Their sweetness in comparison to sucrose is identified in Exhibit 20-2.

Acesulfame Potassium

Description and Uses

Acesulfame potassium (acesulfame K or ace-K) was approved for use in Europe in 1983 and is currently used in more than 3000 products in more than 70 countries around the world. It received FDA approval in 1987 for use in tabletop sweeteners, chewing gums, dry beverage bases, and dry bases for gelatins, puddings, and dairy product analogs.[22] Approval for use in confections (hard and soft candies) was granted in 1993[23] after the FDA altered its decree that low-calorie sweeteners could not be used in confections.[24] Baked goods, refrigerated and frozen desserts, and syrups were approved in 1994.[25] Petitions for other uses including nonalcoholic beverages are pending. It is approved for use in carbonated and noncarbonated sodas and juices and many other food categories in Europe and Canada.

Acesulfame K was discovered in 1967 at Hoechst AG in Germany. It is the potassium salt of an organic substance. Acesulfame K is marketed as Sunett to the food industry by Hoechst Food Ingredients. Hoechst does not produce any foods or the tabletop sweeteners with acesulfame K; other companies purchase the ingredient and manufacture and market the final products.

Applications

Acesulfame K is 200 times sweeter than sucrose, is heat stable, and blends well with other nutritive and nonnutritive sweeteners. Its taste is readily perceptible and described as clean and sweet, with no lingering aftertaste. These attributes contribute to its success in blending with other sweeteners in a variety of food products and beverages. Because it is heat-stable, acesulfame K has been termed the "sweetener you can cook with." Some consumers find that when too much is used, a bitter taste is perceptible.

Exhibit 20-2 Sweetness Intensity of Low-Calorie Sweeteners

Low Calorie Substitute	Sweetness[a]
Currently available in the United States	
Acesulfame K	200
Aspartame	180–220
Saccharin	300–500
Mannitol	0.5
Sorbitol	0.54–0.7
Xylitol	1
Crystalline fructose	1.2–1.8
Glycyrrhizin[b]	50–100
Thaumatin[b]	2000–3000
Under development or regulatory review in the United States	
Alitame	2900
Cyclamate	30
Hydrogenated starch hydrolysates	0.7–0.9
Isomalt	0.45–0.65
Lactitol	0.4
L-sugars	<1
Maltitol	0.85–0.95
Steviosiol	800
Sucralose	600

[a] The sweetness value indicated is an approximation relative to an approximate sweetness index for sucrose of 1.

[b] Approved for use in the United States as a flavorant and outside the United States as a sweetener.

Source: Data from Newsome R. Sugar substitutes. In Altschul AM, ed. *Low Calorie Foods Handbook.* New York: Marcel Dekker; 1993:139–170.

Metabolism

Metabolism studies using both humans and animals have shown that acesulfame K is not metabolized nor does it accumulate in the body. It is rapidly absorbed into the blood after ingestion and rapidly eliminated unchanged in the urine. Because it is not metabolized, it has no caloric value. It has been shown to have no effect on blood glucose, cholesterol, total glycerol, or free glycerol levels.[26]

Safety

No safety concerns have been raised about acesulfame K. It has been tested with animals from conception through their normal lifespan, and then their offspring.[27] No adverse effects were documented even at administered doses 1000s of times higher than anticipated maximum dietary intake by humans. It has been deemed safe for all segments of the population.[3,4]

The amount of potassium in the sweetener is insignificant when compared with amounts in other foods. In one packet of the sweetener, equivalent to the sweetness of 2 teaspoons of sugar, there are only 10 mg of potassium. A medium-sized banana contains 440 mg, and an orange 263 mg.

For those individuals who are allergic to sulfites or sulfa drugs, it is not expected that the sweetener will produce any allergic reactions based on a broad range of safety studies and human experience over the past two decades. The sulfur atom in acesulfame K is not related to sulfites or to sulfa drugs in line with the expectation and experience that an allergic response would not occur.

Aspartame

Description and Uses

Aspartame is a synthetic substance composed of two amino acids (dipeptide), aspartic acid and phenylalanine. It contains 4 calories/g, but because it is 180 to 200 times sweeter than sucrose, it provides very few calories. The NutraSweet Company held the patent for aspartame in the United States until December 1992. Today, other manufacturers, including Holland Sweeteners, sell it to American companies. Aspartame is approved for use in more than 100 countries and in more than 5000 products. Aspartame was responsible for more new products in the 1980s than any other new ingredient.[28]

Aspartame was discovered in 1965 and approved by the FDA as a tabletop sweetener in July 1974.[29] During the review process, formal objections were received by the FDA that required additional review. Seven years later, in July 1981, the FDA Commissioner's Final Decision allowed the use of aspartame in dry food products including tabletop sweeteners and gums.[30,31] In July 1983, aspartame was approved for use in carbonated beverages.[32] Since then, aspartame has received approval for use in many other food categories including the April 1993 approval for use in commercial baked goods and baking mixes.[33] Because aspartame is not stable under extreme temperatures of long duration, some of these applications use an encapsulated form of aspartame, which releases the sweetener during the baking process. The NutraSweet Company has one petition pending with the FDA. It requests approval for aspartame as a general-purpose sweetener and flavor enhancer. This would eliminate the need for future approvals in individual categories.

Applications

Aspartame has a slow onset of a sweet taste that sustains itself over time. It is stable in dry foods but decomposes on prolonged exposure to high temperatures or in liquid form. The stability in liquids was carefully evaluated before the July 1983 approval for use in carbonated beverages.[33] Carbonated beverages stored for 8 weeks at 68°F lost 11 to 16% of their original aspartame. When stored at a higher temperature, 86°F, for 8 weeks, more aspartame (38%) was degraded. The FDA concluded that "although this lack of stability might result in a marginally acceptable product, it would not lead to an unsafe product."[34] There was concern that, when aspartame was exposed to high temperatures, high pH, and a liquid medium, methanol, as a by-product of aspartame breakdown, would accumulate to toxic doses. The amount of methanol potentially available from 1 L of beverage sweetened with aspartame is 58 mg, which is about one-third of the average level found in a similar amount of fruit juice.[34] It has been reported that the methanol content of fruit juices ranges from 12 to 640 mg/L, with an average of 140 mg/L.[35] Some alcoholic beverages have been found to have as much as 1.5 g/L.[34] The amount of methanol available after aspartame ingestion can be estimated at 10% of the weight of the aspartame.[34]

Metabolism

Aspartame is metabolized in the gastrointestinal tract to aspartic acid, phenylalanine, and methanol. The aspartic acid is primarily used for energy through conversion to CO_2 in the Krebs cycle. The phenylalanine is primarily incorporated into body protein, either unchanged or as tyrosine. The methyl group is hydrolyzed by intestinal esterases to methanol.

The metabolism of aspartame is the same as that of its equivalent natural components. The individual components are rapidly metabolized and do not accumulate at recommended intakes.[36] It would be extremely difficult to consume amounts large enough to accumulate to toxic levels because the body continuously clears the by-products from the system.[37,38]

Nehrling et al[37] evaluated the effect of aspartame on blood glucose control and concluded that 2.7 g/d of aspartame does not affect blood glucose control. An interesting finding was that the aspartame group in this study reported four adverse reactions to their capsule, whereas the placebo group reported 15 adverse reactions.

Safety

The safety of aspartame has been questioned for a variety of reasons, including methanol accumulation,[38] brain damage,[39] mental retardation, and endocrine dysfunction.[40] The FDA addressed these concerns before approval and, after subsequent questioning, found them unfounded and deemed the sweetener safe for the general population, including pregnant women and children.[41] After continued questions, the FDA requested that the Centers for Disease Control (CDC) conduct an evaluation of consumer complaints related to aspartame ingestion. After investigators spoke to 517 of 592 persons reporting complaints, the CDC reported that the data "do not provide for the existence of serious widespread, adverse health consequences."[42] The CDC did state, however, that some individuals may have an "unusual sensitivity" to aspartame. In regard to methanol accumulation, no measurable blood levels of methanol (at intakes of 34 mg/kg) or changes in blood formate levels (at intakes of 200 mg/kg) were seen.[43] Methanol levels returned to normal within 24 hours after the larger doses. Formate has been evaluated because methanol is metabolized to formaldehyde, which is converted to formic acid (formate). Brain damage, mental retardation, and endocrine dysfunction have been issues because of aspartame's similar structure to glutamate, which has been shown to cause neurotoxicity. Also, phenylalanine has been linked to behavioral changes when a high-carbohydrate–aspartame diet is ingested.[44] Persons who do not tolerate phenylalanine should avoid aspartame-containing products. More than half of aspartame is phenylalanine. The FDA has concluded that there is no evidence for concern regarding any of these issues, although various groups continue to raise them. Anyone who experiences an adverse reaction to aspartame should document the reaction and discuss it with his or her health care provider(s).

Saccharin

Description and Uses

Saccharin is a white, crystalline powder synthesized from toluene. It is approximately 300 times sweeter than sucrose. Its sole producer in the United States is PMC Specialties Group. It is available in three forms: sodium salt (most commonly used), calcium salt, and the acid form.

Saccharin was discovered accidentally in 1879 by a Johns Hopkins University scientist. An early use of saccharin was as a substitute for sugar in canned vegetables and beverages that were subject to heat damage caused by a lack of refrigeration. During World War I and II, saccharin use increased because of sugar rationing.

In 1972, saccharin was removed from the GRAS list because of its potential link to bladder cancer. (This occurred 2 years after cyclamate was removed.) At that time the FDA concluded that the "continued limited use of saccharin did not constitute a significant risk to public health."[45] This conclusion referred to the 1955 and 1968 statements by the Committee on Food

Protection of the National Academy of Sciences that 1 g/d of saccharin should pose no hazard to an adult. In March 1977, the FDA and the Health Protection Branch in Canada proposed bans on saccharin.

Public hearings across the United States were held to give the consumer a chance to react to the proposed ban. A campaign, spearheaded by the American Diabetes Association and the Juvenile Diabetes Foundation to keep saccharin available for use by persons with diabetes, helped make possible the eventual decision in November 1977 of an 18-month moratorium on the ban. The U.S. Congress repeatedly extended the moratorium in 1979, 1981, 1983, 1985, and 1987, which allowed for saccharin's continued availability. In 1992, the FDA withdrew its proposal to ban saccharin.

Applications

Saccharin continues to be a popular tabletop sweetener despite many claims that it has a bitter aftertaste. Some consumers prefer one of the few available canned, carbonated sodas that does contain saccharin (Tab™) and low-calorie fountain sodas that also contain some saccharin.

Saccharin is only slightly soluble in water and is stable under many conditions. It is synergistic with other sweeteners, such as aspartame. The continued use of saccharin is due at least in part to its long shelf life, low price, and thermal stability.

Metabolism

Saccharin is not metabolized and is excreted unchanged, primarily by the kidneys in the urine.[46]

Safety

The 1977 proposed ban on saccharin was based on research that showed that saccharin caused malignant bladder tumors in second-generation male rats. Since then there has been intensive review of the research protocol, as well as the wording of the Delaney Clause. It has been stated that the saccharin used in the research was impure and that the research design caused the results to be incorrectly interpreted. A retrospective study of persons admitted to 65 hospitals with a primary neoplasm of the lower urinary tract suggested that "as a group, users of artificial sweeteners have little or no excess risk of cancer of the lower urinary tract."[47] In that study, the term artificial sweeteners was used to mean saccharin and cyclamates because both sweeteners were primarily used together until the ban on cyclamates. In 1985, the American Medical Association reviewed experimental data and reaffirmed its stand that saccharin should continue to be available as a food additive.[48] Both the American Dietetic Association and the American Diabetes Association have stated it poses no health hazard.[3,4]

Use of Sweeteners during Pregnancy

The use of low-calorie sweeteners in pregnancy continues to be an issue for some. The most recent position of the American Diabetes Association[3] states that there is no evidence to be concerned about the consumption of the three approved low-calorie sweeteners during pregnancy. The American Dietetic Association acknowledges the safety of aspartame and acesulfame K. However, it notes that some individuals may wish to refrain from consuming saccharin because it does cross the placenta, although no reports of adverse effects exist.[4] Dietitians should be sensitive to hesitations and concerns of pregnant women or other health team members about the use of low-calorie sweeteners during pregnancy; however, they should provide these individuals with the scientifically correct information.

SWEETENERS PENDING FDA APPROVAL

Alitame

Pfizer, Inc. submitted a petition in 1986 for FDA approval of alitame in 16 food categories.[49] The sweetener is a dipeptide-based amide formed from l-aspartic acid and d-alanine. It is reported to have a sweet taste similar to sucrose and is 2000 times as sweet as sucrose. It is stable at high temperatures and over a broad pH range and less stable in lower ranges (acids). It can be used in a wide variety of products including sodas, fruit drinks, baked goods, confections, and tabletop sweeteners.[50]

Alitame is metabolized to its two proteins and other components. The amino acids are metabolized and the remainder excreted unchanged. Alitame is approved for use in Australia (1993), China, Mexico, and New Zealand (1994).

Cyclamate

Cyclamate, a derivative of cyclohexylsulfamic acid, is produced by Abbott Laboratories and is 30 times sweeter than sucrose. It was discovered in 1937 at the University of Illinois but was not introduced into foods until the early 1950s. It was often used in combination with saccharin in a 10:1 blend; saccharin was the smaller portion because it is approximately ten times sweeter than cyclamate.

In 1969, the FDA removed it from the GRAS list and proposed phasing it out of general food use. In 1970, the FDA imposed a ban on all uses of cyclamates because of several studies that indicated it caused cancer in test animals. In 1973, Abbott Laboratories sought permission to remarket the sweetener by submitting 400 toxicologic reports that were completed after 1970. This petition was turned down in September 1980. Abbott Laboratories and the Calorie Control Council repetitioned in 1982 and continue to wait for a response. The current petition requests approval for use of cyclamates in a variety of beverages and food products and as a tabletop sweetener, with a daily intake limit of 1.5 g.[51]

It would be used in combination with other sweeteners because it enhances the sweetness of other sweeteners, is heat stable, mitigates the bitter aftertaste of saccharin when saccharin is the second sweetener, increases the product's stability or shelf life, and usually reduces product cost.[52] Although not available in the United States, cyclamate is presently marketed in more than 50 countries. In Canada, it is allowed in tabletop sweeteners and in pharmaceuticals.

Metabolism and Safety

Cyclamate is metabolized in the digestive tract, and its by-products are secreted by the kidneys. Its primary metabolite is cyclohexylamine, which some scientists believe may be more toxic than cyclamate. Cyclohexylamine is formed from the nonabsorbed cyclamate by bacteria in the gastrointestinal tract. Not all persons are able to metabolize cyclamate and those that do only metabolize a portion of what is consumed.[53] It has been shown that cyclamate has no significant effect on blood glucose.[52]

Cyclamate was removed from the GRAS list in 1969 because bladder tumors developed in rats fed a mixture of cyclamate and saccharin.[54] Abbott's 1982 request, with additional research, was reviewed by the FDA Cancer Assessment Committee.[51] The committee concluded that evidence did not show cyclamate or cyclohexylamine was a cancer-causing agent.[55] The FDA asked the National Academy of Sciences/National Research Council to conduct an independent review of the data. Their report was submitted in January 1985 and also concluded that cyclamate is not a carcinogen.[56] The FDA followed up the NAS suggestion that cyclamate might be a promoter of cancer. An additional report concluded that concept or promotion studies are unsuitable for predicting human carcinogen risk.[57] The FDA continues to review data for other safety issues in addition to carcinogenicity (ie, genetic damage and testicular atrophy).[58] The safety of cyclamate for human use, however, has been supported.[59]

Sucralose

Sucralose is 600 times as sweet as sucrose and was discovered in 1976. It is made from sugar by selectively substituting three chlorine atoms for three hydroxyl groups on the sugar molecule. It has a similar taste profile to sugar with no unpleasant aftertaste and has no calories. It is stable in solutions and at varying pH levels and temperatures. It can be used in cooking and baking. McNeil Specialty Products Company, a Johnson & Johnson company, filed a food additive petition with FDA in 1987 for the use of sucralose in 15 food and beverage categories.[60] This petition is currently under review.

Sucralose is essentially nonmetabolized. It passes rapidly through the body without being broken down. It is not digested in the gastrointestinal tract and only a small amount (about 15% of that ingested) is absorbed through the small intestine. The remainder passes through the digestive system unchanged and is excreted in the feces. Sucralose does not accumulate in any tissues and is not actively transported across the blood-brain barrier to the central nervous system, across the placental barrier, or from the mammary gland into breast milk.[61]

The safety of sucralose was tested and evaluated in more than 100 studies conducted over 18 years.[62] These studies indicate that sucralose can be used safely by everyone, including pregnant and lactating women, children, and persons with type I and type II diabetes.[63] Also, sucralose does not promote tooth decay.[64]

Sucralose has been permitted for use as a food additive in Canada (1992), in Australia (1993), and in Mexico (1994). It is marketed in several countries under the Splenda® brand name.

LOW-CALORIE SWEETENERS UNDER DEVELOPMENT

L-Sugars

L-sugars are mirror images of their "sugar" counterpart and sometimes called left-handed sugars. They are not metabolized and are excreted unchanged, yet provide the sweetness of their counterpart. An additional benefit is that they provide the same bulking properties of their counterpart.

Glycosides

Glycosides are naturally occurring sweet compounds that have been used throughout the world and potentially could be available in the

United States. Stevioside, for example, is 300 times sweeter than sucrose. It is an extract from the leaves of a South American shrub and is approved for use in Japan. Toxicity studies are needed before the FDA can consider its safety.

Glycyrrhizen, also a glycoside, is found in the roots of an Asian and European shrub and is commonly known as licorice. It is 50 to 100 times sweeter than sucrose. Glycyrrhizen has been used as a flavoring in tobacco, root beer, vanilla, and liqueurs and as a foaming agent in soft drinks. It is approved as a natural flavoring on the GRAS list but does not have approval as a low-calorie sweetener.

FAT REPLACERS—THREE CATEGORIES

Fat replacers can be divided into three general categories—carbohydrate-, protein-, and fat-based. Carbohydrate-based fat replacers are currently the most commonly used. Fewer protein and fat-based fat replacers currently exist; however, according to the food technology literature, many more will be developed and approved in the future.[19] It is estimated that fat replacers could potentially replace over 13 billion pounds of traditional fats and oils annually.[65] Product characteristics for the various fat replacers are contained in Table 20-2. Expanded tables are available elsewhere.[19,66]

Carbohydrate-Based Fat Replacers

There are two main categories of carbohydrate-based fat replacers: (1) carbohydrate polymers and (2) polyalcohols.

Carbohydrate Polymers (Modified Food Starches)

These can be collectively referred to as hydrocolloids or water-soluble carbohydrate polymers such as gums, starches, and maltodextrins.[67] This category of carbohydrate-based fat replacers is derived mainly from tapioca, corn, potato, and rice starches. Examples of how they might be listed on a food label are given in Table 20-2.

Complex Carbohydrates. Modified starches provide gelling and thickening properties and are often found in salad dressings, frozen desserts, and baked goods. These hydrocolloids hold three times their weight in water, which adds a "thickness" to a food product.[68]

Gums, Gels, Fiber. Gums, namely, guar, pectin, and xanthan gum, are the oldest fat replacers. Gums assist in replacing fat by acting as stabilizers and emulsifiers and providing structure. These products generally contain 0 to 4 calories/g. Common products with gums and gels are low-fat or fat-free frozen desserts, salad dressings, and yogurts.

Fruit-Based Fat Replacers. Fruit as a fat replacer has been promoted to consumers for use in cooking and baking. Both applesauce and pureed prunes offer bulk and flavor to baked goods in which the fat has been reduced. Fat is reduced, but calories may remain the same due to the needed increase in carbohydrate.[69] This alters the food's impact on blood glucose. The additional carbohydrate and decreased fat foods must be appropriately accounted for in the meal plan.

Polyalcohols/Bulking Ingredients

Sugar alcohols (polyalcohols, polyols) and hydrogenated starch hydrolysates (HSH) fall into this category. They are derived by modifying simple carbohydrates such as sucrose, dextrose, or corn syrup, and contain from 1.6 to 3.0 calories/g because they are only partially metabolized.[70] They provide bulk or volume with a range of sweetness from 40 to 80% of the sweetness of sucrose. They are the ingredients that add volume to the low-calorie sweeteners in some products.

These ingredients can be designed to meet a food's particular needs depending on the originating sugar, the length of the final polymer, and the amount of hydrogen added.

Beyond their functions as bulking ingredients, polyols help replace fat by acting as humectants, meaning they assist in retaining moisture, and texturizers. Reduced-fat foods with these ingredients are ready-to-eat gelatins and puddings, candies (diet), and frozen dairy desserts. The FDA labeling guidelines written in the Code of Federal Regulations stipulate that foods containing certain amounts of bulking ingredients must note that excess consumption may have a laxative effect.[71] Diabetes educators have recognized the need to educate clients about the laxative effect of these ingredients. Because of their increased use today, it is more important to mention this potential. Further discussion of bulking ingredients and sugar alcohols is in Chapter 16 on carbohydrates.

Protein-Based Fat Replacers

Protein-based fat replacers have only been available since 1990, when the NutraSweet Company's product, Simplesse, was given GRAS status by the FDA for use in frozen desserts. Protein-based fat replacements are usually derived from milk, egg, and whey proteins. Individuals with egg and/or cow's milk allergies are likely to have an allergic reaction to foods that contain fat replacers based on egg or cow's milk.[72] The process of microparticulation is one technology for creating these fat replacers. The protein is heated and blended or "sheared" at extremely high temperatures, resulting in microscopic particles. When incorporated into foods, these particles provide the creamy feel of fat without the calories of fat. Protein-based fat replacers have 1 to 5 calories/g versus 9 calories/g for fat. In 1991, the FDA's second GRAS affirmation for Simplesse allowed its use in sour cream, cheese, salad dressings, and several other products. Kraft General Food's product, Trailblazer, is another microparticulated protein that received GRAS approval.[73] Specific product information is in Table 20-2.

Fat-Based Fat Replacers

Currently available fat-based fat replacers are emulsifiers such as the familiar mono- and diglycerides. These emulsifiers can replace up to 50% of the fat in some foods by acting as surface active molecules.[74] Other fat-based fat replacers are quite different, and this group represents the largest potential growth area.[75] Many major food companies hold or are obtaining patents for synthetic fat replacers or oils with hopes for the future; however, none are presently approved for use. The FDA will consider synthetic fats as food additives.[75] Due to their ability to withstand heat, some will be able to be used virtually anywhere that processed fats and oils are used today, such as fried snack foods and commercial and home frying.

Olestra (Olean™) is the only synthetic oil for which a food additive petition has been submitted to the FDA. The proposal, submitted in 1987, has not yet received approval. Olestra has a sucrose core with six to eight fatty acid side chains. Because olestra passes through the digestive tract unchanged, it provides no calories. The revised FDA food additive petition submitted by Procter & Gamble, olestra's manufacturer, is for use as 100% fat replacer in fried snack foods. Because the approval of olestra has taken so long, Congress recently granted a patent extension to Procter & Gamble. The patent extension expires if FDA approval is not granted by January 1996.[76]

Caprenin, manufactured by Procter & Gamble and defined as a structured lipid,[74] has received GRAS approval for use in soft candy and confectionery coatings. Caprenin is categorized as a reduced-calorie triglyceride with a glycerol core composed of the fatty acids caprylic (C8), capric (C10), and behenic (C22). Behenic acid is only partially absorbed and therefore the calories derived from caprenin are only 5 calories/g rather than the usual 9 calories/g for fat.[74]

Research

There is little research on the effects of fat replacers on blood glucose, lipids, and weight as individual foods, within mixed meals, and over time. This is because most are derived from common foods and are not food additives. The most documented research has been done on

Table 20-2 Fat Replacers: How To Identify, Their Use in Foods, and Regulatory Status

Category of Fat Replacer	Examples of Trade Names	Examples of How Identified on Food Label	Types of Food Used In	Examples of Role in Foods and Calorie Content	Regulatory Status
Carbohydrate-based Complex carbohydrates	Maltrin, Lycadex, Paselli SA2, Stellar N-Oil, Sta-Slim Oatrim	Maltodextrin, corn syrup solids, hydrolyzed corn starch, modified food starch	Frozen desserts, cheese, baked goods, sauces, dressings, sour cream, yogurt, baked bread, meats and poultry, cheese	Gelling, thickening, stabilizing, increasing shelf-life, antistaling, adds creaminess and texture; decrease calories, 1 calorie/g when hydrated in product	GRAS approval
Simple carbohydrates/bulking ingredients	Lycasin, Hystar, Neosorb, Litesse	Hydrogenated starch hydrolysate (HSH), hydrogenated glucose syrup, sorbitol, polydextrose, maltitol syrup	Baked goods, confections, chewing gum, frozen dairy desserts, gelatins, puddings, sauces, salad dressings, meat-based products	Adds bulk, aids in retaining moisture, texturizer, lowers freezing point, inhibits crystallization; decreases calories compared to fat—1 to 4 cal/g	GRAS approval; polydextrose approved as food additive
Gums, gels, fiber	Splendid, Viscarin, Sactarin, Gelcarin, Fibrex, Avicel Novagel, Rohodigel, Uniguar, Pycol, Jaquar	Pectin, carrageenan, sugar beet fiber or powder, cellulose gel, locus bean gum, xanthan gum, guar gum	Yogurt, sour cream, salad dressings, bakery products, frozen desserts, cheese spreads, sauces	Binds water, texturizer, thickener, stabilizer, provides mouth-feel of fat; decreases calories—0 to 0.5 calorie/g	GRAS approval
Protein-based	Simplesse, Trailblazer, Lita, Dairy-lo, Veri-lo	Microparticulated egg white and milk protein; whey protein concentrate	Cheese, butter, mayonnaise, salad dressings, sour cream, bakery products, spreads	Provides mouth-feel of fat, cannot be used in fried foods; 1.3 calories/g, ingredients being developed may have higher calories	GRAS approval

Table 20-2 continued

Category of Fat Replacer	Examples of Trade Names	Examples of How Identified on Food Label	Types of Food Used In	Examples of Role in Foods and Calorie Content	Regulatory Status
Fat-based	Caprenin, Olean, Salatrim, all emulsifiers (eg, polyglycer-olesters)	Caprenin; olestra; others being developed not yet deter-mined as to listing	Caprenin, soft candy and confectionery coatings Olestra, pending approval, fried snack foods	Act very similar as "fat," provides creamy texture; Caprenin and Salatrim have 5 calories/g due to decreased absorption, others being developed may have 0 calories due to not being metabolized and they have potential to be used in fried foods	GRAS or food additive approval

Source: Warshaw HS, Franz MJ, Powers MA, Wheeler ML. Fat replacers and their use in foods (technical review). *Diabetes Care*. In press.

olestra[77] and its review can be found elsewhere.[68] Research has centered around gastrointestinal transit time (no effect) and the absorption of fat-soluble vitamins (slight decrease in vitamin A and E).

A study was conducted to determine the metabolic response of a carbohydrate-based bulking agent, HSH, compared with dietary glucose in individuals with and without diabetes.[78] The HSH resulted in decreased glycemia compared with dietary glucose in both populations.

Until more research is conducted, dietitians should encourage clients to use self-monitoring of blood glucose (SMBG) as a tool to determine the effect of these new foods on blood glucose levels. Adding one new food at a time provides the most valuable information and documents the effect of the food for future reference. This type of anecdotal information should also be shared among diabetes educators.

Controlling blood lipids has become an equally important goal to controlling blood glu-cose in an effort to prevent and delay diabetes complications.[3] Therefore, working with clients to reduce total fat and saturated fat intake is a critical part of their diabetes education. Foods with fat replacers may provide clients needed resources to assist them in controlling blood lipids.

GENERAL BENEFITS OF NUTRITION CONSCIOUS FOODS

An important question receiving research attention is whether the use of foods with low-calorie sweeteners and fat replacers actually lower dietary fat and sugar intake, assist with weight loss, and improve other health indicators such as improving glycated hemoglobin and blood lipid profile.

Manufacturers of these foods have used food consumption study figures to project that the use of the new foods will decrease fat and calorie in-take.[5] Unfortunately, recent studies indicate the simple projection analyses do not consider human variables. Several research studies demonstrate that when human subjects are covertly fed fat substitutes, they compensate for dilutions in food energy by increasing energy from other sources.[10,11,79] Rolls et al[11] replaced three different amounts of fat with olestra at the breakfast meal of 24 lean men between 20 and 30 years old. Lunch and dinner were self-selected ad libitum. The results demonstrated a decrease in total fat intake, although carbohydrate intake was increased to provide the missing calories. Total daily calorie intake did not change. The point has been made that the change in macronutrient content of the diet (more carbohydrate and less

---

Exhibit 20-3 Educational Concepts That Relate to the Use of Fat Replacers

Nutrition Therapy Topic	*Concept(s) To Include about Fat Replacers*
1. Consistency in food intake (might be carbohydrate or calorie amounts, number of servings of a food group, etc)	1. Reduced-fat foods may have a higher carbohydrate content.
2. Descriptors on food label	2. Descriptors highlight need to read nutrition facts section of label (total grams fat, carbohydrate). Descriptors include reduced fat; low fat; fat free. *Note:* This does not mean calorie-free.
3. Nutrition facts on food label	3. Compare similar foods with varying amounts of fat to see variation (eg, salad dressings). Total the calories, and fat and carbohydrate grams for a meal or a day and document difference. Discuss impact on nutrition therapy goals for diabetes control, if any.
4. Food impact on blood glucose	4. To measure the impact of a particular food or meal that includes foods with fat replacers, consume a standard meal for 2 to 3 days documenting blood glucose before and after. Then consume the adjusted meal and document blood glucose at same times. Keep other daily activities similar. Record results. Discuss with dietitian.
5. Recommending inclusion or exclusion of specific foods	5. All patients should be clear on their diabetes nutrition therapy goals related to blood glucose, glycated hemoglobin, lipids, and weight. The adjusted food may be a positive inclusion food yet may contribute to other changes in food consumption that are detrimental. For example, if one scoop of reduced-fat ice cream is included, does that lead to actually consuming two scoops because it is reduced fat? Some foods are best avoided. Some foods require greater health team involvement to ensure accurate inclusion. This is an individualized recommendation.
6. Portion control	6. Such foods can be useful when included into an individual's food plan. This means portion control is important. Patients should know what portions are appropriate for their use. Most of these foods are not calorie-free.

Exhibit 20-4 Creative Strategies for Education about Low-Calorie Sweeteners and Fat Replacers

1. Develop a collection of food products/labels; create a professional "garbage collection"; display prominently and use when educating about specific product, fat replacement/ingredient, or food and nutrition labeling.

2. Create a notebook of product labels (especially if educational materials must be transported); laminate labels for preservation; provide notebook to clients overnight (if inpatient); keep in waiting room or office.

3. Do computer nutrient calculations for various foods, demonstrating the percentage of calories as carbohydrate, protein, fat, and nutrition comparisons (include with information on products in above notebook).

4. Request that clients bring in food and nutrition labels from products in question.

5. Make a notebook of clippings about new foods—use newspaper articles, newsletter information (Tufts Diet and Nutrition Letter, Environmental Nutrition, Supermarket Scoop, Supermarket Smarts column from Diabetes Self Management, New Products column from Diabetes Care and Education Newsletter).

6. Develop a handout listing new foods and how they fit into meal planning (eg, exchanges, carbohydrate counting, or USDA Food Guide Pyramid).

7. Create a bulletin board dedicated to sharing information about new food products.

8. Conduct food tastings for clients and staff to try new products or to introduce clients to desirable products (eg, fat-free salad dressing tasting using slices of cucumber, low-sugar jelly or fruit spreads using crackers); provide nutrient and/or exchange information and suggested uses/recipes.

9. Contact food manufacturers to request sample products, information, or coupons (or obtain at professional meetings).

10. Conduct seminars on food and nutrition labeling, new products, and rules of thumb for their use (incorporate tastings); use this format as a way to celebrate National Diabetes Month (November); Diabetes Alert Day (March); Diabetes Educator Week (November); National Nutrition Month (March).

11. Conduct supermarket tours or obtain information/brochures from dietitians who do tours; encourage clients to attend.

12. If you produce a newsletter, include a new products column—profile several new foods, or a category of new food products.

fat) may be beneficial even though total calorie intake remains the same.

Mela[80] notes that most of these studies manipulate the diet in a covert fashion. Mela surmises that lowering fat and calorie intake might be facilitated by consumer knowledge of the manipulation. A feasibility study from the Women's Health Trial to research the effect of a low-fat diet in the prevention of breast cancer found that women had an easier time maintaining the long-term behavior change of substituting specially manufactured low-fat foods versus lowering fat intake from fats and meats.[81] A small amount of weight loss was reported by

Kanders et al[82] with the inclusion of aspartame-sweetened foods in a weight loss program.

EDUCATIONAL POINTS AND CREATIVE STRATEGIES

Food and nutrition labeling has assisted the person with diabetes in identifying the amount of carbohydrate and fat grams in a particular food. Educational concepts about fat replacers that require review and integration into the client's education plan are identified in Exhibit 20-3. Similar concepts relate to the use of low-calorie sweeteners. Exhibit 20-4 lists creative strategies to provide this self-management training to clients. The recommendations to use these foods should be based on an individual's food pattern and preferences as well as diabetes status and nutrition goals. The impact of various foods on blood glucose control should be checked with SMBG.

It is important for diabetes nutrition educators to keep abreast of new food ingredients and products. Suggestions include reading food technology literature, keeping in contact with the food manufacturers, routinely reviewing labels and ingredient lists of new foods, and determining their impact on glycemic, lipid, and weight levels of clients.

REFERENCES

1. Department of Health and Human Services. *Healthy People 2000: National Health Promotion and Disease Prevention Objectives*. Washington, DC: U.S. Government Printing Office; 1990.

2. U.S. Department of Agriculture and U.S. Department of Health and Human Services. *Dietary Guidelines for Americans*. 3rd ed. Washington, DC: US Government Printing Office; 1990. Home and Garden Bulletin no. 232.

3. American Diabetes Association. Position statement: nutrition recommendations and principles for people with diabetes mellitus. *Diabetes Care*. 1994;17(5):519–522.

4. American Dietetic Association. Position Statement. Use of nutritive and non-nutritive sweeteners. *J Am Diet Assoc*. 1993;93(7):816–820.

5. American Dietetic Association. Position statement: fat replacements. *J Am Diet Assoc*. 1991;91(10):1285–1288.

6. American Diabetes Association. Position statement: fat replacers and their use in foods. *Diabetes Care*. In press.

7. Economic Research Service. Sugar and sweeteners. In: *Situation and Outlook Report*. Washington, DC: Department of Agriculture; 1991. Publication no. SSRVI6N4.

8. U.S. Department of Agriculture, Human Nutrition Information Service. *Nationwide Food Consumption Survey: Continuing Survey of Food Intakes by Individuals*. Hyattsville, Md: USDA; 1985. USDA Report nos. 85 and 85-2.

9. National Center for Health Statistics. U.S. Department of Health and Human Services. *National Health and Nutrition Examination Survey III, Phase I, 1988–91*.

10. Foltin RW, Fischman MW, Moran TH, Rolls BJ, Kelly TH. Caloric compensation for lunches varying in fat and carbohydrate content by humans in a residential laboratory. *Am J Clin Nutr*. 1990;52:969–980.

11. Rolls BJ, Pirraglia PA, Jones MB, Peters JC. Effects of olestra, a non-caloric fat substitute, on daily energy intakes in lean men. *Am J Clin Nutr*. 1992;56:84–92.

12. *The Surgeon General's Report on Nutrition and Health*. Washington, DC: U.S. Government Printing Office; 1988. Department of Health and Human Services Publication no. 88-50201.

13. Dexheimer E. On the fat track. *Dairy Foods*. 1992;May: 38–50.

14. Calorie Control Council. Reduced-fat, low-calorie eating more popular than ever. *Calorie Control Commentary*. 1993;15(1):1–2. ISSN 1049-1791.

15. Powers MA. Sweetener blending: how sweet it is! *J Am Diet Assoc*. 1994;94(1):498–500.

16. Ott DB, Edwards CL, Palmer SJ. Perceived taste intensity and duration of nutritive and nonnutritive sweeteners in water using time-intensity evaluations. *J Food Sci*. 1991;56:535–542.

17. Frank RA, Mize SJ, Carter R. An assessment of binary mixture interactions for nine sweeteners. *Chem Senses*. 1989;14:620–632.

18. Powers MA. Sweetening our foods. Blending sweeteners. *Diabetes Educ*. 1994;20(3):243–244.

19. Powers MA, Warshaw HS. Fat replacers. A wide range of choices. *Diabetes Spectrum*. 1992;5(2):72–85.

20. Butchko HH, Kotsonis FN. Acceptable intake vs. actual intake: the aspartame example. *J Am Coll Nutr*. 1991;10:258–266.

21. The Food and Drug Administration. Code of Federal Regulations. Title 21, 101.9: Nutrition Labeling of Food, 1990.

22. *Federal Register*. 1988;53,280379.

23. *Federal Register*. 1992;57(236):57960–57961.

24. Food and Drug Administration: Compliance Policy Guide (CPG), 7105.01, Confectionary use of non-nutritive substances as ingredients.

25. *Federal Register*. 1994;59(230):61538–61545.

26. *Evaluation of Certain Food Additives and Contaminants*. 37th Report of the Joint FAO/WHO Expert Committee on Food Additives. Geneva; 1991. Report no. 806.

27. World Health Organization Expert Committee on Food Additives. *Toxicological Evaluation of Certain Food Additives and Food Contaminants*. Geneva: World Health Organization; no. 16, 1981:11–27, and no. 18, 1983:12–14.

28. O'Brien Nabors L, Lemieux R. History of the commercial development of low-calorie foods. In: Altschul AM,

ed. *Low-Calorie Foods Handbook*. New York, NY: Marcel Dekker, Inc; 1993;91–107.

29. *Federal Register*. July 26, 1974.

30. *Federal Register*. July 24, 1981.

31. *Federal Register*. September 18, 1981.

32. *Federal Register*. July 8, 1983.

33. *Federal Register*. April 19, 1993.

34. Twenty-sixth Report of the Joint FAO/WHO Expert Committee on Food Additives. *Evaluation of Certain Food Additives*. Geneva: World Health Organization; 1981. Technical Report Series 669.

35. Stegink LD, Brummel MC, Filer LJ, et al. Blood methanol concentrations in one-year-old infants administered graded doses of aspartame. *J Nutr*. 1983;113:1600–1606.

36. Stegink LD: Aspartame metabolism in humans: acute dosing studies. In: Stegink LD, Filer LJ Jr, eds. *Aspartame: Physiology and Biochemistry*. New York, NY: Marcel Dekker, Inc; 1984:509–554.

37. Nehrling JK, Kobe P, McLane MP, et al. Aspartame use by persons with diabetes. *Diabetes Care*. 1985;8:415–417.

38. Monte WC. Aspartame: methanol and the public health. *J Appl Nutr*. 1984;36:42–54.

39. Yokogoshi H, Robers CH, Caballero B, et al. Effects of aspartame and glucose administration on brain and plasma levels of large neutral amino acids and brain 5-hydroxyindoles. *Am J Clin Nutr*. 1984;40:1–7.

40. Pardridge WM. Brain metabolism: a perspective from the blood-brain barrier. *Physiol Rev*. 1983;63:1481–1535.

41. Aspartame: Commissioner's final decision. *Federal Register*. 1981;46(Jul 24):38283.

42. FDA. Talk paper: CDC evaluation of aspartame complaints. November 1, 1984. FDA/USDHHS, T84-77.

43. Stegink LD, Brummel MC, McMartin K, et al. Blood methanol concentrations in normal adult subjects administered abuse doses of aspartame. *J Toxicol Environ Health*. 1981;7:281–290.

44. Wurtman RJ. Neurochemical changes following high-dose aspartame with dietary carbohydrates. *N Engl J Med*. 1983;309:429–430.

45. Twenty-fifth Report of the Joint FAO/WHO Expert Committee on Food Additives. *Evaluation of Certain Food Additives*. Geneva: World Health Organization; 1982. Technical Report Series 669.

46. Saccharin and its salts. *Federal Register*. 1977;Dec 9:62209.

47. Morrison AS, Buring JE. Artificial sweeteners and cancer of the lower urinary tract. *N Engl J Med*. 1980;302:537–541.

48. Council on Scientific Affairs. Saccharin—review of safety issues. *JAMA*. 1985;254:2622.

49. *Federal Register*. 1986;51(Sept 29):34503.

50. Hendrick ME. Alitame. In: O'Brien Nabors L, Gelardi RC, eds. *Alternative Sweeteners*. New York, NY: Marcel Dekker, Inc; 1991.

51. Calorie Control Council, Abbott Laboratories. *Food Additive Petition for Cyclamate*. Sept. 22, 1982. 2A3672.

52. Bopp BA, Price P. Cyclamate. In: O'Brien Nabors L, Gelardi RC, eds. *Alternative Sweeteners*. New York, NY: Marcel Dekker, Inc; 1991.

53. Bopp BA, Sonders RC, Kesterson JW. Toxicological aspects of cyclamate and cyclohexylamine. *CRC Crit Rev Toxicol*. 1986;16:213–306.

54. Oser BL, Carson L, Cox GE, Vogin EE, Sternberg SS. Chronic toxicity study of cyclamate: saccharin (10:1) in rats. *Toxicology*. 1975;4:315–330.

55. Cancer Assessment Committee. *Scientific Review of the Long-Term Carcinogenic Bioassays Performed on the Artificial Sweetener, Cyclamate*. Washington, DC: Center for Food Safety and Applied Nutrition, Food and Drug Administration; 1984.

56. National Academy of Sciences/National Research Council. *Evaluation of Cyclamate for Carcinogenicity*. Washington, DC: National Academy Press; 1985.

57. Desso JM, Kelley JM, Fuller BB. MITRE Corporation Report to US Food and Drug Administration. May 1987. FDA Contract no. 223-86-2104.

58. Newsome R. Sugar substitutes. In: Altschul AM, ed. *Low-Calorie Foods Handbook*. New York, NY: Marcel Dekker, Inc; 1993:139–170.

59. O'Brien Nabors L, Miller WT. Cyclamate—a toxicological review. *Comment Toxicol*. 1989;III(4):307.

60. Warshaw HS. Alternative sweeteners—past, present and potential. *Diabetes Spectrum*. 1990;3(5):335.

61. McNeil Specialty Products Company. Sucralose: an introduction to a new low-calorie sweetener. New Brunswick, NJ: McNeil Specialty Products Company; 1994.

62. Sucralose Food Additive Petition 7A3987;765–813.

63. Mezitis N, Koch P, Maggio C, Quddoos A, Pi-Sunyer FX. Glycemic response to sucralose, a novel sweetener, in subjects with diabetes mellitus. *Diabetes*. 1994;43,S1(5):261A.

64. Bower WH, Young DA, Pearson SK. The effects of sucralose on coronal and root-surface caries. J Dent Research. 1990;69(8):1485–1487.

65. Harrigan KA, Breene WM. Fat substitutes: sucrose polyesters and other synthetic oils. In: Altschul AM, ed. *Low-Calorie Foods Handbook*. New York, NY: Marcel Dekker, Inc; 1993;171–180.

66. Warshaw HS, Powers MA. Ingredients that replace fat: their role in today's foods and challenges in educating people with diabetes. *Diabetes Educ*. 1993;19(5):419–430.

67. Frye AM, Setser CS. Bulking agents and fat substitutes. In: Altschul AM, ed. *Low-Calories Foods Handbook*. New York, NY: Marcel Dekker, Inc; 1993:211–251.

68. Warshaw HS, Franz MJ, Powers MA, Wheeler ML. Fat replacers and their use in foods (technical review). *Diabetes Care*. In press.

69. Nutrition Fact Sheet. Reducing the fat in baked goods. *J Am Diet Assoc*. 1995;95(1).

70. Calorie Control Commentary: Low-calorie values may have consumers seeing more polyols soon. Calorie Control Council. 1995;17:4.

71. Food and Drug Administration and Department of Health and Human Services. Code of Federal Regulations (CFR), Chapter 20 (Mannitol, Polydextrose, Sorbitol), Apr. 1, 1990. Washington, DC: U.S. Government Printing Office; 1990.

72. Simpson HA, Cooke SK. Food allergy and the potential allergenicity-antigenicity of microparticulated egg and cow's milk proteins. *J Am Coll Nutr*. 1990;9:410–417.

73. Fat substitute does not need separate GRAS affirmation: FDA. *Food Chemical News*. Aug 17, 1992.

74. Calorie Control Council. *Fat Reduction in Foods*. Atlanta, Ga; 1993.

75. What's new in fat replacement? *Prepared Foods*. July 1992, 73–76.

76. Still no fat city for P & G's olestra. *Business Week*. November 7, 1994.

77. Glueck CJ. Sucrose polyester, cholesterol, and lipoprotein metabolism. In: Akoh CC, Swanson BG, eds. *Carbohydrate Polyesters as Fat Substitutes*. New York, NY: Marcel Dekker, Inc; 1994:169–182.

78. Wheeler ML, Fineberg SE, Gibson R, Fineberg N. Metabolic response to oral challenge of hydrogenated starch hydrolysate versus glucose in diabetes. *Diabetes Care*. 1990;13:733–740.

79. Mattes RD, Caputo FA. Caloric compensation to convert manipulations of dietary fat and carbohydrate intake. *Am J Clin Nutr*. 1991;53(3). Abstract 67.

80. Mela DJ. Nutritional implications of fat substitutes. *J Am Diet Assoc*. 1992;92(4):472–476.

81. Kristal AR, White E, Shattuck AL, et al. Long-term maintenance of a low-fat diet: durability of fat-related dietary habits in the Women's Health Trial. *J Am Diet Assoc*. 1992;92(5):553–559.

82. Kanders BS, Lavin PT, Kowalchuk M, Blackburn GL. Do aspartame (APM) sweetened foods and beverages aid in long-term control of body weight? *Am J Clin Nutr*. 1990;51(3). Abstract 38.

Chapter 21

Fiber Metabolism and Use in Diabetes Therapy

Lesley Fels Tinker
Madelyn L. Wheeler

Consumers became interested in dietary fiber in the 1970s, increased their interest in the 1980s, and have continued their interest into the 1990s. This interest in fiber is, in large part, a response to the dietary guidelines that advise all Americans to increase the fiber content of their diets by selecting foods that are good sources of fiber and starch.[1] These recommendations are also appropriate for persons with diabetes. The American Diabetes Association recommends that for general health, persons with diabetes should consume fiber-containing foods.[2] However, there are many practical application questions that need to be clarified as dietitians counsel their clients with diabetes about implementing these recommendations:

- What is fiber?
- What is soluble and insoluble fiber?
- What does processing (grinding, cooking) do to fiber in a food?
- Where are fiber analysis figures found?
- What effect does fiber have on diabetes control and complications?
- How much fiber is consumed by Americans?
- How much fiber should be in a high-fiber diet?
- Are there federal regulations that control fiber labeling?
- To increase fiber in the diet, should supplements be used, or should the increase come from naturally occurring fiber?

- What are the risks and benefits of increasing fiber in the diet?
- And finally, what are some practical guidelines for increasing fiber in the diet?

The purpose of this chapter is to answer these questions in the context of clinical practice.

FIBER UPDATE FOR DIETITIANS

What Is Fiber?

The term *dietary fiber* was coined by Hipsley[3] in 1953 to include lignin, cellulose, and hemicellulose. Dietary fiber has been redefined, from a human nutrition perspective, as lignin and all plant polysaccharides that are not subject to enzymatic degradation within the human small intestine.[4] Plant polysaccharides include plant cell wall structural components (cellulose), plant cell wall matrix components (eg, some hemicelluloses and pectins), and nonstructural plant cell contents (pectins, hemicelluloses, gums, mucilages, and algal polysaccharides).[5] Although the carbohydrate from fiber cannot be metabolized directly by humans, fiber can be degraded by gastrointestinal microflora to produce short-chain fatty acids that are partially available for absorption by the human intestine.

Chemical Composition

Almost all dietary fiber is considered to be nonstarch polysaccharide and is located within the cell wall (structural polysaccharide). Table

Table 21-1 Classification of Plant Fiber

Major Dietary Fiber Components [a]	Major Monosaccharide Present [b]	Solubility [c]	Food Sources	Probable Physiologic Effects [d]
Structural (cell wall) polysaccharides				
A. Cellulose	None	I	Wheat (whole-wheat flour, wheat bran), vegetables (cabbage, green beans, broccoli, carrots)	A
B. Noncellulosic polysaccharides				
Pectic substances	Rhamnogalacturonans	S	Fruits (citrus, apples), cereals (oats, barley)	B
	Arabinogalactans	?	Vegetables (cauliflower, potatoes)	B
Glucans	ß-Glucans	S	Cereals (oats, barley)	B
Hemicelluloses	Mannans	?	Storage form in many seeds, including legumes	?
	Xylans	I	Cereals (wheat, rye, barley)	A
	Xyloglucans	I	?	?
C. Noncarbohydrate components (lignin) [e]	None	I	Cereal grains (breakfast cereals), older vegetables	A
Nonstructural (cell interior) polysaccharides (gums and mucilages)	Many types	S	Legumes (dried beans), cereal grain (oats, barley), guar gum	B

[a] All plant cell walls are composed of cellulose in the form of microfibrils, which are embedded in a matrix of noncellulosic polysaccharides and protein. As the cell wall matures, the noncarbohydrate polymer, lignin, is formed in the matrix. *Noncellulosic polysaccharide* is a term used for the spectrum of polymers ranging from those rich in uronic acids (pectic fraction) to those poor in uronic acids (hemicelluloses).

[b] Noncellulosic polysaccharide can be classified according to the major monosaccharide present, which usually forms the back-bone chain of the molecule.

[c] S = mainly water-soluble; I = mainly water-insoluble; ? = unknown.

[d] A = increase fecal bulk, speed transit time; B = slow glucose absorption, lower serum cholesterol.

[e] Lignin, by usage, has been regarded as part of dietary fiber, in contrast to the other noncarbohydrate substances—protein, inorganic materials such as silica, and lipid substances such as cutin and waxes.

21-1 identifies the major components of dietary fiber and relates them to selected properties and major food sources. There are two major components of the structural (cell wall) polysaccharides, cellulose and noncellulose, as well as a minor class, the noncarbohydrate components. In addition, a small amount of fiber may be found in the cell body rather than the cell wall, and that fiber is classified as nonstructural polysaccharide.[6,7] Major physiologic responses to fiber may be related to the monosaccharides present and their structural linkages. The chemistry of dietary fibers varies from plant to plant and is affected by growing conditions, as well as age. As the plant matures and cells begin to die, encrusting substances such as lignin make up a greater percentage of the wall. Table 21-2 indicates some of the compositional changes that a

Table 21-2 Composition of Typical Plant Cell Walls

	Immature	Mature
Fiber Component	(percentage of dry cell wall)	
Cellulose	25	38
Noncellulosic polysaccharides	51	43
Lignin	0	17
Waxes, etc	4	0
Protein	9	3

Source: Adapted from *Comprehensive Biochemistry,* Vol. 26A (p 8) by M Florkin and EH Stotz (Eds) with permission of Elsevier Science Publishers B.V., © 1968.

plant cell wall goes through as it develops from the initial immature stages and progresses on to maturity. A general description of the process involved in the chemical analysis of dietary fibers is included in Appendix 21-A.

Physical Properties

The four major physical characteristics of dietary fiber—bacterial fermentation, binding of organic compounds, ion exchange, and water-holding capacity—have an effect on the physiologic response(s) to dietary fiber and are related to the structure and composition of the various dietary fibers.[8] The four physical characteristics and physiologic responses are briefly described below.

Bacterial fermentation occurs in the lower gastrointestinal tract as the result of bacterial degradation of accessible polysaccharides. Soluble dietary fiber (eg, pectin, guar gum) is more accessible to bacteria than insoluble dietary fiber (eg, cellulose, lignin) and hence more fermentable. Fermentation leads to a higher bacterial cell mass in the feces and a somewhat higher fecal mass.

Binding of organic compounds such as bile acids by fiber is related to chemical interactions between dietary fibers and the digestion/metabolic products within the gastrointestinal tract. Some soluble fibers (eg, pectin and psyllium) as well as sources of insoluble dietary fibers (eg,

wheat bran and lignin) have been found to bind bile acids within the small and large intestine and lower their reabsorption.[9] Fibers that form viscous solutions, such as pectin, have been shown to bind bile acids and to lower plasma cholesterol levels.[10–12]

The ion exchange properties of fiber influence mineral metabolism and can potentially create a negative physiologic response to dietary fiber. Phytate, found primarily in cereal grains, can bind a variety of minerals, resulting in higher fecal mineral excretion. However, persons ingesting balanced diets adequate in minerals are probably at minimal risk for negative mineral balance due to dietary fiber intake.[13]

Water-holding capacity is related to the ability of fibers to swell when exposed to water and is characteristic of fibers containing sugar residues with free polar groups, such as pectin.[5] Wheat bran, a source of insoluble fiber and some hemicelluloses, exhibits some water-holding capacity. Wheat bran contributes significantly to fecal bulking.

What Is Soluble and Insoluble Fiber?

The terms *soluble* and *insoluble* dietary fiber were introduced in 1978[14,15] and were based on an analysis method that used water to fractionate dietary fiber. The analytical terms *soluble* and *insoluble* dietary fiber are still commonly, although perhaps inappropriately, used for the categorization of dietary fiber as well as to refer to the food sources of the dietary fibers. Over the years, better knowledge of the chemical composition and the properties of the different types of fibers has influenced the analytical methods used to separate the dietary fibers. Depending on the exact analytical methods used, the amount of total dietary fiber in a sample may vary; furthermore, the amounts of fiber that partition into the soluble and insoluble categories may also vary.[16] This leads to inconsistency in what is meant by "soluble" and "insoluble" dietary fiber. Unfortunately, interpretation of dietary fiber research must include a careful examination of the methods used for determination of the amounts of total dietary and soluble and insoluble dietary fiber.

There are additional objections to the terms *soluble* and *insoluble*. First, fibers are not truly soluble as chemically defined (ie, by physical definition, they form a dispersion rather than a solution). Second, sources of dietary fiber such as fruits or oat bran or wheat bran are a heterogeneous mix of soluble and insoluble fibers and are not simply classified into one or the other category.

The terms *soluble* and *insoluble* remain in use despite the lack of a precise physiologic definition. Analytically, the terms are defined based on the Prosky method of analyzing soluble dietary fiber,[17,18] thus conferring a frame of reference for the terminology. Further, the terms *soluble* and *insoluble* fiber are accepted for food labeling of dietary fiber.[19]

What Is the Effect of Processing (Milling, Cooking) on Fiber?

Most of the dietary fiber found in plant food sources is contained in cell walls. Cooking, freezing, freeze-drying, and chewing a plant destroys its physical structure, but the fiber remains and, in a modified way, still remains hydrated.[20] However, the more the cell walls are disrupted (in other words, the smaller the particle size), the greater the cell wall surface area that is directly accessible to digestive secretions and bacteria and, thus, the more rapid the diffusion, digestion, and metabolism.

The fiber content of cereal grains depends on the fineness of milling. For example, the size of wheat bran particles is determined by the type of mill used.[7] In turn, the size of the particle can affect the physiologic response. Coarse wheat brans and some medium wheat brans have been shown to normalize food transit time through the gastrointestinal tract when transit time had been slow.[21]

Conversely, fine bran can increase fecal bulk but also induces constipation.[22] It has also been shown that a significantly greater percentage of starch is hydrolyzed (ie, split into smaller saccharide units by enzymatic action) with the chemical addition of water when oat, wheat, rye, or rice is milled (ground) as compared with either the rolled product or the whole grain.[23] Hydrolyzed starch is more easily digested than unhydrolyzed starch.

Changes in fiber that occur during food processing have not been well documented.[24] Cooking of starch-rich materials such as cereals and potatoes results in considerable disruption of intracellular adhesion due to the swelling of starch granules. In the legumes category, Golay et al[25] showed that ingestion of beans processed in a manner that maintains the integrity of the cell produced significantly lower glucose and insulin responses in persons with type II diabetes than did ingestion of beans with ruptured cells.

Published fiber analysis reports have indicated little difference in the fiber content of vegetables when processed by cooking, canning, and freezing (Table 21-3). With other plant foods such as prepared cereal products, dietary fiber analysis is complicated by the "resistant starch" (RS) phenomenon. RS can be found in Maillard products, the result of heating food mixtures—toasting to produce cornflakes, for example—containing reducing sugars and amino acids. Reducing sugars are sugars in ring formation with a free hydroxyl group (eg, glucose, galactose, fructose, and ribose) that can act as reducing agents and cause nonenzymatic glycosylation. This process is commonly called "browning." Detailed analysis of the component sugars released in many of these processed starch-rich foods shows that some starch becomes resistant to hydrolysis by the enzymes used in the analysis.[26] Thus, in fiber analysis, this RS in part a product of the browning process, may become a part of the total dietary fiber figure. Muir and O'Dea[27] have developed an in vitro analysis method to measure RS. The crucial question, not yet answered, is whether this phenomenon—resistance to enzymatic hydrolysis in vitro—is also seen in vivo. If not, perhaps some cereal fiber estimates are too high.

Table 21-3 Cooking Effects on Vegetable Fiber Values in Grams

Vegetable	Raw	Raw Cooked	Canned Cooked	Frozen Cooked
		per 100-g serving[a]		
Broccoli	3.2	2.5	0	2.5
Carrots	3.3	3.1	2.9	0
Onions	3.1	2.1	0	0
Spinach	2.4	2.2	2.4	2.1
		per 1/2-cup serving[b,c]		
Broccoli	1.4	2.0	0	2.5
Carrots	1.8	2.4	2.1	0
Onions	2.5	2.2	0	0
Spinach	0.7	2.0	2.6	2.1

[a] *From Plant Fiber in Foods* by JW Anderson, HCF Diabetes Research Foundation, © 1986.

[b] *From Plant Fiber in Foods* by JW Anderson, HCF Diabetes Research Foundation, © 1986; *McCance and Widdowson's The Composition of Foods*, 4th ed by AA Paul and DAT Southgate (Eds), Elsevier Science Publishing Company, Inc, © 1978.

[c] Servings in the 1995 *Exchange Lists for Meal Planning*[45] for raw vegetables are 1 cup not 1/2 cup.

Where Are Fiber Analysis Figures Found?

Most dietitians analyze nutrient intake using food composition tables, publications, or computer programs that access food composition tables. As emphasized earlier, it is essential to be familiar with the sources of data for the fiber values in composition tables because the analytical method used to obtain the data has a profound influence on the values obtained. The dietary fiber literature is replete, with various terms denoting dietary fiber, yet although the terms are analytically defined, they are not synonymous. For example, a few older tables still give values for crude fiber under the heading of "fiber." These values greatly underestimate total dietary fiber according to the analytical method by Prosky et al.[28–31] The Prosky method is an enzymatic gravimetric method currently accepted in the United States by the Association of Official Analytical Chemists for its speed and practicality. The total dietary fiber method by Prosky et al[28–31] includes cellulose, hemicelluloses, pectins, gums, mucilages, and lignin, the primary noncarbohydrate component of dietary fiber. RS is incompletely removed by the total dietary fiber method. Crude fiber, however, refers to the residue left from a food after the food has been extracted with solvent, then acid and base hydrolyzed.[29] Many hemicelluloses, pectins, gums, and mucilages are removed from crude fiber.

The reader should be aware that the terms *crude fiber* and *dietary fiber* are not synonymous. Both terms are correct within their analytical definitions; the terms are simply different. No arithmetical algorithm exists to convert crude fiber values to dietary fiber values because of the complexity and variance of plant compositions. Some dietary fiber data sources give values obtained by one of the detergent fiber methods—neutral detergent fiber (NDF) or acid detergent fiber (ADF). NDF has been used by many authors to signify "insoluble" dietary fiber, not always a correct assumption. The NDF method[32] is a gravimetric procedure that measures cellulose, lignin, some hemicelluloses, and starch. The NDF has been modified by adding an α-amylase treatment to remove starch.[33] The NDF method gives similar values as insoluble fiber for some cereals, especially wheat products that contain significant amounts of cellulose, lignin, or hemicellulose. However, in fruits, vegetables, and cereals containing pectins, some hemicelluloses, gums, mucilages, and algal polysaccharides, the NDF method underestimates significantly the total dietary fiber content.[7]

The ADF method was developed by Van Soest[34] in 1963 and measures cellulose and lignin. The terms *ADF* and *dietary fiber* are not synonymous, although the terms are correct within their respective analytical definitions.

The Southgate procedure[35] determines the noncellulosic polysaccharide (NCP), cellulose, and lignin fractions of dietary fiber by breaking down the fiber and then colorimetrically measuring the component sugars. The procedure relies on a series of steps including extraction of sugars by hot water and alcohol, enzymatic hydrolysis, and acid hydrolysis. The Southgate method is laborious and time-consuming, taking 5 days for the final results. The Southgate procedure does not completely remove resistant starch, for which it has been criticized.

Additional dietary fiber terms with which the reader may be confronted are nonstarch polysaccharides (NSP), insoluble NSP, NCP, and RS. Collaborators in England[36] developed gas-liquid chromatography methods to analyze NSP, insoluble NSP, RS, and NCP. The NSPs are first isolated from the food samples by enzymatic starch hydrolysis. The NSP are then separated into insoluble NSP (cellulose) and NCP. The RS is isolated by modifying the NCP analysis procedure. The NSP classification includes most components of total dietary fiber but does not include lignin.

The physiologic definition of dietary fiber leads to an additional category of dietary fiber, nondigestible oligosaccharides (NDO).[37] Oligofructose is an example of an NDO and is the enzymatic hydrolysis product of inulin. Inulin is found primarily in Jerusalem artichokes, garlic, chicory root, leek, dandelion, globe artichokes, and onions. Consumption in the United States is estimated to be 2 to 8 g/d.[37]

Dietary fiber analysis methodology is complex. The message to the readers, however, is simple—be aware of how the dietary fiber values in the literature were derived. Dietary fiber terms are not interchangeable. Various dietary fiber terms have specific definitions and are not synonymous.

Finally, when making comparisons among fiber values from different sources, it should be remembered that foods are biologic materials and, as such, show biologic variation—age, growing conditions, genetics, etc; many of the differences between values cited by different authors are legitimate and are due, in part, to differences in the samples analyzed. These natural variations reduce the predictive accuracy of all calculations.[7]

Food and Drug Administration (FDA) regulations offer five ways to calculate the energy content of foods.[38] Total carbohydrate may include dietary fiber, or the insoluble fiber may be subtracted from total carbohydrate content before calculating the calorie contribution of the carbohydrate portion of the food. A discrepancy between kilocalories from carbohydrate and total grams carbohydrate in a food suggests that fiber is included in the total carbohydrate listing. For example, one serving of cereal may list 17 g total carbohydrate, with 6 g of this being dietary fiber. Kilocalories would be calculated by multiplying 11 g carbohydrate by 4 kcal/g (equaling 44 kcal per serving) rather than multiplying 17 g carbohydrate by 4 to give 68 kcal per serving.

Where can resources for currently accepted analysis of the fiber content of foods be found? Most total dietary fiber values are in the 1993 *USDA Nutrient Database for Standard References*, release 10, which is the Handbook 8 series in computer-compatible format. The total dietary fiber values are based on the American Association of Analytical Chemists methods. Release 11, in 1995, has all analytical total dietary fiber values analyzed by the American Association of Analytical Chemists methods.

Anderson[39] has published a booklet describing the total dietary fiber and soluble fiber components of more than 300 foods. Some values were determined by the Southgate technique,[35,40] methods of Englyst,[36,41] or the Prosky method.[17,31] The dietary fiber data not directly analyzed were compiled from several published sources.[42–44]

Lanza and Butrum[24] have compiled a list of the dietary fiber content in foods compiled from many sources. This review also critiques various dietary fiber analysis methodologies.

Total dietary fiber values for most of the frequently consumed fiber-containing foods listed in the 1995 edition of the *Exchange Lists for Meal Planning*[45] are given in Appendix 21-B. The fiber values are from the 1993 *USDA Nutrition Database for Standard References*, release 10.

What Effect Does Fiber Have on Diabetes Control and Complications?

When fiber in the diet of an individual with diabetes is increased, the main concern is whether doing so will produce beneficial results: smoothing out blood glucose responses and perhaps decreasing blood lipid levels. The physiologic effects of fiber may be related to several factors, such as the individual fibers present in a food, the nature of the mixture of fibers within a food, the interaction of fibers with other food components, and the maintenance of the physical form of the food.[6] The effects of fiber intake have been extensively studied in persons with diabetes, and both short-term (blood glucose and insulin) and long-term (glycated hemoglobin, cholesterol and triglyceride levels, and weight loss) clinical outcomes have been measured. For additional recent reviews of dietary fiber and diabetes, the reader is referred to the technical review of the nutrition recommendations for persons with diabetes prepared by Franz et al[46] and the review prepared by Nuttall.[47]

Problems Encountered When Interpreting Clinical Trials

It is often difficult to compare results from the multitude of clinical trials that have been reported for the following reasons:

- Source of fiber: different clinical outcomes are produced depending on the source of fiber (eg, wheat bran versus guar versus apple fiber). Soluble-fiber sources, such as guar, seem to produce more desirable lipid lowering and glycemic normalizing responses than insoluble fiber, such as wheat bran.

- Amount of fiber: different amounts of fiber—high dose versus low dose—may produce different outcomes.

- Combinations of fiber: if both soluble and insoluble fibers are combined into a meal, the effects of one fiber may counteract or be synergistic with another fiber present in the same meal.[48]

- Change in macronutrient content: in studies using high-fiber foods, it is difficult to increase the fiber content without changing other macronutrient parameters (ie, increasing carbohydrate or decreasing fat). Few clinical studies have attempted to increase the fiber content of the diet without changing the macronutrient content. One such study was done in a metabolic ward setting and involved high-carbohydrate diets in which both the amount and source of carbohydrate and the source of dietary fiber were constant and only the amount of fiber varied.[49] Also, the polyunsaturated to saturated fatty acid (P/S) ratio and the cholesterol content remained constant. Fiber increase was achieved by changing white bread to whole wheat, fruit juice to whole fruit, refined cereals to whole grain, and adding peanuts as a snack (Table 21-4).

- Length of experimental period(s): the amount of time that fiber is used may affect the outcome of the study. Most of the earlier studies demonstrated changes in glucose control either immediately[50,51] or within the first week of the test diet.[52,53] Jenkins et al[53] found a progressive decrease in insulin requirements for up to 12 weeks with guar supplement but little further change after that for up to 20 weeks.

Table 21-4 Comparison of High Fiber and Normal Fiber 2000-kcal Diets

High Fiber (54 g)		Normal Fiber (22 g)	
Food Items	Weight (g)	Food Items	Weight (g)
Breakfast		**Breakfast**	
Bran flakes 40%	35.0	Rice Krispies	36.8
Orange sections	180.0	Orange juice	130.9
Whole-wheat bread	25.0	White bread	26.3
Low-fat milk	123.0	Low-fat milk	129.4
Butter	5.0	Butter	5.3
Lunch		**Lunch**	
Lean beef	60.0	Lean beef	63.1
Mayonnaise	9.0	Mayonnaise	9.5
Lettuce	10.0	Lettuce	10.5
Whole-wheat bread	50.0	White bread	52.6
Apple slices	165.0	Apple juice	251.4
Nonfat milk	122.5	Low-fat milk	129.4
Snack		**Snack**	
Bran muffin	50.0	Plain muffin	62.1
Applesauce	127.0	Applesauce	128.3
Butter	5.0	Butter	5.3
Dinner		**Dinner**	
Eggnog	74.4	Eggnog	58.3
Turkey breast	60.0	Turkey breast	63.1
Whole corn	169.0	Rice	52.6
Broccoli	92.5	Broccoli	97.3
Butter	5.0	Butter	10.5
Lettuce	55.0	Lettuce	26.3
Whole-wheat bread	50.0	White bread	52.6
Whole banana	200.0	Whole banana	210.4
Snack		**Snack**	
Peanuts	18.0	Raisins	24.1
Raisins	36.2		

These meal plans are examples of a normal fiber (11 g dietary fiber per 1000 kcal) and a high fiber (22 g/1000 kcal) research diets. Fiber increase from normal to high was achieved by changing white bread to whole wheat, fruit juice to whole fruit, refined cereals to whole grain, and adding peanuts as a snack.

Source: Reprinted with permission from *American Journal of Clinical Nutrition* (1986; 43:16), Copyright © 1986, American Society for Clinical Nutrition.

- Compliance with the diet: studies done in a controlled environment (metabolic unit) are more likely to control variability, and short-term studies done using the artificial endocrine pancreas can measure continuous blood glucose change and insulin requirements in persons with insulin-dependent diabetes mellitus (IDDM).[54] In long-term outpatient studies, it is difficult to assess compliance with the diet.

- Other physiologic factors: weight loss, level of control of the diabetes, and the presence of other disease states such as autonomic neuropathy may also affect the clinical results of a fiber trial.

Improvement in Blood Glucose Control

The interest in effects of dietary fiber on blood glucose and insulin levels of individuals with diabetes stems from early work by Anderson[55,56] in the United States and Jenkins in Britain.[57,58] Anderson's studies demonstrated that high-carbohydrate fiber (HCF) diets, containing approximately 70% carbohydrate and 65 g dietary fiber, could produce significantly reduced fasting plasma glucose levels compared with "traditional diabetes diets" (43% carbohydrate, 26 g dietary fiber) in a controlled setting.[55]

Home maintenance HCF diets (55 to 60% carbohydrate, 20 to 25% fat, and 50 g dietary fiber) generally sustained the result in a few patients for up to 4 years.[56] Jenkins et al[57] found that feeding a test meal containing 16 g guar (in bread) and 10 g pectin (in marmalade) significantly diminished the rise of postprandial blood glucose and serum insulin levels in individuals with type II diabetes. Individuals with IDDM showed a reduced mean rise of blood glucose by more than 36%. Vuorinen-Markkola et al[59] observed a mean decrease in fasting and glycosylated hemoglobin levels in persons with type I diabetes consuming 5 g guar gum preprandially four times daily compared with a wheat flour placebo.

Subsequently, many natural food fiber/diabetes studies have been reported, most describing improvement in glucose control; however, it is usually difficult to determine whether this improvement is caused by the fiber component of the diet or by other simultaneous changes in macronutrient content. Anderson[60] indicated that most of the reduction in insulin requirements for lean diabetic patients eating HCF diets may be related to the 70% carbohydrate and 12% fat content, with only a small role assigned to fiber content.

Jenkins et al[58] compared intake of white bread with intake of whole-meal bread; they found identical blood glucose responses and concluded that, at least for cereal products, fiber was not a factor in blood glucose response. Results from Hollenbeck et al[49] support a lack of response due to fiber. In an 8-week study, the amount and source of carbohydrate and source of dietary fiber were held constant. The fiber was either low (11 g/1000 kcal) or high (27 g/1000 kcal). No significant changes were found in glucose control (postprandial values and glycated hemoglobin, or reduction in insulin requirements) in adults with type II diabetes.

By contrast, Riccardi et al[61] studied the effects of three outpatient diets: low carbohydrate (42%) and low fiber (20 g), high carbohydrate (53%) and low fiber (16 g), and high carbohydrate (53%) and high fiber (54 g). Their results indicated that diets high in carbohydrate and low in fiber did not improve metabolic control, whereas the high-carbohydrate, high-fiber diet did. Studies that have included the soluble-fiber supplements guar and pectin have demonstrated improved glucose control. By contrast, insoluble-fiber supplements such as wheat bran and cellulose have usually produced no significant change.

Some evidence suggests fiber may exert its glucose-lowering activity after meals subsequent to when the fiber was initially ingested. For example, Pastors[62] saw a 20% reduction in plasma glucose levels in persons with type II diabetes consuming 6.8 g psyllium/meal after the second meal consumed compared with consuming no psyllium.

Possible mechanisms whereby certain types of fiber may improve glucose metabolic control include increasing the number of insulin receptors on circulating monocytes,[63,64] decreasing postprandial glycemic excursions,[57] and directly influencing hepatic glucose metabolism.[65]

The amounts of dietary fiber were high in studies showing improved glycemic control. These high amounts, often 50+ g/d, would be difficult to achieve for most persons in the Westernized world. The 1994 nutrition recommendations for persons with diabetes[2] do not suggest high-fiber diets for one reason, because the levels necessary to improve glycemic control would be difficult to obtain from foods.

Lipid Changes

A major concern of individuals with diabetes is an increased risk of cardiovascular disease, with one of the risk factors being higher than normal serum cholesterol levels (see Chapter 18). The impetus to look at dietary fiber as a possible method for reducing serum cholesterol levels through increased bile acid losses came from the success of cholestyramine and other ion exchange resins in reducing cholesterol levels.[66] Of the investigated dietary supplemental fibers, only soluble fibers such as pectin, oat bran, and guar gum seem to have a hypocholesterolemic effect.[67]

In studies that have involved the use of fiber-containing foods, rather than fiber supplements, the results have been less clear-cut. Several studies have demonstrated that legumes—lentils, chickpeas, or navy, pinto, or kidney beans—are capable of reducing serum cholesterol levels and, in some instances, also serum triglyceride levels.[68,69] The rise in serum fasting triglyceride concentration normally seen with intake of high-carbohydrate diets[70] can be overcome with incorporation of high amounts of dietary fiber and a restriction in fat.[71,72]

Thus, it appears that the type of fiber ingested determines the hypocholesterolemic action. In general, soluble fibers are more effective than insoluble fibers in lowering blood lipids and flattening the postprandial glucose curve.

Energy Displacement When Adding Fiber-Containing Foods to the Diet

Energy displacement is unavoidable when high-fiber energy-containing foods are used rather than isolated sources of fiber (ie, fiber supplements, which contain little metabolizable energy). For example, switching from a low-fiber to high-fiber diet usually results in an increased carbohydrate intake and decreased fat intake. Stasse-Wolthuis et al[12] reported no change in carbohydrate or protein intakes, an increase in fat intake, and a decrease in alcohol intake when usual diets were compared with experimental diets of subjects participating in a crossover study investigating the effects of high-fiber diets on serum lipids. These investigators concluded that the lower plasma cholesterol level found after a high-fiber diet were only in part due to the high fiber because fat intake was lower during the high-fiber diet.

In conjunction with caloric displacement by the addition of fiber-containing foods is the argument that a lower-fat diet, and not a higher-fiber diet, is the reason for reduced plasma cholesterol levels in persons who have altered their diet by increasing fiber and inadvertently reducing fat intake. Data are plentiful that a lower-fat diet results in a reduced plasma cholesterol level.[73]

Recently, Anderson et al[74] tested the hypocholesterolemic effects of oat bran while controlling for caloric displacement. These researchers showed that with isocalorically distributed diets fed to 20 hypercholesterolemic men and supplemented with oat bran rather than wheat bran, plasma cholesterol, low-density lipoprotein-cholesterol, and apolipoprotein B levels were lower after the oat bran than after the wheat bran. These results support the role of dietary fiber in lowering blood lipid levels beyond the simple displacement of fat intake.

Other Risk Factors

Hypertension is another risk factor for cardiovascular disease in the diabetic syndrome. In one study involving men with diabetes and mild hypertension, a high-fiber diet (65 g/d) produced a significantly lower average blood pressure than did a diet including only 22 g/d; both diets were weight maintaining and had equivalent Na/K ratios.[75]

Most persons with type II diabetes are overweight, and it has been noted that reduction in caloric intake leading to even a small weight loss can produce better blood glucose control.[76] The potential role of fiber-rich foods/supplements in preventing or treating obesity has been reviewed.[77,78] Several mechanisms, including satiety, for explaining the possible effects of dietary fiber in controlling weight or energy metabolism have been suggested. Apple juice (no fiber) can be ingested 11 times faster than whole apples with peel (2 g fiber/100 g) and four times faster than applesauce (1.6 g fiber/100 g), with whole apples rated as providing the greatest satiety.[79] Also, fiber-rich foods usually have a lower caloric density than their refined counterparts, and they may have a bulking effect in the stomach that increases satiety, making low-energy diets acceptable.

Fiber-rich diets may even improve the treatment of persons with diabetes and chronic renal failure. Over a 10-day period, a high-fiber natural food diet (65 g/d) improved blood glucose control compared with a low-fiber diet (27 g/d), with no deleterious effect on blood urea and nutritional status.[80] During this time, the macronutrient content of the diet remained constant.

Foods are complex substances that contain multiple nutrients, which, in general, argues against fiber supplements. Isolated supplements may not have the same metabolic action when taken out of the food matrix or have negative consequences on the metabolism of other nutrients. Yet, circumstances may exist when fiber supplement use is indicated. For example, psyllium seed is often taken for constipation. Soluble-fiber supplements have been shown to improve glucose and lipid blood profiles, as described in this chapter. Careful and individualized client assessment is needed before recommending dietary fiber supplements.

TRANSLATION AND INTERPRETATION TO THE PATIENT/CLIENT/CONSUMER

How Much Fiber Do Americans Consume?

Current evidence indicates that average dietary fiber intakes of adults in industrialized affluent countries are in the range of 15 to 30 g/d.[13] The average American intake of dietary fiber is about 13 g daily for women and 19 g daily for men.[81,82]

Of course, there are considerable individual variations in intake, both in average habitual intake and from day to day. Seasonal variations in dietary fiber intake may also be marked, particularly in rural communities, and vegetarians often have somewhat higher intakes, up to 40 g/d, on the average.[83]

How Much Fiber Should Be in a High-Fiber Diet?

What should be considered a goal to try to achieve in increasing fiber intake? A review of published clinical studies lasting longer than 7 days, and involving high-fiber intake of natural foods, indicated that the average daily amount of dietary fiber was 52 g, with a range of 25 to 35 g/1000 kcal. In Lindsay's study of children with IDDM, 30 g fiber/1000 kcal provided through grains, fruits, vegetables, and high-fiber crackers was apparently close to their limit of acceptability.[84] Investigators using fiber supplements in long-term clinical studies (greater than 7 days) gave an average of 21 g/d in addition to the fiber in usual foods. Mahalko et al[85] regarded the addition of 26 g/d of supplemental fiber—in the form of corn bran, soy hulls, or apple powder—to the diets of persons with type II diabetes as an amount that could reasonably be added to typical Western diets. Because the 26-g supplement had little effect on glucose tolerance or plasma lipids, the amount of added fiber was doubled to 52 g/d. Although this amount improved metabolic parameters, subject tolerance was poor. By contrast, Jones et al[86] gave low-dose guar (10 g/d) for 2 months and found significant reductions in glycated hemoglobin levels.

When a high-fiber diet is indicated, a practical approach for dietitians is to find out what the client's present average intake of fiber is and then to counsel the client with diabetes to increase it gradually, with a goal of perhaps 30 g/d from a variety of food sources.[13] The emphasis is on consuming foods containing dietary fiber rather than consuming grams of fiber. Current recommendations for Americans are to consume five servings of fruits and vegetables daily and six servings of grains daily.[87,88] Even attaining the fruit/vegetable/grain goals may take a period of time to implement as Americans are consuming only about 3-1/2 servings of fruits and vegetables.[89]

Are There Federal Regulations That Control Fiber Labeling?

As of May 1994, dietary fiber information has been included on food labels for foods regulated by the FDA.[19] Total dietary fiber values are to be reported in grams per serving. The daily reference value for dietary fiber is 25 g based on a 2000-kcal diet. A food can claim to contain a "high" amount of dietary fiber if one serving contains 5 g or more of fiber per serving.[90] A food can claim to be a "good source" of dietary fiber if one serving contains 2.5 to 4.9 g per serving.[90] A food can claim to have "more" or "added fiber" if the food has at least 2.5 g more per serving than the reference food.[90] Further, any food making a dietary fiber claim must list the amount of total fat per daily reference amount if the food is not "low fat" (ie, not less than 3 g per serving in general).[90,91]

Certain health claims may appear on food labels.[91] There are two approved health claim areas for fiber-containing foods. First, a food label may make a cancer claim if the food is a grain product, fruit, or vegetable that is a good source of dietary fiber and low fat. Second, a food label may make a coronary heart disease claim if the food is a fruit, vegetable, or grain product, contains at least 0.6 g soluble fiber per daily reference amount, and is low fat, low cholesterol, and low saturated fat.

Fiber values for many foods used in the 1995 edition of the *Exchange Lists*[45] are provided in Appendix 21-B (Total Dietary Fiber Values for Foods).

To Increase Fiber in the Diet, Should Fiber Supplements Be Used or Should the Increase Come from Natural Foods?

Using fiber supplements would seem to be a very simple way to incorporate fiber into the diet: take x grams one to four times per day and forget about having to decide which foods are high in fiber. Clinical studies involving such supplements as guar and pectin have shown an improvement in glycemic control. However, fiber supplement use is not without problems. There is some evidence that the method of incorporation of such supplements as guar is a factor in determining response. Supplements are probably more effective in altering the pattern of glucose and insulin response (delay in peak response) if given with a meal, rather than before it, and if mixed with the liquid portion of the meal, such as soup, rather than put into a bread.[92] Also, adding an effective amount of fiber supplement into foods in a palatable way has been difficult. Fiber supplements may come from further processing foods that are a normal part of the diet, such as tomato flour, dried prune products, apple and pear fibers, or washed orange pulp, or from fibers that have not been traditionally a part of the eating pattern of humans (eg, wood lignins, tobacco fiber, lignin, or shellfish aminopolysaccharides).[93] As fiber continues to be a health issue, manufacturers may incorporate more of these unusual sources in commercially available fiber supplements and foods made with supplements without toxicity testing or proof of physiologic claims, thereby misleading the public.[94] Also, some fiber supplements may have microbiologic contamination, and others, such as bagasse, a residue from sugar cane, may disintegrate into sharp needlelike particles on grinding. Also, concentrated hydrophilic sources—plant gums and mucilages—can form viscous solutions on hydration. If concentrated dry portions are consumed, subsequent hydration and swelling in the gastrointestinal tract can lead to blockage.[20,95] Thus, clients should be advised to increase their normal consumption of fluid. Finally, adding supplements to a diet that is perhaps nutritionally deficient does not address one of the primary goals of the diabetic diet, that of nutritional adequacy.

Therefore, current recommendations are that fiber in the diet be increased by use of natural foods rather than supplements wherever possible.[2] The issue remains whether supplements

Table 21-5 Risk versus Benefit of Increasing Fiber Intake

Risks	Benefits
Gastrointestinal side effects: flatulence, abdominal discomfort	Earlier satiety
Intestinal blockage/ bezoars (rare)	Possible weight reduction
Possible vitamin and mineral malabsorption, especially in the elderly	Possible reduction of cholesterol serum levels
Possible hypoglycemia if taking insulin	Possible smoothing out of blood glucose response

added to natural foods, such as guar gum incorporated into spaghetti, should be considered fiber supplements or high-fiber natural foods.

What Is the Risk versus Benefit of Increasing Fiber in the Diet?

Individuals need to assess the risks versus benefits of increasing fiber intake (Table 21-5). A bothersome problem when increasing consumption of high-fiber foods is abdominal discomfort, cramping, and flatulence. This problem can be minimized by starting with small servings of fiber-rich foods and gradually increasing fiber intake. Another problem that has bothered researchers is possible vitamin and mineral malabsorption caused by a high-fiber diet. Many factors influence the relationship of fiber to vitamin and mineral absorption, such as type of food, type of added fiber, and effect of complexing agents (phytic acid, oxalic acid). Fiber ions might bind calcium.[96] After 6 to 12 months of taking 14 to 26 g/d of a guar supplement, Jenkins et al[97] found no evidence of mineral (zinc, copper, calcium) deficiency in their patients. Anderson et al,[98] following 15 patients on a HCF diet (25 to 35 g dietary fiber/1000 kcal) for approximately 21 months, found that average values for serum calcium, phosphorus, alkaline phosphatase, iron, total iron-binding capacity, mag-

nesium, hemoglobin, vitamin B_{12}, and folic acid concentrations were normal. Although deficiencies have not been detected, a multivitamin and mineral supplement is routinely prescribed with the HCF diets as a safeguard.[56] In the elderly, who may already be deficient in calcium and vitamin D and have bone disease, routine addition of fiber and phytate in the form of bran, without supplementary minerals, seems premature. Until studies are undertaken to ensure that elderly persons adapt adequately and do not have prolonged mineral malabsorption, fiber should be added cautiously.[96] The few clinical studies involving fiber and children with diabetes[84,99,100] or pregnant women with diabetes[101,102] have shown no harmful effects of fiber. Appetites of children should be monitored to ensure that fibrous foods are not so filling that they limit other nutrient intakes. Adding fiber to the diet of persons taking insulin might cause hypoglycemic reactions if insulin is not reduced. Also, fiber may be contraindicated in persons who have gastric manifestations of diabetic autonomic neuropathy.[103]

Incorporating Fiber into the Diet

Although the benefits of high-fiber diets may be demonstrated in a controlled setting, their usefulness will remain limited unless patients comply with diet changes when at home.

Not everyone is a candidate for long-term high-fiber diets. For example, of 37 nonobese men with diabetes, 9 were considered to be unsuitable candidates—because of schizophrenia and well-documented gastric emptying problems—for long-term follow-up on the highly structured HCF diet regimen.[56]

How can the dietitian/nutrition counselor help willing-to-try clients make changes in their diet patterns and eating behaviors to incorporate more fiber? Specifically, how can clients be encouraged to increase their fiber intakes from the present average of 13 to 22 g/d to 30 g/d? How can clients be encouraged to increase their intake of grains, vegetables, and fruits? The Five-a-Day program encourages increased fruit and vegetable servings; results are not yet available.[104]

- Increasing fiber content of the diet usually requires altering the macronutrient composition of the diet (more carbohydrate and less fat and meat). Convince individuals that it is "good" to eat more of the "right kind" of carbohydrate as a first step!
- Develop palatable diets that contain high-fiber foods that are readily available in the grocery store: whole-grain breads and cereals, dry beans, and common vegetables and fruits. However, a cup of salad containing only iceberg lettuce is not a high source of fiber. Table 21-4 and Exhibit 21-1 show typical daily menus that have been included in high-fiber clinical research studies.
- Convince individuals to be consistent in the amount of fiber eaten from day to day and to try to increase the amount gradually over a period of weeks. Doing so helps prevent flatulence and diarrhea and makes it easier for the client to reach the final goal amount per day.
- Process food to maintain its cellular integrity. For example, use rolled or whole grain rather than ground cereals and legume products. Have clients choose foods that are cooked for the least amount of time that are acceptable to them.
- Include daily a variety of sources of fiber foods in the diet to achieve a good balance of soluble and insoluble fiber, such as wheat bran and legumes, as well as nutrients.

SUMMARY AND APPLICATIONS TO PRACTICE

The dietitian is challenged with understanding the variety of terminologies used in the dietary fiber field, keeping up with food labeling requirements, and keeping up with the dietary fiber research that directs clinical care. These

Exhibit 21-1 Sample 1500-kcal High-Fiber (33.6 g) Maintenance Menu

		Fiber/Serving (g)
Breakfast	8 oz skim milk	—
	1/4 cup Grapenut cereal	4.7
	1 whole-wheat English muffin	2.6
	2 pats margarine	—
	1/2 cup orange juice	0.1
Noon Meal	2 slices whole-wheat bread	2.6
	1 oz ham	—
	1/2 cup tomatoes	1.4
	1/2 large carrot	1.2
	1 cup spinach	1.9
	4 tsp salad dressing	—
	8 oz skim milk	—
Evening Meal	1 whole-wheat dinner roll	1.7
	3 oz baked chicken	—
	1/2 cup green peas	4.1
	1/2 cup cooked carrots	2.2
	1/2 cup zucchini	2.0
	1/2 cup red cabbage	1.5
	3 pats margarine	—
Snack	6 cups popcorn	5.6
	1 small apple	2.0
Total		**33.6**

Note: This day's meal plan is an example of a 1500-calorie HCF home maintenance diet used by Anderson and includes approximately 55% carbohydrate, 20% protein, 25% fat, 20 to 25 g dietary fiber/1000 kcal, 200 mg cholesterol, and a high P/S ratio. Approximately 27% of the total dietary fiber is from soluble sources. Although not shown in this specific example, the HCF diet contains dry beans and oats in abundance.

Source: L Story et al. Adherence to high carbohydrate, high fiber diets: long-term studies of nonobese diabetic men, Copyright The American Dietetic Association. Reprinted by permission from *Journal of The American Dietetic Association*, Vol. 85:1105, 1985.

knowledge challenges come before the challenge of guiding clients to make changes, or not, in their dietary intakes. Despite significant research showing improvements from dietary fiber supplementation in blood and lipid profiles of persons with diabetes, current recommendations are to increase fiber from food sources. Food sources of fiber certainly preserve the whole food matrix and coexistent nutrients. Dietitians are encouraged to assess the health needs of each individual client when determining whether to rely on food sources of dietary fiber or add fiber supplements.

REFERENCES

1. *Dietary Guidelines for Americans.* 3rd ed. Washington, DC: U.S. Department of Agriculture, US Department of Health and Human Services; 1990.

2. American Diabetes Association. Nutrition recommendations and principles for persons with diabetes. *Diabetes Care.* 1994;17:519–522.

3. Hipsley EH. Dietary fiber and pregnancy toxaema. *BMJ.* 1953;2:420–422.

4. Trowell H, Southgate DAT, Wolever TMS, et al. Dietary fibre redefined (letter). *Lancet.* 1976;1:967.

5. Schneeman BO. Physical and chemical properties, methods of analysis, and physiological effects. *Food Technol.* 1986;40:104–110.

6. Selvendran R. The plant cell wall as a source of dietary fiber: chemistry and structure. *Am J Clin Nutr.* 1984;39:320–337.

7. Southgate DAT, Englyst H. Dietary fibre: chemistry, physical properties and analysis. In: Trowell H, Burkitt D, Heaton K, eds. *Fibre, Fibre-Depleted Foods and Disease.* New York, NY: Academic Press; 1985:31–56.

8. Schneeman BO. Soluble vs insoluble fiber—different physiological responses. *Food Tech Fed Eur Biochem Soc Lett.* 1987; February:81–82.

9. Story J, Watterson JJ, Matheson HB, Furumoto EJ. Dietary fiber and bile acid metabolism. In: Furda I, Brine CJ, eds. *New Developments in Dietary Fiber.* New York, NY: Plenum Press; 1990:43–48.

10. Miettenen TA, Tarpila S. Effect of pectin on serum cholesterol, fecal bile acids and biliary lipids in normolipidemic and hyperlipidemic individuals. *Clin Chim Acta.* 1977;79:471–477.

11. Kay RM, Truswell AS. Effect of citrus pectin on blood lipids and fecal steroid excretion in man. *Am J Clin Nutr.* 1977;30:171–175.

12. Stasse-Wolthuis M, Albers HFF, van Jerveren JGC, et al. Influence of dietary fiber from vegetables and fruits, bran, or citrus pectin on serum lipids, fecal lipids, and colonic function. *Am J Clin Nutr.* 1980;33:1745–1756.

13. Committee on Diet and Health, Food and Nutrition Board Commission on Life Sciences, National Academy of Sciences. Dietary fiber. In: *Diet and Health. Implications of Reducing Chronic Disease Risk.* Washington, DC: National Academy Press; 1989:291–310.

14. Southgate DAT, Hudson GJ, Englyst H. The analysis of dietary fiber—the choices for the analyst. *J Sci Food Agric.* 1978;29:979–988.

15. Southgate DAT. The definition, analysis and properties of dietary fiber. *J Plant Food.* 1978;3:9–19.

16. Marlett JA, Chesters JG, Longacre MJ, Bogdanske JJ. Recovery of soluble dietary fiber is dependent on the method of analysis. *Am J Clin Nutr.* 1989;50:479–485.

17. Prosky L, Asp N, Schweizer TF, DeVries JW, Furda I. Determination of insoluble, soluble and total dietary fiber in foods and food products: interlaboratory study. *J Assoc Off Anal Chem.* 1988;71:1017–1023.

18. Prosky L. Collaborative study of a method for soluble and insoluble dietary fiber. *Adv Exp Med Biol.* 1990;270:193–203.

19. Part 101 Food Labeling. *Federal Register.* 1993;58:2176.

20. Eastwood MDRP. A new look at dietary fiber. *Nutr Today.* 1984;19:6–11.

21. Payler DK, Pomare EW, Heaton KW, et al. The effect of wheat bran on intestinal transit. *Gut.* 1975;16:209–213.

22. Wrick KL, Robertson JB, Van Soest PJ, et al. The influence of dietary fiber source on human intestinal transit and stool output. *J Nutr.* 1983;113:1464–1479.

23. Snow P, O'Dea K. Factors affecting the rate of hydrolysis of starches in foods. *Am J Clin Nutr.* 1981;34:2721–2727.

24. Lanza E, Butrum RR. A critical review of food fiber analysis and data. *J Am Diet Assoc.* 1986;86:732–743.

25. Golay A, Coulston AM, Hollenbeck CB, et al. Comparison of metabolic effects of white beans processed into two different physical forms. *Diabetes Care.* 1986;9:262–266.

26. Southgate DAT. *The Measurement and Characterisation of Cereal Dietary Fibre.* Brussels: Proceedings of the Brood en Gezondheid; 1985. No. 1-17-27.

27. Muir JG, O'Dea K. Measurement of resistant starch: factors affecting the amount of starch escaping digestion in vitro. *Am J Clin Nutr.* 1992;56:123–127.

28. Prosky L, Asp N, Furda I, et al. Determination of total dietary fiber in foods and food products: interlaboratory study. *J Assoc Off Anal Chem.* 1984;67:1044–1052.

29. Prosky L, Harland B. Dietary fiber methodology. In: Trowell H, Burkitt D, Heaton K, eds. *Dietary Fibre, Fibre-Depleted Foods and Disease.* New York, NY: Academic Press; 1985.

30. Prosky L. Analysis of total dietary fibre: the Collaborative Study. In: Vahouny GV, Kritchevsky D, eds. *Dietary Fiber.* New York, NY: Plenum Publishing Corp; 1985:1–16.

31. Prosky L, Asp N, Furda I, et al. Determination of total dietary fiber in foods and food products: collaborative study. *J Assoc Off Anal Chem.* 1985;68:677–679.

32. Van Soest PJ, Wine RH. Use of detergents in the analysis of fibrous feeds. IV. Determination of plant cell-wall constituents. *J Assoc Off Anal Chem.* 1967;50:51–55.

33. Trowell H, Burkitt D Heaton K, eds. *Dietary Fibre, Fibre-Depleted Foods and Disease.* London: Academic Press; 1985.

34. Van Soest PJ. Use of detergents in the analysis of fibrous feeds. II. A rapid method for the determination of fiber and lignin. *J Assoc Off Anal Chem.* 1963;46:829–835.

35. Southgate DAT. Determination of carbohydrates in foods. II. Unavailable carbohydrates. *J Sci Food Agric.* 1969;20:331–335.

36. Englyst H, Wiggins HS, Cummings JH. Determination of the non-starch polysaccharides in plant foods by gas-liquid chromotography of constituent sugars as alditol acetates. *Analyst.* 1982;107:307–318.

37. Roberfroid M, Gibson GR, Delzene N. The biochemistry of oligofructose, a nondigestible fiber: an approach to calculate its caloric value. *Nutr Rev.* 1993;51:137–146.

38. Part 101 Food Labeling. *Federal Register.* 1993;58:2175.

39. Anderson JW. *Plant Fiber in Foods.* Lexington, Ky: HCF Nutrition Research Foundation, Inc; 1990. No. 1-32.

40. Southgate DAT. *Determination of Food Carbohydrates.* London: Applied Science Publishers; 1976.

41. Englyst HN, Hudson GJ. Colorimetric method for routine measurement of dietary fibre as nonstarch polysaccharides. A comparison with gas-liquid chromotography. *Food Chem.* 1987;24:53–76.

42. Anderson JW, Bridges SR. Dietary fiber content of selected foods. *Am J Clin Nutr.* 1988;47:440–447.

43. Englyst H, Bingham SA, Runswick SA, Collinson E, Cummings JH. Dietary fibre (non-starch polysaccharides) in fruit, vegetables, and nuts. *J Hum Nutr Diet.* 1988;1:247–286.

44. Englyst H, Bingham SA, Runswick SA, Collinson E, Cummings JH. Dietary fibre (non-starch polysaccharides) in cereal products. *J Hum Nutr Diet.* 1989;2:257–276.

45. American Diabetes Association, American Dietetic Association. *Exchange Lists for Meal Planning.* New York, NY: American Diabetes Association; 1995.

46. Franz MJ, Horton ES, Bantle JP, et al. Nutrition principles for the management of diabetes and related complications (Technical Review). *Diabetes Care.* 1994;17:490–518.

47. Nuttall FQ. Dietary fiber in the management of diabetes. *Diabetes.* 1993;42:503–508.

48. Wahlquist ML, Morris MJ, Littlejohn GO, Bond A, Jackson RVJ. The effects of dietary fibre on glucose tolerance in healthy males. *Aust NZ J Med.* 1979;9:154–158.

49. Hollenbeck CB, Coulston AM, Reaven GM. To what extent does increased dietary fiber improve glucose and lipid metabolism in patients with non–insulin-dependent diabetes mellitus (NIDDM)? *Am J Clin Nutr.* 1986;43:16–24.

50. Goulder TJ, Alberti KGMM, Jenkins DJA. Effect of added fiber on the glucose and metabolic response to a mixed meal in normal and diabetic subjects. *Diabetes Care.* 1978;1:351–355.

51. Jenkins DJA, Wolever TMS, Hockaday TDR, et al. Treatment of diabetes with guar gum. Reduction of urinary glucose loss in diabetics. *Lancet.* 1977;2:779–780.

52. Jenkins DJA, Wolever TMS, Nineham R, et al. Guar crisp bread in the diabetic diet. *BMJ.* 1978;2:1741–1747.

53. Jenkins DJA, Wolever TMS, Nineham R, et al. Dietary fiber and diabetic therapy. A progressive effect with time. *Adv Exp Med Biol.* 1979;119:275–279.

54. Christiansen JS, Bonnevie-Nielsen V, Svendsen PA, et al. Effect of guar gum on 24-hour insulin requirements of insulin-dependent diabetic subjects as assessed by artificial pancreas. *Diabetes Care.* 1980;3:659–662.

55. Anderson JW, Ward K. Long-term effects of high carbohydrate, high-fiber diets on glucose and lipid metabolism. A preliminary report on patients with diabetes. *Diabetes Care.* 1978;1:77–82.

56. Story L, Anderson JW, Chen WL, et al. Adherence to high-carbohydrate, high-fiber diets: long-term studies of non-obese diabetic men. *J Am Diet Assoc.* 1985;85:1105–1110.

57. Jenkins DJA, Goff DV, Leeds AR. Unabsorbable carbohydrates and diabetes: decreased postprandial hyperglycemia. *Lancet.* 1976;2:172–174.

58. Jenkins DJA, Wolever TMS, Jenkins AL, et al. Glycemic response to wheat products: reduced response to pasta but no effect of fiber. *Diabetes Care.* 1983;6:155–159.

59. Vuorinen-Markkola H, Sinisalo M, Koivisto VA. Guar gum in insulin-dependent diabetes: effects on glycemic control and serum lipoproteins. *Am J Clin Nutr.* 1992;56:1056–1060.

60. Anderson JW. The role of dietary carbohydrate and fiber in the control of diabetes. *Adv Int Med.* 1980;26:67–96.

61. Riccardi G, Rivellese A, Pacioni D, et al. Separate influence of dietary carbohydrate and fibre on the

metabolic control in diabetes. *Diabetologia.* 1984;26:116–121.

62. Pastors JG. Psyllium fiber reduces rise in postprandial glucose and insulin concentrations in patients with non–insulin-dependent diabetes. *Am J Clin Nutr.* 1991;53:1431–1435.

63. Pedersen O, Hjollund E, Lindskov HO, et al. Increased insulin receptor binding to monocytes from insulin-dependent diabetic patients after a low-fat, high-starch, high fiber diet. *Diabetes Care.* 1982;5:284–291.

64. Hjollund E, Pedersen O, Richelsen B, et al. Increased insulin binding to adipocytes and monocytes and increased insulin sensitivity of glucose transport and metabolism in adipocytes from non–insulin-dependent diabetics after a low-fat/high-starch/high-fiber diet. *Metabolism.* 1983;32:1067–1075.

65. Kirby RW, Anderson JW, Sieling B, et al. Oat-bran intake selectively lowers serum low-density lipoprotein cholesterol concentrations of hypercholesterolemic men. *Am J Clin Nutr.* 1981;32:824–829.

66. Story J, Kritchevsky D. Comparison of the binding of various bile acids and bile salts in vitro by several types of fiber. *J Nutr.* 1976;106:1292–1294.

67. Van Horn LV, Liu K, Parker D, et al. Serum lipid response to oat product intake with a fat-modified diet. *J Am Diet Assoc.* 1986;86:759–764.

68. Anderson JW, Story L, Sieling B, et al. Hypocholesterolemic effects of oat-bran or bean intake for hypercholesterolemic men. *Am J Clin Nutr.* 1984;40:1146–1155.

69. Jenkins DJA, Wong GS, Patten R, et al. Leguminous seeds in the dietary management of hyperlipidemia. *Am J Clin Nutr.* 1983;38:567–573.

70. Anderson JW. Effect of carbohydrate restriction and high carbohydrate diets on men with chemical diabetes. *Am J Clin Nutr.* 1977;30:402–408.

71. Anderson JW. High-fiber diets for diabetic and hypertriglyceridemic patients. *Can Med Assoc J.* 1980;123:975–979.

72. Anderson JW, Chen WL, Sieling B. Hypolipidemic effect of high-carbohydrate, high-fiber diets. *Metabolism.* 1980;29:551–558.

73. Committee on Diet and Health, Food and Nutrition Board Commission on Life Sciences, National Academy of Sciences. Atherosclerotic cardiovascular diseases. In: *Diet and Health. Implications of Reducing Chronic Disease Risk.* Washington, DC: National Academy Press; 1989:529–548.

74. Anderson JW, Gilinsky NH, Deakins DA, et al. Lipid responses of hypercholesterolemic men to oat-bran and wheat-bran intake. *Am J Clin Nutr.* 1991;54:678–683.

75. Anderson JW. Plant fiber and blood pressure. *Ann Intern Med.* 1983;98:842–846.

76. Henry RR, Schaeffer L, Olefsky JM. Glycemic effects of intensive caloric restriction and isocaloric refeeding in noninsulin-dependent diabetes mellitus. *J Clin Endocrinol Metab.* 1985;61:917–925.

77. Anderson JW, Sieling B. High fiber diets for obese diabetic patients. *Obes/Bariatric Med.* 1980;9:109–113.

78. Bjoemtorp P, Vahouny GV, Kritchevsky D. *Dietary Fiber and Obesity.* New York, NY: Alan R Liss, Inc; 1985.

79. Haber GB, Heaton KW, Murphy D, et al. Depletion and disruption of dietary fibre. Effects on satiety, plasma glucose, and serum-insulin. *Lancet.* 1977;2:679–682.

80. Rivellese A, Parillo M, Giacco A, et al. A fiber rich diet for the treatment of diabetic patients with chronic renal failure. *Diabetes Care.* 1985;8:620–621.

81. *Physiological Effects and Health Consequences of Dietary Fiber.* Rockville, Md: Life Sciences and Research Office, Federation of American Societies for Experimental Biology; 1987.

82. Lanza E, Jone DY, Block G, Kessler L. Dietary fiber intake in the U.S. population. *Am J Clin Nutr.* 1987;46:790–797.

83. Bingham S. Dietary fibre intakes: intake studies, problems, methods and results. In: Trowell H, Burkitt D, Heaton K, eds. *Dietary Fibre, Fibre-Depleted Foods and Disease.* New York, NY: Academic Press; 1985:77–104.

84. Lindsay AN, Hardy S, Jarrett L, et al. High-carbohydrate, high-fiber diet in children with type I diabetes mellitus. *Diabetes Care.* 1984;7:63–67.

85. Mahalko JR, Sandstead HH, Johnson LK, et al. Effect of consuming fiber from corn bran, soy hulls, or apple powder on glucose tolerance and plasma lipids in type II diabetes. *Am J Clin Nutr.* 1984;29:25–34.

86. Jones DB, Slaughter P, Lousley S, et al. Low-dose guar improves diabetic control. *J R Stat Soc Series.* 1985;78:546–548.

87. *The Food Guide Pyramid.* Washington, DC: U.S. Department of Agriculture, Human Nutrition Information Service; 1992.

88. Department of Health and Human Services. *Healthy People 2000.* Washington, DC: Public Health Service; 1990.

89. Subar AF, Heimendinger J, Krebs-Smith SM, et al. *5 a Day for Better Health: A Baseline Study of American's Fruit and Vegetable Consumption.* Rockville, Md: National Cancer Institute; 1992.

90. Stehlin D. A little "lite" reading. Washington, DC: Food and Drug Administration; 1994; May:32. FDA Consumer Special Report: Focus on Food Labeling.

91. Brown MB. *Label Facts for Healthful Eating— Educator's Resource Guide.* Chicago, Ill: The American Dietetic Association; 1993.

92. Wolever TMS, Jenkins DJA, Nineham R, et al. Guar gum and reduction of post-prandial glycaemia. Effect of incorporation into solid food, liquid food, and both. *BMJ.* 1979;41:505–510.

93. Furda I. *Unconventional Sources of Dietary Fiber.* Washington, DC: American Chemical Society; 1983.

94. *Report of the Expert Advisory Committee on Dietary Fiber to the Health Protection Branch, Health and Welfare Canada.* Ontario: National Health and Welfare; 1985.

95. Mullin JD. Dietary fiber sources for human studies. *Am J Clin Nutr.* 1978;31S:103–106.

96. James WPT, Branch WJ, Southgate DAT. Calcium binding by dietary fibre. *Lancet.* 1978;1:638–639.

97. Jenkins DJA, Wolever TMS, Taylor RH, et al. Diabetic glucose control, lipids, and trace elements on long term guar. *BMJ.* 1980;1:1353–1354.

98. Anderson JW, Ferguson SK, Karounos D, et al. Mineral and vitamin status of high-fiber diets: long-term studies of diabetic patients. *Diabetes Care.* 1980; 3:38–40.

99. Baumer JH, Drakeford JA, Wadsworth J, et al. Effects of dietary fibre and exercise in mid-morning diabetic control. A controlled trial. *Arch Dis Child.* 1982;57:905–909.

100. Kinmouth AL, Angus RM, Jenkins PA, et al. Whole foods and increased dietary fibre improve blood glucose control in diabetic children. *Arch Dis Child.* 1982;57:187–194.

101. Kuhl C, Molsted-Pedersen L, Hornnes PJ. Guar gum and glycemic control of pregnant insulin-dependent diabetic patients. *Diabetes Care.* 1983;6:152–154.

102. Ney D, Hollingsworth DR, Cousins L. Decreased insulin requirement and improved control of diabetes in pregnant women given a high-carbohydrate, high-fiber, low-fat diet. *Diabetes Care.* 1982;5:529–533.

103. Canivet B, Creisson G, Freychet P, et al. Fibre, diabetes, and risk of bezoar. *Lancet.* 1980;2:862.

104. Havas S, Heimendinger J, Reynolds K, et al. 5 a day for better health: a new research initiative. *J Am Diet Assoc.* 1994;94:32–36.

SUGGESTED READING

Anderson JW, Smith BM, Geil PB. High-fiber diet for diabetes. Safe and effective treatment. *Postgrad Med.* 1990;88:157–168.

Franz MJ, Horton ES, Bantle JP, et al. Nutrition principles for the management of diabetes and related complications (Technical Review). *Diabetes Care.* 1994;17: 490–518.

Nuttall FQ. Dietary fiber in the management of diabetes. *Diabetes.* 1993;42:503–508.

Prosky L, DeVries JW. *Controlling Dietary Fiber in Food Products.* New York, NY: Van Nostrand Reinhold; 1992:161.

Riccardi G, Rivellese AA. Effects of dietary fiber and carbohydrate on glucose and lipoprotein metabolism in diabetic patients. *Diabetes Care.* 1991;14:1115–1125.

Spiller GA, ed. *CRC Handbook of Dietary Fiber in Human Nutrition.* Boca Raton, Fla: CRC Press; 1993:648.

Tinker LF. Dietary fiber: variables that affect its nutritional impact. *Diabetes Spectrum.* 1990;3(3):191–196.

Vinik AI, Wing RR. The good, bad, and the ugly in diabetic diets. *Endocrinol Metab Clin North Am.* 1992;21: 237–279.

Analysis of Dietary Fiber

A major barrier to the understanding of the nutritional significance of dietary fiber has been problems associated with its analysis. The complexity of physiologic actions of dietary fiber within the gastrointestinal tract leads to difficulty of analysis because analysis relies on chemical processes, not physiologic processes. Dietary fiber has biologic actions, but no bioassay exists. Also, dietary fiber is a heterogeneous group of compounds, each with differing responses to chemical analysis. In the United States, and several other countries, an enzymatic gravimetric assay for total dietary fiber[1] has been accepted as the recommended method for dietary fiber analysis and food labeling.[2] Criticism of this method includes the fact that it does not measure resistant starch, which is not digested in the human small intestine, and hence physiologically acts as dietary fiber.[3] Thus, consensus for a universally accepted method of dietary fiber analysis does not yet exist, and the reader of dietary fiber research is cautioned to carefully read the method(s) used to analyze dietary fiber when comparing results from several studies. Various dietary fiber analysis methods are reviewed in a recently published conference proceedings text.[4]

In 1988, an enzymatic gravimetric procedure was developed and tested at multiple laboratory sites across the United States to analyze soluble and insoluble dietary fiber.[1,5] Good correlation was found between total dietary fiber analyzed by the Prosky method[6,7] and summing the amounts of soluble and insoluble dietary fiber analyzed in the Prosky method for soluble and insoluble dietary fiber.[1]

Among the methods currently available to measure the individual components of dietary fiber, the Southgate chemical fractionation procedure,[8] supplemented with gas or liquid chromatography, seems to be the most popular one. As do other fiber methods, the Southgate method continues to evolve and is quite complicated and time-consuming. A quick method that yields a complete analysis of all components is needed but is still far from being realized.

REFERENCES

1. Prosky L. Collaborative study of a method for soluble and insoluble dietary fiber. *Adv in Exper Med Biol.* 1990;270:193–203.

2. Schweizer TF. Dietary fiber analysis and nutrition labelling. *Adv Exper Med Biol.* 1990;270:265–272.

3. Englyst HN, Trowell H, Southgate DAT, Cummings JH. Dietary fiber and resistant starch. *Am J Clin Nutr.* 1987;46:873–874.

4. Furda I, Brine CJ. *New Developments in Dietary Fiber.* New York, NY: Plenum Press; 1990.

5. Prosky L, Asp N, Schweizer TF, DeVries JW, Furda I. Determination of insoluble, soluble and total dietary fiber in foods and food products: interlaboratory study. *J Assoc Off Anal Chem.* 1988;71:1017–1023.

6. Prosky L, Asp N, Furda I, et al. Determination of total dietary fiber in foods and food products: interlaboratory study. *J Assoc Off Anal Chem.* 1984;67:1044–1052.

7. Prosky L. Analysis of total dietary fibre: the Collaborative Study. In: Vahouny GV, Kritchevsky D, eds. *Dietary Fiber.* New York, NY: Plenum Publishing Corp; 1985:1–16.

8. Southgate DAT. Determination of carbohydrates in foods. II. Unavailable carbohydrates. *J Sci Food Agric.* 1969;20:331–335.

Total Dietary Fiber Values for Foods

STARCH: BREADS, CRACKERS, SNACKS

Food	Quantity	Total Dietary Fiber (g)
Bagel	0.5 Bagel	0.7
Bread, pita	0.5 Pita bread	0.5
Bread, pumpernickel	1.0 slice	1.9
Bread, raisin	1.0 slice	1.1
Bread, rye	1.0 slice	2.0
Bread, white (including French and Italian)	1.0 slice	0.6
Bread, whole-wheat	1.0 slice	2.0
Bread sticks	2.0 Bread sticks	0.6
Crackers, oyster	24.0 Crackers	0.5
Crackers, animal	8.0 Crackers	0.5
Crackers, graham	3.0 Crackers	0.6
Crackers, saltines	6.0 Crackers	0.5
Crispread	2.0 slices	3.2
Croutons	1.0 cup	0.9
English muffins	0.5 English muffin	0.8
Frankfurter roll	0.5 Frankfurter roll	0.6
Hamburger bun	0.5 Hamburger bun	0.6
Matzos	0.8 oz	0.6
Melba toast	5.0 slices	1.6
Popcorn, popped, no salt/fat added	3.0 cups	3.6
Pretzels, sticks/rings	0.8 oz	0.7
Roll, plain bread	1.0 Roll	0.8
Rye crisp	4.0 Rye crisps	2.7
Tortilla, corn	1.0 Tortilla	1.3
Tortilla, flour, 7–8 in. diameter, RTC	1.0 Tortilla	1.1

STARCH: CEREAL

Food	Quantity	Total Dietary Fiber (g)
40% Bran flakes cereal	0.5 cup	4.7
All bran dry cereal	0.5 cup	10.0

Sources: Foods: *Exchange Lists for Meal Planning* (pp 6–12), the American Diabetes Association, Inc., and The American Dietetic Association, Copyright 1995. Primary fiber source: USDA/ARS—Beltsville Human Nutrition Research Center, *1993 USDA Nutrition Database for Standard References*, release 10, Hyattsville, Md. (Most values are based on the AOAC methods for total dietary fiber.) Secondary fiber source (foods not in HB8): *Plant Fiber in Foods* by JW Anderson, HCF Nutrition Research Foundation, Inc, 1990.

Food	Quantity	Total Dietary Fiber (g)
Bran buds dry cereal	0.3 cup	10.7
Cheerios oats dry cereal	0.75 cup	1.6
Cornflakes dry cereal	0.75 cup	0.6
Cream of rice, cooked	0.5 cup	0.1
Cream of wheat cereal, cooked	0.5 cup	0.9
Grapenuts dry cereal	3.0 Tbsp	1.9
Grapenut flakes dry cereal	0.75 cup	2.9
Kix dry cereal	0.75 cup	0.3
Oatmeal, cooked cereal	0.5 cup	2.0
Product 19 dry cereal	0.75 cup	0.9
Puffed rice dry cereal	1.5 cups	0.4
Puffed wheat dry cereal	1.5 cups	0.9
Raisin bran dry cereal	0.5 cup	3.5
Rice Krispies dry cereal	0.75 cup	0.3
Shredded wheat dry cereal	0.5 cup	2.5
Wheaties, wheat dry cereal	0.75 cup	2.1
Whole-wheat hot natural cereal, cooked	0.5 cup	1.9

STARCH: DRIED BEANS, GRAINS, PASTA

Food	Quantity	Total Dietary Fiber (g)
Beans, baked	0.3 cup	3.2
Beans, kidney, canned, solids and liquids	0.3 cup	2.8
Beans, white, cooked	0.3 cup	3.8
Bulgur	0.5 cup	4.1
Cornmeal, dry, degermed, enriched	2.5 Tbsp	1.6
Grits, cooked	0.5 cup	0.2
Lentils, cooked	0.3 cup	5.2
Macaroni, cooked firm	0.5 cup	0.9
Noodles, enriched egg, cooked	0.5 cup	0.9
Peas, blackeyed, cooked	0.3 cup	3.7
Peas, split, cooked	0.3 cup	5.4
Rice, brown, cooked	0.3 cup	1.2
Rice, white, long-grain, cooked, hot	0.3 cup	0.2
Spaghetti, cooked firm	0.5 cup	1.2
Wheat germ, toasted	3.0 Tbsp	2.7

STARCH: STARCHY VEGETABLES

Food	Quantity	Total Dietary Fiber (g)
Beans, lima, canned, solids and liquids	0.5 cup	4.0
Beans, lima, frozen, cooked	0.5 cup	6.1
Corn on cob, cooked	1.0 Corn on cob	2.2
Corn, frozen, cooked	0.5 cup	2.0
Corn, whole kernel, vacuum pack	0.5 cup	6.0
Peas, green, canned, drained	0.5 cup	3.5
Peas, green, frozen, cooked	0.5 cup	4.4

Food	*Quantity*	*Total Dietary Fiber (g)*
Plantain, cooked slices	0.5 cup	1.8
Potato, baked with skin	3.0 oz	2.0
Potato, mashed, flakes (milk and fat added)	0.5 cup	2.4
Potato, sweet, canned, vacuum pack, pieces	0.3 cup	2.0
Potato, white, boiled, peeled	3.0 oz	1.5
Squash, winter	0.75 cup	5.3

STARCH: STARCH + 1 FAT

Food	*Quantity*	*Total Dietary Fiber (g)*
Biscuit, baked	1.0 Biscuit	0.6
Cornbread, baked	2.0 oz	1.4
Crackers, round butter-type	6.0 Crackers	0.4
French fries, oven heated, no salt	10.0 French fries	1.6
Muffin, plain, baked	1.0 Muffin	1.2
Noodles, chow mein	0.5 cup	0.9
Pancakes, made from mix, prepared	2.0 Pancakes	1.0
Stuffing, bread, prepared	0.3 cup	1.5
Taco shells	2.0 Taco shells	2.1
Triscuits	6.0 Triscuits	1.5
Waffle, prepared, from mix	1.0 Waffle	0.7

VEGETABLES: COOKED

Food	*Quantity*	*Total Dietary Fiber (g)*
Artichoke	0.5 Artichoke	3.2
Asparagus, frozen	0.5 cup	2.8
Asparagus, spears, canned, drained	0.5 cup	1.9
Beans (green, wax), canned, drained	0.5 cup	1.3
Beans, snap, frozen	0.5 cup	2.2
Beets, canned, drained, sliced	0.5 cup	1.5
Broccoli, spears, frozen	0.5 cup	2.8
Brussels sprouts, frozen	0.5 cup	3.3
Cabbage, fresh	0.5 cup	2.1
Carrots, canned, drained	0.5 cup	1.1
Carrots, fresh	0.5 cup	2.6
Cauliflower, frozen	0.5 cup	2.0
Collard greens, fresh	0.5 cup	1.3
Eggplant, fresh	0.5 cup	1.2
Mushrooms, canned, drained	0.5 cup	1.9
Mushrooms, fresh	0.5 cup	1.7
Mustard greens, fresh	0.5 cup	1.4
Okra, frozen	0.5 cup	2.6
Onions, fresh, chopped	0.5 cup	1.5
Pea pods, fresh	0.5 cup	2.2
Peppers, green, fresh	0.5 cup	0.8

Food	Quantity	Total Dietary Fiber (g)
Sauerkraut, canned	0.5 cup	3.0
Spinach, canned, drained	0.5 cup	2.6
Spinach, frozen	0.5 cup	2.8
Squash, summer, fresh	0.5 cup	1.3
Tomatoes, canned, solids and liquids	0.5 cup	1.2
Turnip greens, fresh	0.5 cup	2.2
Turnips, fresh, cubed	0.5 cup	1.6
Zucchini squash, fresh	0.5 cup	1.3

VEGETABLES: RAW, JUICE

Food	Quantity	Total Dietary Fiber (g)
Bean sprouts, raw	1.0 cup	1.9
Broccoli, raw, chopped	1.0 cup	2.6
Carrots, raw, ep	1.0 cup	3.3
Cauliflower, raw, ep	1.0 cup	2.5
Onions, raw, ep	1.0 cup	2.9
Pepper, green, raw, ep	1.0 cup	1.8
Squash, summer, raw, ep	1.0 cup	2.5
Tomato juice	0.5 cup	0.5
Tomatoes, raw, ep	1.0 cup	2.0
Vegetable juice	0.5 cup	1.0

FRUITS: FRESH, CANNED, DRIED

Food	Quantity	Total Dietary Fiber (g)
Apple, unpeeled	1.0 Apple	2.9
Apples, dried	4.0 slices	2.3
Applesauce, unsweetened	0.5 cup	1.5
Apricots, canned, juice pack	0.5 cup	1.6
Apricots, dried	7.0 slices	2.2
Apricots, fresh	4.0 Apricots	3.4
Banana, fresh	0.5 Banana	1.4
Blackberries, fresh	0.75 cup	5.4
Blueberries, fresh	0.75 cup	2.9
Cantaloupe, fresh	1.0 cup	1.3
Cherries, canned, juice pack, sweet	0.5 cup	0.9
Cherries, sweet, fresh	12.0 Cherries	1.9
Dates	2.5 Dates	1.6
Figs, dried	1.5 Figs	2.6
Figs, fresh	2.0 Figs	3.3
Fruit cocktail, canned, juice pack	0.5 cup	1.4
Grapefruit, canned	0.75 cup	0.7
Grapefruit, fresh	0.5 Grapefruit	1.3
Grapes, fresh seedless	15.0 Grapes	0.8
Honeydew melon, fresh	1.0 cup	1.0

Food	Quantity	Total Dietary Fiber (g)
Kiwi, fresh	1.0 Kiwi	3.1
Mandarin oranges, canned, juice pack	0.75 cup	1.3
Mango, fresh	0.5 Mango	1.9
Nectarine, fresh	1.0 Nectarine	2.2
Orange, fresh	1.0 Orange	3.1
Papaya, fresh	1.0 cup	2.5
Peach, fresh	1.0 Peach	2.6
Peaches, canned, juice pack	0.5 cup	1.2
Pear, fresh	0.5 Pear	2.0
Pears, canned	0.5 cup	2.5
Persimmon, fresh	2.0 Persimmons	1.0
Pineapple, canned, juice pack	0.3 cup	0.6
Pineapple, fresh	0.75 cup	1.4
Plums, fresh	2.0 Plums	2.0
Pomegranate, fresh	0.5 Pomegranate	0.5
Prunes, dried, uncooked	3.0 Prunes	1.8
Raisins, dark, seedless	2.0 Tbsp	0.7
Raspberries, black, fresh	1.0 cup	8.4
Strawberries, fresh	1.25 cups	4.3
Tangerine, fresh	2.0 Tangerines	3.9
Watermelon, fresh	1.25 cups	1.0

FRUITS: JUICES

Food	Quantity	Total Dietary Fiber (g)
Apple juice/cider, canned/bottled	0.5 cup	0.1
Cranberry juice cocktail, bottled	0.3 cup	0.0
Grape juice, bottled	0.3 cup	0.1
Grapefruit juice, canned	0.5 cup	0.1
Orange juice, canned	0.5 cup	0.2
Orange juice, fresh	0.5 cup	0.2
Orange juice, frozen, reconstituted	0.5 cup	0.2
Pineapple juice, canned	0.5 cup	0.1
Prune juice, bottled	0.3 cup	0.9

FATS: NUTS, SEEDS

Food	Quantity	Total Dietary Fiber (g)
Almonds, dry roasted	6.0 Almonds	1.1
Cashews, salted	1.0 Tbsp	0.3
Peanuts, dry roasted, no salt	10.0 Peanuts	0.7
Pecans	2.0 Pecans	0.5
Pine nuts	1.0 Tbsp	0.5
Pumpkin seeds, roasted	2.0 tsp	0.5
Sunflower seeds, dry roasted	1.0 Tbsp	0.7

Food	Quantity	Total Dietary Fiber (g)
Walnuts, English	2.0 Walnuts	0.4
Avocado, fresh	0.1 Avocado	1.5
Coconut, shredded, dried, sweetened	2.0 Tbsp	2.6
Olives, ripe	5.0 Large	1.2

FREE FOODS: VEGETABLES

Food	Quantity	Total Dietary Fiber (g)
Cabbage, Chinese, raw	1.0 cup	0.8
Cabbage, raw, green	1.0 cup	1.6
Celery, raw	1.0 cup	2.0
Cucumber, raw	1.0 cup	0.8
Endive/escarole, raw	1.0 cup	1.5
Lettuce, iceberg, raw	1.0 cup	0.8
Mushrooms, raw	1.0 cup	0.8
Onion, green, raw	1.0 cup	2.6
Parsley, raw	0.5 cup	1.0
Pepper, hot green chili, raw	1.0 cup	2.3
Radishes	1.0 cup	1.9
Romaine, raw	1.0 cup	1.3
Spinach, raw	1.0 cup	1.5
Watercress, raw	1.0 cup	0.4
Zucchini, raw	1.0 cup	1.6

Note: Portion sizes are consistent with their exchange serving sizes. RTC = ready to cook; ep = edible portion.

Part V

Making Food Choices

Chapter 22

Guidelines to Enhance Food Selection

Carolyn Leontos

Nutrition therapy is the most challenging aspect of diabetes care and education.[1] Adhering to principles of healthy eating requires that the person with diabetes be knowledgeable about those principles and have the skills to practice them daily. Eating occasions are important to all people and frequently connected to significant events in their lives. The registered dietitian (RD), well versed in current aspects of diabetes therapy, is the team member who can best help clients acquire the skills they need to integrate eating habits and diabetes management.[2] The nutrition assessment determines the many factors of how and why a person makes food choices. The RD needs to explore these carefully to integrate all factors into the intervention (Exhibit 22-1).

START IN THE GROCERY STORE

Selecting food begins in the grocery store. According to the Food Marketing Institute, an average supermarket in a medium-sized city carries approximately 30,000 items. *New Product News* reported 12,897 new food products appeared daily in 1993. Assessing a client's ability to make appropriate choices in the grocery store is an important part of medical nutrition therapy. It is helpful to determine why clients make the food choices they do in a grocery store. Reasons may include cost, time, familiarity, and impulse.

If food preparation time is of primary importance, they may be willing to pay for convenience. Many persons, however, may have more time than money and need money-saving tips. It

is usually less expensive to do food preparation at home rather than to have someone do it for you. For example, boneless, skinless chicken breast is more expensive per pound than a whole chicken. However, if your client cannot resist cooking and eating the skin of the chicken when it is in their kitchen, then the more expensive skinless cut of chicken might be the best choice for them. It is important to know your clients well so that recommendations are based on individual client needs.

Other factors may be that shopping time is limited and that this time is not used efficiently. This can lead to impulse buying. The most basic change for an impulse shopper may be making a grocery list and purchasing only the items on that list.

Simple strategies such as shopping once a week rather than more frequently can help control impulse buying. The grocery list should contain ample food from all the food groups to pre-

---

Exhibit 22-1 Nutrition Assessment

Nutrition assessment should include

- Food Purchasing
- Food Preparation
- Food Budget
- Label Knowledge
- Portion Size
  - –measuring skills
  - –estimating skills

Exhibit 22-2 Shopping List

Starches/Breads	*Vegetables*	*Fruit*
Pasta	Raw	Fresh
Rice	Lettuce	Apples
Cereal	Tomatoes	Oranges
Hot _____	Potatoes	Grapefruit
Cold _____	Onions	Bananas
Bread	Peppers	_____
Dinner Rolls	Celery	Canned/Frozen
_____	Radishes	Peaches
_____	Carrots	Pineapple
_____	_____	Pears
_____	Canned/Frozen	_____
	Broccoli	
Poultry, Fish, Meat	Cauliflower	*Staples*
Chicken	Carrots	Coffee
Turkey	Zucchini	Tea
Tuna	_____	Salt
Ground Round		Pepper
_____	*Milk Products*	Spices
_____	Fluid Milk	_____
_____	Skim/Nonfat	Condiments
	1%	_____
Fats	2%	Other
Margarine	Yogurt	_____
Vegetable Oil	_____	Occasional Foods
Olives	_____	_____
_____		

pare a week's worth of meals. Some educators use sample shopping lists to teach this skill and help clients get started (Exhibit 22-2). Suggest that clients avoid impulse buying by shopping after a meal when they are not hungry. Another tactic is suggesting a "field trip" to the produce department to discover different fruits and vegetables.

Consider organizing grocery store tours for small groups of clients. All this takes is the consent of the store manager and organizational skills on the part of the RD. Select a slow time of day on a typically slow day for the store. Be very familiar with the store and decide the key points you wish to make. This setting is ideal to demonstrate cost comparisons between store and name brands; fresh, frozen and canned items; large and small containers; and specially prepared foods versus the "do-it-yourself" versions.

Is cost of food an issue? If the food budget is severely limited, identify alternative sources of food, such as the local food bank. Become familiar with the resources in your area.

NUTRITION LABELING

Although laws regulating misleading labeling have been in existence since the early 1900s

Exhibit 22-3 Important Dates in History of Food/Nutrition Labels

1906	Food and Drug Administration prohibited misleading and false statements on food and drug labels.
1907	Federal Meat Inspection Act gave USDA authority to inspect meat and prevent false labeling.
1938	Federal Food, Drug and Cosmetic Act replaced the 1906 act. This established a foundation for current food labeling requirements.
1957	Poultry Products Inspection Act gave USDA authority to inspect and regulate poultry.
1966	Fair Packaging and Labeling Act.
1972	The FDA published regulations for the enforcement of the Federal Food, Drug and Cosmetic Act and Fair Packaging and Labeling Act. Established voluntary nutrition labeling effective in 1975.
1982	Sodium regulations proposed.
1986	Effective date for compliance with sodium regulations.
1990	Nutrition Labeling and Education Act (NLEA). Proposed FDA nutrition labeling regulations published.
1993	Final NLEA rules published. Health claims effective on May 8, 1994. Nutrition labeling and nutrient content effective on May 8, 1994. USDA's Food Safety and Inspection Service issues regulations for labeling of meat and poultry effective July 6, 1994.
1994	Nutrition labeling regulations mandatory.

(Exhibit 22-3), consistent information on food labels is a result of the Nutrition Labeling and Education Act of 1990.[3] This act made food labeling mandatory for processed foods regulated by the Food and Drug Administration (FDA). About 90% of processed foods will be labeled. Examples of exempt foods include plain coffee, tea, some spices, and other foods that do not contain a significant amount of nutrients. Bulk foods and ready-to-eat foods such as deli items are also exempt.

Processed meats and poultry products are regulated by the U.S. Department of Agriculture's (USDA) Food Safety and Inspection Service. They are covered by mandatory nutrition labeling regulations consistent with those of FDA. These regulations took effect on July 6, 1994.

Both USDA and FDA have voluntary labeling programs for fresh foods. USDA's voluntary program covers raw poultry and meats. FDA's voluntary program covers the top 20 most commonly consumed varieties of fresh fish, fruits, and vegetables. If voluntary compliance by retailers is not adequate, the regulating agencies may move for mandatory regulations.

After much exploration as to the best and most useful design of a food label, the current format was selected. It consists of four parts: the nutrition panel entitled *Nutrition Facts* (Exhibit 22-4), nutrient content claims, health claims, and ingredient labeling. This label became mandatory on May 8, 1994. Manufacturers were given 2 years from that date to incorporate the label on all products.

The nutrition panel on the label is titled *Nutrition Facts* and provides both the professional and the person with diabetes with precise information on the nutrient content of processed foods. Consistent serving sizes allow easy comparisons between different brands and types of products. An example of this is salad dressing. Since the introduction of *Nutrition Facts,* the serving size on the label must reflect the amount of food customarily consumed. Thirty grams, approximately 1 oz, is the reference size serving for salad dressing. Thus, it is easy to compare the caloric and nutrient content of Brand X Creamy Dressing with Brand Y Cheese Dressing.

Goal-directed recommendations for nutrition therapy in managing diabetes mandate that advice be tailored to individual needs of clients. The *Nutrition Facts* panel on the label helps professionals by providing consistent specific information. Put together a collection of food labels

Exhibit 22-4 Reading the Nutrition Facts Panel

The food label can help you make informed food choices. You can use the label to understand how all foods—including your favorites—fit into a healthy diet that includes a variety of foods in moderate amounts.

Nutrition Facts Title
The new title "Nutrition Facts" signals the new label.

Calories & Calories from Fat
In addition to the total calories contained in a serving of the food, the panel also lists how many of the calories come from fat. These amounts alone are not enough to see how the food fits in a total diet. The rest of the nutrition panel, including "% Daily Value," will help you better understand.

Serving Size
Serving size is based on a typical portion as determined through consumer surveys conducted by the U.S. government. All the other information on the panel about the food relates to this serving size.

Amount per Serving
The numbers next to the nutrients listed in this part of the panel are simply weights, measured in grams (g) or milligrams (mg). They show how much of each nutrient a serving contains.

Vitamins & Minerals
All labels must include the % Daily Value for four key vitamins and minerals: vitamin A, vitamin C, calcium, and iron. If other vitamins or minerals have been added or if the product makes a claim about other vitamins or minerals, their % Daily Values also must be listed.

Nutrition Facts

Serving Size 1 cup (248g)
Servings Per Container 4

Amount Per Serving

Calories 150   Calories from Fat 35

                                    % Daily Value*

Total Fat 4g	**6%**
Saturated Fat 2.5g	**12%**
Cholesterol 20mg	**7%**
Sodium 170mg	**7%**
Total Carbohydrate 17g	**6%**
Dietary Fiber 0g	**0%**
Sugars 17g	
Protein 13g	

Vitamin A 4%	•	Vitamin C 6%	
Calcium 40%	•	Iron 0%	

* Percent Daily Values are based on a 2,000 calorie diet. Your daily values may be higher or lower depending on your calorie needs:

		Calories:	2,000	2,500
Total Fat	Less than		65g	80g
Sat Fat	Less than		20g	25g
Cholesterol	Less than		300mg	300mg
Sodium	Less than		2,400mg	2,400mg
Total Carbohydrate			300g	375g
Dietary Fiber			25g	30g

% Daily Value
For a balanced diet, there are recommended daily amounts you should have of each nutrient. The % Daily Value tells you how much of the recommended amount of each nutrient is in a serving of the food. *It is important to note, however, that the % Daily Value on all labels is based on a sample diet of 2000 calories a day.* If you need more than that, the food would add a lower % Daily Value to your diet. If you need less than 2000 calories, the food would add a higher % Daily Value to your diet. You should view the % Daily Value listed on labels as a guide.

Recommended Total Daily Amounts
This section is always the same when it appears on labels. It shows the recommended amount, in grams or milligrams, of each nutrient for two different sample diets—one based on 2000 calories a day, the other on 2500.

Why do some food packages have a shorter or abbreviated nutrition label?
Foods that have only a few of the nutrients required on the standard label can use a short label format. What is on the label depends on what is in the food. Small- and medium-sized packages with very little label space can also use a short label.

Source: Courtesy of the Food and Drug Administration.

Table 22-1 Comparison of Label Serving Sizes with Exchange List for Meal-Planning Serving Sizes

Food	FDA Reference Amount[a]	Exchange Amount
Bread	50 g	1 slice (28 g, 1 oz)
Potatoes, plain, fresh, canned, or frozen[b]	110 g	1/2 cup (90 g)
Rice, cooked[b]	140 g	1/3 cup
Pasta, cooked[b]	140 g	1/2 cup
Meat, ready-to-eat	55 g (2 oz)	1 oz (28 g)
Vegetables, cooked[b]	85 g	1/2 cup
Vegetable juice	240 ml (1 cup)	1/2 cup (120 ml)
Fruit, canned or frozen[b]	140 g	1/2 cup
Fruit juice	240 ml (1 cup)	1/2 or 1/3 cup (120 or 80 ml)
Margarine or butter	14 g (1 Tbsp)	1 tsp (5 g)
Vegetable oil	14 g (1 Tbsp)	1 tsp (5 g)
Milk	240 ml (1 cup)	8 oz (240 ml)

[a] FDA reference amount is serving size customarily consumed; however, only the term *serving size* will appear on the label. Individual units such as one slice of bread may be declared a serving if they weigh between 50 and 200% of the reference amount.

[b] Cooked rice, pasta, vegetables, and fruit may vary in volume; therefore, reference amount is based on weight rather than a common household measurement.

to assess client education needs and to teach label reading skills. The nutrient content of a specific serving of food will be easily available. Thus, if carbohydrate counting is the food planning approach of choice, the food label becomes an invaluable tool. The same is true if fat gram counting or calorie counting is used to help manage blood glucose or weight. **If your clients use the Exchange Lists for Meal Planning, it is crucial they understand that the serving size listed on *Nutrition Facts* does not necessarily correspond with that of the Exchange Lists** (see Table 22-1).

Probably the most important concept to emphasize when teaching both meal planning and label reading is accurate portion size. A dietitian's pre-eminent skill is teaching. An example of a lesson plan for a hands-on activity that teaches skills necessary for accurate estimation of portion size is outlined in Exhibit 22-5.

The format of the *Nutrition Facts* panel is consistent from product to product, allowing for ease in comparison. Nutrients in food will be listed in terms of amount per serving and in Percent Daily Value (%DV). Daily Value (DV) is a term that is specific to the *Nutrition Facts* panel—a reference made up of daily reference values (DRVs) and reference daily intakes (RDIs). DRVs address nutrients for which no set standards exist. These are fat, saturated fat, cholesterol, total carbohydrate, fiber, sodium, and potassium. RDIs refers to vitamins, minerals, and protein previously described by the U.S. RDAs (U.S. recommended daily allowances). The U.S. RDAs are based on the National Academy of Sciences' recommended dietary allowances (RDAs). They were introduced in 1973 as a reference for voluntary nutrition labeling. Their numbers were generous as they were based on the recommendations for the age group (older than the age of 4) with highest need, usually adolescent boys. The DVs are not recommended intakes of any specific nutrient. They are used as a reference point to provide perspective on overall dietary needs.

DVs on the label are calculated on a 2000-calorie reference. Many people require fewer or more than 2000 calories daily. On labels, DV is based on fat as 30% of calories, saturated fat as 10% of calories, carbohydrate as 60% of calories, and protein as 10% of calories.

Medical nutrition therapy requires that the percentage of calories from carbohydrate, protein, and fat be determined through nutrition assessment. American Diabetes Association Nutrition Recommendations for 1994 state that protein should not be lower than the RDA or 0.8 g/kg. Percentage of fat is also variable based on individual client factors such as weight and

biochemical profile (see Chapter 3 for in-depth explanation of these concepts). It is necessary to calculate DVs for clients based on their specific needs. Table 22-2 gives examples of individualized DVs.

Nutrient content descriptors are specific terms that may be used to describe the level of a nutrient in a food (see Table 22-3).

In addition to mandating the information on the *Nutrition Facts* section of the label, FDA set specific criteria regarding health claims on other parts of the label. These address relationships between a food or a specific nutrient and the risk of a condition or a disease. FDA has established strict requirements about when and how these claims may be used. For example, any health claim about calcium and osteoporosis must state those at greatest risk for developing osteoporosis in later life are white and Asian teenage and young adult women who are in their bone-forming years. Health claims cannot be targeted toward audiences who are not generally consid-

---

Exhibit 22-5 Lesson Plan—Measuring Foods

Objective—Client will become familiar with average portions and demonstrate ability to measure food accurately using common household utensils.

Key facts—Accurate measurement skills are essential to consistent food intake. This lesson teaches clients to estimate food portions correctly.

Activity:
1. Provide a box of dry cereal and a bowl.
2. Have client pour an average portion into the bowl.
3. Client then measures the cereal with a dry measuring cup.
4. Discuss with client how to fit this serving into their food plan.

Activity:
1. Use colored water to simulate juice.
2. Ask client to pour a 4-oz portion.
3. Have client pour contents of glass into liquid measuring cup.
4. Discuss with client how to fit this serving into their food plan.

Evaluation suggestion:
Client improves ability to estimate accurately one serving of dry cereal and juice.

Note: This skill needs to be periodically evaluated.

Table 22-2 Individualizing Daily Values

		I	II	III
Carbohydrate		57%	50%	60%
Protein		13%	15%	10%
Fat		30%	35%	30%
Total Fat	Less than	51 g	58 g	65 g
Saturated Fat	Less than	17 g	17 g	20 g
Cholesterol	Less than	300 mg	300 mg	300 mg
Sodium	Less than	2400 mg	2400 mg	2400 mg
Total Carbohydrate		214 g	188 g	300 g
Dietary Fiber		20 g	20 g	25 g
Protein[a]	At least	50.9 g	72.7 g	50 g

Note: Columns I and II illustrate DVs for two different 1500-calorie diets with macronutrients determined according to individual needs. Column III gives DVs for the 2000-calorie label reference.

[a] Protein for plan I based on 140-lb person; plan II, 160-lb person.

ered at risk for the condition the claim addresses. Health claims currently allowed are listed in Table 22-4.

There are no health claims allowed for any food or nutrient and diabetes. The American Diabetes Association states that individual foods should be eaten as part of a healthful diet and that no food should be prohibited. It specifically discourages manufacturers from advertising foods as beneficial to persons with diabetes and maintains that the label statement "Diabetics: this product may be useful in your diet on the advice of a physician. This is not a reduced-calorie food" should be deleted from federal regulations.[4] However, under current law, manufacturers may continue to target foods for segments of the market, specifically persons with diabetes.

Therefore, it is particularly important to provide clients with accurate information on the role of sucrose, fructose, other nutritive sweeteners, and nonnutritive sweeteners in the food/meal plan of the person with diabetes. Current scientific evidence does not justify the use of one caloric sweetener over another.[2]

This has some important ramifications for the diabetes educator. If we compare preserves sweetened with sucrose, preserves sweetened with a noncaloric sweetener, and spreadable fruit, we must look at carbohydrate and caloric content as well as price. The portion size of these products will be consistent on the *Nutrition Facts* panel. Table 22-5 illustrates the differences in the three items. Because we are aware that the amount of carbohydrate rather than the source of carbohydrate is the important[5] factor in affecting blood glucose control, our clients' choice of product should depend on personal taste or cost rather than source of sweetener. If portion size is the most important factor *Nutrition Facts* provides the consistent information necessary to make this choice.

The *Nutrition Facts* panel lists sugars as a part of total carbohydrate on the food label. All sugars—sucrose, lactose, maltose, galactose, glucose, and fructose—are included in this total. Sugar's place on the label reinforces the concept that they, regardless of their source, are a part of total carbohydrate in the diabetic diet.

In addition to the specific claims listed, FDA allows *healthy* to be used on a food label if a food is low in fat and saturated fat and does not contain more than 60 mg of cholesterol or 480

Table 22-3 Nutrient Content Descriptors

Descriptor	Definition
Free:	None or physiologically inconsequential amounts of fat, saturated fats, cholesterol, sodium, sugars, calories
Reduced:	≤ 25% of nutrient or calories of reference product (reduced-calorie mayonnaise would have ≤ 25% fewer calories than regular mayonnaise)
Less:	≤ 25% of nutrient or calories of reference product (pretzels can claim less fat than potato chips)
Light:	1/3 the calories or 1/2 the fat of reference food, sodium content of low-calorie, low-fat food reduced 50% or can be used to describe color or texture
More:	≥ 10% of DV
High:	≥ 20% DV
Good source:	10–19% of DV
Calorie free:	≤ 5 calories
Low calorie:	≤ 40 calories
Sodium free:	≤ 5 mg
Very low sodium:	≤ 35 mg
Low sodium:	≤ 140 mg
Sugar free:	≤ 0.5 g
Fat free:	≤ 0.5 g
Low fat:	≤ 3 g
Low saturated fat:	≤ 1 g
Low cholesterol:	≤ 20 mg and ≤ 2g saturated fat
Lean and extra lean (meat, poultry, seafood, and game meat)	
Lean:	≤ 10 g fat, ≤ 4 g saturated fat ≤ 95 mg cholesterol/100 g
Extra lean:	≤ 5 g fat, ≤ 2 g saturated fat ≤ 95 mg cholesterol/100 g

Note: All amounts refer to one serving.

Source: Reprinted from *Federal Register* (1993;58:632–691;2066–2964).

Table 22-4 FDA-Approved Health Claims

Nutrient/Condition	Criteria	Model Claim
Calcium and osteoporosis	• Food must contain ≥20% of DV for calcium (200 mg) per serving • Target group most in need of calcium (teen and young adult white and Asian women) • Must state need for exercise and healthy diets	"Regular exercise and a healthy diet with enough calcium helps teen and young adult white and Asian women maintain good bone health and may reduce their high risk of osteoporosis later in life."
Fat and cancer	• Food must be low-fat or extra lean	"Development of cancer depends on many factors. A diet low in total fat may reduce the risk of some cancers."
Saturated fat and cholesterol and coronary heart disease (CHD)	• Food must be low-saturated fat, low-cholesterol, and low-fat or extra lean	"While many factors affect heart disease, diets low in saturated fat and cholesterol may reduce the risk of this disease."
Fiber-containing grain products, fruits and vegetables and cancer	• Food must contain grain products, fruits, or vegetables • Food must be low-fat • Food must be a good source (at least 5 g per serving) of dietary fiber (without fortification)	"Low-fat diets rich in fiber-containing grain products, fruits, and vegetables may reduce the risk of some types of cancer, a disease associated with many factors."
Fruits, vegetables, and grain products that contain fiber and risk of CHD	• Food must contain fruits, vegetables, and grain products, low-saturated fat, low-fat, and low-cholesterol • Contain ≥0.6 g soluble fiber per serving (without fortification)	"Diets low in saturated fat and cholesterol and rich in fruits, vegetables, and grain products that contain some types of dietary fiber, particularly soluble fiber, may reduce the risk of heart disease, a disease associated with many factors."
Sodium and hypertension	• Food must be low-sodium	"Diets low in sodium may reduce the risk of high blood pressure, a disease associated with many factors."
Fruits and vegetables and cancer	• Foods must be low-fat, good source of dietary fiber or vitamin A or C	"Low-fat diets rich in fruits and vegetables (foods that are low in fat and may contain dietary fiber or vitamin A or C) may reduce the risk of some types of cancer, a disease associated with many factors. Broccoli is high in vitamins A and C, and it is a good source of dietary fiber."

Source: Reprinted from *Federal Register* (1993;58:632–691;2066–2964).

Table 22-5 Comparison Chart

Item	Serving Size	Carbohydrate[a]	Calories[a]	Price[a]
Strawberry preserves	1 Tbsp, 14 g	12 g	48	.07
Strawberry spreadable fruit	1 Tbsp, 9 g	9 g	36	.10
Light strawberry preserves	1 Tbsp, 14 g	6 g	24	.11

[a] Carbohydrate, calories, and price listed refer to serving size of 1 tablespoon.

mg of sodium. The USDA allows this descriptor if the food is "lean" and contains no more than 480 mg of sodium. The 60 mg of cholesterol and 480 mg of sodium represent 20% of the DV of these nutrients.

RECIPE MODIFICATION

A recipe can be defined as a list of ingredients and directions for preparing a dish. Recipe modification usually involves changing either amounts or types of ingredients. We are most concerned about reducing fat, sugar, and salt; we also usually want to increase the fiber. It is important to consider the function of the ingredient before attempting to change the amount of that ingredient in a recipe.

Fat adds flavor to foods, increases tenderness of baked goods, contributes to a fine texture in baked goods and ice cream, and separates the starch granules to prevent lumpiness in sauces and gravies. It also prevents food from sticking to the pan. Sugar contributes sweet flavor, tenderness, texture, moisture, browning, and volume in baking. It provides food for yeast during the fermentation process, thereby helping yeast bread to rise. Sugar acts as a preservative in sweet spreads such as jellies and jams as well as some types of pickles. Nonnutritive sugar substitutes can easily replace the sweetening power of sugar but do not provide other qualities. Salt is used primarily for flavor, yet also acts to inhibit excess yeast growth in breads and rolls. It also improves the texture of yeast dough products. Salt is essential for certain types of pickles.

Consider the function of the ingredient and its effect on product outcome before modifying the recipe. If the primary function of added fat is to prevent sticking to the pan, nonstick cookware or cooking spray will eliminate the need for the fat. If flavor is the primary concern, additional ingredients such as spices or herbs may be necessary. In many instances, ingredients can be reduced without sacrificing flavor. Adjusting recipes is an experimental process. Some changes work very well, whereas others are unsuccessful. Exhibit 22-6 gives some suggestions for ingredient modifications and substitutions.

A variety of cookbooks with modified recipes are available in most bookstores. They include classic gourmet-type foods, ethnic specialties, and "American" cuisine. The dietitian can provide guidance in modifying individual favorite or traditional family recipes. This nutrition intervention may be the key motivator in adhering to a modified meal plan.

PACKING LUNCHES TO GO

If your client with diabetes works outside the home, a discussion of meals eaten at work is in order. Many worksite food service facilities consist of vending machines or fast-food with limited choices. The expense incurred with purchasing lunch may be a concern. Bringing lunch from home is a viable alternative to either scenario.

Find out what facilities are available at the worksite. A refrigerator and microwave oven often expand choices. Frozen entrees, "planned-overs," or easily reconstituted dried or canned foods are all possible. It is important to emphasize food choices, as well as convenience and food safety.

Sandwiches are the traditional standby when it comes to packing a lunch. Make them more appetizing by suggesting that they be prepared on a wide variety of breads, rolls, bagels, tortillas, or pita pockets. They can be prepared weekly and frozen. Fillings made with mayonnaise do not freeze as well as plain poultry, meat, or fish. Lean roast meats, poultry, and fish usually contain less sodium than cured or processed meats, such as ham or luncheon meats. Deli meats such as turkey and roast beef frequently have salt added. Suggest that clients cook on the weekend, and slice, label, and freeze lunch-size portions of home-prepared meats in small plastic bags. This suggestion works equally well with left-overs. Low-fat refried beans can be spread in a pita pocket for a vegetarian sandwich. Freezing fillings or prepared sandwiches ahead can help alleviate that early-morning-time-crunch that may be a barrier to packing lunch. Raw vegetables and condiments do not freeze well and should be added to sandwiches at mealtime.

Fruits and vegetables are nature's original fast foods. They will complement the entree or sandwich and round out the lunch. Broccoli; carrot sticks; cauliflower; red, yellow, green, or orange bell pepper rings; cherry tomatoes; alfalfa sprouts; and celery sticks all pack easily.

Exhibit 22-6 Scrumptious Substitutions

Ingredient	Suggested Alteration
Fat	✓ Limit fat to 2 Tbsp for each cup of flour in cakes, muffins, or quick breads.
	✓ Reduce fat by 1/3. If the recipe calls for 3/4 of a cup, use 1/2 cup.
	✓ Substitute fruit puree for some of the fat.
	✓ Use 2 egg whites or 1/4 cup egg substitute in place of 1 whole egg.
	✓ Use 2/3 cup vegetable oil in place of 1 cup butter (fat content is the same but is unsaturated rather than saturated).
	✓ Use 1 cup skim milk for 1 cup whole milk.
	✓ Use 1 cup evaporated skim milk in place of cream.
	✓ Use yogurt in place of sour cream. Even whole milk yogurt has only about 25% of fat of sour cream.
Sugar	✓ Limit sugar to 1 Tbsp for each cup of flour in quick breads and muffins.
	✓ Reduce sugar by 1/3. If the recipe calls for 3/4 of a cup, use 1/2 cup.
	✓ Cinnamon, nutmeg, or vanilla will enhance sweetening power.
	✓ Use a nonnutritive sweetener when appropriate.
Salt	✓ Reduce salt by 1/2 or omit entirely.
	✓ Spices and herbs will substitute flavor.
	✓ Do not eliminate from yeast breads or rolls.
Fiber	✓ Use 1/2 whole-wheat flour in recipe.
	✓ Grind bran cereals in food processor and substitute for 1/4 of all-purpose flour in recipe.
	✓ Use brown or wild rice instead of white rice.

Fat-free or low-fat dressing makes a convenient dip. Individual containers of canned juice-packed fruit can provide variety throughout the year. Many persons find that taking fresh fruit for lunch is a good way to be sure it is included in their diets.

Food safety is especially important for persons with diabetes. The nausea and diarrhea that accompany food poisoning will interfere with good metabolic control. Safe food handling is a simple precaution to help prevent these problems.

- Keep food in a safe temperature range—below 40° or above 140°F.
- Pack lunches in insulated containers with a cold pack.
- Freeze foods to serve as a cold pack (ie, sandwiches or juice box).
- Use insulated containers to maintain hot or cold temperatures.
- Cook food thoroughly. Meat, poultry, and fish should be cooked to safe temperatures.
- Make sure that everything that touches food is kept clean.
- Use new, clean brown bags. Used bags can carry insects or bacteria from previous contents. Keep recyclable lunch containers clean.

These same basics of appropriate choices and food safety apply to picnics, barbecues, camping trips, or hikes. Dried fruit a safe easy snack choice for hikers. Individually packaged foods with long shelf life such as packages of cheese and crackers or beef jerky also work well.

REFERENCES

1. Lockwood D, Frey ML, Gladish NA, Hiss RG. The biggest problem in diabetes. *Diabetes Educ.* 1986;12:30–33.
2. American Diabetes Association. Position statement: nutrition principles and recommendations: 1994. *Diabetes Care.* 1994;17:519–522.
3. Office of the Federal Register. *Federal Register.* Vol. 58. Washington, DC: National Archives and Records Administration; January 6, 1993:632–691 and 2066–2964.
4. American Diabetes Association. Position statement: food labeling. *Diabetes Care.* 1994;17:488–489.
5. American Diabetes Association. Technical review: nutrition principles and recommendations: 1994. *Diabetes Care.* 1994;17:490–518.

SELECTED READINGS

Bantle JP, Swanson JE, Thomas W, Laine DC. Metabolic effects of fructose in diabetic subjects. *Diabetes Care.* 1992;15:1468–1476.

Franz MJ. Avoiding sugar: doesn't research support traditional beliefs? *Diabetes Educ.* 1994;19:144–150.

Powers MA. Facilitating nutritional changes in "difficult" patients. *Diabetes Spectrum.* 1991;4:186–192.

RESOURCES

Reading Food Labels: A Handbook for People with Diabetes. American Diabetes Association, American Heart Association, American Association of Diabetes Educators, May 1994.

Label Facts for Healthful Eating: Educator's Resource Guide. Mona Boyd Browne, R.D., The American Dietetic Association, 1993.

Chapter 23

Adjusting Nutrition Therapy for Special Situations

Karmeen D. Kulkarni

Through nutrition therapy, the client with diabetes learns how to manage the many nutrition-related variables that arise during the course of a typical day. Also, nutrition therapy helps the client plan for those occasions outside routine daily activities. This chapter addresses a variety of nutrition-related situations that are essential components of diabetes nutrition therapy, some of which may be part of an individual's typical day whereas others may happen only occasionally.

The registered dietitian (RD) is responsible for presenting this information as it all involves adjustments to the basic meal plan. Providing self-management training on these topics takes time and is critical to achieving glucose control. Adequate nutrition therapy sessions must be provided to ensure accurate and safe decision making.

Topics covered are

1. *Alcohol:* its metabolism and physiology, the nutritional content and calorie level of various types of alcohol, and appropriate food exchanges for alcoholic beverages

2. *Eating away from home:* guidelines for dining at restaurants, food substitutes, adapting one's meal pattern when dining out

3. *Traveling:* how to adjust the meal plan for domestic and international travel

4. *Hypoglycemia:* what is hypoglycemia, why it occurs, foods used for its treatment,

the carbohydrate (CHO) and calorie content of foods used to treat hypoglycemia

5. *Sick day management:* conversion of the meal plan to adjust for altered appetite, and the purpose of maintaining carbohydrate intake

6. *Schedule changes:* how to adjust the meal plan; swing shift

ALCOHOL

The alcohol in beverages is ethanol. This is the molecule that is intoxicating in liquor such as whiskey, gin, brandy, beer, and wine. These contain ethanol in different concentrations. One alcohol equivalent or drink is usually defined as a 5-oz glass of wine, 1.5 oz of distilled spirits (whiskey, gin, vodka), or 12 oz of beer. Each of these contains approximately 0.5 oz or 12 g of alcohol.[1] Alcohol is absorbed rapidly by the stomach and small intestines and appears in the bloodstream within 5 minutes after ingestion. The alcohol concentration in the blood reaches its highest level 30 to 90 minutes after ingestion. Foods high in fat and protein may slow the alcohol absorption rate by delaying the gastrointestinal emptying time.

The body does not store alcohol; it is metabolized by the liver via three different pathways. The main pathway is the alcohol dehydrogenase (ADH) system. The second pathway is the microsomal ethanol oxidizing system. The third pathway involves the enzyme catalase, but an insignificant amount of alcohol is metabolized this way. The initial step in the ADH system is the conversion of alcohol to acetaldehyde by the enzyme, ADH. Acetaldehyde is further reduced by the enzyme acetaldehyde dehydrogenase to carbon dioxide, water, and acetyl coenzyme A (CoA). Both carbon dioxide and water are eliminated from the body, whereas acetyl CoA is subsequently converted to fatty acids that are stored by the body and used for energy.

This is similar to fat metabolism, in which the initial step is the breakdown of triglyceride to glycerol and fatty acid. The fatty acids are then converted into two carbon units in complex with acetyl CoA. Almost all tissues are able to use fatty acids for energy, whereas glycerol is oxidized in only a few tissues. Most of the glycerol is carried to the liver where it can be oxidized for energy, or it can be used for synthesizing new triglycerides.

Alcohol and Hypertriglyceridemia

Hypertriglyceridemia is more evident in persons with diabetes than in those without diabetes and may play a significant role in cardiovascular disease. Persons with diabetes have a greater predisposition toward cardiovascular disease than persons without diabetes.[2]

Untreated diabetes is one of the most common causes of severe hypertriglyceridemia of the secondary type, either by itself or in combination with another secondary cause, alcohol. Obesity is the most common primary cause. The primary type of hypertriglyceridemia is the familial type.[3]

In a person who is fasting, alcohol consumption may cause a brief rise in the plasma triglyceride level. In susceptible persons with hypertriglyceridemia, even two to three 4-oz glasses of wine can cause a further increase in the triglyceride levels, which can persist even after alcohol intake is stopped. It is not clear how long this elevation lasts. However, in some individuals with hypertriglyceridemia who have drunk large amounts of alcohol and have a temporary rise in triglycerides, the triglyceride level returns to normal after the alcohol is discontinued. Alcohol should be avoided or consumed with caution by persons who have elevated triglyceride levels.

Physiologic Impact of Alcohol on Blood Glucose Levels

Alcohol intake may cause hypoglycemia because the enzyme most common in alcohol metabolism, ADH, inhibits gluconeogenesis in the liver. In a fasting person, 2 oz of distilled liquor may result in hypoglycemia. In a fed person, with well controlled diabetes, moderate alcohol intake of either 8 oz of regular beer, 4 oz of dry wine, or 2 oz of distilled liquor along with a meal does not seem to affect the blood glucose level dramatically.[4] Individuals who have had just a small food intake may experience hypoglycemia within 6 to 36 hours after alcohol ingestion.[5] Self-monitoring blood glucose (SMBG) levels before and after alcohol intake and a meal enables the person to predict potential hypoglycemia and prevent it from occurring.

Alcohol has been shown to cause hyperglycemia in the fed state due to glycogenolysis in the liver and peripheral insulin resistance.[6] The rise in blood glucose is dependent on the quantity of alcohol consumed and the amount of liver glycogen stores available.[1]

Use of Alcohol in Cooking

The amount of alcohol used in cooking rarely exceeds 2 to 3 Tbsp per serving. It is a creative way of flavoring foods. Alcohol evaporates at a low temperature of 172.4°F. It has been assumed that when it evaporates, the flavor is left, and the remaining calories are so minimal that they do not have to be calculated into the meal plan. This assumption is not always accurate because the preparation method determines the amount of alcohol that is retained in the cooked foods. However, because the amount of alcohol used in cooking is so minimal, the amount of calories contributed per serving will be minimal. It is a gourmet flavoring method with negligible calories.

A consideration for some clients is that some cooking wines contain sodium; unfortunately, not all cooking wines have the sodium content listed on their label. One of the brands of cooking wine with the sodium content listed is "Fancy Foods." Its sodium content is 1.5% of the total volume in the bottle, so multiply total grams of volume by 1.5% to obtain grams of sodium. For example:

$$3 \text{ oz} = 90 \text{ g}; 90 \text{ g} \times .015 = 1.35 \text{ g sodium}.$$

When using vinegar wine, clients can check the ingredient list to see if sodium is added and the Nutrition Facts label for the amount. A recent visit to the grocery store found Holland House™ brand of cooking vinegar wine had 190 mg sodium per 2 tablespoons (1 oz; 30 g; or 1/8 c).

Nutritional Content and Use of Alcohol

A drink is defined as 12 oz of regular beer, 1.5 oz of distilled liquor, or 5 oz of wine.[7] Dry wines and low-calorie wines that are lower in CHO should be recommended over sweeter wines, as should reduced-calorie beer. Low-CHO wines contain less than 2% residual sugar (Exhibit 23-1). The residual sugar content of wines can be learned by writing directly to the winery. Wine labels provide the alcohol content of the wine. Labels on distilled liquor indicate the proof; 50% of the proof is equal to the alcohol content. Beer labels provide the calorie content and no other information. A liquor merchant

who is knowledgeable may be able to provide additional information if needed.

Because alcohol has a high calorie content (7 calories/g) and is metabolized in a similar way to fat, it usually is planned into the meal plan in exchange for fat. If alcohol is consumed daily, some dietitians calculate it separately from CHO, protein, and fat because alcohol does not contribute any essential nutrients to the diet. Distilled liquors have no nutrient value. Beer and wine contain minimal amounts of calcium, magnesium, iron, and vitamin B and are high in potassium such that they may be restricted for a person on a low-potassium diet. Beer and wine also contain some CHO that should be appropriately exchanged for fruit or starch exchanges or counted as grams of CHO, if CHO counting, as well as fat for the alcohol. Table 23-1 provides the composition and food exchange values of alcoholic beverages.

The American Diabetes Association 1994 Nutrition Principles and Recommendations recommend that the same precautions regarding the use of alcohol that apply to the public are also applicable to persons with diabetes.[7] When a person's diabetes is well controlled, their blood glucose level will not be impaired by moderate alcohol use when consumed with a meal.

Persons with diabetes should be cautioned that mixed alcoholic beverages contain additional calories and CHO which will affect the blood glucose level. If a beverage mix is needed, it should be planned as part of the meal (orange juice as a mixer—subtract fruit or the amount of CHO from the total CHO from the meal plan). Calorie-free mixes—listed in Exhibit 23-2—can be used in place of calorie-dense mixes.

Patients should be instructed about the following guidelines when consuming alcohol:

- Drink only when diabetes is well controlled and with the advice of the medical team (RD, RN, MD).
- Drink only with a meal or snack, not on an empty stomach.
- Try to use unsweetened drinks with noncaloric mixers, and avoid beer and sweet

---

Exhibit 23-1 Wines with Less Than 2% Carbohydrate Content

White	Red
Chablis	Burgundy
Dry Chenin Blanc	Cabernet Sauvignon
Chardonnay	Claret
French Colombard	Gamey Beaujolais
Dry Riesling	Dry Rose
Dry Sauterne	Dry Champagne
Dry Sauvignon Blanc	Dry Sherry
White Burgundy	

Table 23-1 Alcoholic Beverages: Calorie, Carbohydrate, and Food Exchange Values

Beverage	Serving Size (oz)	Calories (per serving)	Carbohydrate (g/serving)	Alcohol (g/serving)	Food Exchange
Distilled Liquors					
Whiskey	2	138	0	21.8	3 fat
Vodka (80 proof)	2	128	0	15	3 fat
Rum (80 proof)	1.5	96	0	15	2 fat
Wines					
Red, Table	4	84	0.5	11.2	2 fat
Rose, Table	4	84	0.4	11.2	2 fat
White, Table	4	80	0.8	11.2	2 fat
Beer					
Regular	8	96	8.8	8.7	1/2 starch + 1 1/2 fat
Light	12	100	4.8	11.6	2 fat
Cocktails					
Daiquiri	4	224	8	28.1	1/2 starch + 4 fat
Manhattan	4	256	3.6	37	5 1/2 fat
Martini	4	252	0.3	18.5	5 1/2 fat

Source: USDA Agriculture Handbook, No. 8-14, *Composition of Foods: Beverages, Raw, Processed, Prepared*, U.S. Department of Agriculture, 1987.

---

wines. Light dry wines are preferable to almost any other type of alcohol.

- Count alcohol calories as fat calories in the diet.

- Try to limit alcohol intake.

- Avoid alcohol if hypertriglyceridemia is present.

- Never drink before driving.

Exhibit 23-2 Calorie-Free and Calorie-Dense Mixers

Calorie Free	*Calorie Dense*
Water	Regular carbonated
Club soda	beverages
Diet carbonated beverages	Fruit juice
Lemon juice	Premade mixes
Diet tonic	Tonic
Mineral water	
Tonic	

- Do not jeopardize your health by giving in to social pressures to drink.

- Avoid hypoglycemia the morning after drinking alcohol by keeping the same schedule: get up at the same time, do a fasting blood glucose, and eat breakfast.

Persons Requiring Insulin and Alcohol Intake

For individuals on insulin, two or fewer drinks of alcohol can be part of and in addition to their usual food intake.[7] It is recommended that alcohol be consumed with a meal or soon after. Even small amounts of alcohol can cause hypoglycemia and make a person appear drunk; symptoms include stuttering, light-headedness, and anxiousness. If a person with diabetes is considered drunk, the appropriate treatment for hypoglycemia may be denied or delayed. If weight control is a concern, the appropriate alcohol calories should be incorporated into the meal plan so that the day's total caloric intake remains the same. Otherwise, limited alcohol intake may not require any meal plan modification when consumed with a meal.

Persons Requiring Oral Hypoglycemic Medication and Alcohol Intake

Some persons taking the oral hypoglycemic agent (OHA) chlorpropamide may experience mild Antabuse-like symptoms—flushing of the face and neck, nausea, impaired speech within 3 to 10 minutes of drinking alcohol, and heart palpitations. The effects can last for 1 hour or more. Other OHAs do not produce these symptoms.

When alcohol calories are added to the meal plan or added on to an already increased calorie intake, weight control for the overweight individual with type II diabetes may be more difficult to achieve. Therefore, the primary concern about alcohol consumption of a person with type II diabetes is the ingestion of extra calories. For that reason, alcohol is often planned into the diet as calories and/or fat.

****

Case Study: Use of Alcohol

Marcy is a 26-year-old single woman who likes to end her workweek on Friday with a glass of wine at a local bar with some friends. Marcy's usual meal plan is three meals (7:30 A.M., 12 noon, 6:00 P.M.) and two snacks (10:00 A.M. and 8:00 P.M.) with a split mixed dose of regular and NPH insulins one-half hour before breakfast and supper.

Marcy had two questions for her dietitian regarding alcohol intake:

1. When to test her pre-supper blood glucose level because she needed that test to determine how much regular insulin to take? She knew that the alcohol in the wine that she drank between 5:00 and 5:30 might be giving her a lower reading than on other days of the week.

2. Should she eat something when she drank the wine? Her preference was not to because she was struggling with her weight.

General alcohol intake guidelines state that a person with type I diabetes, like Marcy, can add one to two drinks to a meal without any adjustments. Noting that all guidelines need to be carefully individualized, the dietitian reviewed Marcy's blood glucose record and insulin peak times. She saw the following:

Day/Time	Blood Glucose	Insulin
Tuesday		
7:00 A.M.	123	10 R/8 NPH
12 noon	132	
5:30 P.M.	149	6 R/10 NPH
7:30 P.M.	110	
Wednesday		
7:00 A.M.	112	10 R/8 NPH
12 noon		
5:30 P.M.	101	5 R/10 NPH
7:30 P.M.	94	
Thursday		
7:00 A.M.	95	10 R/8 NPH
12 noon	112	
5:30 P.M.	136	6 R/10 NPH
7:30 P.M.	120	

Goals

1. Avoiding hypoglycemia was the primary goal of Marcy's dietitian: Marcy's morning NPH insulin would be peaking about 5:00 P.M.; the alcohol would be lowering her blood glucose level; she would be eating a later supper; and she would be driving home alone.

2. Marcy's goal was to not gain weight while enjoying social time with her friends.

Intervention

The following nutrition therapy guidelines were agreed on. Marcy would test her blood glucose level at 5:00 P.M.

1. If her blood glucose level was greater than 130 mg/dL, she would meet her friends, have her glass of wine, then retest before she ate dinner at 6:30 P.M. She would adjust her evening regular insulin dose based on this test.

2. If her blood glucose level was less than 130 mg/dL, she would deduct CHO from her evening meal and eat it before meeting her friends for a drink. She would retest her blood glucose 30 minutes later. If her blood glucose level had increased to 130 to 150 mg/dL, she would meet her friends, have the wine, and retest before her evening meal at 6:30 P.M. This would enable Marcy to prevent a possible hypoglycemic episode and also not to increase her daily calories and thereby deal with her concern regarding weight gain.

Follow-Up

Marcy would monitor her blood glucose levels several additional times the next day (Saturday)—after breakfast and lunch as well as before these meals. She would record the test results along with her insulin doses, food intake, and activity. If she had unexplained hypoglycemia, she was to call her physician immediately. Otherwise, she was to contact her dietitian before the following Friday to discuss the event, evaluate intervention results, and plan for future social events. Longer-term evaluation was to include this component of nutrition therapy in reviewing HbA$_{1c}$ values and weight.

****

EATING AWAY FROM HOME

Dining out is on the rise. Americans eat more than 30% of their meals away from home, which averages one meal a day. With so much of a person's nutrition coming from a restaurant kitchen, the art of eating out needs to come close to being a science for the person with diabetes. For many clients with diabetes, working meals purchased away from home into their meal plan is a priority. Eating at a friend's home or buying a meal to bring home may provide similar challenges.

During the initial nutrition assessment, the dietitian should determine the immediacy of information about eating away from home. The "eating out" profile is identified by documenting how often the client eats away from home, where he or she eats, and foods most often ordered (Exhibit 23-3). This enables the RD to focus on teaching clients skills to eat out and yet meet their goals of diabetes management.[8]

Initially persons will need to decide on their attitude toward eating out. If it is an occasional, special occasion-type event, then there would be more give in their food choices. But if they eat out five or more times a week, then the attitude focus should be on healthy choices being the norm.[8]

Following a meal plan at home and in a controlled environment prepares persons with diabetes to enjoy eating out. They can eat out with less hesitation if they know which foods they should eat, the portion sizes, and how to substitute appropriately. It is the dietitian's responsibility to help in this preparation. Carrying one's meal plan on a small card that fits in a wallet helps the person remember food choices or exchanges. If the person is not using the exchange system, specific individualized guidelines on choosing food can be written on the card.

Nutrition therapy goals related to glucose control, fat, sodium, and calorie intake may be compromised if adequate self-management training is not provided. Education and training focusing on having patients be assertive and curious regarding the foods they order prepares them to make appropriate food selections.

Exhibit 23-3 Assessment of Dining Out Pattern

1. Per week, how often do you eat away from home?

   Number of times in a restaurant _____

   Carry out _____

2. List which meals or snacks are the most frequently eaten away from the home.

   _____

   _____

   _____

3. List the restaurants or take-out places that you frequent (some examples, fast-food, fine dining, family-style, specify ethnic favorites).

   _____

   _____

   _____

4. Describe the most commonly ordered foods:

   _____

   _____

   _____

The dietitian can, along with the client,

- role-play a restaurant scene or encourage the person to do so with a friend
- review a collection of restaurant menus of varying types—fast-food, buffets, sit-down, ethnic
- discuss food preparation and review portion sizes
- call the restaurant in advance to obtain more information about the menu and how the food is prepared

Meal plan adjustments and food selection suggestions include:

- Saving fat calories/exchanges for the day and use them at the meal that they plan to eat out. Doing so will not dramatically affect the blood glucose level.
- Decreasing CHO from starch or fruit servings in order to include the "extra" CHO found in sauces, gravies, and other food items served at restaurants.
- Requesting lower-sugar, -fat, and -calorie items. Some restaurants may provide diet jams and jellies and diet syrups on request.
- Share an entree if portion sizes are large, or order side dishes, appetizer and a salad, or request a container for leftovers.

Exhibit 23-4 provides additional suggestions to help the restaurant diner select food wisely and Table 23-2 has suggested food items for eating at a friend's home. Many book stores have books that provide nutrient information for a variety of restaurants. Some restaurants, especially the fast-food type, provide this information to their customers. Many dietitians have this information readily available to use during nutrition therapy.

Empowering clients with all these new skills increases their confidence in eating out. Also strongly recommended is the use of SMBG to see the effect of specific foods on blood glucose levels.

Ethnic Food Exchanges

The United States is a melting pot with a variety of ethnic cuisines that the person with diabetes can work into his or her meal plan. See Appendix 12-B for a list of common Mexican, Chinese, East Indian, Italian, and Jewish foods and their exchange values. Making this information available helps the person with diabetes comfortably enjoy a variety of ethnic foods. Appendix 15-A lists additional resources for ethnic foods.

Adjusting Meal Times

It is not always possible to eat meals at the same time each day, especially when eating away from home. Following are examples of

Exhibit 23-4 Guidelines for Eating at Restaurants

Appetizer: Choose unsweetened fruit juice or vegetable juice; vegetables, such as carrots, celery, or radishes; broth—fat-free, chicken or beef; vegetable soups; fruits, such as melons or strawberries.

Salad: Choose vegetable salads with vinegar or lemon juice. (Combining a sugar substitute with lemon juice provides a calorie-free sweet and sour dressing.) Because low-calorie dressings are not frequently available at restaurants, carrying one's own dressing in a small container is usually accepted.

Soup: Choose bouillon, broth, or consomme; vegetable cream soups are high in fat.

Sandwiches: Avoid salad-type fillings as they are often high in fat. Chicken, turkey, low-fat cheese, and lean meat are acceptable fillings. Request that bread not be buttered and that mayonnaise or dressing be served separately.

Meat: Specify that no fat be added. Choose roast beef, roast veal, small lean steak (tenderloin or sirloin), veal chop or pork chop cutlet, roast lamb, lamb chop, and poultry (remove skin). Remove all visible fat and request that meat be served without gravy or sauce. Eat only the number of ounces allowed on your meal plan, and bring the remainder home in a "doggie bag." Use the leftover meat at another meal.

Eggs: Choose boiled or poached; avoid fried or creamed.

Fruit: Select fresh fruit or unsweetened fruit juices in portion sizes based on the meal plan.

Vegetable: Choose any vegetable prepared without sauce, butter, or margarine. Use lemon juice or vinegar. If the vegetable is buttered, count it as a fat exchange.

Bread: Choose plain breads and rolls, soda crackers, rye krisp, or melba toast. French bread and English muffins count as a starch exchange. Eat plain or with butter from allowed fat exchanges. Avoid rich muffins, sweet rolls, and doughnuts.

WAYS TO REDUCE FAT WHEN DINING OUT
- Request that salad dressing, butter, margarine, mayonnaise, or sour cream be served separately on a side dish.
- Check if broiled, grilled, or baked meat, fish, or poultry has been prepared in a large amount of oil.
- Check if vegetables are cooked in large amounts of butter/margarine. If they are, request that the amount be reduced or eliminated.
- Check if the bean salads, tuna salads, chicken salads, pasta salads, or potato salads have fat added to them. If so, avoid ordering them.

---

several situations that require additional attention.

If the person with diabetes is anticipating eating a larger evening meal at a later time than usual, a blood glucose test should be done at the time of the person's regularly scheduled evening meal. If the blood glucose level is 60 to 120 mg/dL, then the evening snack should be eaten at the time of the evening meal and the delayed meal can be eaten at the time of the snack. If the blood glucose level is 150 mg/dL, or greater, a snack is not necessary, and the evening meal can usually be delayed up to 2 hours. If the person is taking insulin and the type of insulin is regular, it can be taken premeal. If it is a combination of short-acting and intermediate-acting insulin, it can also be taken premeal. If the person is on an OHA in the evening, it can be taken premeal.

If the evening meal and evening snack are to be combined, a premeal dose of supplemental short-acting insulin may be indicated if the person usually takes insulin. This should be discussed with the person's health care team. Before eating the evening meal, a blood glucose test is again recommended. If the level is 150 mg/dL or greater, extra regular insulin, a reduction in the meal's CHO, or an increase in activity may be indicated. A blood glucose test before bedtime is also recommended. If the level is 150 to 180 mg/dL or lower, an evening snack, in addition to the one eaten with supper, may be indicated. Clinical observation and review of SMBG records will help determine the ideal snack. The snack should always contain CHO and may or may not need to contain a protein source. If the blood glucose level is 180 mg/dL or greater, usually no snack is indicated. Persons taking a long-acting insulin at bedtime could adjust that dosage based on their bedtime blood glucose level and desire for a snack.

TRAVEL AND THE PERSON WITH DIABETES

The stresses of travel can cause difficulties in diabetes management. However, dietitians can help alleviate these situations by helping their clients plan ahead and work through some problem-solving activities.

It is recommended that the person with diabetes carry a food kit at all times when traveling. Examples of foods appropriate for an emergency food kit include

- canned fruit or vegetable juice, boxed fruit juice, dried fruit
- crackers, cereal
- peanut butter
- peanut butter and crackers, cheese and crackers
- canned meat and fish
- popcorn, pretzels, graham crackers, vanilla wafers

- jars of cheese spread
- nuts
- Lifesavers, hard candies, or other glucose source to treat hypoglycemia (tablet or liquid form)

Along with an emergency food kit, individuals should be reminded to carry their blood glucose testing equipment, insulin and syringes, other medications, and medical identification. These items should be kept with the person at all times and not be placed in baggage that is stored way from them, which may get lost. When traveling by car, insulin should be kept with the person at all times and not be put in the glove compartment or be exposed to extremely high temperatures or allowed to freeze.

Table 23-2 Menu Suggestions When Entertaining Friends with Diabetes

Foods	Recommended	Not Recommended
Salads	Vegetables or fresh salads without dressing already added; use lemon wedge or vinegar; sugar-free gelatin	Salad mixtures with dressing Regular gelatin mixtures
Vegetables	Stewed, steamed, or boiled or seasoned with herbs/spices	Creamed, fried, au gratin, escalloped
Potatoes and substitutes	Mashed, baked, boiled, or steamed; rice or noodles	Fried, escalloped, french fried, browned, creamed
Breads	Hard or soft rolls, plain muffins, biscuits, crackers or corn bread, bagels, tortillas, tacos	Sweet rolls, coffee cakes, danish, doughnuts, rich muffins
Meat, fish, poultry	Roasted, baked, grilled, broiled, or boiled; trim off excess fat	Fried, breaded, cooked in a high-fat gravy, meats in cream sauce
Eggs	Soft, hard-cooked, or poached	Fried, scrambled, or cream
Dessert [a]	Fresh fruit, angel food cake, desserts made with a minimum amount of sugar or fat	Pudding, custard, pastry, pie, doughnuts, danish roll, cake, sundaes

[a] Sugar-free gelatin and sugar-free pudding can be used as dessert items. Low-calorie sweeteners can be used to sweeten cooked or raw food items. Some persons with diabetes might substitute cake, ice cream, or high-sugar dessert items for other CHO foods in the meal; however, they are not the most nutritious choices.

Table 23-3 Sample of Airline Food Choices*

Airline	Special Meals	Most Popular Meal	Advance Notice (h)
American	22	Vegetarian	4–24
Continental	12	Vegetarian	24
Delta	19	Low-cholesterol/low-fat	6–12
Northwest	22	Low-fat/Kosher	12–24
TWA	30	Kosher	24
United	25	Travelers Lighter Choice	24
USAir	22	Vegetarian	24

* Data subject to change.

Car Travel

When traveling by car or train, it may be expensive to eat every meal in a restaurant. These economic, time-saving meals can be brought from home:

- Breakfast: fresh fruit, wheat bread, bagel, or English muffin, with low-fat cheese or peanut butter, dry cereal, tea or coffee, low-fat or skim milk (a thermos can be used for milk, or powdered milk can be used)
- Lunch or supper: low-fat cheese or lean meat sandwiches, fresh fruit, raw vegetables, milk, or diet soda

Airline Travel

Airlines provide a variety of special meals depending on the duration of the flight and the destination. Whether such a meal is available on a specific flight should be determined with the airlines before the reservation is made, and the meal should be requested when the reservation is made (see Table 23-3). The availability of the meal should be reconfirmed when the person's seat assignment is provided. When boarding the plane, the person should remind the airline attendants about the meal and give them his or her seat number and name. An example of a "diabetic meal" served by one airline is

- sunshine salad (mixed greens, carrots, cucumber)
- low-calorie Italian dressing (served in individual packets)
- chicken breast, baked, with skin, no breading
- broiled fresh mushrooms, no fat added
- broccoli, no fat added
- crusty roll with margarine (individual servings)
- fresh grapes
- beverages available: diet sodas, fruit juice, 2% milk

Some may also find it useful to call the airline in advance to find out what is served for a diabetic meal versus a regular meal and then make a decision as to which one would be preferred. Appropriate choices from a regular meal could also be selected, but as the following highlights, "regular" meals can be varied. Eating away from home guidelines may be useful. An airline diabetic meal does not have sugar, dessert, or foods that contain sugar as an ingredient. Other meal choices include vegetarian, kosher, low-cholesterol/low-fat, seafood, and a fruit platter. On international flights, many airlines offer choices such as halal, the Muslim equivalent of kosher, and Japanese.

Airlines have recently revised and expanded their menu selections, making them more attractive to their consumers. Weight Watchers' meals are now a standard third choice on American Airlines' transcontinental flights. One of Americans' most popular dishes, pizza, is available on all flights.

Northwest Airlines offers a la carte meals, fashioned after buffet-style restaurants. Passengers choose entrees from a serving cart flight attendants roll down the aisle. Northwest also offers meals based on dishes from popular restaurants in cities it serves, such as Leeann Chin Chinese cuisine of Minneapolis-St. Paul and Seattle and Corky's Barbecue in Memphis, and special food items such as Lloyd's Barbeque and Colombo's Frozen Yogurt.

Northwest and KLM Royal Dutch Airlines also have enhanced the menu for their joint World Business service on international flights. To make it easier for passengers to work or sleep during the flight, they are serving meals earlier and quicker. They are also letting passengers choose when they want their snacks and what kind they want. About 20% of the meals stored on board represent the national cuisine in the flight's destination.

Air France, which serves 100 countries, sometimes offers special courtesies. Japanese food is served on flights to Japan. The airline celebrates holidays such as New Year's Eve with special menus and gourmet foods in all seating classes. On Thanksgiving, passengers on flights to the United States get turkey with cranberry sauce and pumpkin pie. It also serves meals to celebrate other countries' holidays.

Tips: if a flight is delayed, milk, fruit juice, nuts, and crackers are usually available at airport vending machines. On an international flight, do not carry fresh fruit or vegetables through Customs, as they may be quarantined and definitely confiscated. Drink plenty of fluids, especially on long flights, to prevent dehydration. On international flights, water is often served between meals. Hypoglycemia may not occur while traveling by air as food is served frequently and activity is minimal. However, individuals with diabetes should be encouraged to walk in the aisle of the airplane to provide some activity and pro-

mote circulation. They should test their blood glucose level to determine food intake, activity, and insulin needs.

Cruise/Boat Travel

If a client is planning a cruise or travel by ship, there is a never-ending supply of food from 6 A.M. to midnight. There are all-you-can-eat buffets and meals. It is definitely a challenge to not overeat. Suggestions include eating "free" food between meals, switching to a different meal plan such as CHO counting, and not eating late-night meals and the in-between fare. A variety of exercise opportunities and equipment are available to help expend excess calories. Frequent SMBG will guide the traveller as to what changes might be needed in the meal plan, activities, or medication.[9] A discussion with the physician and dietitian about anticipated situations will help make the trip safer and less anxiety-prone. At that time, a revised meal plan and medication regimen for the cruise may be established.

****

Case Study: Cruise Ship Travel

Jim and his wife planned a 5-year anniversary boat cruise. Jim's height was 5'9", weight 210 lb, weight loss 20 lb, present weight 190 lb. The weight loss has enabled Jim to discontinue his OHA. He is maintaining his weight on an 1800-calorie meal plan, and does not want to gain weight on the cruise.

Goals

1. To maintain his weight and his blood glucose levels in the optimal range so he did not have to resume his OHA.
2. To enjoy the cruise without too much pressure of managing his diabetes.

Intervention

1. An exercise regimen was established for weight maintenance and extra exercise

planned if additional calories were consumed.

2. A list of menus, restaurants, and snack foods available on the cruise were requested by Jim and the dietitian in advance. A "free" food list was made from this information.

3. CHO counting was the meal-planning option that was to be used to provide for flexibility.

4. Blood glucose was monitored before each meal and at bedtime.

Examples of Guidelines for Exercise

• 1/2 hour modest exercise: additional 10 g CHO.

• A limit of 45 g CHO per 3 hours.

Follow-Up

Jim and his wife would follow the guidelines established with his dietitian. His physician provided him with medical information that a physician might need in an emergency. After the cruise, Jim was to contact his dietitian, and further follow-up plans were to be established.

****

Traveling through Different Time Zones

When a person with diabetes is traveling into a different time zone, the timing and the amount of diabetes medication may need to be adjusted on the day of actual travel. The person should find out the type and timing of the meals served on the airline so the medication dose can be adapted to the meal pattern. When east to west or west to east travel is involved, the time change will cause a disruption of the eating and sleeping pattern. A smooth transition of the new schedule with the medication dose can be achieved by maintaining both meal plan and medication schedules to the person's "own clock" for the first 12 to 24 hours after arrival and then gradu-

ally changing to the new time. Those on diet alone would not need to make such detailed transition adjustments.

One of the best methods to approach the transition is to draw two time lines, one above the other. On the first, note the current schedule (wake-up, meals, medication, sleep), and on the other one, note the times that correspond to the current schedule (if 2-hour time change, first line would possibly begin with 6 A.M., the bottom line would begin with 8 A.M.). This can usually help plan for a day or two of transition before or at the beginning of a trip and also on the return. Adjusting medication an hour either way usually does not complicate management. Greater time changes should be discussed with the traveler. Some people who travel frequently or take short business trips prefer to remain on their "home" time.

Food Choices in Other Countries

When traveling to Africa, Asia, or South America, it is recommended that dairy products, milk, peeled fruits, leafy vegetables, raw meats, or seafood be avoided as they may cause gastrointestinal problems. Ice cubes and unboiled drinking water should also be avoided, although boiled beverages, such as coffee, tea, or hot chocolate, are safe to drink. Nonalcoholic beverages and diet beverages may not be readily available in all countries outside the United States and Canada, and canned fruit juices may not be available. Bottled water is becoming more popular.

The traveler should check the label for the ingredients to see how the food can fit into the meal plan. Because labeling laws may be different in other countries and the beverage may contain nutritive sweeteners, persons should feel free to ask about food preparation and the ingredients in products. In addition to the above discussion regarding travel preparation, the most basic preparation is to emphasize that the person with diabetes knows his or her meal plan and therefore is able to make appropriate food choices (refer to the section on eating out).

HYPOGLYCEMIA

Hypoglycemia, also known as insulin reaction, insulin shock, and low blood sugar, occurs when there is either more insulin in the bloodstream than necessary, decreased food intake, or increased activity. A blood glucose level of 60 mg/dL or less indicates that hypoglycemia is present.[10] Diabetes educators usually advise treating blood glucose levels of 70 mg/dL or less as hypoglycemic reactions. Hypoglycemia usually only occurs in persons taking insulin but has been documented in persons taking OHAs.

The dietitian should review signs and symptoms, treatment, and prevention of hypoglycemia with all clients taking a diabetes medication. This should be included in the diabetes self-management training. It fits in with the topic areas that the dietitian would be discussing (eg, portion sizes, effect of certain foods or meals on blood glucose levels, changes in meal times, balancing food intake with activity and diabetes medication). Family members or significant others should be part of this discussion (Exhibit 23-5).

Initial warning signs of hypoglycemia include shakiness, sweating, confusion, and irritability. Advanced symptoms of hypoglycemia include headaches, blurred vision, lack of coordination, confusion, or anger. Table 23-4 details varying signs and symptoms of hypoglycemia.

Hypoglycemia may be difficult to notice and may occur more frequently in a person with diabetes who has been using insulin for a few years.[11] This could be because the two main counterregulatory systems do not function normally after a 1- to 5-year duration of insulin dependency.[11] The immediate physiologic response of glucagon to hypoglycemia is absent when persons with diabetes receive exogenous insulin. There is also a deficiency of epinephrine response after several years of having diabetes.[11] Persons with an inadequate epinephrine response demonstrate the following symptoms of hypoglycemia: drowsiness, temporary loss of memory, and confusion.[12] Some individuals with diabetes of more than 5 years' duration

have hypoglycemia unawareness and may not even have the above symptoms. Therefore, in these persons, frequent SMBG is critical in helping to avoid or identify hypoglycemia and treating it appropriately.

Eating an adequate amount of food at the recommended times is important to help avoid a hypoglycemic reaction. When a person is on one to two insulin injections per day (conventional therapy), meals and snacks should be planned to cover the peak times of a person's insulin dose. Intensive therapy is defined as three or more insulin injections per day or on an insulin pump. The matching up of the grams of CHO to regular insulin during meals and snacks should be as accurate as possible to help prevent hypoglycemia. In the Diabetes Control and Complications Trial (DCCT), the risk of severe hypoglycemia occurred approximately three times more during intensive therapy than during conventional therapy.[12]

Activity-Related Hypoglycemia

Increased activity lowers blood glucose levels, and the insulin dose may need to be reduced by one-third or more, depending on a person's insulin sensitivity. If the insulin dose is not adjusted and the activity is increased, then the blood glucose level should be tested after the activity. If it is 70 mg/dL or less, the low blood glucose should be treated appropriately, as dis-

---

Exhibit 23-5 Checklist for RD Regarding Client Management Training for Hypoglycemia

✓ Causes

✓ Signs and symptoms, mild/moderate, advanced

✓ Treatment
    Blood glucose < 70 mg/dL
    15 g CHO, wait 15 minutes—15/15 rule
    Retest, monitor symptoms

✓ Hypoglycemia unawareness

✓ Glucagon, if type I and some with type II

Table 23-4 Examples of Symptoms and Treatment of Hypoglycemia

Client	Type and Duration of Diabetes	Therapy	Symptoms	Treatment
Sam	Type II, 2 years	Nutrition, OHA	Headache	SMBG to document low blood glucose. One 6-oz can apple juice. Wait 15 minutes and retest. If blood glucose within 100 m/dL range, no retreatment and wait until the next meal
Mary	Type II, 25 years	Nutrition, exercise, OHA	Dizzy, light-headed	Same procedure as Sam but treatment of choice is 8 oz of skim or low-fat milk
Susan	Type I, 30 years	Nutrition, exercise, insulin pump	Conversation does not make sense. Thought process muddled	Uses 15/15 rule. Frequent retesting. May require two to three 15/15 treatments before blood glucose stabilizes. A third choice would include protein

cussed later in this section. The effect of exercise can sometimes last up to 24 hours. Therefore, frequent blood glucose monitoring can help the person avoid hypoglycemia.

Patient education/self-management training on the prevention of hypoglycemia should be a part of the nutrition education by the dietitian. In the teaching sessions, the dietitian should provide a set of guidelines for the prevention of hypoglycemia.

Signs and Symptoms

Some of the common symptoms for mild to moderate and advanced hypoglycemia have been described earlier. Each individual should become aware of their own specific signs and symptoms of hypoglycemia. Prevention of hypoglycemia is important for all persons with diabetes, but particularly for individuals with hypoglycemia unawareness, in whom prevention is even more important.[13]

Timing of meals and consistency of CHO content of meals (eating an adequate amount of food at the recommended times) is important to help avoid a hypoglycemic episode. But realistically, individuals will never adhere to a structured meal plan completely. The task for the dietitian is to provide patients with the knowledge and skills to make food and medication adjustments so that flexibility with meals and snacks is possible. Individualized insulin dosage ranges can be provided for flexibility for individuals on insulin.[14]

Self-Monitoring Blood Glucose Levels

It is essential to educate patients to use SMBG, to keep blood glucose records, and to interpret the results for their diabetes management. This should be emphasized even more to the person with hypoglycemia unawareness.

Treatment

Hypoglycemia has to be treated immediately with some form of glucose (not only should the person rely on the symptoms but also on an immediate blood glucose test) (Exhibit 23-6). Fifteen grams of CHO are recommended for treatment; this amount raises the blood glucose by 50 to 100 mg/dL in 15 to 30 minutes. The response, of course, varies from person to person and is possibly influenced by how low the blood glucose actually is and the cause of the reaction. Food items that provide 15 g of CHO are listed in Exhibit 23-7. A blood glucose test is recommended 15 minutes after treatment.

The 1994 Nutrition Recommendations from the American Diabetes Association provides us with the information that all CHO are created equal, whether they are simple or complex. For example, one-half cup of fruit juice (simple) versus one slice of wheat bread (complex), both provide 15 g of CHO. Either one can be used for the treatment of hypoglycemia. The source of the CHO does not matter. It is the amount of CHO and also what the person can tolerate the best during the hypoglycemic episode. Exhibit 23-7 provides suggested amounts of CHO to take for varying levels of hypoglycemia.

If the blood glucose level is at or less than 50 to 80 mg/dL, the initial CHO should be followed by an additional 15 g of CHO and then another blood glucose test 15 minutes after treatment. After treatment, if the blood glucose has risen to a normal range of 80 to 120 mg/dL and it is still 1 hour or more until the next meal or snack, 15 g of additional CHO should be consumed. Some clinicians recommend protein with the CHO which could be one-half sandwich, 1 cup milk, six crackers, and 1 to 2 oz of cheese. Monitoring the

results of varying treatments for similar reactions will help determine the specific amount and type of CHO that is required and whether protein is needed.

Testing again in 15 minutes is useful to confirm the reaction is over. If the blood glucose level still remains less than 80 mg/dL, additional CHO should be consumed.

Glucagon

Glucagon is used to treat hypoglycemia in a person who has passed out or cannot swallow. Most persons who take insulin should have glucagon available in case of a severe reaction. Some clinicians do not recommend it to all their clients with type II diabetes.

Glucagon is extracted from beef and pork pancreas and causes an increase in blood glucose concentration and is used in the treatment of hypoglycemia. It is effective in small doses, and no evidence of toxicity has been reported with its use. Glucagon acts only on liver glycogen and converts it to glucose. The half-life of glucagon in plasma is approximately 3 to 6 minutes, which is similar to that of insulin. A physician's prescription is required to purchase glucagon. Periodically review with clients the directions for use and have them check the expiration date.

Glucagon should *not* be mixed in anticipation of hypoglycemia because it is only stable when mixed for approximately 1 month; the shelf life of unmixed glucagon is several years. When mixing and administering glucagon, it is important that the following steps are followed. The following are directions for mixing glucagon that requires mixing in two vials:

1. Flip the tops off the vials. Wiping with alcohol is not necessary.

2. Pull back the plunger of a 100-U syringe to approximately 100, and push the needle through the rubber top of the vial marked *1*. Push the plunger down until all the air is in the vial.

3. Invert the vial and withdraw all the fluid (with a child younger than 8, only one-

---

Exhibit 23-6 General Treatment of Hypoglycemia—15/15 Guideline

If blood glucose is <70 mg/dL eat 15 g of carbohydrate; blood glucose should increase 50 mg/dL in 15 to 30 minutes

In 15 minutes, retest blood glucose
If blood glucose is <80 mg/dL eat additional 15 g of carbohydrate
If blood glucose is >80 mg/dL eat if next meal is >1 hour—15 g carbohydrate

In 15 minutes, retest if unsure if reaction is over. Treat as above.

half of the vial or 50 U). The vial contains approximately 100 U.

4. Inject all the fluid into the vial marked *2* (the one with the powder tablet).

5. Shake the vial until the tablet dissolves (within seconds).

6. Withdraw all the dissolved solution from this vial (2).

7. Inject the glucagon into an insulin injection site in the same manner as insulin (review insulin injection technique).

8. Because vomiting is a common side effect of glucagon administration, turn the person's head to the side to avoid aspiration.

9. When the individual is awake and able to swallow, feed him or her some form of carbohydrate to prevent a recurrence of the hypoglycemia.

10. The individual should notify his or her physician after receiving glucagon to determine why the hypoglycemia occurred and to make any necessary changes in the diabetes management regimen.

Another type of glucagon emergency kit contains a syringe already filled with diluting fluid which is injected into one vial. The vial is then shaken and made ready to use. The solution should only be used if it is clear and water-like in consistency.

Other Tips

In the Winter 1993 issue of the *Diabetes Care and Education* newsletter, Double Perspectives column, RDs with diabetes were surveyed regarding the prevention and treatment of hypoglycemia to help provide RDs with the practical information in this critical area of medical nutrition therapy.[15] With regard to the treatment of hypoglycemia, most of the individuals surveyed used the 15/15 rule but modified this based on how low their blood glucose level was and what they were going to do after the hypoglycemia episode. Some examples that were cited:

Exhibit 23-7 Advanced Treatment of Hypoglycemia

If blood glucose is:	51–70 mg/dL	41–50 mg/dL	≤40 mg/dL
Amount of carbohydrate recommended for treatment	15 g	20 g	30 g
Apple or orange juice	4 oz	6 oz	8 oz
Grape juice	3 oz	4 oz	6 oz
BD Glucose Tablets (5 g CHO per tablet)	3 tablets	4 tablets	6 tablets
Dex-4 (4 g CHO per tablet)	4 tablets	5 tablets	7 tablets
Milk	10 oz	14 oz	20 oz
Lifesavers—1 piece per serving, all flavors (3 g CHO per piece)	5 Lifesavers	7 Lifesavers	10 Lifesavers

Source: Courtesy of the Diabetes Health Center, Salt Lake City, Utah.

- blood glucose 60–65 mg/dL: a form of glucose

- blood glucose 65 mg/dL: 1/2 to 3/4 cup juice or 4 to 6 Lifesavers

If the next meal was going to be sooner than 45 minutes, then 10 g of CHO were used. If the meal following the reaction was going to be delayed, then more than 15 g of CHO would be consumed.

About half of the individuals reported a tendency to overtreat. They then ate less at the following meal to balance out calories. Some said proportioned forms of treatment such as commercial glucose preparations or proportioned amount of fruit juices helped avoid overtreatment. It was noted that record keeping helped identify the overtreatment and increased calorie intake.[15]

Overtreatment of hypoglycemia can occur very easily if a person only relies on symptoms and not on blood glucose results. Overtreating with additional food can cause an increased caloric intake resulting in weight gain as well as a greater than desired rise in blood glucose levels. It is, however, a very natural tendency to overeat. Therefore, it is crucial to discuss in detail this area of self-management because repeated hypoglycemic episodes, weight gain, and elevated blood glucose levels influence diabetes control and quality of life.

Some persons with diabetes tend to want to eat such foods as ice cream or chocolate to treat hypoglycemia. They would like to make an unpleasant experience "pleasant" with foods that they seldom eat. However, these foods, in addition to being a source of increased calories, are also high in fat, which is absorbed at a slow rate. They therefore are not an appropriate form of treatment for hypoglycemia because low blood glucose has to be treated immediately with a food source that is primarily carbohydrate. The dietitian is responsible for providing very specific instructions about the treatment of hypoglycemia. The food items used to treat hypoglycemia are in addition to the meal plan

and are not deducted from the food usually consumed at the next meal.

With regard to hypoglycemia unawareness, frequent SMBG during the day, with a bedtime and 3 A.M. blood glucose are recommended. Other practical recommendations include SMBG during the peak time of insulin, before driving, and pre- and postexercise. With regard to the symptoms of hypoglycemia, it was reported that hypoglycemic symptoms from short-acting insulin were more specific and fast than the symptoms from intermediate-acting insulin.[15]

To translate these personal/professional experiences to assisting the patient with diabetes; self-management training should include discussions of:

1. time of meals, snacks
2. eating planned meals, snacks
3. exercise in relation to time of food intake
4. onset, peak, duration of insulin or OHA
5. self-monitoring of blood glucose as part of the daily regimen
6. premeasured hypoglycemia treatment in a survival kit
7. glucagon use by significant others

Follow up with the patient to analyze the cause of hypoglycemia, any pattern in the time of day, peak action of insulin, and exercise. This may help prevent hypoglycemia in the future.

SICK DAY MANAGEMENT

Four main rules for sick day management are that patients should

1. Take their insulin or OHA. Even when eating less, additional insulin may be needed.
2. Test their blood glucose frequently.
3. Test their urine for ketones.
4. Keep eating or drinking fluids even when blood glucose levels are elevated. Try to eat usual amount of CHO, divided into smaller meals and snacks if necessary; if

Exhibit 23-8 Carbohydrate Content of Foods Appropriate for Sick Day Use

	Carbohydrate Content (g)
Starch Exchanges	
1 slice bread	15
1/2 cup hot cereal	15
6 saltine crackers (2-in. squares)	15
4 soda crackers (2 1/2-in. squares)	15
3 graham crackers (2 1/2-in. squares)	15
1/2 cup ice cream	15
1 cup broth soup	15
1 cup soup, cream	
(reconstituted with water)	15
(reconstituted with milk)	25
Meat Exchanges	
1/4 cup low-fat cottage cheese	0
1 oz American or Swiss cheese	0
1 poached or soft-boiled egg	0
Vegetable Exchanges	
1/2 cup tomato juice	5
1/2 cup vegetable juice	5
Fruit Exchanges	
1/2 twin popsicle	10
Fruit juices (unsweetened):	
1/3 cup cranberry, grape	15
1/3 cup prune juice	15
1/2 cup apple, pineapple	15
1/2 cup apricot	15
1/2 cup cherry, grapefruit, orange, or	
peach juice	15
Milk Exchanges	
1 cup milk	12
1 cup yogurt	12
1/4 cup plain pudding	12
Other Carbohydrates	
1/2 cup ice milk	15
1/2 cup regular gelatin	15
1/4 cup sherbet	15
4 oz regular carbonated beverage, cola-type	15

their blood glucose is 250 mg/dL or higher, all the usual amount of CHO is not necessary. Protein and fat intake is based on the person's tolerance. Protein suggestions are in Exhibit 23-8. Frequent fluid intake is also recommended.

Ketones in the urine and an elevated blood glucose level indicate that additional insulin, particularly regular or short-acting insulin, may be needed. When the body is unable to use glucose, it breaks down fats for energy, and the by-products of the fat breakdown are ketones. Along with elevated blood glucose levels, the presence of ketones in the urine indicates the potential for ketoacidosis. The individual's physician should be informed immediately.

The individual with diabetes who does not use insulin should monitor his or her blood glucose levels very closely. If the blood glucose level is 250 mg/dL or greater continuously for 24 hours, the physician should be informed. Individuals with non–insulin-dependent diabetes mellitus may lapse into a coma without any sign of ketones in their urine.

Consuming fluids and taking an adequate dose of insulin are critically important during an illness. If nauseated, sipping one to two tablespoons of any caloric or noncaloric fluid every 15 to 30 minutes should be attempted. If an individual is able to eat, soft, semisolid foods such as soups, custard, and yogurt in small amounts are often well tolerated. The person should be encouraged to follow the CHO portion of their meal pattern if possible. This plan should be detailed before becoming ill and can be part of a "sick day" kit that the client keeps. Other items in the kit may be a can of regular carbonated beverage, box of regular gelatin, ketone urine test strips, health care team's telephone numbers, and clients's own telephone number. Also include a check list of steps to manage the illness, and manage guidelines for testing blood glucose and urine for ketone levels. Foods from the "Free Food List" can be used after the caloric and CHO contents of the person's meal plan have been met. Vomiting and diarrhea cause loss of potassium and sodium. Broth, vegetables, or tomato juice help replace some of the lost sodium.

If unable to tolerate solids or semisolids, the person should drink liquids with appropriate amounts of carbohydrate (Exhibit 23-8; a general guideline is 10 to 15 g CHO per 1/2 to 1 hour and 8 oz liquid every hour). A sample menu, which is based on the individual's meal pattern, for managing a sick day is helpful to the person with diabetes (Exhibit 23-9).

MEAL PLAN AND INSULIN ADJUSTMENT WHEN SCHEDULES CHANGE

Diabetes management can be difficult when work schedules change, especially when insulin is required. It is helpful if the dietitian and patient can detail the schedule changes, carefully outlining meal times and activity and management possibilities. The physician needs to approve medication changes, so including him or her in this process is beneficial.

Persons with type I diabetes who work the night shift, from 11 P.M. to 7 A.M., 5 days a week, usually should take two or more injections of insulin a day. For two injections, a general guideline is to take two-thirds of the dose for the day in the evening before going to work and to take the rest (one-third) after coming home the next day in the morning. On the person's day off, half of the daily dose can be taken in the morning and the other half before the evening meal. A meal plan schedule during workdays can look like the one in the case study described below.

****

Case Study: Swing Shift Employment

Susan works a swing shift at a factory. She has learned to make the following adjustments with her dietitian's help. She and the dietitian have reviewed her insulin requirements, calorie level, food preferences and availability, and social schedule to develop a practical management plan. During the initial implementation of this schedule, Susan had close telephone follow-up

---

Exhibit 23-9 Sample Menu for a 1200-Calorie Exchange Pattern Useful during Sick Days

	Meal Pattern/ Exchanges	Sample Menu
Breakfast	1 skim milk	1 cup skim milk
	2 starch	1/2 cup cooked oatmeal
		1 whole wheat toast
	1 fruit	1/2 cup unsweetened canned peaches
Lunch	2 medium-fat meat	2 oz swiss cheese
	2 vegetable	1 cup "V8" juice
	2 starch	6 saltine crackers
		1/4 cup sherbet
	1 fruit	1/2 cup apple juice
Midafternoon Snack	1 starch	1 cup cream soup
Dinner	2 medium-fat meat	1/2 cup cottage cheese
	2 vegetable	1 cup tomato juice
	2 starch	12 soda crackers
	1 fruit	1/2 cup unsweetened canned pears
Bedtime Snack	1 starch	2/3 cup tapioca pudding
	1 meat	
	1 fruit	1/2 cup unsweetened canned apricots

with her dietitian. Susan faxed blood glucose, food, and activity records and insulin doses. These were used for adjustments if needed.

1. 10:00 P.M.: Takes insulin
2. 10:30 P.M.: Eats a meal
3. 11:00 P.M.: Goes to work
4. 3:00 A.M.: Eats a meal at work
5. 8:00 A.M.: Returns home, takes insulin, eats an 8:30 A.M. meal at home
6. 9:00 A.M.: Goes to bed
7. 5:00 P.M.: Eats a snack
8. 8:00 P.M.: Eats a snack (optional, depends on glucose level)

SMBG is recommended before each meal.

The meal plan schedule during non-workdays is as follows:

1. 8:00 A.M.: Takes insulin
2. 8:30 A.M.: Eats a meal
3. 12:30 P.M.: Eats a meal
4. 4:00 P.M.: Eats a snack (optional, depends on blood glucose level)
5. 6:00 P.M.: Takes insulin
6. 6:30 P.M.: Eats a meal
7. 9:00 to 10:00 P.M.: Eats a snack (optional, depends on blood glucose level)

SMBG is recommended before each meal.

****

For a change in activity on workdays and off days for persons with type I working swing shifts, the following basic information should be emphasized:

• The site of the insulin injection should be selected depending of the type of work activity. Activity within a half-hour of insulin injection increases the rate of insulin ab-

sorption from the site of the injection. This rapid absorption results in a faster utilization of glucose, which could lower blood glucose and lead to hypoglycemia. More frequent SMBG on high-activity workdays helps prevent hypoglycemia.

• An increase in food intake or a reduction in insulin is recommended during times of increased activity. To decide how much more food is necessary, blood glucose levels should be monitored before and after the activity.

When activity on a workday is much greater than on a day off, insulin adjustment may need to be made on workdays. The total insulin dose may need to be decreased by 10 to 20%. For example:

Insulin dose:
  6 regular 26 NPH before breakfast
  4 regular 8 NPH before evening
    meal
Total dose = 6 + 4 + 26 + 8 = 44

10% of total dose: 4.4 U (44 x 0.10)
  or, can round to 4 or 5 U
15% of total dose: 6.6 units (44 x
  0.15) or can round to 7 U
20% of total dose: 8.8 U (44 x 0.20) or
  can round to 9 U

Some individuals can be on multiple daily injections of premeal short-acting insulin and a long-acting insulin such as ultralente to act as a basal dose of insulin. The premeal short-acting insulin and long-acting insulin can vary based on the person's shift schedule.

CONCLUSION

The dietitian, because of his or her training and expertise in the area of medical nutrition therapy and diabetes, has the skills, knowledge, and expertise to adjust and adapt the diabetes meal plan to fit any situation that the client is faced with.

Using data from blood glucose, food, exercise, and medication records, the dietitian can provide the client with critical diabetes self-management skills.

REFERENCES

1. American Diabetes Association. Technical review: nutrition principles for the management of diabetes and related complications. *Diabetes Care.* 1994;17(5):490.

2. Santen RJ, Willis PW, Fajans SS. Atherosclerosis in diabetes mellitus. Correlations with serum lipid levels, adiposity, and serum insulin level. *Arch Intern Med.* 1972;130:833–842.

3. Franz MJ. Alcohol and diabetes. Part 2. Its metabolism and guidelines for its occasional use. *Diabetes Spectrum.* 1990;3:210–216.

4. Walsh DJ, O'Sullivan DJ. Effect of moderate alcohol intake on control of diabetes. *Diabetes.* 1974; 23:440–442.

5. Franz MJ. Diabetes mellitus: consideration in the development of guidelines for the occasional use of alcohol. *J Am Diet Assoc.* 1983;83:148–149.

6. Menze R, Metel DC, Brunstein U, Heinke P. Effect of moderate ethanol ingestion on overnight diabetes control and hormone secretion in type 1 diabetic patients. *Diabetologia.* 1991;34:A188.

7. American Diabetes Association. Position statement: nutrition recommendations and principles for people with diabetes mellitus. *Diabetes Care.* 1994;17(5):519.

8. Warshaw H. Eating away from home: teaching creatively and successfully. Nutrition update. *Diabetes Educ.* 1992;18:21–28.

9. Diabetes Care and Education Practice Group. Double perspectives. *Newsflash.* 1993;14(3):13–15.

10. American Diabetes Association. Technical review: hypoglycemia. *Diabetes Care.* 1994;17:734–755.

11. Holmes DM. The person and diabetes in the psychosocial context. *Diabetes Care.* 1986;9:2.

12. DCCT Research Group. Epidemiology of severe hypoglycemia in the DCCT. *Am J Med.* 1991;90:450–459.

13. Anderson E. Diabetes care and education. Challenges and lessons from the DCCT. Hypoglycemia: prevention and treatment. *On The Cutting Edge.* 1994;15(2):12.

14. DCCT Research Group. Nutrition intervention for intensive diabetes therapy in the DCCT. *J Am Diet Assoc.* 1993;93:768–772.

15. Diabetes Care and Education Practice Group. Double perspectives. *Newsflash.* Double perspectives. 1993;14 (1):14–16.

Chapter 24

Eclectic Issues in Diabetes Nutrition Therapy

Melinda Downie Maryniuk

Research regarding the roles of minerals and vitamins in the etiology, management, and treatment of diabetes has been appearing prominently in both the lay and scientific literature.[1,2] In particular, magnesium, chromium, and vitamin E are being more thoroughly studied. At the same time, questions are raised about how nonfood items such as tobacco, caffeine, over-the-counter medications, and recreational drugs affect glycemic control. This chapter presents current information on the relationships between these substances and diabetes control.

MINERALS AND VITAMINS

Magnesium

Magnesium, the second most abundant intracellular cation, plays an important role in cellular metabolism. It is found primarily in bone and muscle tissue, with only about 1% in extracellular fluid. Normal serum concentrations are 1.5 to 2.0 mEq/L. Magnesium is important for cardiac contractility and conductivity and the maintenance of normal intracellular calcium, potassium, and perhaps sodium levels. A deficiency of magnesium has been linked with several disorders including insulin resistance, carbohydrate intolerance, cardiac arrhythmias, high blood pressure, accelerated atherosclerosis, dyslipidemia, and adverse outcomes of pregnancy.

Hypomagnesemia has been observed in patients with both insulin-dependent diabetes mellitus (IDDM) and non–insulin-dependent diabetes mellitus (NIDDM). Although many factors may lead to low levels of magnesium, the most common reason for persons with diabetes is diabetic ketoacidosis and increased urinary excretion due to glycosuria. A second cause of a deficiency is due to decreased intestinal absorption, and the third is due to decreased dietary intake. Hypermagnesemia may develop in patients with renal insufficiency. The levels of toxicity are not clearly defined, but central nervous system depression appears at levels of about 8 to 10 mEq/L.

Researchers are looking at the role of magnesium in several different functions as related to diabetes. First, magnesium may play a role in insulin resistance and carbohydrate intolerance. Second, there may be a relationship between hypomagnesemia and retinopathy. Significantly lower serum magnesium levels are observed in diabetic patients with proliferative retinopathy than with patients without retinopathy.[3] However, other research has shown no significant difference in 24-hour urinary levels of magnesium in IDDM patients both with and without retinopathy.[4]

Because magnesium is largely an intracellular cation, it is difficult to measure magnesium levels. Serum and urine magnesium levels only measure a fraction of the total body magnesium and, although not completely accurate, give a generally useful clinical indication of magnesium status. Other methods for assessing magnesium status that may better reflect total body magnesium levels, such as ion selective electrodes or phosphate nuclear magnetic resonance spectroscopy, are research-based and not generally available for clinical use. Routine evaluation of magnesium status is not warranted in otherwise healthy individuals with diabetes. However, it is appropriate to measure the serum magnesium in patients at risk for deficiency, including patients with congestive heart failure, ketoacidosis, ethanol abuse, long-term parenteral nutrition, pregnancy, or deficiency of potassium or calcium.

The recommended dietary allowance (RDA) for magnesium is 280 mg for women and 350 mg for men. Magnesium occurs in a wide variety of foods, particularly in the following: nuts (1 oz almonds = 77 mg), meats and fish (3 oz = approximately 30 mg), milk (1 cup = 30 mg), fruit (1 banana = 33 mg), and vegetables (1/2 cup spinach = 57 mg). Although a balanced diet should provide adequate amounts of magnesium, a study of 50 patients with NIDDM who had received instruction on a standard exchange system diabetic diet showed that only 20% of the group met the RDA for magnesium.[5]

A consensus statement from the American Diabetes Association[6] concluded that only diabetic patients at high risk of hypomagnesemia should have total serum magnesium assessed, and such levels should be repeated only if hypomagnesemia can be demonstrated (generally defined as <1.25 mEg/L of magnesium). If supplementation is recommended, an oral preparation of magnesium chloride (MgC_{12}) should be administered until serum levels of magnesium return to normal or the condition causing the deficiency is reversed. The recommended dose is 20 to 130 mg of elemental magnesium.[2] In patients with renal insufficiency and diminished glomerular filtration, oral magnesium replacement therapy must be carefully monitored because of the risk of hypermagnesemia.

Chromium

Chromium, an essential trace mineral, has been studied both as a cause of diabetes and a treatment. It has been shown in both animal models and in humans that, if a chromium deficiency develops, impaired glucose tolerance occurs. Chromium is found in a variety of foods in both an inorganic and an active form as part of a complex that has been termed *glucose tolerance factor* (GTF). Experimental chromium deficiency has been shown to result in impaired glucose tolerance, reduction of body growth and longevity, elevated serum cholesterol levels, and decreased sensitivity of peripheral tissues to exogenous or endogenous insulin. It has been hypothesized that, when a chromium deficiency occurs, the body requires more insulin to control the blood glucose level.

The benefits of this nutrient as related to diabetes have been overemphasized at times. Because chromium is a nutrient and not a drug, supplementation can have practical importance only if a deficiency can be expected to exist. A chromium deficiency is not common; however, it has been noted that tissue chromium levels of elderly persons may be exceptionally low in this country.

One study did find significant improvements in glucose tolerance and total lipids in elderly subjects when their diets were supplemented with 9 g of chromium-rich brewer's yeast. This group was compared with a similar population who received a 9-g supplement of chromium-poor torula yeast. Groups both with and without diabetes were compared. The results support the thesis that the elderly may have a low level of chromium and that an effective source of chromium repletion may improve their carbohydrate tolerance.[7]

Chromium picolinate is a chelated form of chromium that has enhanced absorption and bioavailability. In a research study conducted in Israel, this form of chromium was used and found to have a hypoglycemic effect on 47% of the 243 persons with diabetes who took the supplement for a brief study period. Chromium reduced insulin, sulfonylurea, or metformin requirements in 115 patients, but the NIDDM group showed greater improvements. The placebo was ineffective.[8] Because chromium picolinate has received much media attention, many patients have been asking about the benefits of taking supplements. However, until further research confirming the benefits are available, the American Diabetes Association does not recommend supplementation with chromium unless a deficiency is documented.[1]

The 1989 RDA recommends an intake of 50 to 200 µg/d of chromium for adults. Sources of chromium, in addition to brewer's yeast, include meats, especially liver; whole grains; potatoes and apples with skins; wheat germ; oysters; and cheese. Supplementing diets with chromium or with chromium-rich foods may have some benefit in those persons who have a deficiency in this nutrient (the elderly) and who have some available endogenous insulin (Exhibit 24-1). There is some evidence that the failure of some humans to respond to chromium is due to a lack of nicotinic acid to serve as a substrate for GTF synthesis. Either dietary or supplementary nicotinic acid is necessary for effective utilization of chromium.[9] Although research shows that additional chromium may be beneficial in some patients, cautious administration is important. The concentration range within which chromium is stimulatory is narrow, and excess amounts of it depress insulin activity.[10]

Zinc

Zinc is an essential trace mineral directly involved in the physiology and action of insulin. Insulin is stored as zinc crystals in the ß-cells of the human pancreas, as well as in that of most mammals. Zinc is added to insulin preparations to retard the absorption of injected insulin. It has been suggested that abnormal zinc metabolism may play a role in the pathogenesis of diabetes and some of its complications. Although serum zinc levels in persons with diabetes has not been correlated with blood glucose levels, the lower serum zinc levels that have been observed are probably the result of diabetes-related hyperzincuria and impaired intestinal zinc absorption.[11,12] It has also been demonstrated that pharmacologic doses of supplemental zinc had no effect on glycated hemoglobin levels in diabetic patients.[13] A low serum level of zinc is generally considered to be less than 70 µg/dL.

Zinc supplementation may have beneficial effects for some individuals. In a study of elderly subjects, those who received zinc supplements had faster healing venous leg ulcers than those with lower serum zinc levels.[14] Zinc deficiency in children with insulin-dependent diabetes may contribute to poor growth, and supplementation has been shown to increase height velocity.[15] One side effect of supplementation is that a pharmacologic dose of zinc (>250 mg of elemental zinc daily) has resulted in increased levels of low-density lipoprotein-cholesterol (LDL-C) and decreased levels of high-density lipoprotein-cholesterol.[16]

As is the case with so many micronutrients, it is very difficult to get an accurate assessment of zinc nutritional status. Many factors affect the plasma or serum zinc levels such as the time of day of the assessment, a fasting or fed state, pregnancy, or the presence of inflammatory conditions. It is important to recognize that a change in the level of zinc needs to be correlated with other abnormal biochemical and physiologic functions to demonstrate that altered zinc status reflects deficiency or excess. At present, no clear guidelines exist for diagnosis and treatment of marginal zinc status in persons with diabetes.[1]

Vanadium

There is a growing body of research investigating vanadium, a trace element and common constituent of the earth's crust. Two oxidative forms of vanadium, vanadate and vanadyl, ap-

Exhibit 24-1 Chromium Content of Selected Foods (µg dry weight)

Oysters	2.16
Liver	1.77
Brewer's yeast	1.17
Spinach	1.03
Carrots	0.78
Wheat bran	0.42
Chicken breast	0.37

Source: Adapted with permission from *Journal of Agricultural and Food Chemistry* (1979;27;490), Copyright 1980, American Chemical Society.

pear to have insulin-like properties in a number of isolated cell systems and in animal models of type I and type II diabetes. Vanadium is widely distributed in nature and is an essential element in goats, but its nutritional significance in humans remains unclear.[17] The average human total body pool of vanadium is about 100 µg depending on local soil concentrations. Most tissues contain intracellular vanadium at concentrations between 0.1 and 1 µm. It appears to have effects on cellular regulation and as an endogenous constituent of most mammalian tissue. Studies of vanadium salts in animal models of diabetes show a significant reduction in blood glucose levels.[18,19] The efficacy and mechanism of vanadate as a potential oral hypoglycemic agent in humans is beginning to be investigated. One small study concluded that oral supplementation with sodium metavanadate improved insulin sensitivity in some subjects with IDDM and more strikingly, in NIDDM. It may also have independent lipid lowering effects.[20]

There are several commercially available preparations of vanadyl sulfate, mainly available at health food stores and it is also a component of several multivitamin preparations. The dose taken usually ranges from 7.5 to 130 mg/d as vanadyl sulfate. There is no apparent major toxicity of therapy except for some gastrointestinal intolerance. It will be interesting to watch for further research to uncover the mechanisms and potential benefits of vanadium supplementation.

Antioxidants: ß-carotene, Vitamin C, and Vitamin E

Antioxidants have received a great deal of attention in the literature in recent years especially related to their potential role in cardiovascular and cancer risk reduction. As antioxidants, ß-carotene, in combination with other nutrients including vitamin E and vitamin C, can diminish the negative impact of the highly reactive free radicals that can cause cell injury. Therefore, it is being explored whether antioxidant supplementation can prevent or reduce this cell injury, thereby reducing the risks of some long-term complications. Long-term studies are necessary in this area as there

can be risks from large-dose supplementation if there is not a proven benefit. For example, epidemiologic evidence indicates that diets high in ß-carotene and vitamin E are associated with reduced risks of lung cancer. However, a recent study of 29,133 male smokers, some of whom took ß-carotene (20 mg/d), some of whom took vitamin E (α-tocopherol 50 mg/d), and some who took both, who were studied for 5 to 8 years, showed no reduction in the incidence of lung cancer. In fact, the group taking ß-carotene had significantly more cases of lung cancer.[21]

Research has shown that vitamin E may have a role in reducing the risks of complications by inhibiting nonenzymatic glycosylations of protein. In a study that included 15 subjects with NIDDM, vitamin E supplements (900 mg/d for 4 months) were shown to be useful in improving insulin action.[22] A second study of NIDDM patients that also supplemented vitamin E in doses of 900 mg/d demonstrated minimal but significant improvement in metabolic control.[23]

Despite the fact that vitamin E is a fat-soluble vitamin, research has indicated that its toxicity level is low. In human studies with double-blind protocols and in large population studies, oral vitamin E supplementation resulted in few side effects even at doses as high as 3200 mg/d.[24]

Research at the Joslin Diabetes Center is examining whether supplemental vitamin E can prevent the functional changes in retinal blood vessels induced by diabetes, which can lead to retinopathy. The effectiveness of vitamin E treatment in preventing the hyperglycemia-induced biochemical and physiologic dysfunctions in vascular tissues of diabetic rats has already been demonstrated.[25] Patients with both IDDM and NIDDM are being studied.

Another study concluded there was no significant association between glycohemoglobin and intake of vitamin E, vitamin C, and ß-carotene in people with diabetes.[26] However, the doses of the nutrients studied were not pharmacologic doses as used in the above-mentioned studies. The RDA for vitamin E is 30 mg/d, the vitamin C RDA is 60 mg, and for vitamin A it is 1000 µg retinol equivalents for men and 800 µg for women.

Despite the newness of this research, exaggerated health claims are increasingly being made for antioxidant vitamins. In a commentary by noted nutrition expert and consumer advocate Victor Herbert, readers are warned about the "antioxidant myth."[27] He points out that the effect of these nutrients are not consistently antioxidant but may be pro-oxidant as well. The effect also may be influenced by a variety of factors, including the nutritional status of the individual (particularly the blood iron status) and the source of the nutrient (food or supplement). Although further research may confirm a role for supplementation with particular nutrients, at this point, there is not enough information to advocate their use or to determine appropriate dosage levels.

Additional Vitamins and Minerals

Whether or not individuals with diabetes should routinely take multivitamin and mineral supplements remains controversial.[28] Although it is true that a well-balanced diet will provide the Recommended Dietary Allowances, a recent survey concluded that 25% of the U.S. population do not eat vegetables and 43% do not eat fruit on any given day.[29] It is well acknowledged that there are many population groups who may benefit from nutritional supplementation, including dieters who consume less than 1200 kcals/day, vegetarians, the elderly, pregnant and lactating women, inpatients in the critical care environment, persons with uncontrolled diabetes, and those who hate taking medications that may affect their vitamin or mineral status.[1]

In addition to the nutrients previously mentioned, there are many others being studied that may have an impact on diabetes. Table 24-1 summarizes selected macronutrients, their relation to diabetes, food sources, the RDA or estimated safe and adequate daily dietary intake (ESADDIs), and citations for research studies.

Fish Oils

Fish oils containing omega-3 fatty acids have been reported to be linked with reducing the risk for cardiovascular disease. These fatty acids have been shown to reduce serum lipids and lipoproteins, to impair platelet aggregation, and to decrease blood pressure. They are particularly effective in reducing triglycerides. However, because early reports demonstrated a worsening on glycemic control, the use of these oils in diabetes needs further study.

It has been observed that as little as 30 g of fish per day reduces the incidence of coronary heart disease. If this is valid and can be extended to persons with diabetes, the antiatherogenic effects of omega-3 fatty acids may be obtained with much lower doses than previously recognized and therefore not cause as much of a deterioration on glycemic control. It is also interesting to note that the hyperglycemic effects of fish oil concentrates are not likely to make control worse than the elevations that may be expected from nicotinic acid, a drug used to treat hypertriglyceridemia.[30]

Research has also shown that persons who supplement their diets with daily doses of omega-3 fatty acids show improvement in blood pressure. Supplemental doses studies were between 2.7 and 15 g/d. In these studies, not only did glycemic control worsen but so did lipids as measured by increases in total and LDL-C. Some argue that these worsening effects are not as common in IDDM patients. Interestingly, no additional benefits were noted when 6 g/d of fish oil was given to people who ate fish three times a week or more.[31]

Therefore, more fish in the diet seems safer and just as effective as fish oil supplements in protecting the cardiovascular system. Supplementation with commercial fish oil preparations for the treatment of severe hypertriglyceridemia must only be undertaken with medical and dietary supervision and cannot be recommended in general for persons with diabetes.

NONFOOD ITEMS

A dietitian completing a thorough nutritional assessment not only should ask questions regarding usual food and beverage intake but should also be aware that certain nonfood items

Table 24-1 A Review of Selected Vitamins and Minerals in Relation to Diabetes

Nutrient	Relation to Diabetes	Source	RDA or ESADDI
Copper[1,2]	• deficiency is associated with impaired glucose tolerance in animals • deficiencies are rarely seen in adults • elevated serum Cu levels have been noted in the following groups: NIDDM, elderly, with complications	organ meats, seafood, nuts, seeds	1.5–3 mg[b]
Manganese[3,4]	• deficiency in animals causes impaired glucose tolerance, which is normalized after Mn supplementation • elevated serum Mn levels are common in diabetes • supplementation in NIDDM does not have glucose-lowering effects	whole grains, vegetables, fruit	2.0–5.0 mg[b]
Iron[5,6]	• iron excess found in hemochromatosis is commonly associated with glucose intolerance • one study showed improved glycemia after therapy with deferoxamine and corresponding reductions in iron levels • iron metabolism may be altered in diabetes	meats, eggs, fortified grains	10 mg (men) 15 mg (women)[a]
Selenium[7–9]	• antioxidant; parallels many functions of vitamin E • deficiency has been related to certain forms of cardiomyopathy • not well studied in diabetes • no reason to believe persons with diabetes are at risk for deficiency	seafood, organ meats, whole grains	70 µg (men) 55 µg (women)[a]
Thiamine[10,11]	• the occasional patient with neuropathy may respond to pharmacologic doses	cereals, pork	1.5 mg (men) 1.0 mg (women)[a]
Niacin[12–14]	• nicotinic acid and chromium may improve glucose tolerance • suggestions that nicotinamide may protect the pancreatic ß-cell function in new-onset diabetes and improve diabetes control need further research • nicotinic acid is used to treat hyperlipidemia but has hyperglycemic effects	fish, meat, grains, milk	13–20 µg
Vitamin B$_{12}$[15–17]	• associated with IDDM in the context of polyglandular autoimmune diseases • prevalence of NIDDM and pernicious anemia increases with age • no causal relationship between diabetes and B$_{12}$ deficiency • one study showed leg parasthesias improved after intrathecal injections of high-dose methylcobalamin	meats, animal products	2.0 µg

Table 24-1 continued

Nutrient	Relation to Diabetes	Source	RDA or ESADDI
Vitamin D[18,19]	• functions as a regulator of calcium and phosphate metabolism • changes in vitamin D metabolism and bone mass have been noted in IDDM, particularly prepubertal children • women with NIDDM may have reduced bone mineral content; however, risk of fracture does not appear to be greater	fortified milk, eggs, butter	5 µg[a]
Biotin[20]	• serum biotin levels lower in persons with NIDDM; oral doses of 9 mg biotin daily corrected hyperglycemia in these patients	liver, milk, mush-rooms, vegetables	100–200 µg[b]

[a] RDA
[b] ESADDI

REFERENCES FOR TABLE 24-1

1. Cohen AM, Teitelbaum A, Miller E, Bentor V, Hirt R, Fields M. The effect of copper on carbohydrate metabolism. *Isr J Med Sci.* 1982;18:840–844.

2. Noto R, Alicata R, Sfogliano L, Neris S, Bifarella M. A study of cupremia in a group of elderly diabetics. *Acta Diabetol Lat.* 1983;20:81–85.

3. Everson GJ, Shrader RE. Abnormal glucose tolerance in manganese deficient guinea pigs. *J Nutr.* 1968;94:89–94.

4. Walter RM, Aoki T, Keen CL. Acute oral manganese does not consistently affect glucose tolerance in nondiabetic and type II diabetic humans. *J Trace El Exp Med.* 1991;4:73–79.

5. Cutler P. Deferoxamine therapy in high ferritin diabetes. *Diabetes.* 1989;38:1207–1210.

6. Redman JB, Pyzdrowski KL, Robertson P. No effect of deferoxamine therapy on glucose homeostasis and insulin secretion in individuals with NIDDM and elevated serum ferritin. *Diabetes.* 1993;42:544–549.

7. Van Rij AM, Thomson CD, McKenzie JM, Robinson MF. Selenium deficiency in total parenteral nutrition. *Am J Clin Nutr.* 1979;32:2076–2085.

8. Asayama K, Kooy NW, Burr IM. Effect of vitamin E deficiency and selenium deficiency on insulin secretory reserve and free radical scavenging systems in islets: decrease of islet manganosuperoxide dismutase. *J Lab Clin Med.* 1986;107:459–464.

9. Strain JJ. Disturbances in micronutrient and antioxidant status in diabetes. *Proc Nutr Soc.* 1991;50:591–604.

10. Mooradian AD, Morley JE. Micronutrient status in diabetes mellitus. *Am J Clin Nutr.* 1987;45:877–895.

11. Saito N, Kimura M, Kuchiba A, Itokawa Y. Blood thiamine levels in outpatients with diabetes mellitus. *J Nutr Sci Vitaminol.* 1987;33:421–430.

12. Urberg M, Parent M, Hill D, Zemel M. Evidence for synergism between chromium and nicotinic acid in normalizing glucose tolerance. Abstract. *Diabetes.* (suppl) 1986;34:147A.

13. Mendola G, Casamitjana R, Gomis R. Effect of nicotinamide therapy upon ß-cell function in newly diagnosed type I diabetic patients. *Diabetologia.* 1989;32:160–162.

14. Garg A, Grundy SM. Nicotinic acid as therapy for dyslipidemia in non–insulin-dependent diabetes mellitus. *JAMA.* 1990;264:723–726.

15. Trence DL, Morley JE, Handwerger BS. Polyglandular autoimmune syndromes. *Am J Med.* 1984;77:107–116.

16. Reed RL, Mooradian AD. Nutritional status and dietary management of elderly diabetic patients. *Clin Geriatr Med.* 1990;6:883–901.

17. Ide H, Jujiya S, Asanuma Y, Tsuji M, Sakai H, Agishi Y. Clinical usefulness of intrathecal injection of methylcobalamin in patients with diabetic neuropathy. *Clin Ther.* 1987;9:183–192.

18. Rodland O, Markestad T, Aksnes L, Aarskog D. Plasma concentrations of vitamin D metabolites during puberty of diabetic children. *Diabetologia.* 1985;28:663–666.

19. Weinstock RS, Goland RS, Shane E, Clemens TL, Lindsay R, Bilezikian JP. Bone mineral density in women with type II diabetes mellitus. *J Bone Miner Res.* 1989;4:97–101.

20. Maabashi M, Makino Y, Furukawa Y, Ohinata K, Kimura S, Sato T. Therapeutic evaluation of the effect of biotin on hyperglycemia in patients with NIDDM. *J Clin Biochem Nutr.* 1993;14:211–218.

may affect diabetes control. Some forms of tobacco, certain over-the-counter medications, and recreational drugs may have a hyperglycemic effect in the patient with diabetes who is a chronic abuser of these substances.

Cornstarch

Nocturnal hypoglycemia in children with glycogen storage disease has been successfully averted when uncooked cornstarch is given. Studies have shown that in 15 to 46% of the cases of hypoglycemia a cause cannot be identified. Also, nearly 40% of 285 episodes of hypoglycemia in children occurred during sleep.[32] With the focus on intensive insulin therapy, there is keen interest in identifying ways to reduce the risks of hypoglycemia. This has been tested in children with diabetes and was found to significantly lessen the frequency of hypoglycemic episodes in children who are intensively managed and who had a history of low blood sugars through the night.[33] In the study, 25 to 50% of the bedtime snack carbohydrate was administered as cornstarch added to milk (one tsp of cornstarch contains about 7 g of carbohydrate). Improvements were demonstrated without increasing the mean fasting blood glucoses or altering overall glycemic control. Although this may be a useful treatment, one should not initiate the treatment without investigating the cause and working to normalize glycemia.

Tobacco

The total sugar content in tobacco varies widely among the different forms (pouch, plug, snuff, pipe, cigar), the different brands, and the different states where the leaves are dried, cured, and processed. One analysis revealed that pouch tobacco, commonly used for chewing, contains a mean level of 34.4 g of glucose per 100 g of tobacco (34%). Plug tobacco, at 24%, has the next highest level. Some forms of pouch tobacco, however, were found to contain more than 60% glucose.[34]

The significance of this level of glucose for a person with diabetes depends on several factors, including the size of the "pinch" or "chew" of tobacco (a typical chew is about 2 g of tobacco), the frequency with which new tobacco is added to the mouth, and whether the person spits or swallows the juice. A new pinch could be added as often as every 20 minutes. A large amount of tobacco would need to be chewed for it to have much influence on blood glucose because 2 g of a highly sugared tobacco may contain only 1.2 g of glucose, and 10 g (five chews) will contain only 6 g of glucose.

However, a case example of how chewing tobacco affected diabetes control was reported in the *New England Journal of Medicine*.[35] A 56-year-old man with IDDM was being carefully monitored in the hospital with a controlled diet and insulin regimen, but his hyperglycemia continued. Only after the patient was observed closely for 48 hours was it recognized that the patient chewed a "candified" brand of tobacco and swallowed the juice. Although the patient refused to stop chewing the tobacco, he did agree to stop swallowing the juice, and with no further changes in therapy, glycemia returned to more normal ranges.

Medications

Many medications contain some form of sugar to enhance their palatability. Persons with diabetes are usually cautioned that antacids, cough syrups, and alcohol-based elixirs may contain significant amounts of carbohydrate. However, these are usually not ingested for a long enough time or in large enough quantities to affect diabetes control. A study that compared the effects of two cough syrup formulations (one with sugar and one without) on the control of NIDDM found no differences between products.[36]

The *New England Journal of Medicine* reports that 15 mL of some liquid antacids contain more than 2000 mg sugar, and some tablets contain between 500 mg and 1000 mg.[37] Although a typical dose of the antacid—not more than 30 mL every other hour—would create a relatively minor glycemic response, some persons may be particularly sensitive to the higher-sugar antacids.

Physicians advise some patients to take certain drugs along with a particular food or beverage. For example, hypertension medications may be taken with a banana, or iron supplements may be swallowed with a glass of orange juice. It is important in meal planning to make sure that the patient recognizes these other sources of calories in the diet even though they may not be recalled as part of a typical meal or snack. The dietitian must incorporate the calories and/or carbohydrate contributed from these foods into the overall meal plan.

Acarbose

"Starch blockers" or α-amylase inhibitors received much publicity several years ago as an aid to weight reduction. These α-amylase inhibitors, isolated from certain legumes or beans, were shown to bind amylases in vitro and enhance fecal energy and excretion in rats. However, a review of clinical studies that examined the action of commercial starch blockers revealed them to be ineffective in the reduction of starch digestion.[38] Because starch blockers were originally marketed as a food supplement, they had not undergone the rigorous testing to which new drugs are subjected by the Food and Drug Administration (FDA). The FDA has since declared starch blockers to be drugs, and all were recalled from the market for appropriate research and testing.

One type of starch blocker, acarbose, is currently in clinical use outside the United States and is under review in this country. Acarbose, an α-glucoside hydrolase inhibitor, has hypoglycemic effects by blocking the digestion of starches, sucrose, dextrin, and maltose to absorbable monosaccharides. Absorption of glucose and other monosaccharides is not affected. The net result is a decrease in the postprandial rise in plasma glucose levels. It may be useful in patients with both type I or type II diabetes.[39] Acarbose does not cause weight reduction, because no significant malabsorption occurs with

appropriate pharmacologic doses. It also does not cause hypoglycemia by itself. However, if hypoglycemia occurs due to its being combined with another antidiabetic agent, the treatment of choice should be glucose, as the absorption of sucrose or other carbohydrates would be inhibited by the acarbose.[40]

The ideal dose range is being investigated. In a multicenter, double-blind placebo controlled trial of persons with NIDDM, acarbose-treated patients had statistically significant reductions in mean HbA_{1c} levels of 0.78, 0.73, 1.10% (relative to placebo) in the 100, 200, and 300 mg (three times daily) groups respectively when studied for a 16-week period.[41] Generally, patients who receive acarbose at these higher doses also exhibit side effects including flatulence, abdominal distension, and diarrhea. However, one study that administered a low dose of acarbose as a powder along with meals instead of a tablet showed subjects having no side effects with the 25 mg three-times-a-day dose, yet beneficial results were still achieved.[42]

Recreational Drugs

Little data are available on the effects of controlled and illicit drugs on diabetes management. All the adverse effects of such drugs as marijuana, central nervous system (CNS) stimulants, depressants, hallucinogens, and opiates on overall health are not known. Their specific effects on glycemia are even less well defined.

The major problem posed by most of the recreational drugs is that they can alter the patient's perception of reality and time, judgment, and behavior and thus result in poor self-care and poor regulation of blood glucose. Such drugs as marijuana are often used in conjunction with alcohol, which further impairs clear thinking and interferes with diabetes management. Some drugs can affect the appetite. CNS stimulants, such as amphetamines and cocaine, and hallucinogens cause decreased appetite or anorexia; other drugs trigger eating, such as the frequent snacking or "munchies" associated with marijuana. Many CNS stimulants are chemically

Exhibit 24-2 Sources of Caffeine

Food	mg/100 ml
Instant coffee	44
Dripolated coffee	97
Decaffeinated coffee	0.5–6
Tea, brewed 1–5 min	20–33
Carbonated beverages	
Coke	18
Pepsi	12
RC Cola	9
Dr Pepper	17
Mountain Dew	15
Instant cocoa	6
Medications	**mg/unit**
Analgesics	
Cafergot	100
Excedrin	65
Midol	32
Anacin	32
Stimulants, such as	
NoDoz, Vivarin	100–200

Sources: Handbook of Clinical Dietetics by The American Dietetic Association, Yale University Press, 1981; *Psychosomatics* (1980; 21:411), Copyright © 1980, Cliggott Publishing Company.

similar to catecholamines and stimulate glycogen breakdown in the liver, leading to hyperglycemia.[43]

Opiate (morphine, heroin) addicts are reported to have increased HbA_{1c} levels and impaired glucose tolerance as compared with non–drug-taking healthy males.[44] Patients with diabetes who are abusing recreational drugs should, of course, be referred to specialists in the treatment of drug problems. They should also be encouraged to do self-monitoring of blood glucose to see the specific effect that the drug has on their diabetes control and to make appropriate management adjustments.

Caffeine

Caffeine is one of several methylxanthine derivatives that occur naturally and are found in coffee beans, tea leaves, kola nuts, and cocoa beans. Theophylline and theobromine are also xanthines. It has been estimated that the average

American adult ingests more than 200 mg caffeine per day from dietary sources. Persons consuming medications containing caffeine may receive 30 to 200 mg of additional caffeine per tablet (Exhibit 24-2). Ingested caffeine is rapidly absorbed, metabolized, and excreted in the urine as methylxanthine derivatives. Within a few minutes after consumption, caffeine enters all tissues, and after 1 hour it is distributed in proportion to tissue water content. The metabolic half-life of caffeine in the plasma and most organs is about 3 hours.[45]

Caffeine is probably most noted for its effects as a cardiac muscle stimulant, a stimulant of gastric acid secretion, and a diuretic. However, the diabetes educator should be aware of its potential to elevate blood glucose. This hyperglycemic effect occurs from caffeine's ability to potentiate the effects of epinephrine and glucagon.[46] One research study concluded that the hyperglycemic effect of caffeine could be seen only after consumption of pure caffeine and not after drinking coffee or other caffeine-containing beverages.[47]

The clinical significance of the hyperglycemic effect of caffeine needs further investigation. Although an endocrine response has been shown in humans at levels of 500 mg of caffeine administered at one time, few persons would ingest this much caffeine at once. It does not seem necessary to restrict caffeine because of its hyperglycemic characteristics, but dietitians should be aware that this drug may be related to high blood glucose levels in persons who consume several cups of strong coffee in a short time.[48]

Jerusalem Artichokes

Special properties have been attributed to the Jerusalem artichoke, leading some to believe that it is a particularly good food for persons with diabetes to consume. The chief carbohydrate of this tuberous, starchy root vegetable is inulin, a fructose polymer. It has erroneously been claimed that, once ingested, inulin turns to insulin and thus alleviates the need for the medi-

Exhibit 24-3 Myoinositol Content of Selected Foods

Food	Amount	Myoinositol Content (mg)
Green beans, shelled fresh	1/2 cup	193
Spinach, fresh	1/2 cup	8
Cantaloupe, fresh	1/4	355
Raisins	1 Tbsp	4
Wheat bread, stone ground	1 slice	287
Wheat bread, Roman meal	1 slice	9
Beans, Great Northern, canned	1/2 cup	440
Corn, yellow, canned	1/3 cup	19

Source: Adapted with permission from *American Journal of Clinical Nutrition* (1980;33:1954), Copyright © 1980, American Society for Clinical Nutrition.

cation. Another erroneous claim is that, because the carbohydrate is a form of fructose, it contains virtually no calories. For this reason, its use was reportedly encouraged in the preinsulin era.[49] The Jerusalem artichoke, which bears little resemblance to the more popular globe artichoke, contains 57 calories, 13 g carbohydrate, and 1.5 g protein per 75 g or one-half cup slices.[50] Although the Jerusalem artichoke may produce a lower glycemic response than a potato or similar root vegetables due to its fructose content, this hypothesis is yet to be tested.

Myoinositol

Myoinositol, a six-carbon cyclic polyalcohol, may play an important role in the function of peripheral nerves. Some researchers have shown that an increase in the daily dietary intake of myoinositol significantly improves sensory nerve function in patients with diabetic neuropathy. Myoinositol is present in measurable amounts in all living cells but is most prevalent in fruits, beans, grains, and nuts. Some researchers hypothesize that increased myoinositol intake may delay the onset of diabetic peripheral neuropathy.[51] Others, however, have been unable to reproduce the improved nerve function potential.[52] An analysis of 487 foods for myoinositol revealed that the best sources are

foods from plant sources. Foods from animals—meats, milk, cheese, eggs—contain low amounts of myoinositol. Notice in Exhibit 24-3 the wide variation of myoinositol content of foods even within the same food group.

REFERENCES

1. Mooradian AD, Failla M, Hoogwerf B, Maryniuk M, Wylie-Rosett J. Selected vitamins and minerals in diabetes. *Diabetes Care.* 1994;17:464–479.

2. Baker DE, Campbell RK. Vitamin and mineral supplementation in patients with diabetes mellitus. *Diabetes Educ.* 1992;18:420–426.

3. McNair P, Christiansen C, Madsbad S, et al. Hypomagnesemia, a risk factor in diabetic retinopathy. *Diabetes.* 1978;27:1075.

4. Yang XY, Redmond GP, Castellani WJ, et al. Trace element levels in blood and 24-hour urine of insulin dependent diabetic individuals with and without retinopathy. *Diabetes.* 1985;34(suppl 1):207A.

5. Schmidt L, Heins J. Low magnesium intake among NIDDM patients: a call for concern. *Diabetes.* 1993;42 (suppl 1):49a.

6. American Diabetes Association. Magnesium supplementation in the treatment of diabetes. *Diabetes Care.* 1992;15:1065–1067.

7. Offenbacher EG, Pi-Sunyer X. Beneficial effect of chromium-rich yeast on glucose tolerance and blood lipids in elderly subjects. *Diabetes.* 1980;29:919.

8. Ravina A, Slezak L. Chromium in the treatment of clinical diabetes. *Harefuah.* 1993;125(5-6):142–145.

9. Urberg M, Parent M, Hill D, et al. Evidence for synergism between chromium and nicotinic acid in normalizing glucose tolerance. *Diabetes.* 1986;35(suppl 1):37A.

10. Goodhart R, Shils M. *Modern Nutrition in Health and Disease*, 6th ed. Philadelphia, Pa: Lea & Febiger; 1980.

11. Kinlaw WB, Levine AS, Morley HE, Silbis SE, McClain CJ. Abnormal zinc metabolism in type II diabetes mellitus. *Am J Med.* 1983;75:273–277.

12. Song MK, Mooradian AD. Intestinal zinc transport: influence of streptozotocin induced diabetes, insulin and arachindonic acid. *Life Sci.* 1988;42:687–694.

13. Pai LH, Prasad AS. Cellular zinc in patients with diabetes mellitus. *Nutr Res.* 1988;8:889–897.

14. Hallbook T, Lanner E. Serum-zinc and healing of venous leg ulcers. *Lancet.* 1972;2:780–782.

15. Nakamura T, Higashi A, Nishiyama S, Fujumoto S, Matsuda I. Kinetics of zinc status of children with IDDM. *Diabetes Care.* 1991;14:533–557.

16. Hooper PL, Visconti L, Garry PJ, Johnson GE. Zinc lowers high-density lipoprotein cholesterol levels. *JAMA.* 1980;244:1960–1961.

17. Harland BF, Harden-Williams BA. Is vanadium of human nutritional importance yet? *J Am Diet Assoc.* 1994;94:891–894.

18. Meyerovitch J, Rothernberg P, Shechter Y, Bonner-Weir S, Kahn CR. Vanadate normalizes hyperglycemia in two mouse models of non-insulin dependent diabetes mellitus. *J Clin Invest.*1991;87:1286–1294.

19. Shechter Y. Insulin mimetic effects of vanadate. *Diabetes.* 1990;39:1–5.

20. Goldfine AB, Folli F, Patti ME, Simonson DC, Kahn CR. Clinical trials of vanadium in human diabetes mellitus. Abstract. Vanadium: Biochemistry, physiology, and potential use in diabetes therapy. 1994 Satellite Symposium of the XIIth IUPHAR Congress. Montreal, Canada.

21. Alpha-Tocoperhol, Beta Carotene Cancer Prevention Study Group. The effect of vitamin E and beta carotene on the incidence of lung cancer and other cancers in male smokers. *N Engl J Med.* 1994;330:1029–1035.

22. Paolisso G, D'Amore A, Guigliano D, Ceriello A, Varricchio M, D'Onofrio F. Pharmacologic doses of vitamin E improve insulin action in healthy subjects and non–insulin-dependent diabetic patients. *Am J Clin Nutr.* 1993;57:650–656.

23. Paolisso G, D'Amore A, Galzerano D, et al. Daily vitamin E supplements improve metabolic control but not insulin secretion in elderly type II diabetic patients. *Diabetes Care.* 1993;16:1433–1437.

24. Bendich A, Machlin L. Safety of oral intake of vitamin E. *Am J Clin Nutr.* 1988;48:612–619.

25. Kunisaki M, King G. Vitamin E treatment prevents the hyperglycemia induced biochemical and physiological dysfunctions in vascular tissues of diabetic rats. *Diabetes.* 1994;43:111a.

26. Shoff SM, Mares-Perlman JA, Cruickshanks KJ, Klein R, Klein B, Ritter LL. Glycosylated hemoglobin concentrations and vitamin E, vitamin C, and beta-carotene intake in diabetic and nondiabetic older adults. A*m J Clin Nutr.* 1993;58:412–416.

27. Herbert V. The antioxidant supplement myth. *Am J Clin Nutr.* 1994;60:157–158.

28. Campbell RK, Thom SL. Micronutrients and diabetes: The supplementation controversy. *Diabetes Spectrum.* 1995;8:238–243.

29. National Livestock and Meat Board. Eating in America Today (EAT): A Dietary Pattern and Intake Report. Chicago, Ill: MRCA Information Services; 1994.

30. Malasanos TH, Stacpoole PW. Biological effects of ω-3 fatty acids in diabetes mellitus. *Diabetes Care.* 1991;41:1160–1179.

31. Tjoa HI, Kaplan NM. Nonpharmacological treatment of hypertension in diabetes mellitus. *Diabetes Care.* 1991;14:449–460.

32. Devgan S, Kaufman FR. The use of uncooked cornstarch to avert nocturnal hypoglycemia in young patients with type I diabetes mellitus. *Diabetes.* 1994;43 (suppl 1):97a.

33. Ververs MTC, Rouwe C, Smit GPA. Complex carbohydrates in the prevention of nocturnal hypoglycemia in diabetic children. *Eur J Clin Nutr.* 1993;47:268–273.

34. Going RE, Hsu SC, Pollack RL, et al. Sugar and fluoride content of various forms of tobacco. *J Am Dent Assoc.* 1980;100:27.

35. Pyles ST, Van Voris LP, Lotspeich FJ, et al. Sugar in chewing tobacco. *N Engl J Med.* 1981;304:365.

36. LeMar HJ, Georgitis WJ. Effect of cold remedies on metabolic control of NIDDM. *Diabetes Care.* 1993; 16:426–428.

37. Stolinsky DC. Sugar and saccharin content of antacids. *N Engl J Med.* 1981;305:166.

38. Starch blockers do not block starch digestion. *Nutr Rev.* 1985;43:46.

39. Balfour JA, McTavish D. Acarbose. An update of its pharmacology and therapeutic use in diabetes mellitus. *Drugs.* 1993;46:1025–1054.

40. Toeller M. Nutritional recommendations for diabetic patients and treatment with alpha-glucosidase inhibitors. *Drugs.* 1992;44(suppl 3):13–20.

41. Coniff RF, Shapiro JA, Robbins D, et al. Reduction of glycosylated hemoglobin and postprandial hyperglycemia by acarbose in patients with NIDDM. *Diabetes Care.* 1995;18:817–824.

42. Jenny A, Proietto J, O'Dea K, Nankervis A, Traianedes K, D'Embden H. Low-dose acarbose improves

glycemic control in NIDDM patients without changes in insulin sensitivity. *Diabetes Care*. 1993;16:499–502.

43. Campbell RK, Ruhlman GG. Recreational drugs and diabetes, part 3: controlled substances. *Pract Diabetol*. 1985;4:10.

44. Ceriello A. Increased glycosylated proteins in opiate addicts. *Diabetes Care*. 1984;7:104.

45. Graham DM. Caffeine—Its identity, dietary sources, intake and biological effects. *Nutr Rev*. 1978;36:97.

46. Katims JJ, Murphy KMM, Snyder SH. Xanthine stimulants and adenosine. In: Creese I, ed. *Stimulants: Neurochemical, Behavioral and Clinical Perspectives*. New York, NY: Raven Press; 1983.

47. Cheraskin E, Ringsdorf WM, Setyaadinadja ATSH, et al. Effect of caffeine versus placebo supplementation on blood glucose concentrations. *Lancet*. 1967;1:1299.

48. Dews PB. *Caffeine: Perspectives from Recent Research*. New York, NY: Springer-Verlag; 1984.

49. Ney D, Hollingsworth DR. Nutritional management of pregnancy complicated by diabetes: historical perspective. *Diabetes Care*. 1981;4:627.

50. U.S. Department of Agriculture: *Composition of Foods: Vegetables and Vegetable Products*. Agriculture Handbook No. AH-8-11. Washington, DC: Government Printing Office; 1984.

51. Clements RS, Darnell B. Myoinositol content of common foods: development of a high myoinositol diet. *Am J Clin Nutr*. 1980;33:1954.

52. Gregersen G, Borsting PT, Servo C. Myoinositol and function of peripheral nerves in human diabetes. *Acta Neurol Scand*. 1978;58:241.

Part VI

Life Stages

Chapter 25

Children and Adolescents

Lea Ann Holzmeister

Optimal care of children and adolescents with insulin-dependent diabetes mellitus (IDDM) is complex and requires a coordinated approach to management. A team approach is necessary for optimal treatment. Education about the disorder is critical to establish the groundwork for future success of the child and family in self-management.

The education process is based on a structured diabetes education curriculum adapted to the individual child and family.[1] Providing information about meal planning and eating is an intregal component of self-management training.[2] The process of educating parents and children in diabetes care begins at the time of diagnosis. Initially, however, parents and children may be too upset to assimilate the large body of information needed. Therefore, the education process is staged to provide essential survival skills at the time of diagnosis. In-depth education is provided during the weeks and months following when the families' grief reaction subsides and they are more ready to learn the skills required to implement the management program.

Food and feeding issues are important in the physical and psychological growth of children. The education about food and nutrition must take into consideration the child's developmental level. The educational curriculum for the child must be concordant with the child's level of cognitive development and adapted to the learning style and intellectual ability of the individual child and family.[3,4] Appropriate meal plan education must be provided to promote a positive attitude toward eating and food.

CLASSIFICATION AND PREVALENCE

Criteria for Diagnosis

IDDM in children is characterized by clinical signs and/or symptoms of polyuria, polydipsia, ketonuria, and weight loss. The weight loss may be associated with a decrease in the rate of growth and physical development.

Prevalence

IDDM accounts for approximately 3% of all new cases of diabetes diagnosed each year in the United States.[5] The prevalence of IDDM in children is about 1 in 600 children younger than 16.[6] IDDM prevalence appears to vary according to race and among different countries, with rates lower among blacks, Hispanics, and Asians compared with whites. The risk of developing IDDM is higher than virtually all other severe chronic diseases of childhood such as cystic fibrosis, peptic ulcer, and leukemia. The age-specific incidence rises from very low levels in the early months of life and peaks around 10 to 13 years of age in girls and 1 to 2 years later in boys. By the age of 50, approximately 10% of siblings of individuals with IDDM will develop IDDM.[7] There is a significantly higher risk of diabetes among children of diabetic fathers (6%)[8] than among children of diabetic mothers (2%).[9]

In some parts of the world, the incidence of IDDM appears to be increasing. The changes in the incidence and prevalence of IDDM can be explained only on the basis that environmental

Exhibit 25-1 Other Types of Diabetes in Childhood

Type	Characteristics
Non–Insulin-Dependent Diabetes Mellitus	• With or without obesity • Seldom develop ketosis, except under stress • May require insulin for treatment of symptomatic hyperglycemia • Defects of insulin cell receptor function or abnormalities of post-receptor insulin action
Maturity Onset Diabetes of Youth of Youth (MODY)	• Autosomal dominant • Usually associated with obesity • Onset in first two decades of life • Resistant to development of long-term complications • Seem to make a structurally abnormal insulin molecule with poor biological activity • May be insulin dependent at onset, but may progress to a non–insulin-dependent course

factors play a important role in determining the incidence of IDDM.

Seasonal variability in diagnosis of IDDM has been postulated.[10] However, since IDDM has a long subclinical period, the seasonal pattern in diagnosis may result from the seasonal occurrence of factors (such as common infections) that precede the appearance of symptoms.[7]

Types of Diabetes in Childhood

In addition to IDDM, a few children may develop some other type of diabetes (Exhibit 25-1). Different management strategies may be required, depending on the characteristics. Exhibit 25-2 lists some of the more frequently secondary causes of diabetes in childhood.[11]

PATHOGENESIS

IDDM is an autoimmune disorder in which ß-cell destruction occurs in a genetically susceptible host.[12] Clinical onset may be preceded by an extensive asymptomatic period during which ß cells are continuously destroyed. When ongoing destruction has reduced ß-cell mass by 80 to 90%, overt diabetes ensues.

The evolution of IDDM is thought to begin with genetic predisposition followed by precipitating events of uncertain type and progressive autoimmune destruction of pancreatic ß cells.[13] Genetic features of IDDM include the histocompatibility leukocyte antigen (HLA) complex, located on chromosomes,[6] which consists of a cluster of genes that code for transplantation antigens and regulation of the immune response.[5] Certain HLA types, principally the DR_3 and DR_4 loci, are present in approximately 95% of patients with IDDM. It is hypothesized that genes creating diabetes susceptibility appear to act at the level of the immune system.[14]

The autoimmune process is strongly implicated in ß-cell destruction.[13] This is evidenced by presence at diagnosis of inflammatory cells around islets and of anti-islet cell and anti-insulin antibodies and activation of T-lymphocytes. Also, there is an association of IDDM with other autoimmune disorders.

Environmental factors may also play a role in the initiation of autoimmune ß-cell destruction. This is evidenced by the worldwide regional differences in its incidence and the discordance between monozygotic twins. Viruses may play a role in the pathogenesis of IDDM through direct

Exhibit 25-2 Secondary Causes of Diabetes in Childhood

Cause	*Characteristics*
Pancreatic trauma, disease or resection	85 to 90% removal of pancreas
Hormone-induced	eg, Acromegaly, Cushing syndrome
Drugs and chemical agents	eg, Glucocorticoids and antileukemic (L-asparaginase)
Genetic syndromes	eg, Cystic fibrosis—mild ketosis resistant
Insulin receptor abnormalities	eg, Acanthosis nigricans, leprechaunism

ß-cell cytotoxicity, by triggering autoimmunity to islets by the infection of ß-cells or lymphocytes.[14]

Various dietary factors have also been implicated in the incidence of IDDM. Replacing proteins with amino acids in the diets of non-obese diabetic mice, an animal model for the study of IDDM, decreases the incidence of diabetes.[15] A recent study reported an increased risk of IDDM among children with a diabetes susceptibility gene who had early exposure to cow's milk.[16] A critical overview of clinical evidence relating cow's milk exposure and IDDM reports early cow's milk exposure may be an important determinant of subsequent IDDM and may increase the risk approximately 1–5 times.[17] Though these studies are inconclusive, breastmilk remains the preferred feeding during the first year of life.

GOALS OF THERAPY

Glycemic control is an important factor in the genesis of diabetic complications as evidenced by the Diabetes Control and Complications Trial.[18] Thus, the goal of therapy for persons with diabetes is to maintain glycemic status as close to the normal range as safely possible. However, the attempt to define therapeutic goals for children is complicated by data that suggest that the prepubertal years of diabetes may contribute minimally to long-term prognosis.[19] Additionally, children who develop diabetes at a young age may be at increased risk for the development of cognitive impairment due to multiple

episodes of severe hypoglycemia.[20,21] Therefore, maintaining very tight control of glucose levels in very young children may be harmful.

The glycemic goals for children must then be placed in a broader context of realistic management goals which include

- prevention of diabetic ketoacidosis and severe hypoglycemia
- relief of symptoms and elimination of signs of uncontrolled diabetes such as polydipsia, polyuria, weight loss, and hyperlipidemia
- maintenance of normal growth, sexual development, and ideal body weight; accommodation of periods of strenuous activity
- promotion of a sense of physical and emotional well-being

These goals must be individualized according to patient and family needs.

INSULIN THERAPY

Insulin regimens in children and adolescents range from one to two daily injections of insulin (conventional insulin therapy) to three or four injections each day (intensive insulin therapy) or continuous subcutaneous insulin infusion.

Generally, children with newly diagnosed IDDM require an insulin dose of 0.6 to 1.0 U/kg per day.[22] However, if the patient is diagnosed before the onset of ketonuria the initial dose may be lower. Adolescents who may be less sensitive to insulin may require 1.0 to 1.5 U/kg per day.[23] Insulin doses are adjusted based on the results of blood glucose measurements over 2 to 3 days.

Within a few weeks after diagnosis, approximately two-thirds of children[24] will experience the "honeymoon" phase, which is a partial recovery of ß-cell function. The "honeymoon" phase or remission occurs less frequently in children younger than 2 years old and is more common in the late teenage years and in adults.[5] Insulin requirements may be considerably less (<0.5 U/kg per day) to maintain glycemic control and some individuals may even temporarily cease to require insulin. The "honeymoon" phase may last for more than several months to one year.

Human insulin is used for newly diagnosed children unless there is difficulty with control due to the more rapidly developing peak effect and the shorter duration of action of human intermediate-acting insulin.[22] This may require a change to animal-source insulin as it peaks later and has longer duration.

Conventional Insulin Therapy

Conventional insulin therapy in children involves the use of twice-daily injections of insulin, usually a mixture of rapid- (regular) and intermediate-acting (NPH/isophane or lente) insulin given before breakfast and before the evening meal or at bedtime.[25] The rapid-acting insulin before breakfast and supper provides a peak level of plasma insulin to match nutrient absorption. The intermediate-acting insulin given at breakfast provides a more slowly developing peak that occurs at the time of the midday meal. The intermediate-acting insulin given at dinner should provide sufficient basal insulin required to suppress hepatic glucose production overnight. The intermediate-acting insulin, given before dinner, may peak during the early morning hours (midnight to 4 A.M.), the time when normal insulin requirements are at their lowest.[26] This mismatch between insulin delivery and insulin requirements frequently causes nocturnal and/or early morning hypoglycemia.[27] This may be followed by prebreakfast hyperglycemia "dawn phenomenon."[28] This may require a three-injection regimen consisting of a mixed dose before breakfast, rapid-acting insulin before the evening meal, and intermediate-acting insulin at bedtime.[29] For young children who retire early and/or are unwilling to take three injections a day, a trial of ultra-lente insulin replacing NPH before supper may be used.[30]

A single daily injection of intermediate-acting insulin may be used for children diagnosed very early and having persistent substantial endogenous insulin secretion or during the honeymoon phase.

Of the total daily dose on twice-daily injections of a mixture of short-acting and intermediate-acting insulin regimen, usually 60 to 75% is given before breakfast and 25 to 40% is given before supper. Approximately 25 to 35% of the morning dose and 30 to 50% of the presupper dose is regular insulin.[22] However, the optimal ratio required for each patient is influenced by the relative size and composition of meals and must be adjusted according to self-monitoring of blood glucose (SMBG).

Intensive Insulin Therapy

Alternative insulin delivery regimens such as multiple daily injections (MDI) or continuous subcutaneous insulin infusion (CSII) using a portable insulin pump mimic the normal pattern of physiologic insulin but are not commonly used with children and adolescents.[31] Consistent and long-term sustained improvement in glycemic control using CSII has not been observed in children and adolescents and young adults (8 to 26 years old).[32] Intensive insulin therapy requires intensification of all aspects of diabetes management which may be unacceptable or unsafe for children and adolescents. In the effort to strive for normoglycemia, more frequent and more severe hypoglycemia may occur which is unsafe in children.[20,21] Therefore, considerable care must be taken in the selection of children or adolescents for MDI or CSII regimens, and intensive education and supervision are required to achieve the benefit of this form of management.

NUTRITION THERAPY

Nutrition therapy is essential in the management of diabetes in children and adolescents. However, adherence to nutrition and diet is one of the most challenging parts of diabetes care for many patients, especially adolescents.[33,34] Many children (and their parents) do not possess the knowledge and skill required for good dietary adherence, regardless of their motivation.[35] The key to effective nutrition therapy is an individualized approach, which includes a thorough assessment, patient (and parent) participation in goal setting, selection of an appropriate nutrition intervention, and evaluation of the effectiveness of the nutrition care plan.[36] A registered dietitian with training and experience in the treatment of diabetes in children and adolescents can contribute valuable expertise to the diabetes management team by using these four key components when providing nutrition therapy for diabetes.[37]

Assessment

The main purpose of the nutrition assessment of the child or adolescent with diabetes is to gather valuable information needed to make future decisions about the nutrition care plan.[38] The assessment phase allows the dietitian the opportunity to establish a trusting relationship with the patient and family, which is essential for successful diabetes management. The nutrition assessment of a child or adolescent with diabetes includes the following: pattern of growth; food history and activity patterns; monitoring results of blood glucose; insulin regimen; lipids; glycosylated hemoglobin; psychosocial situation; and urine testing.[39]

Growth

Pattern of growth is related closely to the general health and nutrition during childhood. For children and adolescents with diabetes, a major goal in the nutritional care is maintenance of normal weight gain and growth. When insulin is not available in sufficient amounts, pattern of growth is affected.[40,41] Five to ten percent of children with IDDM will experience growth ab-

normalities. Children most likely to be affected are those with the earliest onset of diabetes and those with poor glycemic control.[42]

Growth and weight gain should be assessed at each office visit by plotting the child's height and weight on the National Center for Health Statistics (NCHS) percentile growth charts.[43] Ideally, data should be recorded at least every 3 to 4 months, but at least annually.[42] Growth deviations should be evaluated to determine the origin. Exhibit 25-3 outlines possible diabetes- and non–diabetes-related growth deviations.[44]

An extreme example of the effects of insulin deficiency is the relatively rare Mauriac syndrome (diabetic dwarfism). These children are markedly delayed in linear growth and sexual maturation and appear pale and chronically ill. Laboratory analysis includes hyperglycemia, hyperlipidemia, and elevated glycohemoglobin.

The assessment of growth deviations should begin by confirming the accuracy of previous height and weight plots by re-plotting them and discussing the family's subjective assessment of the child's current weight and height status. After the verification of the growth and weight gain status, an assessment of energy intake should be made. Growth deviations with nutrition-related causes require appropriate nutrition intervention and therapy that focuses on improving caloric and nutrient intake.[44]

Monitoring

SMBG is the widely accepted and preferred method of metabolic monitoring for children.[45] Monitoring schedules vary depending on the intensity of control and the needs and goals of the patient. A reasonable frequency for testing is for the patient to perform SMBG before each dose of insulin, with additional tests before lunch and at bedtime twice each week (once during the school week and once on the weekend) and at 2 to 3 A.M. once or twice each month. Bedtime testing is important for children who have had strenuous or increased exercise during the day to determine the size of the bedtime snack needed to prevent delayed hypoglycemia.[46] SMBG, when used in conjunction with intensified insu-

Exhibit 25-3 Possible Growth Deviations in Children with IDDM

1. **Possible causes of poor weight gain**
   - Diabetes-Related
     Poor glycemic control
     Underinsulinization
     Suboptimal energy intake due to poor
        appetite or over-restriction of calories
   - Non–Diabetes-Related
     Hyperthyroidism
     Malabsorption
     Suboptimal energy intake due to poor
        appetite or over-restriction of calories
     Poor appetite
     Psychosocial dwarfism
     Abnormal eating behaviors

2. **Possible causes of poor linear growth**
   - Diabetes-Related
     Poor glycemic control
     Underinsulinization
     Suboptimal energy intake due to poor
        appetite or over-restriction of calories
   - Non–Diabetes-Related
     Malabsorption
     Psychosocial dwarfism
     Hypothyroidism or other endocrine disorders
     Suboptimal energy intake due to poor
        appetite or over-restriction of calories

3. **Possible causes of excessive weight gain**
   - Diabetes-Related
     Excessive energy intake
     Overtreatment of hypoglycemia
     Excessive fear of hypoglycemia
     Overinsulinization
   - Non–Diabetes-Related
     Hypo-activity
     Excess "hunger" or appetite
     Hypothyroidism (*always* accompanied by
        poor linear growth)

lin regimens and adjustments in insulin and diet, is a valuable tool that enables children and adolescents to improve their glycemic control and to have greater flexibility in their lives.[47]

Target ranges for blood glucose levels before meals and before the bedtime snack are 70 to 180 mg/dL. Because of the risk of hypoglycemia in an infant and toddler, it is advisable to keep blood glucose values in a slightly higher range, between 100 and 200 mg/dL.

The nutrition assessment should include a review of the child's SMBG records to identify frequent low and/or high results. If consistent high or low readings are found, the diet can be reviewed to evaluate correlations with food eaten and blood glucose results. Blood glucose test results can be useful in evaluating types and amounts of food eaten in a meal or snack, meal spacing, and body weight changes. For example, hypoglycemia before lunch might indicate that the breakfast is too small or of the wrong composition, a skipped morning snack, inadequate adjustment for exercise, a delayed lunch, or too much insulin. Consistent low readings with excessive weight gain might indicate excessive calorie intake from treatment of hypoglycemia. Appropriate adjustments in the diet and/or insulin can be recommended.

Glycated Hemoglobin

Glycated hemoglobin (HbA$_1$ or HbA$_{1c}$) is an accurate reflection of long-term glycemic control and can be used to assess the accuracy of blood glucose records. The level of glycated hemoglobin is directly proportional to the integrated blood glucose concentration over the preceding 2 to 3 months. Normal glycated hemoglobin ranges are 4.0 to 6.0% for HbA$_{1c}$ and 5.0 to 8.0% GHb, however, fewer than 5% of children treated with conventional insulin therapy have levels within the normal range.[22]

Urine Testing

Urine testing is an indirect and semiquantitative assessment of the blood glucose level and has many limitations as a means of optimally monitoring control of diabetes in children. However, urine should always be tested for the presence of ketones whenever the child is sick or when the blood glucose level exceeds 240 mg/dL.[5]

Lipids

Diabetes is a major risk factor for morbidity and mortality due to coronary heart disease, cerebrovascular disease, and peripheral vascular disease.[48,49] Furthermore, young persons with IDDM are more likely to die from cardiovascular disease (CVD) than their age- and sex-matched nondiabetic counterparts.[50] CVD risk in girls with IDDM is similar to that found in nondiabetic boys while the risk in boys with IDDM is even greater.[48] Therefore, reducing the risk factors associated with CVD in children and adolescents with IDDM is essential.

The risk factors associated with the risk for CVD in IDDM include hypertension, smoking, and lipoprotein abnormalities.[48] It appears that the lipoprotein profiles of persons with IDDM may be directly influenced by blood glucose control.[51] When adolescents with IDDM are treated with adequate insulin therapy and diet, lipoprotein profiles are similar to that of teenagers without IDDM.[52]

The National Cholesterol Education Program (NCEP) Expert Panel on Blood Cholesterol Levels in Children and Adolescents and the American Academy of Pediatrics have recommended selective cholesterol screening of children and adolescents who have a family history of premature CVD or at least one parent with high blood cholesterol.[53,54] Selective screening by the practicing physician may also be appropriate for children and adolescents with other risk factors such as smoking, hypertension, obesity, and IDDM. Such annual screenings should include fasting lipid profile, including total cholesterol, triglycerides, high-density lipoprotein-cholesterol (HDL-C),[54] and calculated:

$$\text{LDL-cholesterol} = \text{Total cholesterol} - \text{HDL-C} - \frac{\text{triglycerides}}{5}$$

(See Tables 25-A-1 through 25-A-4 in Appendix 25A for serum total cholesterol, LDL-C, HDL-C, and triglyceride levels in U.S. children and adolescents.[53])

Psychosocial Issues

Diabetes management affects the family in many ways. To meet the demands of manage-ment that are placed on eating, physical activity, finances, and time require major adjustments in life style. To provide successful nutrition therapy it is essential to assess the family dynamics and evaluate barriers to these life-style changes. It is important to identify how the responsibilities for diabetes management are defined and supported within the family, how these treatment responsibilities are shared among family members, and how and when responsibilities are transferred from parents(s) to child as the child develops. If the sole assumption of diabetes responsibilities is by one parent, is there an option to address education to both parents? If this is a single-parent family, is there another adult such as a grandparent who could be encouraged to participate as a support for the primary person? If the child lives between two separate families, all caregivers should be included in assessment and self-management training.

Food/Activity Patterns

The nutrition assessment includes obtaining a nutrition and activity history to determine usual food intake and activity patterns as well as information about attitudes toward nutrition and health. For children and adolescents, it is important to obtain information about[39]

- Daily schedules on weekdays and weekends

- Frequency of meals and snacks consumed away from home (eg, at school, with friends or relatives, at day care, in restaurants)

- Exercise-related questions (type, duration, time of day, frequency, intensity, and treatment of hypoglycemia)

- Child's/family's expectations and general attitude toward diabetes; do other family members have diabetes and what is their experience and knowledge from previous exposure?

- What nutrition intervention stage (basic nutrition intervention or in-depth nutrition intervention) is indicated at this time?

- Developmental stage (how to balance independence and dependence in diabetes self-care between the child and parent)

- To whom should the self-management training be directed (ie, parent and/or child); what style of learning does the person learn best, and what is the learning and reading ability?

NUTRITION GOAL SETTING

Nutrition recommendations for children and adolescents with diabetes should be individualized to promote life-long healthy eating habits while maintaining a sense of normalcy for the child and family.

Energy Requirements

The total intake of energy (calories) and nutrients must balance the daily expenditure of energy and satisfy the requirements for normal growth. The energy requirements vary considerably with age, weight, sex, height, stage of sexual development, and level of physical activity. The appetite of most children is the best indicator of energy needs.[56]

A newly diagnosed child with IDDM may present with negative energy balance due to the weight loss caused by inadequate insulin supply. When insulin therapy is initiated the child will be very hungry and will regain the lost weight. Approximately 10 to 25% more calories than usual will be required. Once the weight and growth pattern return to normal, the child will usually become less hungry, and a decrease in insulin dose and food intake will occur.

Assessment of a child's actual daily food intake using a 24-hour dietary recall or 3-day diet history is the primary indicator of daily caloric needs. Theoretical guidelines for estimating energy requirements for children are available if the daily food intake is inconclusive[57,58] but are difficult to translate into practical use. Table 25-1 outlines the recommended dietary allowances (RDAs) for energy and protein requirements which can be used as a guide to reinforce the actual estimate.[59] Caloric needs change continuously in children, especially during growth spurts (before the age of two and the adolescent growth spurt) or as activity level varies and, therefore, food intake should be evaluated every 3 to 6 months.[39] The amount of food should be adjusted up or down depending on the child's appetite over a few days. When adjusting the caloric level, the effect on the child's blood glucose levels must be evaluated. Insulin adjustments may be necessary to avoid hyperglycemia or hypoglycemia.

Parents should be discouraged from withholding food if a child's blood glucose levels are high. Adequate energy intake for normal growth and development are of primary importance. Instead, insulin dose adjustments should be used.

Carbohydrate

The American Diabetes Association recommends that the percentage of energy from carbohydrate will vary according to the individual's eating habits and glucose and lipid goals. Following general guidelines to reduce fat in the diet of children older than the age of 2 will lead to a diet rich in carbohydrate.[59] Sucrose-containing foods can be incorporated into the diet of children and adolescents on a regular basis with adjustments in insulin doses as necessary. However, excessive use of high-sucrose-containing foods may promote dental caries[60] as well as replace nutrient dense foods. Use of sucrose-containing foods such as cookies, donuts, and sweetened beverages may be included after adequate intake from all essential food groups.

Fiber

Dietary fiber may be advantageous in treating or preventing several gastrointestinal disorders, and soluble fibers seem to show modest reductions on serum lipids.[61] However, the effect of dietary fiber on glycemic control is probably insignificant. For adults with diabetes the fiber in-

Table 25-1 National Research Council RDAs—1989: Median Heights and Weights and Recommended Energy and Protein Intakes

	Age in Years	Weight		Height		Calories		Protein
		kg	lb	cm	in	/kg	/day	g
Infants	0–0.5	6	13	60	24	108	650	13
	0.5–1.0	9	20	71	28	98	850	14
Children	1–3	13	29	90	35	102	1300	16
	4–6	20	44	112	44	90	1800	24
	7–10	28	62	132	52	70	2000	28
Males	11–14	45	99	157	62	55	2500	45
	15–18	66	145	176	69	45	3000	59
	19–24	72	160	177	70	40	2900	58
Females	11–14	46	101	157	62	47	2200	46
	15–18	55	120	163	64	40	2200	44
	19–24	58	128	164	65	38	2200	46

Note: From birth to age 10 years, no distinction between sexes is made regarding energy requirements. Separate allowances are recommended for boys and girls older than 10 years because of differences in the age of onset of puberty and patterns of physical activity. Considerable variability is seen in the timing and magnitude of the adolescent growth spurt and in activity patterns. Consequently, the range of the recommendation for children older than 10 years is wider, and energy allowances should be adjusted individually to take into account body weight, physical activity, and rate of growth.

Source: Data from *Recommended Dietary Allowances*, ed.10, National Academy Press, 1989.

take recommendations are the same as for the general population (20 to 35 g/d from a wide variety of food sources).

A high-fiber diet for children and adolescents is advantageous; however, there is concern that high fiber intake may affect caloric intake.[62] High-fiber foods tend to be more bulky and lower in calories, thus reducing the satiety level for additional calories. Therefore, when following general guidelines to decrease the level of fat in the diet that increases the level of carbohydrate and fiber, it is important to evaluate the ability of the child to take the volume of food necessary to accommodate caloric requirements.

Protein

At present, the recommendations for protein intake for people with diabetes is the same as for the general population.[59] For children, adequate protein is essential to ensure normal growth, development, and maintenance of body protein stores. However, children in the United States commonly eat diets that are at least twice the RDAs.[63] Therefore, intake of protein at 12 to 20% (0.9 to 2.2 g/kg body weight per day) of total daily calories may require an initial decrease from the usual diet (see Table 25-1 for RDAs for protein intakes for children and adolescents).

Fat

The American Diabetes Association recommends a diet low in total fat, with saturated fat less than 10% of calories for children and adolescents to promote overall health and reduce cardiovascular risk factors.[59]

The NCEP Expert Panel on Blood Cholesterol Levels in Children and Adolescents recommends a Step 1 diet for children and adolescents older than the age of 2 with borderline or high LDL-C levels (see Table 25-A-2). A Step 1 diet maintains an intake of less than 300 mg cholesterol daily and no more than 30% of total calories as fat. Of the total fat, less than 10% should be provided from saturated fat, up to 10% by polyunsaturated, and the remainder by monounsaturated fat. If a reduction of LDL-C is not obtained after at least 3 months on a Step 1 diet, implementation of the Step 2 diet is indicated. The Step 2 diet requires the reduction to less than 7% of total calories from saturated fat and 200 mg cholesterol per day with the other parameters remaining the same. Drug therapy is considered in children ages 10 years and older if, after an adequate trial of diet therapy (6 months to 1 year), LDL-C remains greater than160 mg/dL and there is a family history of CVD with two or more CVD risk factors.[53]

Sodium

Sodium sensitivity varies greatly among individuals. There is no conclusive evidence that high sodium intake in persons with IDDM is detrimental to health or specifically associated with hypertension.[37] Therefore, sodium intake recommendations are the same as for the general population (2400-3000 mg/d).[63,64] This recommendation should be balanced with consideration of the other nutrition changes required. The reduction of added salt to food consumed should be advised as a good nutritional principle for the child and family.[37]

Blood pressure should be monitored every 6 to 12 months[37] and if hypertension develops, a sodium-restricted diet should be recommended. For adults with mild or moderate hypertension, 2400 mg or less of sodium per day is recommended.[65] However, in younger children sodium intake of 2400 mg/d may not, in fact, be a restriction. A recommended sodium intake based on body weight may be more appropriate.

Nonnutritive Sweeteners

Children are more likely than adults to ingest large doses of nonnutritive sweeteners per kilogram of body weight due to their smaller body size. Also, children with diabetes are more likely to consume foods sweetened with nonnutritive sweeteners. This results in a greater concern over the issue of safety and its relationship to dose in children.[37]

Three nonnutritive sweeteners (saccharin, aspartame, and acesulfame K) have been approved for use in the United States. Acceptable daily intake (ADI) which includes a 100-fold safety factor for all three nonnutritive sweeteners, has been established. Actual intake is much less than the ADI in adults and children.[59] Excessive consumption of nonnutritive sweeteners may be due to the overuse of low calorie foods in an attempt to satisfy a child's appetite and need for additional calories. It is important to assess the use of nonnutritive sweeteners in the context of the entire diet. The availability and use of three nonnutritive sweeteners decreases the risk for potential problems associated with excessive consumption of any one sweetener.[66] A method for estimating aspartame consumption in children is available when the diet appears to have excessive amounts.[67]

Alcohol

Because alcohol may increase the risk for hypoglycemia in people treated with insulin, alcohol should only be ingested with a meal. Because children as young as 11 years may drink alcoholic beverages, it is essential to teach safe, moderate, alcohol consumption to preteenagers. Specific signs which might indicate alcohol use by teens includes changes in behavior, school performance, and relationships with parents. Erratic blood glucose values on weekends might also indicate alcohol use.

Meal/Snack Timing and Composition

Eating patterns in children usually require three meals and two to three snacks per day. A meal plan should be designed based on the individual's usual food intake and activity patterns and insulin therapy integrated into this pattern. Consistent meal times are important to synchronize with time-actions of insulin. This may be difficult for families with irregular schedules and mealtimes. Often times, a weekday schedule and a weekend schedule are needed. Flexibility in schedules can be obtained by use of planned snacks. For example, if dinner will be delayed due to a late afternoon piano lesson, an additional afternoon snack may be needed. The amount of the mixture of insulin at dinner can be decreased, especially for children watching their weight.

Two to three snacks per day are often required on conventional and intensive insulin therapy in children. However, when children reach junior high school, the morning snack may not be needed due to more consistent activity habits and fewer recess periods. A careful review of morning activity patterns as well as time and composition of breakfast and lunch are required to determine if the midmorning snack is necessary.

The best composition of snacks is not known. However, it has been suggested[37] that the bedtime snack consist of a protein and starch source to promote a slower and more prolonged glycemic effect. The snack should not be decreased or omitted if the blood glucose is high before bed, as blood glucose can drop during sleep due to NPH insulin peak action. If the blood glucose before bed continues to be high for several days, the regular insulin before dinner may need to be increased or the amount or types of food before dinner may need to be adjusted. The bedtime snack should be increased if blood glucose levels before bedtime are low, or if there is extra evening activity.

Specific guidelines for adjusting the bedtime snack are as follows: If the blood glucose is less than 80 mg/dL, double the bedtime snack and retest the blood glucose 2 hours later. If the bedtime blood glucose is between 80 and 120 mg/dL, give an additional one-half snack.

Children with IDDM need a consistent level of food intake, which is often the most difficult adjustment for families to make.[68] Children's daily food intake varies day to day according to their appetite.[56] Therefore, when determining a meal plan for children, it is important to obtain a diet history for several days to determine average daily intake. Because intake and eating patterns on weekends may vary from weekdays, a typical weekend daily food intake should be obtained as well.

Schooltime

School schedules, physical education and recess, and after-school activities require special considerations when designing a meal plan for children with IDDM. Parents must be given snack and mealtime guidance to help children feel confident and be more compliant with their diabetes management plan.[69] Determining school rules regarding snacking and discussing with the child where the snack will be eaten and what the child feels comfortable eating at school are important. Some children are most comfortable eating quietly in the classroom than risk being noticed leaving the room to go to the nurses' office. A quick snack such as juice might be an easier snack choice than crackers which make noise when crunching. Keeping extra snack items with the school nurse and in a backpack will provide protection if a snack is forgotten or if hypoglycemia occurs while walking to and from school or riding the bus. Parents should be encouraged to obtain the school lunch menus and talk with the school cafeteria personnel about their child's diet needs. A valuable component of nutrition intervention and evaluation by the registered dietitian is a discussion and review of the school lunch menus. It is important to identify what foods are offered at lunch and between meals in the cafeteria or in vending machines. Often, school lunches provide the quantity and composition in a typical meal plan for that child's age.

Activity and Exercise

Developing active life-style habits during childhood and adolescence is an essential component of good health. The potential benefits of

Exhibit 25-4 Components To Assess in the Child's
Current Eating and Activity Patterns

- Child's favorite activities (sedentary and active)
  (eg, television viewing habits)
- Physical education activities and time of class
- After-school activities (inside or outside play)
- Extracurricular activities (team sports, seasonal
  activities, camps) and duration/intensity of activity
- Blood glucose testing schedule and frequency
- Type/amount of food used to treat hypoglycemia

regular physical activity for the person with IDDM are to improve cardiovascular fitness and insulin sensitivity, decrease blood pressure, improve blood lipids levels, prevent obesity, and improve emotional well-being.[70–72] However, longitudinal studies on exercise training in children and adolescents with IDDM show conflicting results regarding overall improvements in glycemic control.[71,73,74] The inability to improve glycemic control may have been due to the inappropriate increases in food intake or decreases in insulin dose to prevent exercise-induced hypoglycemia.

Although activity and exercise for children with IDDM offer many important social and developmental experiences that help "normalize" the life style of the child, exercise provides the potential challenges of hypoglycemia and hyperglycemia. Hypoglycemia can occur during or after an exercise as a result of peak insulin action coinciding with timing of exercise. For children and adolescents, this may occur more frequently in late spring when longer days allow children more outside play. Hyperglycemia may worsen if exercise is started during poor metabolic control. To prevent and/or treat these potential complications, it is essential that parents and children are educated about appropriate management strategies to encourage continued participation in activity and exercise.

Each child's glycemic response to a specific exercise is individual. Therefore, the appropriate amount and type of food and/or reduction in insulin must be determined on an individual trial-and-error basis.[68] Daily activity patterns of children are often unpredictable, therefore, maintaining a three meal/three snack pattern is often helpful in preventing hypoglycemia.[75] Components to assess in the child's current eating and activity patterns are found in Exhibit 25-4.[75]

Blood glucose monitoring before, during, and after the activity is essential, especially when adding a new activity. However, this may not be practical in some instances when the child is left to perform the testing independently and make judgments from the results. Food can be added before and/or after the exercise, depending on blood glucose levels. If exercise is of short duration and testing of blood glucose can be done after the activity, it is often best to delay consumption of extra food until after the exercise. This will help determine how much extra carbohydrate, if any, is needed. In general, for each 45 to 60 minutes of physical activity 10 to 15 g of carbohydrate should be eaten in addition to the regular snack. More strenuous and/or exercise of long duration (greater than 60 minutes) may require an extra 10 to 15 g of carbohydrate every half hour.[59] Adjustments based on blood glucose levels is essential to avoid overfeeding or underfeeding the active child.[59] Examples of food that contains 10 to 15 g of carbohydrate that children might find palatable are listed in Exhibit 25-5. It is essential that parents inform teachers, coaches, recess monitors, and others who might supervise their children during physical activity regarding food adjustments during exercise and treatment of hypoglycemia.[75] For parents not comfortable providing this information, the registered dietitian could provide an annual seminar for the school staff involved or for the school system. When frequency and duration of physical activity increase consistently, as occurs when a child attends summer camp, it is often appropriate to reduce insulin dose by 10 to 20% to avoid severe hypoglycemia.[22]

Hypoglycemia

Hypoglycemia is the most frequent acute complication of IDDM.[76] Occasional, mild hypoglycemia is an inevitable consequence to good metabolic control.[77] However, repeated or prolonged severe hypoglycemia can cause permanent damage to the central nervous system in very young children.[20,21] Following a severe episode of hypoglycemia, fear of hypoglycemia may become a barrier to maintaining optimal glycemic control. Prevention and treatment of hypoglycemia are discussed in Chapter 23.

Sick Days

The objective of sick day management is to minimize deterioration of metabolic control and to prevent hospitalization due to diabetic ketoacidosis (DKA).[78] If the child is unable to consume solid foods, liquids that contain a source of carbohydrate (eg, fruit juices, popsicles, regular gelatin, or sweetened carbonated beverages) should be used. For children experiencing decreased appetite and intake due to illness with blood glucose values less than 150 mg/dL a decrease of short-acting and intermediate-acting insulin may be required. For children experiencing illness with moderate to

large ketones an increase in the short-acting insulin will be required.

Eating disorders

The prevalence of eating disorders in individuals with IDDM is 7 to 35%, exceeding the range of 1.3 to 5% reported in the general population.[79] This is presumably due to factors such as the focus on diet, exercise, and guilt over diet indiscretions. Unexplained poor metabolic control (skipped insulin or severely reduced insulin) and unexplained severe hypoglycemia (restrictive dieting) may be indicative of an eating disorder.[80] Prevention should begin by understanding the child/teenager and family characteristics associated with disordered eating patterns and avoid being too restrictive.[37] An overview of obesity in adolescents with diabetes is available.[81]

Intervention

Nutrition intervention is determined by the information obtained from the nutrition assessment and the established goals of the patient. To avoid overwhelming the family or attempting to provide all the information during one session, nutrition intervention must be provided in two stages, basic nutrition intervention and in-depth nutrition intervention.[36] (See Chapters 3 and 9 for further description of nutrition intervention stages.)

Components of effective nutrition intervention and meal planning for children and adolescents include adequate calories and nutrition, individualization, and regular eating patterns. Successful implementation of the meal plan requires that the responsibility of the child and parent in the feeding relationship be considered.[82,83] Various meal-planning approaches and resources are available that allow an individualized approach based on the knowledge and skills necessary for changing or maintaining eating habits.[38]

The Exchange System for Meal Planning is the most widely used method of meal planning.[84] Use of the exchange system in children is a

---

Exhibit 25-5 Examples of Foods To Add for Exercise

Food	Amount
Chewy granola bars	1/2 bar
Dried fruit	1/4 cup
Fig bars	1 bar
Fruit/cereal bars	1/2 bar
Fruit rolls	1
Fruit snacks	1/2 pouch
Grapes	15
Raisins	2 Tbsp or 1 small box
Beverages	
Juice	4 oz
Regular soft drinks	4 oz
Sports drink (ie, Gatorade)	8 oz

Note: Each food in the serving size listed provides 10 to 15 g of carbohydrate.

method that provides a solid knowledge base for understanding foods, food composition, and foods' effects on blood glucose. Specific benefits of using the exchange system as well as considerations for use with different age groups have been outlined.[85] Although the exchange system is the most widely used meal-planning approach, no long-term studies have evaluated the effectiveness in children. Dietary knowledge, skills, and adherence may improve by use of active learning versus didactic.[86]

Carbohydrate exchange counting has also been used in the pediatric population to teach meal planning.[87] This method of nutrition intervention is based on the principle that carbohydrate is the main dietary determinant of insulin requirements.[88] Initially, the basics of the exchange system are taught, followed by information on the total carbohydrate exchanges. The benefits to this meal-planning approach in the pediatric population include increased flexibility for variations in appetite and food preferences, expanded food choices, and basic balanced diet knowledge. However, carbohydrate exchange counting may not be appropriate for the overweight child or the child with elevated cholesterol because it does not focus on fat and protein. Specific use of carbohydrate counting for managing feeding problems and fussy toddlers has been outlined.[87]

A variety of meal-planning approaches must be used according to the individual needs of the family. Selected resources (cookbooks, meal planning resources, and audiovisuals) for use in self-management training with the child and family with IDDM are outlined in Appendix 25-B.

Evaluation

The fourth stage in medical nutrition therapy for diabetes is evaluation of the goals and determination of the effect of the intervention. At this phase, it is important to judge whether the nutrition intervention led to incorporation of new behaviors and whether new goals are needed.[36] Children and adolescents need ongoing follow-up to provide support for developmental and life-style changes and gradual shifting of re-

sponsibility for diabetes care. Follow-up is recommended every 3 to 6 months.

Child Development

At each developmental stage of childhood, diabetes management requires a team approach to consider the normal developmental needs (physical, behavioral, and cognitive) of the child and how diabetes has an effect on these stages. Guidelines for determining age-appropriate diabetes management tasks are available.[1,3] A developmentally staged curriculum for children 5 to 18 years of age with IDDM is available in Appendix 25-C.

During infancy, the parents take total responsibility for learning and maintaining diabetes care. The management of diabetes is complicated by the difficulty in administration and adjusting small insulin doses. Insulin administration must be coordinated with erratic, spontaneous appetites and sleep schedules of the baby. The risk of unrecognized hypoglycemia, along with the psychosocial issues seen in families with very young children with chronic illness, is an additional management concern. Specific management goals for the infant with diabetes include achieving and maintaining acceptable blood glucose control while avoiding hypoglycemia reactions and diabetic ketoacidosis. Of equal importance is maintenance of normal growth, development, and emotional well-being of the child.[89]

Prevention of hypoglycemia and establishment of a flexible meal plan based on developmental milestones and individual tolerances is paramount. Cellular injury to the nervous system is more likely to occur with hypoglycemia in the infant; therefore, early recognition and treatment of hypoglycemia is important. Parents must be taught to recognize symptoms such as grouchiness, irritability, and unexplained crying as hypoglycemia instead of typical hypoglycemic symptoms which are not always readily perceived. A fully conscious infant with mild to moderate hypoglycemia is treated with 2 to 4 ounces of fruit juice or 4 ounces of 5% glucose water by bottle.

One to two teaspoons of Karo Syrup or glucose gel product applied inside of the infant's mouth (on the gums) can be used if the infant is unable to drink from a bottle. Severe hypoglycemia should be treated with glucagon (0.5 mg).

Infants with diabetes generally require very small amounts of injected insulin making it difficult to measure even in low-dosage syringes. Therefore, diluted insulin (U10, U25, or U50) permits these small insulin doses to be more easily measured.

Blood glucose monitoring of infants is recommended four times a day (before meals and at bedtime). Parents may feel more reassured when the bedtime blood glucose value is obtained at 10 or 11 P.M. than at the infant's actual bedtime. Blood glucose testing sites for the infant include finger, toes, and earlobes. Parents are encouraged to perform the test or injection quickly while holding the infant securely and comforting the child afterward.

Meal planning for infants with diabetes must take into consideration the rapid rate of growth and nutritional demands during the first year of life. A flexible meal plan based on developmental milestones and individual tolerances is essential to promote a positive environment for eating. Periodic assessment (one to two times per month) of the child's growth, nutritional status, appetite system, and blood glucose control can determine if the meal plan is appropriate for the child's needs.

Children during toddlerhood establish a sense of autonomy and explore their surroundings. Toddlers do not have the cognitive skills to understand the need for consistent eating habits and schedules or the intrusive painful procedures necessary for diabetes care. Thus, meal times and injections or finger sticks for blood glucose monitoring may become a battleground. Parents need information, reassurance, support, and flexible meal-planning guidelines.[39] Feeding guidelines for toddlers are outlined in Exhibit 25-6.[90]

Elementary school-age children (ages 5 to 12 years) are characterized by growth in intellectual, athletic, and artistic skills and a sense of gender identity. Entrance into school is one of the initial situations in which parents and children must cope with the social meaning of diabetes and the tasks of educating others about the disease. Therefore, many families need assistance from their health-care team to educate school personnel, coaches, and scout leaders about such topics as school lunch choices, hypoglycemia prevention and management, and snack schedules. At this stage of development children are also more aware of differences between themselves and others and are anxious for peer approval. Children at this age may be able to become more involved in diabetes self-care tasks at home such as selecting among several appropriate snack choices. During the later elementary school years, it is important to emphasize this as a skill-building phase and encourage participation and build self-esteem.

During adolescence many changes in physical development, school experiences, cognitive development, social networks, and family dynamics occur. Teenagers are eager to question authority and demonstrate independence. For most females, the onset of a menstrual cycle during adolescence does not cause difficulty with metabolic control of diabetes. However, close observation of blood glucose values during this time is warranted. Puberty has also been associated with insulin resistance and the challenge of achieving metabolic control.[91] This is complicated when parents attempt to transfer more of the responsibility of diabetes care to the teenager. To influence teenagers, it is important for health professionals to identify what is important in the client's life. For example, if a teenager is working toward playing on the football team but is not willing to properly monitor blood glucose values and make proper adjustments in snack patterns, it might be helpful to discuss the ability to excel in the sport with considerations for diabetes management. During the later teenage years (ages 16 to 19 years) when the individual becomes more able to handle the responsibilities of self-care, it is important to review current nutrition therapy for diabetes and prepare the teenager to live independently.

Exhibit 25-6 Toddler Feeding Guidelines

1. **If your child wants to drink more fruit juice** than the 4-oz serving allowed,
   - dilute the juice with water or diet soda pop
   - offer a piece of fruit instead, which takes longer to eat and is more filling

2. **If your child doesn't like milk,**
   - flavor the milk with sugar-free Nestle's Quick
   - offer other high-calcium foods such as cheese, plain or sugar-free pudding, or sugar-free fudgesicle

3. **If your child won't eat vegetables,** don't make an issue of it. Vegetables are so low in carbohydrates that they have minimal effect on blood glucose levels. Similar nutrients are found in fruit, juice, or vitamin and mineral supplements.

4. **If your child won't eat fruit,**
   - offer fruit juice (limit to one 4 oz serving per day)
   - use vitamin and mineral supplements

5. **If your child won't finish his or her meal or snack,** don't force the issue. Instead,
   - offer beverages (milk provides both carbohydrates and proteins)
   - serve child-size portions

6. **If your child wants more food,** offer "free" foods such as sugar-free popsicle, Kool Aid, Jello, and nonstarchy vegetables; foods containing less than 20 calories and 5 g carbohydrates per serving can generally be eaten freely.

7. **If your child goes on a food jag** (requesting one food often), don't object because boredom will eventually lead to change.

8. **If your child takes a long time to eat,**
   - offer child-size portions (your expectations of how much your child can eat may be too high)
   - ask your health care provider for guidance

9. **If your child doesn't like eating breakfast,**
   - vary food offered (eg, different cereals, bagels, English muffins, frozen waffles)
   - mix sugar-free Carnation Instant Breakfast in milk for a meal in itself
   - try non-traditional breakfast foods (eg, sandwiches, pizza, leftovers)

DIABETES CAMP

There are over 70 diabetes camps throughout the United States that provide children with the opportunity to meet other children with diabetes and learn the importance of nutrition, exercise, insulin, and blood glucose monitoring. Much of the learning takes place through positive experiences and activities the children participate in. The first-hand experiences at camp provide a much stronger impression than learning it from a professional or family member.

Children of all ages can attend camp; however, parents and professionals must evaluate if the child is ready to make the separation for a residential program. Usually, this happens when the child reaches the first or second grade. When the child is ready to attend camp, it is important to find the camp most suited to the child's needs. There are camps with general recreation programs as well as camps with an emphasis in a particular activity such as canoeing, backpacking, bicycling, etc. Parents can research the camps and their philosophy for diabetes management by meeting the camp leadership, visiting the camp site, and speaking with parents and children who have already attended camp. Parents should identify what the camp team will provide in terms of diabetes management and diabetes education as well as the expertise of the staff. A complete directory of diabetes camps in the United States can be obtained from the American Diabetes Association (1-800-232-3472).

The American Diabetes Association and the American Camping Association have developed standards for diabetes camps which should be used for any camp hosting children with diabetes. However, each camp should have established goals and objectives as well as a defined plan for recreation, diabetes care, and education. Common goals which most programs establish are as follows:[92]

- Ensure an atmosphere for the physical and emotional well-being of young people and of their families.

- Provide opportunities to learn more about diabetes by active participation and experiences.

- Provide opportunities to develop a positive attitude about diabetes by working with adults who also have diabetes and serve as positive role models.

- Gain motivation and form habits that contribute to a positive and more stable diabetes management program.

- Learn new recreation skills.

- Develop an appreciation for nature and the camp environment.

- Participate in democratic living and learn more skills necessary to live with and relate to others.

- Make friendships and learn to share with others.

- Provide professionals the opportunity to work with, observe, and learn more about young people with diabetes.

REFERENCES

1. Committee on Youth Education, American Diabetes Association. *Curriculum for Youth Education.* Alexandria, Va: American Diabetes Association, 1983.

2. Franz M. The dietitian: a key member of the diabetes team. *J Am Diet Assoc.* 1981;79:302–305.

3. Kohler E, Hurwitz LS, Milan D. A developmentally staged curriculum for teaching self-care to the child with insulin-dependent diabetes mellitus. *Diabetes Care.* 1982;5:300–304.

4. Johnson SB, Pollak T, Silverstein JH, et al. Cognitive and behavioral knowledge about insulin dependent diabetes among children and parents. *Pediatrics.* 1982;69:708–713.

5. American Diabetes Association. *Physician's Guide to Insulin-Dependent (Type I) Diabetes Diagnosis and Treatment.* Alexandria, Va: ADA; 1988:3.

6. American Diabetes Association. *Diabetes 1991 Vital Statistics.* Chicago, Ill: American Diabetes Association; 1991.

7. Warram JH, Rich SS, Krolewski AS. Epidemiology and genetics of diabetes mellitus. In: Kahn CR, Wier GC, eds. *Joslin's Diabetes Mellitus.* Philadelphia, Pa: Lea & Febiger; 1994:201–215.

8. Warram JH, Krolewski AS, Gottlieb MS, Kahn CR. Differences in risk of insulin-dependent diabetes in offspring of diabetic mothers and diabetic fathers. *N Engl J Med.* 1984;311:149–152.

9. Warram JH, Krolewski AS, Kahn CR. Determinants of IDDM and perinatal mortality in children of diabetic mothers. *Diabetes.* 1988;37:1328–1334.

10. Gamble DR. The epidemiology of insulin-dependent diabetes, with particular reference to the relationship of virus infection to its etiology. *Epidemiol Rev.* 1980;2:49–70.

11. Lebovit HE. Etiology and pathogenesis of diabetes mellitus. *Pediatr Clin North Am.* 1984;31:521–530.

12. Nerup J, Mandrup-Poulsen T, Molvig J, et al. Mechanisms of pancreatic B-cell destruction in type I diabetes. *Diabetes Care.* 1988;11(suppl 1):16–22.

13. Eisenbarth GS. Type I diabetes mellitus: a chronic autoimmune disease. *N Engl J Med.* 1986;314:1360–1368.

14. Eisenbarth GS, Ziegler AG, Colman PA. Pathogenesis of insulin dependent (type I) diabetes mellitus. In: Kahn CR, Weir GC, eds. *Joslin's Diabetes Mellitus.* Philadelphia, Pa: Lea & Febiger; 1994:216–239.

15. Coleman DL, Kuzava JE, Leiter EH. Effect of diet on incidence of diabetes in non-obese diabetic mice. *Diabetes.* 1990;39:432–436.

16. Kostraba JN, Cruickshanks KJ, Lawler-Heavner J, et al. Early exposure to cow's milk and solid foods in infancy, genetic predisposition and risk of insulin dependent diabetes mellitus. *Diabetes.* 1993;42:288–295.

17. Gerstein HC. Cow's milk exposure and type I diabetes mellitus. *Diabetes Care.* 1994;17(1):13–19.

18. Diabetes Control and Complications Trial Research Group. The effect of intensive treatment of diabetes on the development and progression of long-term complications in insulin-treated diabetes mellitus. *N Engl J Med.* 1993;329:977–986.

19. Kostraba JN, Dorman JS, Orchard TJ, et al. Contribution of diabetes duration before puberty to development of microvascular complications in IDDM subjects. *Diabetes Care.* 1989;12:686–693.

20. Ryan C, Vega A, Drash A. Cognitive deficits in adolescents who developed diabetes early in life. *Pediatrics.* 1985;75:921–927.

21. Rovert JF, Ehrlich RM, Hoppe M. Intellectual deficits associated with early onset of insulin-dependent diabetes mellitus in children. *Diabetes Care.* 1987;10:510–515.

22. Wolfsdorf JI, Anderson BJ, Pasquarello C. Treatment of the child with diabetes. In: Kahn CR, Weir GC, eds. *Joslin's Diabetes Mellitus.* Philadelphia, Pa: Lea & Febiger; 1994:530–551.

23. Mann NP, Johnston DI. Improvement in metabolic control in diabetic adolescents by the use of increased insulin dose. *Diabetes Care.* 1984;7:460–464.

24. Sochett EB, Daneman D, Clarson C, Ehrlich RM. Factors affecting and patterns of residual insulin secretion

during the first year of type 1 (insulin-dependent diabetes mellitus) in children. *Diabetologia*. 1987;30:453.

25. Langdon DR, James FD, Sperling MA. Comparison of single- and split-dose insulin regimens with 24-hour monitoring. *J Pediatr*. 1981;99:854–861.

26. Clark WL, Haymond MW, Santiago JV. Overnight basal insulin requirements in fasting insulin-dependent diabetes. *Diabetes*. 1980;9:78–80.

27. Shalwitz RA, Farkas-Hirsch R, White NH, Santiago JV. Prevalence and consequences of nocturnal hypoglycemia among conventionally treated children with diabetes mellitus. *J Pediatr*. 1990;116:685–689.

28. Bolli GB, Gerich JE. The "dawn phenomenon"—a common occurrence in both non–insulin-dependent and insulin-dependent diabetes mellitus. *N Engl J Med*. 1984;310:746–750.

29. Francis AJ, Home PD, Hanning I, et al. Intermediate acting insulin given at bedtime: effect on blood glucose concentrations before and after breakfast. *BMJ*. 1983;286:1173–1176.

30. Wolfsdorf JI, Laffel LMB, Pasquarello C, et al. Split-mixed insulin regimen with human ultra lente before supper and NPH (isophane) before breakfast in children and adolescents with IDDM. *Diabetes Care*. 1991;14:1100–1106.

31. Kaye R. Research and practice in the treatment of insulin dependent diabetes: a survey of 53 pediatric diabetologists. *Pediatrics*. 1984;74:1079–1085.

32. Brink SJ, Stewart C. Insulin pump treatment in insulin-dependent diabetes mellitus: children, adolescents, and young adults. *JAMA*. 1986;255:617–621.

33. Anderson BJ, Miller JP, Auslander WF, Santiago JV. Family characteristics of diabetic adolescents: relationships to metabolic control. *Diabetes Care*. 1981;4:586–594.

34. Lockwood D, Frey ML, Gladish NA, Hiss RG. The biggest problem in diabetes. *Diabetes Educ*. 1986;12:30–33.

35. Lorenz RA, Christensen NK, Pichert JW. Diet related knowledge, skill, and adherence among children with insulin dependent diabetes mellitus. *Pediatrics*. 1985;75:872–876.

36. Diabetes Care and Education, a practice group of the American Diabetic Association, Tinker LF, Heins JM, Holler HJ. Commentary and translation: 1994 nutrition recommendations for diabetes. *J Am Diet Assoc*. 1994;94:507–511.

37. Committee on Nutrition. *Nutritional Management of Children and Adolescents with Insulin Dependent Diabetes Mellitus*. Elk Grove Village, Ill: Academy of Pediatrics; 1985.

38. Holler HJ, Pasters JG, eds. *Meal Planning Approach for Diabetes Management*. Chicago, Ill: American Diabetic Association; 1994.

39. Connell JE, Thomas-Dobersen D. Nutritional management of children and adolescents with insulin-dependent diabetes mellitus: a review by the Diabetes Care and Education dietetic practice group. *J Am Diet Assoc*. 1991;91:1556–1564.

40. Jackson RL. Growth and maturation of children with insulin dependent diabetes mellitus. *Pediatr Clin North Am*. 1984;31(3):545–566.

41. Wise JE, Kolb EL, Sauder SE. Effect of glycemic control on growth velocity in children with IDDM. *Diabetes Care*. 1992;15(7):826–830.

42. Sperlin MA. Growth. In: *Physician's Guide to Insulin Dependent (Type I) Diabetes: Diagnosis and Treatment*. Alexandria, Va: American Diabetes Association; 1988:135–136.

43. National Center for Health Statistics. *NCHS Growth Curves for Children Birth–18 Years*. Hyattsville, Md: National Center for Health Statistics; 1977. U.S. Vital and Health Statistics. Ser. 11, no. 165.

44. Steranchak L. Growth in children with IDDM. Selected aspects of diabetes nutrition—prevention and management in infants and children. *Diabetes Care Educ*. 1993;14(4):9–10.

45. Daneman D, Siminerio L, Transue D, et al. The role of self-monitoring of blood glucose in the routine management of children with insulin-dependent diabetes mellitus. *Diabetes Care*. 1985;8:1–4.

46. Whincup G, Milner RDG. Prediction and management of nocturnal hypoglycemia in diabetes. *Arch Dis Child*. 1987;62:333–337.

47. Carney RM, Schechter K, Homa M, et al. The effects of blood glucose testing versus urine sugar testing on the metabolic control in insulin-dependent diabetic children. *Diabetes Care*. 1983;6:378–380.

48. American Diabetes Association. Consensus statement. Role of cardiovascular risk factors in prevention and treatment of macrovasular disease in diabetes. *Diabetes Care*. 1989;12:573–579.

49. American Diabetes Association. Consensus statement. Detection and management of lipid disorders in diabetes. *Diabetes Care*. 1993;16(suppl 2):106–112.

50. Dorman JS, LaPorte RE, Kuller LH, et al. The Pittsburgh insulin-dependent diabetes mellitus (IDDM) morbidity and mortality study: mortality results. *Diabetes*. 1984;33:271–276.

51. Dunn FL. Plasma lipid and lipoprotein disorders in IDDM. *Diabetes*. 1992;41(suppl 2):102–106.

52. DCCT Research Group. Lipid and lipoprotein levels in patients with IDDM. *Diabetes Care*. 1992;15:886–894.

53. National Cholesterol Education Program. *Report of the Expert Panel on Blood Cholesterol Levels in Children and Adolescents*. Bethesda, Md: U.S. Department of Health and Human Services; 1991. National Heart, Lung and Blood Institute Publication 91-2732.

54. American Academy of Pediatrics. Statement on cholesterol. *Pediatrics*. 1992;90:469–473.

55. Nucci A. Lipid levels and cardiovascular risk—a review. Selected aspects of diabetes nutrition—prevention and management in infants and children. *Diabetes Care Educ*. 1993;14(4):17–21.

56. Birch LL, Johnson SL, Anderson G. The variability of young children's energy intake. *N Engl J Med*. 1991;324:232–235.

57. Powers MA, ed. *Nutrition Guide for Professionals*. Alexandria, Va: American Diabetes Association and the American Dietetic Association; 1988.

58. National Research Council: *Recommended Dietary Allowances*. 10th ed. Washington, DC: National Academy Press; 1989.

59. American Diabetes Association. Position statement. Nutrition recommendation and principles for people with diabetes mellitus. *Diabetes Care*. 1994;17:519–522.

60. Glinsmann WH, Irausquin H, Park YK. Evaluation of health aspects of sugars contained in carbohydrate sweetener; report of Sugars Task Force, 1986. *J Nutr*. 1986;116:S1–S216.

61. National Research Council, Committee on Diet and Health, Food and Nutrition Board. *Diet and Health: Implication for Reducing Chronic Disease Risk*. Washington, DC: National Academy Press; 1989.

62. American Academy of Pediatrics, Committee on Nutrition. Plant fiber intake in the pediatric diet. *Pediatrics*. 1981;67:572–575.

63. American Heart Association Nutrition Committee. Rationale of the diet heart statement of the American Heart Association. *Circulation*. 1993;88:3009–3029.

64. National High Blood Pressure Education Program. *Working Group Report on Primary Prevention of Hypertension*. Bethesda, Md: U.S. Department of Health and Human Services, National Institutes of Health; 1993.

65. American Diabetes Association. Treatment of hypertension in diabetes (consensus statement). *Diabetes Care*. 1993;16:1394–1401.

66. American Dietetic Association. Position statement: appropriate use of nutritive and non-nutritive sweeteners. *J Am Diet Assoc*. 1987;87:1689–1694.

67. Thomas-Dobersen D. Calculation of aspartame intake in children. *J Am Diet Assoc*. 1989;89:831–833.

68. Brink SJ. Pediatric, adolescent and young adult nutrition issues in IDDM. *Diabetes Care*. 1988;11:192–200.

69. Thomas-Dobersen D. School time: snack and meal guidelines. Selected aspects of diabetes nutrition—prevention and management in infants and children. *Diabetes Care Educ*. 1993;14(4):14.

70. Armstrong JJ. A brief overview of diabetes mellitus and exercise. *Diabetes Educ*. 1991;17(3):175–178.

71. Austin A, Warty V, Janosky J, et al. The relationship of physical fitness and lipoprotein(a) levels in adolescents with IDDM. *Diabetes Care*. 1993;16(2):421–425.

72. American Diabetes Association. Position statement: diabetes mellitus and exercise. *Diabetes Care*. 1990;13:804–805.

73. Landt KW, Campaigne BW, James FW, et al. Effects of exercise training on insulin sensitivity in adolescents with type I diabetes. *Diabetes Care*. 1985;8:461–465.

74. Huttunen NP, Laukela S, Snip M, et al. Effects of once-a-week training program on physical fitness and metabolic control in IDDM. *Diabetes Care*. 1989;12:737–740.

75. Canterbury MM. Activity and exercise in children with diabetes. Selected aspects of diabetes nutrition—prevention and management in infants and children. *Diabetes Care Educ*. 1993;14(4):15–17.

76. Frier BM. Hypoglycemia and diabetes. *Diabetic Med*. 1986;3:513–525.

77. Goldstein DE, England JD, Hess R, et al. A prospective study of symptomatic hypoglycemia in young diabetic patients. *Diabetes Care*. 1981;4:601–605.

78. Schade DS, Eaton RP. Prevention of diabetic ketoacidosis. *JAMA*. 1979;242:2455–2458.

79. Stancin T, Link DL, Reuter JM. Binge eating and purging in young women with IDDM. *Diabetes Care*. 1989;12:601–603.

80. Rodem GM, Johnson LE, Garfinkel PE, et al. Eating disorders in female adolescents with insulin dependent diabetes mellitus. *Int J Psychiatry Med*. 1986;16(1):49–57.

81. American Dietetic Association. Obesity in adolescents with diabetes. *Diabetes Care Educ*. 1989;10(4):1–13.

82. Satter E. *Child of Mine. Eating with Love and Good Sense*. Palo Alto, Calif: Bull Publishing Co.; 1983.

83. Satter E. *How to Get Your Kid To Eat ... but Not Too Much*. Palo Alto, Calif: Bull Publishing Co.; 1987.

84. Green J, Wheeler M, Roseth JW. Survey of dietitians opinions and use of food exchange lists and alternative approaches. *Diabetes*. 1986;35(suppl 1):44A.

85. Bertorelli AM. Pros of food exchange list. Selected aspects of diabetes nutrition—prevention and management in infants and children. *Diabetes Care Educ*. 1993;14(4):24–27.

86. Delamater AM, Smith JA, Kurtz SM, et al. Dietary skills and adherence in children with type I diabetes mellitus. *Diabetes Educ*. 1988;14:33–36.

87. Held NA. Pros of carbohydrate exchange counting. Selected aspects of diabetes nutrition—prevention and management in infants and children. *Diabetes Care Educ*. 1993;14(4):27–30.

88. Halfon P. Correlation between amount of carbohydrate in mixed meals and insulin delivery by artificial pancreas in seven IDDM subjects. *Diabetes Care*. 1989;12(6):427–429.

89. Holzmeister LA. Caring for infants with diabetes. Selected aspects of diabetes nutrition—prevention and management in infants and children. *Diabetes Care Educ.* 1993;14(4):11–13.

90. Connell J. Pizazz in the pediatric population. *Diabetes Educ.* 1991;17(4):251–256.

91. Amiel SA, Sherwin RS, Simonson DC, et al. Impaired insulin action in puberty: a contributing factor to poor glycemic control in adolescents with diabetes. *N Engl J Med.* 1986;315:215–219.

92. Madden PB. Diabetes camps. Selected aspects of diabetes nutrition—prevention and management in infants and children. *Diabetes Care Educ.* 1993;14(4):32–33.

Serum Total Cholesterol, LDL-C, HDL-C, and Trigylceride Levels in U.S. Children and Adolescents

Table 25-A-1 Serum Total Cholesterol Levels in U.S. Children and Adolescents (mg/dL)

			BOYS						
			Percentiles						
Age (Years)	*Number*	*Overall Mean*	*5*	*10*	*25*	*50*	*75*	*90*	*95*
0-4	238	159	117	129	141	156	176	192	209
5-9	1253	165	125	134	147	164	180	197	209
10-14	2278	162	123	131	144	160	178	196	208
15-19	1980	154	116	124	136	150	170	188	203

			GIRLS						
			Percentiles						
Age (Years)	*Number*	*Overall Mean*	*5*	*10*	*25*	*50*	*75*	*90*	*95*
0-4	186	161	115	124	143	161	177	195	206
5-9	1118	169	130	138	150	168	184	201	211
10-14	2087	164	128	135	148	163	179	196	207
15-19	2079	162	124	131	144	160	177	197	209

Note: All values have been converted from plasma to serum. Plasma values x 1.03 = serum value.

Source: Data from National Cholesterol Education Program. *Report of the Expert Panel on Blood Cholesterol Levels in Children and Adolescents*. Bethesda, Md: U.S. Department of Health and Human Services; 1991. National Heart, Lung and Blood Institute Publication 91-2732.

Table 25-A-2 Serum LDL-C Levels in U.S. Children and Adolescents (mg/dL)

WHITE BOYS

Age (Years)	Number	Overall Mean	Percentiles						
			5	10	25	50	75	90	95
5-9	131	95	65	71	82	93	106	121	133
10-14	284	99	66	74	83	97	112	126	136
15-19	298	97	64	70	82	96	112	127	134

WHITE GIRLS

Age (Years)	Number	Overall Mean	Percentiles						
			5	10	25	50	75	90	95
5-9	114	103	70	75	91	101	118	129	144
10-14	244	100	70	75	83	97	113	130	140
15-19	294	99	61	67	80	96	114	133	141

Note: All values have been converted from plasma to serum. Plasma values x 1.03 = serum value. The number of children 0 to 4 years of age who had LDL-C and HDL-C measure was too small to allow calculation of percentile in this age group. However, note that the percentile for total cholesterol (Table 25-1) for ages 0 to 4 and 5 to 9 are similar.

Table 25-A-3 Serum HDL-C Levels in U.S. Children and Adolescents (mg/dL)

WHITE BOYS

Age (Years)	Number	Overall Mean	Percentiles						
			5	10	25	50	75	90	95
5-9	142	57	39	43	50	56	65	72	76
10-14	296	57	38	41	47	57	63	73	76
15-19	299	48	31	35	40	47	54	61	65

WHITE GIRLS

Age (Years)	Number	Overall Mean	Percentiles						
			5	10	25	50	75	90	95
5-9	124	55	37	39	48	54	63	69	75
10-14	247	54	38	41	46	54	60	66	72
15-19	295	54	36	39	44	53	63	70	76

Note: All values have been converted from plasma to serum. Plasma values x 1.03 = serum value. The number of children 0 to 4 years of age who had LDL-C and HDL-C measure was too small to allow calculation of percentile in this age group. However, note that the percentile for total cholesterol (Table 25-1) for ages 0 to 4 and 5 to 9 are similar.

Table 25-A-4 Serum Triglyceride Levels in U.S. Children and Adolescents (mg/dL)

BOYS

Age (Years)	Number	Overall Mean	Percentiles						
			5	10	25	50	75	90	95
0-4	238	58	30	34	41	53	69	87	102
5-9	1253	30	31	34	41	53	67	88	104
10-14	2278	68	33	38	46	61	80	105	129
15-19	1980	80	38	44	56	71	94	124	152

GIRLS

Age (Years)	Number	Overall Mean	Percentiles						
			5	10	25	50	75	90	95
0-4	186	66	35	39	46	61	79	99	115
5-9	1118	30	33	37	45	57	73	93	108
10-14	2087	78	38	45	56	72	93	117	135
15-19	2079	78	40	45	55	70	90	117	136

Note: All values have been converted from plasma to serum. Plasma values x 1.03 = serum value.

Selected Resources for Use in Self-Management Training with the Child and Family with IDDM

MAGAZINES

Countdown
Juvenile Diabetes Foundation International (JDFI)
Dylak S., Editor
432 Park Avenue South
New York, NY 10016-8013
(800) 223-1138

Kids Corner
American Diabetes Association
National Service Center
P.O. Box 25757
1616 Duke Street
Alexandria, VA 22314
(703) 549-1500

Newsnotes (Barbara Davis Center for Childhood Diabetes)
Children's Diabetes Foundation
777 Grant Street, Suite 302
Denver, CO 80203
(800) 695-2873

BOOKS

A Guide for Parents of Children and Youth with Diabetes
Hollerorth HJ, EdD.
Joslin Diabetes Center
One Joslin Place
Boston, MA 02215
(617) 732-2400

An Instructional Aid on Juvenile Diabetes Mellitus, 9th Edition (1993)
Travis L, MD, FAAP.
Century Business Communications
P.O. Box 200633
Austin, TX 78720-0633
(210) 832-0611

Children with Diabetes (1986)
American Diabetes Association
National Service Center
P.O. Box 25757
1616 Duke Street
Alexandria, VA 22314
(800) 232-3472

Everyone Likes To Eat, 2nd Edition (1993)
Hollerorth HJ, EdD; Kaplan D, MS, RD; with
Bertorelli AM, RD, CDE.
Joslin Diabetes Center
One Joslin Place
Boston, MA 02215
(800) 232-3472

Grilled Cheese at Four O'Clock in the Morning (1988)
Miller J.
American Diabetes Association
National Service Center
P.O. Box 25757
1616 Duke Street
Alexandria, VA 22314
(800) 232-3472

It's Time To Learn about Diabetes: A Workbook on Diabetes for Children (1991)
Betschart J, MN, RN, CDE.
Chronimed Publishing
13911 Ridgedale Drive
Minnetonka, MN 55305
(800) 848-2793

The Joy of Snacks (1991)
Cooper N, RD.
Chronimed Publishing
13911 Ridgedale Drive
Minnetonka, MN 55305
(800) 848-2793

The Kids, Food, and Diabetes Family Cookbook
(1991)
Loring G.
Juvenile Diabetes Foundation International
14755 Ventura Boulevard, Suite 1-744
Sherman Oaks, CA 91403
(310) 842-6742

Sugar Free ... Kid's Cookery (1987)
Majors JS.
Apple Press
5536 S.E. Harlow
Milwaukee, OR 97222
(503) 653-0895

Parenting a Diabetic Child: A Practical,
Empathetic Guide To Help You and Your Child
Live with Diabetes (1993)
Loring G.
Juvenile Diabetes Foundation International
14755 Ventura Boulevard, Suite 1-744
Sherman Oaks, CA 91403
(310) 842-6742

Understanding Insulin Dependent Diabetes, 7th
Edition (1992)
Chase HP, MD.
Children's Diabetes Foundation at Denver
700 Delaware Street
Denver, CO 80204
(800) 695-2873

Whole Parent, Whole Child: A Parent's Guide to
Raising a Child with a Chronic Illness (1991)
Moynihan PM, RN, PNP, MPH; Haig B, RD,
   CDE.
Chronimed Publishing
13911 Ridgedale Drive
Minnetonka, MN 55305
(800) 848-2793

Teenagers with Insulin-Dependent Diabetes (1992)
A Curriculum for Adolescents, Families, and
   Health Professionals Media Library
The University of Michigan Medical Center
1327 Jones Drive, Suite 104
Ann Arbor, MI 48105
(313) 998-6140

In Control: A Guide for Teens with Diabetes
(expected in Fall 1995)
Thom S and Betschart J.
Chronimed Publishing
13911 Ridgedale Drive
Minnetonka, MN 55305
(800) 848-2793

**BOOKLETS, BROCHURES, AND
PAMPHLETS**

Diabetes Day-by-Day: Just for Teens
Diabetes Day-by-Day Parent's Quick Guide to
Kids with Diabetes
American Diabetes Association
Order Department
c/o PBD
1650 Bluegrass Lakes Parkway
Alpharetta, GA 30239
(800) 232-6733

Diabetes: A Book for Children (1992)
Parker LR, RN, BSN.
Media Library
The University of Michigan Medical Center
1327 Jones Drive, Suite 104
Ann Arbor, MI 48105
(313) 988-6140

Making Choices: Teenager with Diabetes (1986)
Anderson BJ, PhD; Burkhart MT, RN, MA;
   Charron-Prochownik D, RN, MS.
Media Library
The University of Michigan Medical Center
1327 Jones Drive, Suite 104
Ann Arbor, MI 48105
(313) 988-6140

Diabetes: A Book for Parents (1992)
Parker LR, RN, BSN.
Media Library
The University of Michigan Medical Center
1327 Jones Drive, Suite 104
Ann Arbor, MI 48105
(313) 988-6140

Healthy Eating for Healthy Growing (1983)
American Association of Diabetes Educators
444 N. Michigan Avenue, Suite 1240
Chicago, IL 60611
(312) 644-2233 or (800) 338-3633

Nutrition for Children with Diabetes (1987)
American Diabetes Association
National Service Center
P.O. Box 25757
1616 Duke Street
Alexandria, VA 22314
(703) 549-1500 or (800) 232-3472

Snack Ideas (1986)
Joslin Diabetes Center
One Joslin Place
Boston, MA 02215
(617) 732-2400

Teddy Ryder Rides Again (1990)
American Diabetes Association
National Service Center
P.O. Box 25757
1616 Duke Street
Alexandria, VA 22314
(703) 549-1500

*Treatment of Hypoglycemic Reactions in Infants
(1992)*
Barr P, Funnell MM.
Media Library
The University of Michigan Medical Center
1327 Jones Drive, Suite 104
Ann Arbor, MI 48105
(313) 988-6140

*Your Child Has Diabetes ... What You Should
Know (1986)*
American Diabetes Association
National Service Center
P.O. Box 25757
1616 Duke Street
Alexandria, VA 22314
(703) 549-1500

When a Family Gets Diabetes (1990)
Heegaard M, MA, ATR; Ternard C, MD.
Chronimed Publishing
13911 Ridgedale Drive
Minnetonka, MN 55305
(800) 848-2793

Single Topic Diabetes and Nutrition Resources:
Children with Diabetes (birth to 5 years)
Children with Diabetes (6–11 years)
Teens, Food and Making Choices
American Diabetes Association
The American Dietetic Association
Order Department
c/o PBD
1650 Bluegrass Lakes Parkway
Alpharetta, GA 30239
(800) 232-6733

AUDIOVISUALS

*It's Time To Learn about Diabetes: A Video on
Diabetes for Children (1993)*
Betschart J, MN, RN, CDE.
Chronimed Publishing
13911 Ridgedale Drive
Minnetonka, MN 55305
(800) 848-2793

Josh (1993)
American Diabetes Association
National Service Center
P.O. Box 25757
1616 Duke Street
Alexandria, VA 22314
(703) 549-1500

Just Like Me (1992)
Baker K.
Scottish Rite Children's Medical Center
Education Department
1001 Johnson Ferry Road NE
Atlanta, GA 30342
(404) 250-2148

*Putting the Pieces Together: Teenagers and
Diabetes (1986)*
Burkhart MT, RN, MA; Anderson BJ, PhD.
Media Library
The University of Michigan Medical Center
R4440 Kresge 1
Ann Arbor, MI 48109-0518

*The Nuts and Bolts of Diabetes: (1) Ketoacidosis,
(2) Low Blood Sugar Reactions (1984)*
Carey Chase V, RN.
Barbara Davis Center for Childhood Diabetes
Office of Educational Services
University of Colorado Health Sciences Center
Box A-066
Denver, CO 80262

Diabetes in Your School or Child Care Center
International Diabetes Center
5000 West 39th Street
Minneapolis, MN 55416
(612) 927-3393

*Care of Children with Diabetes in Child Care and
School Settings*
University of Colorado School of Nursing
Learner Managed Designs, Inc.
2201-K West 25th Street
Lawrence, Kansas 66047
(913) 842-9088

Curriculum Content

**CURRICULUM CONTENT—STAGE I, INITIATIVE:
KINDERGARTEN THROUGH SECOND GRADE (AGES 5–8)**

Content	Activities
Insulin administration	
1. Measuring dose	Count by ones and twos
	Read numbers
	No simple addition
2. Asepsis, germs	Do not touch sterile parts of syringe
	Cleans bottle top and skin
3. Drawing up insulin	Rotate bottle
	Draw insulin into syringe
	Clear air bubbles
	Check accurate dose with adult
4. Injection technique	Select and prepare site
	Stabilize needle, draw back for blood
	Inject self
5. Care of equipment	Discard in safe place
	Store safely
6. Importance of injection	Learn name of own insulin
Timing of dose	Arrange clock hands to injection time
Insulin = medicine; never inject for fun (pets, siblings, etc)	Inject doll for practice
Urine testing	
1. Urine test strips are poisonous	Safe handling and storage of urine test strips
2. How to test	Test own urine, recognize colors, record results
Diabetes physiology	
1. Low sugar symptoms and needs for quick sugar snack	Watch puppet show on symptoms of high and low sugar, how to treat, and who to tell
2. High sugar symptoms	
3. Need to tell adult any symptoms	
Hygiene and health	
Cleanliness	Wash hands
Clothes protect from weather	Color in appropriate clothes for weather

Source: Adapted from Kohler E, Hurwitz LS, Milan D. A developmentally staged curriculum for teaching self-care to the child with insulin–dependent diabetes mellitus. *Diabetes Care*. 1982;5(3):300-304. Copyright © 1982, American Diabetes Association.

CURRICULUM CONTENT—STAGE II, INDUSTRY:
THIRD THROUGH SIXTH GRADE (AGES 9–12)
Basic Skills: Injection Techniques and Insulin Administration, Urine Testing

Content	Activities
What is diabetes?	
1. Principles of diabetes and purpose of insulin	Review content on diabetes from 6- to 8 yr-old class
2. Words: hyperglycemia, hypoglycemia, ketoacidosis a. Meaning	Introduce terms and causes for each Describe how each feels and relate the words to own feelings Describe appropriate treatment for each
Insulin	
1. Time of action of own insulin	Graph insulin, meals, and sugars
2. Balance of food and insulin	Discuss insulin action as it relates to own daily schedule
Home testing	
1. Interpretation of test results in relation to insulin, diet, and exercise	Interpret meaning of N-5%, and what is % and volume Have normal blood sugars
2. Dose adjustment from looking at record sheet	Question/answer session related to the effect of insulin, diet, exercise Review record sheets
3. Home blood testing	Test blood with instant fingerstick method
4. Normal blood sugars	Learn normal and dangerous blood sugar ranges
Relationships of:	
1. Insulin, diet, exercise	Discuss effects of exercise, diet, and insulin on blood sugar Have child solve simple everyday situations

CURRICULUM CONTENT—STAGE III, IDENTITY:
JUNIOR-HIGH SCHOOL (AGES 12–14)

Basic Skills: Insulin Administration, Urine Testing, Knows What Diabetes Is and Symptoms of
High and Low Sugar, Knowledge of Insulin and Equipment Used

Content	Activities
Physiology of diabetes	
1. Difference between hyper-glycemia and ketoacidosis	Recognize signs and symptoms of each
2. Effects of hormones, stress, growth on diabetes	Plot own growth and insulin doses Identify stress circumstances
Monitoring diabetes	
1. Normal blood sugar	Do instant sugar on self and plot on graph
2. Urine sugar, concept of 1% and volume	Calculate grams sugar in urine
a. How to test testing equipment	Check Ketostix with nail polish remover and sugar tests with Coke vs table sugar
3. Relationship of urine spill to blood sugar	Plot blood and urine tests and review lag time for urine
4. Glycohemoglobin	Review normal range
Management of diabetes	
1. Time of action of different types of insulin	Problem solve insulin dose needs on basis of urine and/or blood tests
2. Effect of insulin, diet, exercise	Record and plan activities and intake
Complications	
1. Long-term problems of diabetes, current concepts of etiology, and prevention	Discuss microvascular, large vessels, polyol pathway using simple terms
2. Rationale for lab tests including cholesterol, triglycerides, glycohemoglobin	Tour laboratory Discuss importance of exercise, foot care, and regular eye checks
Diabetes management	
1. Special situation: partying, dates, social activities	Plan meal in restaurant Plan party, fast foods with exchanges
2. Schedule changes, illness, part-time jobs	List sample activities, identify problem times

CURRICULUM CONTENT—STAGE IV, IDENTITY-INTIMACY:
HIGH SCHOOL (AGES 15–18)

Basic skills: Injection, Urine and Blood Testing, Basic Understanding of Diabetes and Its
Management, Knowledge of Insulin and Equipment Used, Knowledge of Normal Blood Sugars

Content	Activities
Diabetes: management	
1. Problem-solving situations for balance of insulin, diet, exercise, and stress	Adjust insulin and diet with health staff for stimulated extra activities, work, sports, schedule changes, and on basis of sample urine or blood glucose record
2. Sharing your diabetes	Initiate role playing on how to tell whom
Complications	
1. Prevention of complications of diabetes	Discuss role of sugar balance and specific preventive measures
2. Signs, symptoms, and recognition of complications of diabetes	Describe early symptoms of complications as well as clinical and laboratory monitoring for each complication
3. Appropriate treatment for them	Discuss treatment of each complication with guest specialist
Resources	
1. How to get emergency and specialty care	Find medical resources in phone book
2. Roles of various health professionals and medical specialists	Initiate role playing of appointment making and relating to physicians and other health professionals
3. Importance of regular health care	
Future planning	
1. Risks and disadvantages of diabetes in long-living situations	Invite guest speakers who are diabetic adults
2. Discussion of new research	Demonstrate pumps and other new modalities of care
3. Genetic transmission; reproduction	Discuss with geneticist and obstetrician
4. Job possibilities: what information is necessary to give employer	Fill out sample forms
5. Driving, insurance, medical costs	Budget for diabetic care items, shop for bargains

Chapter 26

Pregnancy and Diabetes

Boyd E. Metzger

The improved expectations for pregnancies in women with diabetes mellitus constitute one of the "success stories" in worldwide diabetology.[1] There are few situations in clinical diabetes in which comparable improvements have been achieved. Perinatal losses in pregnancies complicated by diabetes were reduced from an incidence of 33% in the late 1920s to 6.5% by the end of the 1970s.[2] Indeed, in the past decade, many centers have reported perinatal mortality figures for the offspring of women with insulin-dependent diabetes mellitus (IDDM) that approximate those found in the general population.[3,4] Moreover, the frequencies of other complications, such as toxemia, hydramnios, macrosomia, and neonatal hypoglycemia, have also been diminished to a striking extent.

Multiple factors have contributed to these laudable developments.[1-5] Historically, emphasis on team care, liberal use of hospitalization for the metabolic regulation of the mother, and obstetric monitoring of the fetus have been implicated. The improvements have also paralleled increased sophistication in the techniques for assessing fetal maturation, estimating gestational age, and providing neonatal intensive care. However, the refinements in the management of the diabetes and the growing emphasis on "tight metabolic regulation" throughout pregnancy may well transcend all other considerations. This is because all the complications seem to be linked to maternal metabolism rather than more occult factors. For example, all the late complications of diabetic pregnancies can be replicated in rhesus monkeys by rendering the mothers diabetic with streptozotocin during the first trimester, thus affirming that these problems are related to the metabolic rather than the genetic or immunologic aspects of the mother's diabetes.[6] Moreover, the complications do not occur when the father rather than the mother is diabetic, thereby providing further evidence for intrauterine rather than genetically determined metabolic factors. In view of the above, any management strategies in pregnancies complicated by diabetes must be based on a sophisticated understanding of (1) the metabolic changes that occur normally in the mother due to pregnancy per se and (2) how these changes induce an altered requirement for insulin. Such an understanding of metabolic pathophysiology becomes particularly important for the health care professional who is responsible for the dietary aspects of the patient's management.

ACKNOWLEDGMENT: The research from the Northwestern University Diabetes in Pregnancy Center cited in this report has been supported in part by grants DK10699, MRP-HD11021, RR48, HD19070, HD62903, and HD23141 and training grant DK07169 from the National Institutes of Health.

I would like to express appreciation to Margaret A. Powers, MS, RD, CDE who was the senior contributing author to this chapter for the first edition. Many of her contributions are retained in the material for the second edition.

METABOLIC ADAPTATIONS IN NORMAL PREGNANCY

General Features of Maternal Metabolism during Pregnancy

Hytten and Leitch[7] reported that women "eating to appetite" gain approximately 24 to 28 lb (11 to 13 kg) of body weight during pregnancy. The weight gain in early gestation occurs largely through an accumulation of maternal body fat and accounts for about 3.5 kg. Most of the remaining increase in weight is gained in the second half of pregnancy and can be ascribed to the increasing mass of the products of conception, the growth of the uterus, the development of breasts, and the expansion of maternal blood volume and interstitial fluids.[7]

Together with the increase in the mass of the conceptus, an increasing resistance to insulin action occurs in the second half of pregnancy. In women with normal insulin-secretory reserves,

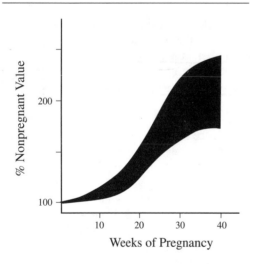

Figure 26-1 The Effect of Pregnancy on Stimulated Insulin Secretion. The increments in circulating insulin above basal values after challenge with glucose have been summated to derive an index of stimulated secretory response. The figure compares range of published value during pregnancy with similar estimates secured in nongravid subjects. *Source:* Reprinted with permission from *Diabetes* (1980;29: 1025), Copyright 1980, American Diabetes Association Inc.

this is usually offset by an increase in plasma insulin in the basal state and by an increased secretion of insulin in response to nutrient challenge (Figure 26-1). However, in women with marginal or absent insulin reserves, this endogenous compensation for the normal "diabetogenic effect" of pregnancy may not be possible. Thus, intrinsic secretory limitations may result in the emergence of gestational diabetes mellitus (GDM) as the pregnancy progresses (see below) or in an increase in the requirements for insulin in the women in whom known diabetes antedated the pregnancy (ie, pregestational diabetes mellitus [PGDM]). The pregnancy-related changes in carbohydrate and insulin economy are reversed in the immediate postpartum period. Their parallel action with the growth of the conceptus during pregnancy and their subsidence after expulsion of the conceptus render it likely that all these changes are linked to some properties of the conceptus.

Metabolic Contributions of the Conceptus

Increase in Hormones of Pregnancy

As the conceptus arises de novo and develops throughout gestation, two properties warrant particular attention. First, the conceptus may function as an added site for the removal of maternal hormones and for the biosynthesis of endocrine principles. Goodner and Freinkel[8] first established that maternal insulin does not cross the placenta, although some may be sequestered, bound, and degraded there. However, estrogens, progesterone, human chorionic somatomammotropin (HCS), also called human placenta lactogen (HPL),[9] and such novel metabolically active peptides as corticotropin-releasing hormone[10] are synthesized and released by the placenta in a fashion that tends to parallel the growth of the conceptus. Each hormone has been shown to augment the responsiveness of the mother's pancreatic islets to secretory stimulation and to alter her sensitivity to insulin action in the periphery, although the status of estrogens remains somewhat controversial.[11,12] For example, HCS (HPL) can exert lipolytic effects and may engender insulin resistance in non-gravid subjects when infused overnight in amounts designed to simulate the plasma levels that are obtained during late gestation.[13] Similarly, administration of progesterone to nongravid subjects can increase both stimulated and basal insulin secretion and augment such metabolic processes as gluconeogenesis.[14] Thus, these hormones, which appear in ever-increasing amounts in the maternal circulation in parallel with increase in placental mass, create a metabolic setting in which insulin action is blunted and islet secretory performance is augmented.

Use of Maternal Fuels

Second, the conceptus may function as an additional site for the removal of maternal fuels.[11] Within the constraints of placental blood flow, fat-derived fuels such as ketones, glycerol, and the non–protein-bound fraction of free fatty acids (FFA) traverse the placenta in direct proportion to their concentration in maternal blood (ie, in a concentration-dependent fashion). Moreover, less expendable maternal fuels such as glucose and certain amino acids are also transferred across the placenta in accordance with their concentrations in the maternal circulation. All these fuels can be used for the continuing growth and oxidative needs of the conceptus so that the conceptus may be viewed as a continuously feeding boarder within an intermittently eating host. The net unidirectional fluxes of nutrients to the conceptus are not inconsiderable: glucose use by the term human fetus has been estimated to approximate 6 mg/kg per minute[15] in contrast to the glucose turnover of 2 to 3 mg/kg per minute in the normal human adult.[16] Growth of the human fetus during the third trimester requires the net transfer of 54 μmol/d of nitrogen across the placenta.[17] Consequently, maternal mechanisms for conserving 3- to 6-carbon nutrients may be compromised meaningfully as the pregnancy progresses and the fuel needs of the conceptus increase.

The hyperinsulinemia of normal late pregnancy does not seem to reduce the number of insulin receptors on cells.[18] Thus, the insulin resistance of pregnancy seems to be mediated at the postreceptor level.[11,12] The underlying factors have not been elucidated fully. However, a good case can be made for the combined action of the increasingly available hormones of pregnancy, as well as the increasing siphonage of maternal fuels.[11,12] Precise replication of the insulin resistance of pregnancy has not been achieved experimentally with either component alone.

Modifications of the Fed and Fasted States

Every aspect of maternal fuel economy is altered by the integrated actions of the growing conceptus.[11,12] Because of the continuous removal of glucose, amino acids, and related 3- to 6-carbon nutrients by the fetus, especially during the period of most active fetal development in late pregnancy, the pregnant mother cannot conserve endogenous fuels in the fasted state with the same parsimony that characterizes starvation under nongravid conditions. Three decades ago, consideration of these factors prompted Freinkel[19] to suggest that pregnant women should experience the normal adaptations to dietary deprivation more rapidly and more profoundly in late pregnancy ("accelerated starvation"). Within the context of accelerated starvation, a heightened shift to the products of fat metabolism would "spare" glucose and amino acids in the mother for use by the fetus while minimizing the insult to maternal nitrogen and carbohydrate reserves. Subsequent experimental and clinical observations have been consistent with this proposition.[11,12] It has been demonstrated that even minor dietary deprivations elicit enhanced mobilizations of fat and greater rises in plasma and urinary ketones during the latter half of pregnancy. A greater fall in maternal blood glucose is also seen coincident with a greater activation of the processes by which new glucose is formed in the liver (gluconeogenesis) and ammonia is produced (ammoniogenesis) in the course of glucose production by the kidney.[20] The reduction in blood glucose in humans,[21] as well as in primates[22] and rats,[20] may progress to frank hypoglycemia. This fasting hypoglycemia of pregnancy has been viewed as a "substrate deficiency syndrome"[23] because it is attended by an excessive fall in plasma glucogenic amino acids (especially alanine) and presumably by an inability of amino acid mobilization for new glucose formation to "keep up" with the rates of glucose removal.

There has been some question whether accelerated starvation occurs under conditions of an ordinary clinical setting. Our observations of pregnant women from whom food was withheld from dinner at 6:00 P.M. to lunch time the next day have indicated that their midmorning increases in plasma FFA, glycerol, and ketones and their reductions in plasma glucose and amino acids are significantly greater than the changes that occur in these same circulating fuels when nonpregnant women are subjected to identical periods of dietary deprivations.[24,25] Thus, the common clinical practice of "skipping breakfast" for laboratory tests or other clinical procedures may not be without major metabolic implications in late normal pregnancy.

In this setting of accelerated starvation and heightened intracellular diversion to the products of fat metabolism, significant deviations from normal nongravid patterns are also seen whenever food is ingested (ie, the fed state). Ingestion of oral glucose after an overnight fast in late normal pregnancy elicits a greater and more prolonged increase in blood glucose, greater increments in plasma of very low-density lipoprotein, and a greater concurrent fall in plasma glucagon. Freinkel and colleagues[26] designated these modifications of the fed state that occur in normal gestation as "facilitated anabolism." Because glucose crosses the placenta in a concentration-dependent fashion, it has been suggested that the exaggerated hyperglycemia after glucose feeding in late pregnancy would ensure the availability of a greater proportion of the dietary glucose for transplacental transfer.[26] The increased plasma triglycerides could abet this objective by substituting for some of the circulating glucose as a maternal oxidative fuel and thereby sparing this glucose for transplacental flux.[26] Finally, the greater suppression of glucagon after glucose ingestion could also facilitate anabolism because, at least in theory, it would attenuate any persistently ongoing contributions of glucagon to such intrahepatic aspects of accelerated starvation as glycogenolysis, gluconeogenesis, and ketogenesis.[26] The integrated consequences of accelerated starvation and facilitated anabolism result in a wholly different pattern for normal fuel homeostasis in late pregnancy.[11,12]

The metabolic profile of normal late gestation is characterized by lower values for fasting plasma glucose and greater and more prolonged postprandial increments in glucose than under nongravid conditions.[27] These factors account for the somewhat different normal values for oral glucose tolerance during gestation.[28] Similarly, the normal plasma values for most amino acids are lower during the fed as well as the fasted state during normal pregnancy,[23,27] plasma cholesterol is increased and unaffected by dietary excursion,[27] plasma triglycerides are increased and subject to further mild augmentation during carbohydrate ingestion,[26,27] and FFA values are greater following 14 or more hours of dietary deprivation.[24,25] In association with these altered fuel patterns, basal levels of plasma insulin levels are increased modestly, and insulin secretion in response to glycemic stimulation is increased two- to threefold[11,12] (see Figure 26-1). Thus, as summarized above, the diurnal patterns of ambient fuels are substantially different in late gestation than under nongravid conditions. The oscillations between the fed and the fasted state are characterized by greater amplitude; the resultant demands for flexibility with regard to acute and chronic insulin secretion are therefore much greater.

IMPLICATIONS OF MATERNAL METABOLISM FOR THE CONCEPTUS

Implications for Fetal Development and Neonatal Life

These changes in maternal metabolism assume perhaps greatest significance with regard

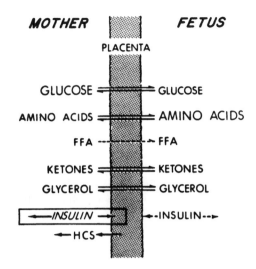

Figure 26-2 Placental Permeability and the Relationships between Maternal and Fetal Fuels. Maternal insulin is the potent arbiter of the fuels available for transfer. *Source:* Reprinted with permission from *Diabetes* (1980;29:1028), Copyright 1980, American Diabetes Association Inc.

to their implications for the conceptus. Maternal fuels are the building blocks from which all embryogenesis and subsequent fetal development must take place. Appreciation of this relationship prompted Freinkel and Metzger[11,12,29] to suggest that the metabolic aspects of pregnancy should be viewed as a "tissue culture experience." The tissue culture formulation stresses that the placenta and fetus develop in an incubation medium derived from maternal fuels (Figure 26-2). As summarized in more detail elsewhere[11,12,29] and discussed in the preceding section, maternal glucose traverses the placenta freely by facilitated diffusion, neutral and basic amino acids are transported actively in a concentration-dependent fashion, ketones and glycerol gain ready access to the fetus in proportion to maternal blood levels, and unbound FFA appear to cross the placenta in sufficient amounts to provide at least the necessary essential fatty acids. Some biotransformations may arise within the placenta (eg, the abundant gen-

eration of lactic acid from glucose) or the fetus (eg, gluconeogenesis in some species). Additional rate-limiting determinants may also influence the incubation medium, such as uterine and/or placental blood flow, mechanical and/or biochemical restrictions to placental transfer, and even "genetic factors." Nonetheless, in view of the parallelism between the circulating levels of nutrients in mother and fetus, the mother's fuels may provide a valid sample of the tissue culture medium.[11,12,29]

Influence of Maternal Insulin

The role of maternal insulin warrants particular emphasis. All the above fuels in the mother, during the fasted as well as the nonfasted state, are affected quantitatively and qualitatively by maternal insulin. Thus, although maternal insulin does not cross the placenta[8] (Figure 26-2), it is the ultimate arbiter of the whole system.[11,12,29] First, it may regulate the quantitative aspects of the incubation medium. Whenever maternal insulin is laggard or insufficient, insulin-dependent nutrients will persist longer and more abundantly in the circulation of the mother. They will thus have greater opportunity for concentration-dependent delivery to the conceptus. Second, maternal insulin may also influence the qualitative features. For example, the mother's insulin critically affects the generation of endogenous fuels, such as ketones, which are not contained in the maternal dietary mixture but which also seem to cross the placenta according to maternal blood levels.

Fetal Insulin Response

Finally, more indirect effects on developing fetal tissues must be considered. For example, although maternal insulin does not cross the placenta it may play a key role in the maturation of the insulin-secreting capabilities of the ß-cells in the fetal pancreas. It is firmly established that increased exposure of fetal islets to ambient nutrient secretagogues can result in their premature proliferation and functional maturation.[30] Thus, an increased delivery of nutrients from the mother will cause the relatively unresponsive fe-

Maternal   Placental   Fetal

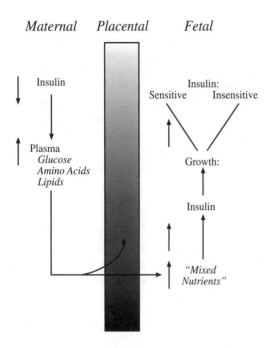

Figure 26-3 Fetal Development According to the Modified Pedersen Hypothesis. *Source:* Reprinted with permission from *Diabetes* (1980;29:1030), Copyright 1980, American Diabetes Association Inc.

tal ß-cells to assume more adult patterns and to release more insulin so that the fetus can retain an even greater proportion of the nutrients within fetal insulin-responsive tissues.

The latter dynamic interplay may explain the increased incidence of macrosomia and neonatal hypoglycemia in the offspring of diabetic mothers.[11,12,29,31] As shown in Figure 26-3, the tendency in such offspring to increased weight and disproportionate growth of insulin-sensitive tissues such as fat may be related to the increased delivery of fuels from the mother and the consequent enhancement of fetal insulin secretion. The persistently increased secretion of insulin by these islets during the neonatal period may play a major role in the neonatal hypoglycemia. Fetal hyperinsulinism may also profoundly influence the functional maturation of important metabolic or developmental pathways of other organs (eg, liver, heart, and lung).

Long-Range Implications

A more subtle aspect of maternal metabolism during pregnancy and the tissue culture formulation has also received attention. Freinkel[11] suggested that the potential effects of the fuels in the incubation medium during pregnancy should be considered from a pharmacologic as well as nutritional perspective. He postulated that the ambient fuels that are available during embryogenesis and fetal life may exert permanent impact on the offspring by influencing genetic expression of terminally differentiating, poorly replicating cells during critical phases of intrauterine development. This pharmacologic possibility was designated "fuel-mediated teratogenesis."[11] The late manifestations of the process would depend on the developmental events that are going on at the time of the disturbance in maternal fuel metabolism. For example, inappropriate maternal hyperglycemia or hyperaminoacidemia, or both, during the third trimester when fetal adipocytes, muscle cells, pancreatic ß-cells, and the neuroendocrine axis are undergoing maximal proliferation and differentiation might result in a greater propensity to later obesity or non–insulin-dependent diabetes mellitus (NIDDM) ("anthropometric or metabolic teratogenesis")[11]; abnormal fuel mixtures during the second trimester when brain cells are being formed might find expression in altered intellectual or psychological patterns ("behavioral teratogenesis")[11]; and disturbances during the early part of the first trimester might compromise normal organogenesis and so produce congenital lesions ("organ teratogenesis").[11]

Increasing evidence now supports the intrinsic assumption of fuel-mediated teratogenesis that nurtures (as exemplified by the intrauterine metabolic environment), and that may modify nature, as represented by genetic endowment.[32–36] Maternal diabetes (exclusively type II) is associated with an increased risk of both obesity and the development of NIDDM in young adults in the highly inbred Pima Indian population.[32] Among women with GDM, maternal histories of diabetes have been observed more frequently than expected.[34] Cross-sectional epidemiologic studies in Britain[37] and France[38] have demonstrated that individuals with NIDDM more often have had a diabetic mother than a diabetic father. The development of diabetes in the offspring of diabetic rats is influenced by perturbed maternal carbohydrate metabolism, as well as by genetic factors.[39,40]

At the Northwestern University Diabetes in Pregnancy Center, we have investigated, in a prospective study, the relationships between insulin secretion in the fetus, and glucose tolerance in adolescence, in offspring of diabetic mothers and have found a high prevalence of both obesity[35] and impaired glucose tolerance (IGT)[36] in our cohort of children. Both are independently linked to the presence of fetal hyperinsulinism as reflected in amniotic fluid insulin concentrations in late gestation. Our data suggest the following sequence of events: maternal hyperglycemia is associated with fetal hyperinsulinism (the Pedersen hypothesis[31]); fetal hyperinsulinism predisposes to obesity in childhood and IGT in adolescence (the Freinkel hypothesis[11]). Offspring of diabetic mothers with normal amniotic fluid insulin had an incidence of IGT similar to the general population. But those offspring of mothers with the highest concentrations of amniotic fluid insulin in utero have a 13-fold increased risk of developing IGT by early adolescence.[36] Rhesus monkeys made hyperinsulinemic but euglycemic in utero by infusion of insulin into the fetus, develop abnormal glucose tolerance as pregnant adults.[41] Together, these data from humans and primates implicate exposure to excess insulin action in utero in the predisposition to diabetes mellitus.

Importantly, the implications of fuel-mediated teratogenesis may extend far beyond the isolated problems of pregnancy complicated by diabetes. Maternal insulin regulates most fuels in the maternal circulation in all pregnancies and thereby always delimits the metabolic mixtures that are available for transplacental transfer. Conceivably, therefore, fuel-mediated effects on embryo or fetal development may be anticipated in any situation or with any agent that can modify maternal insulin production, release, and/or action during pregnancy.[11] Thus, the nutritional and metabolic lessons to be learned from the pregnant diabetic patient may have fruitful relevance for the management of all pregnancies, whether or not they are attended by concomitant disease.

MEDICAL MANAGEMENT

Classification

Current reports suggest that diabetes mellitus diagnosed before conception (ie, PGDM) complicates 0.2 to 0.3% of all pregnancies[42] and that "glucose intolerance of variable severity with onset or first recognition during the present pregnancy" (ie, GDM) may be present in an additional 2 to 3% of the population.[43–46] The latter potentially constitutes an appreciable public health problem, because there are more than 3 million live births in the United States each year.

We[5] and others[47] have recently departed from the traditional classification for women with PGDM devised several decades ago by White.[48] In the White classification, age at onset and duration of diabetes in combination with micro- or macrovascular complications served as the predictors of perinatal risk. In the present era, fetal losses are uncommon. However, the degree of metabolic control throughout pregnancy and the presence or absence of vascular complications, independent of maternal age or duration of diabetes mellitus, are more specific predictors of maternal or fetal morbidities. In patients with PGDM, we attempt to distinguish those with type I diabetes from those with type II diabetes.[43] Each group is then subdivided, based on whether diabetic complications are known to be present. As shown in Exhibit 26-1, abbreviations are added for specific complications as postscripts.

In keeping with recommendations of the National Diabetes Data Group and three international workshop-conferences on GDM, we define GDM as "carbohydrate intolerance with onset or first recognition during the present pregnancy."[43–46] We also adhere to the screening

Exhibit 26-1 Classification of Carbohydrate Intolerance during Pregnancy[a]

Class	*Classification Criteria*
Gestational diabetes mellitus (GDM)	Carbohydrate intolerance of varying severity with onset or first recognition during the present pregnancy. Diagnosis as per Exhibit 26-2. Antepartum subclassification on basis of values for fasting glucose
GDM Class A₁	Fasting glucose normal for pregnancy: venous plasma <105 mg/dL (5.8 mmol/L)
GDM Class A₂	Fasting glucose exceeds normal for pregnancy: Venous plasma ≥105 mg/dL (5.8 mm/L); on at least two occasions
	Postpartum reclassification
	Evaluation by 75 g oral glucose tolerance test to classify according to the criteria of NDDG as: "Previous abnormality of glucose tolerance (GDM)" if glucose tolerance normal at this time, or impaired glucose tolerance (IGT), or diabetes mellitus
Previous GDM	Abnormality of glucose tolerance in a previous pregnancy, without diabetes mellitus having been diagnosed postpartum (postpartum glucose tolerance test normal, impaired, or not performed)
Class A₁—Previous GDM	(see above for fasting blood glucose parameters)
Class A₂—Previous GDM	
Pregestational diabetes mellitus	Diabetes mellitus diagnosed according to NDDG criteria when not pregnant
Diabetes mellitus—type I	
Uncomplicated	Absence of retinopathy, nephropathy, neuropathy, coronary artery disease, or hypertension
Complicated	Presence of one or more of the above (see below for designation and definitions)[b]
Diabetes mellitus—type II	
Uncomplicated	As for type I diabetes
Complicated	As for type I diabetes

[a] Classification is based on prevailing practices in author's center and the recommendations of the National Diabetes Data Group (NDDG),[43] and the First, Second, and Third Workshop-Conferences on Gestational Diabetes.[44-46]

[b] ***BDR***, Background diabetic retinopathy; ***PDR***, proliferative diabetic retinopathy; ***NEPH***, diabetic nephropathy defined as ≥ 0.5 g protein in 24-hour urine collection, and/or serum creatine consistently ≥1.2 mg/dL (106 mmol/L); ***NEUR***, neuropathy, defined as known gastroparesis when not pregnant, orthostatic hypotension, or sensory abnormalities in lower extremities detected at bedside examination; ***CAD***, coronary artery disease diagnosed by history, ECG, or stress ECG; ***HTN***, hypertension, defined as blood pressure ≥140/90 consistently.

(Designations are appended to primary diagnosis as appropriate [eg, Diabetes Mellitus—type II—uncomplicated; Diabetes Mellitus—type I—BDR, NEPH; etc]).

Source: Reprinted from Metzer BE, Purdy LP, and Phelps RL, Diabetes Mellitus and Pregnancy. In DeGroot LJ, ed, *Endocrinology*, ed 3 with permission of WB Saunders, Copyright 1994; 1464-1481.

and diagnostic procedures and criteria for GDM recommended by the workshop-conferences. Further, we subdivide GDM on the basis of the severity of metabolic disturbances[11,29,49–51] and use fasting plasma glucose (FPG) as the distinguishing characteristic (Exhibit 26-1). Thus, we designate pregnant women as GDM class A_1 when values for FPG are within the normal range for pregnancy[28] (ie, <105 mg/dL, 5.8 mmol/L) and as GDM class A_2 when values equal or exceed this limit.

General Principles of Treatment

The primary goal for a pregnancy complicated by diabetes is the delivery of a healthy baby at term. Complications for mother or baby may arise from medical, obstetric, or neonatal factors. Thus, team management by the internist (diabetologist), obstetrician (perinatologist), pediatrician (neonatologist), nurse-educator, dietitian, and others as needed, continues to be essential to achieve this goal optimally.[1–5] Women with good metabolic control and an adequate understanding of the principles of intensive diabetes management do not undergo routine hospitalization at any time during pregnancy. Those with PGDM who have not achieved stable, good metabolic control before conception are often hospitalized soon after they are referred for care. Our goals during this hospitalization are to (1) establish control of diabetes as rapidly as possible; (2) expand the education of the patient regarding diet, self-glucose monitoring, obstetric course, and fetal monitoring; and (3) perform ophthalmologic examinations and tests of renal function to assess the severity of any diabetic complications that may be detected. Medical, psychosocial, financial, and other implications of diabetes in pregnancy are also reviewed with the patient and her family. Aside from this, we do not routinely hospitalize women with PGDM during pregnancy. However, we do not hesitate to hospitalize patients if metabolic control deteriorates or other medical or obstetric complications arise. Women with GDM are not hospitalized before the onset of labor unless hospitalization is necessary to initiate treatment with insulin.

Pregestational Diabetes Mellitus

Prepregnancy Counseling

Women with diabetes who are contemplating pregnancy should have the benefit of early counseling.[1,3–5] It is not warranted to discourage pregnancy solely on genetic grounds because the risk of diabetes in the offspring of insulin-dependent parents is considerably less than previously thought. Long-term follow-up of offspring born between 1928 and 1934 has demonstrated the presence of IDDM in 1.3% of those whose mothers had IDDM, whereas the figure is 6.1% among those whose fathers had IDDM.[52] With regard to perinatal risks, current evidence suggests that metabolic control during gestation rather than the duration of diabetes is the major determinant.

By contrast, the presence of advanced complications of diabetes mellitus has important implications. Both mother and fetus are at high risk in the presence of serious nephropathy[53,54] or ischemic vascular disease.[53] In addition, although laser photo coagulation therapy can be used effectively during pregnancy, diabetic retinopathy not infrequently worsens during gestation, particularly in women with pre-existing severe background retinopathy or proliferative changes.[55,56] The potential for such acceleration of retinopathy is greatest when metabolic control is initially poor and is restored most rapidly.[55,56] In the Diabetes Control and Complications Trial[57] and other studies of shorter duration,[58,59] similar transient worsening of retinopathy has been observed in nongravid subjects during the first few months to 1 year after the initiation of "tight" control of diabetes. Thus, although it is not clear whether pregnancy per se contributes to acceleration of retinopathy, women with pre-existing preproliferative retinopathy and those with proliferative changes should be aware of the potential for deterioration during pregnancy.

*Humalog (Lispro)
is now available
(onset 0–¼ hr
extremely fast)*

Beyond the immediate ramification for pregnancy, women with advanced nephropathy, proliferative retinopathy, or arteriosclerotic vascular disease should be aware that further visual impairment, renal failure, or symptomatic vascular disease would compromise the care of a young family. In such cases, pregnancy should be considered only with full understanding of the medical and psychosocial implications.

Finally, the clinical and experimental evidence that congenital malformation in pregnancies complicated by diabetes may be linked to disturbances in maternal metabolism[11,60,61] and that control of maternal diabetes during the period of organogenesis in the embryo[62] may reduce the prevalence of birth defects in the offspring[61] make a compelling case for establishing "tight" control of diabetes before conception. However, we do not know precisely what mediates the teratogenic effects of maternal diabetes nor the duration of the metabolic disturbance that can put the embryo at risk.[61] From epidemiologic and clinical studies, it appears that the risk of birth defects in pregnancies complicated by diabetes is reduced to near normal when metabolic control, as judged by glycohemoglobin concentrations measured in early pregnancy, is within 4 to 6 standard deviations of normal.[61] Premeal capillary blood glucose levels of 100 to 120 mg/dL will generally result in glycated hemoglobin concentrations within this range. Even lower levels may be optimal if a patient can achieve such results without frequent or severe hypoglycemic reactions. However, glycated hemoglobin concentration is an imperfect index of risk to the infant. Therefore, it should not be used to assure subjects that they are at no increased risk or as a specific indication for elective termination of pregnancy.

Insulin

Optimal therapy must be individualized. Because of the exaggerated metabolic oscillations that characterize normal metabolism in pregnancy, combinations of intermediate and regular insulin are usually used. In early pregnancy, tight control can often be accomplished with injections twice daily. However, by the time the contrainsulin factors in pregnancy reach peak intensity after 24 to 28 weeks' gestation, most women with IDDM are treated in our center with regular insulin three times daily before meals and additional smaller amounts of intermediate-acting insulin at breakfast and supper, or bedtime.[1,3-5] Data from normal pregnant women studied at our center[27] and several others[63-65] indicate that fasting and premeal plasma glucose levels range from 70 to 90 mg/dL and that peak postprandial values rarely exceed 140 mg/dL in late gestation. Our goal is to maintain maternal plasma glucose in all pregnant diabetic patients within these limits throughout gestation but not at the expense of recurrent severe hypoglycemia. However, in contrast to the potential risk of adverse effects of hypoglycemia during embryogenesis in early pregnancy,[66] maternal hypoglycemia during the latter two-thirds of pregnancy does not seem to be associated with deleterious consequences for the fetus.[67]

Monitoring Control of Diabetes *?same rec for preconcep*

We[1,3-5] recommend self-monitoring of capillary blood glucose for all women who are treated with insulin during pregnancy unless it is precluded by physical limitations or other factors. At a minimum, subjects are asked to test their blood before each meal, at bedtime daily, and whenever hypoglycemia is suspected. Twice weekly, subjects are asked to obtain values 1 hour after each meal as well. At clinic visits, patients monitor capillary blood at the time that venous blood is drawn for plasma glucose determinations to verify the accuracy of their monitoring techniques. A lesser dependence on in-hospital care is the major change that has occurred since such monitoring is routinely performed in an outpatient setting.

Although monitoring urine glucose adds little to the information obtained from capillary glucose monitoring, urinary ketone measurements are useful to detect inadequate dietary intake, particularly of carbohydrate, and to provide early warning of impending decompensation of metabolic control. Thus, <u>our patients monitor their morning specimen each day and at any time that premeal capillary blood glucose values exceed 150 mg/dL</u>.

Measurements of glycosylated hemoglobin are obtained at enrollment and monthly until term to supplement the information obtained from blood glucose monitoring.[1,3–5] When such values from late first or early second trimester are elevated substantially, they may predict a higher likelihood for the presence of major malformations in the fetus.[61] The serial assessments of glycated hemoglobin often reassure patients that their efforts to achieve better control of diabetes have been effective. Occasionally, the failure to see a good correlation between glycated hemoglobin concentration and the reported results of capillary glucose monitoring may provide a clue to unsuspected falsification of monitoring results and other forms of noncompliance. Measurements of fructosamine or glycated albumin can provide an alternate method of assessing metbolic control when estimates of glycated hemoglobin may not be reliable, such as in the presence of hemoglobinopathies or hemolysis.

Obstetric Surveillance

Serum screening and ultrasound as surveillance are used for the detection of fetal anomalies. Measurement of maternal serum α-fetoprotein between 15 and 18 weeks of gestation can detect 80 to 90% of open neural tube defects.[68] The risk of diverse fetal anomalies in these pregnancies warrants a comprehensive fetal anatomic survey by ultrasound, which is is best performed after 18 weeks when the size of the fetus is sufficient to facilitate sonographic examination of all fetal structures.

Ultrasound examinations during pregnancy can also confirm estimated due date and provide an assessment of the pattern of fetal growth. Confirmation of gestational age is performed early in gestation; whereas, evolving fetal macrosomia can be detected by serial measurements of fetal head and abdominal size in the late second and third trimesters of pregnancy.[69–71]

Intrauterine fetal death (IUFD) in late gestation was a relatively common event before the time that good maternal metabolic control throughout pregnancy was the standard of care for women with pregnancy complicated by diabetes mellitus.[1] Presently, the risk of fetal death may not be appreciably increased over background rates in pregnancies attended by excellent metabolic control, particularly in the absence of vascular disease or pregnancy complications. The etiology of IUFD has not been firmly established in human gestation. However, data from animal models suggest that sustained fetal hyperglycemia, increased placental lactate production, increased fetal uptake of glucose and lactate, and stimulated fetal oxygen consumption ultimately lead to fetal hypoxemia.[72–74]

Several biophysical methods of fetal assessment can be used to provide objective reassurance of fetal well-being.[75] The contraction stress test is one in which the fetal heart rate pattern is evaluated in response to induced uterine contractions. Although highly predictive of fetal well-being, it is time-consuming and has largely been replaced by the nonstress test. This requires only the observation of fetal heart rate in response to spontaneous fetal activity. The biophysical profile by ultrasound assesses fetal activity, fetal muscle tone, fetal breathing activity, and the volume of amniotic fluid volume, in addition to the nonstress test. A weighted score is determined. This is sometimes referred to as the "intrauterine Apgar score." The nonstress test is used as the primary means of fetal surveillance in our center. Although routine testing is usually initiated by 32 weeks of gestation, earlier testing is indicated for pregnancies complicated by significant hypertension or other medical complications that may place the woman at increased risk of fetal death. Amniocentesis to evaluate pulmonary maturation is not performed routinely when pregnancy is carried to term.[1,3–5] As a result of the changes summarized above, obstetric monitoring is fully integrated into an outpatient program, and patients are not hospitalized until delivery unless good metabolic control is not being maintained or obstetric complications develop.

Delivery and Puerperium

The objectives of medical management during labor are to establish and maintain euglycemia on the one hand and to prevent the appearance of ketosis on the other. To achieve these objectives, we administer glucose intravenously as 10% dextrose in water (50 to 60 g every 6 hours), together with sufficient regular insulin by subcutaneous bolus or intravenous drip to maintain capillary blood glucose concentrations (measured every 1 to 4 hours throughout labor) in the range of 70 to 120 mg/dL. Almost without exception, insulin requirements decline dramatically after parturition (often 50% or more). Women who wish to breastfeed are maintained at or above their predelivery diet. Those who do not breastfeed are returned immediately to a diet appropriate for nongravid women (usually 30 to 32 calories/kg ideal body weight [IBW]). All are encouraged to apply the diabetes management skills acquired during gestation.

Gestational Diabetes Mellitus

Definition and Magnitude of the Problem

The prevalence of GDM, defined as "carbohydrate intolerance of variable severity with onset or first recognition during the present pregnancy,"[43–45] was reported in 2 to 6% of pregnancies at centers in the United States,[28,51,76–78] with even higher figures in some populations.[78,79] As such, it is several-fold more common than pregnancy in women with PGDM[42] and represents a major public health problem.[44–46]

Many have found that perinatal losses are increased when GDM is undetected or treated casually (for review, see refs. 4 and 5). In most centers, pregnancies complicated by GDM are classified as "high-risk," and such designation leads to more intensive obstetric supervision, which of itself represents a form of intervention.

Consequently, current reports[44–46] generally show little if any increased perinatal loss in GDM. By contrast, patients with GDM continue to be at increased risk for fetal macrosomia,[51,80] birth trauma, and operative delivery,[80–82] and offspring have more frequent morbidities (hypoglycemia, hypocalcemia, polycythemia, and hyperbilirubinemia). Offspring of mothers with GDM may experience increased risk of obesity[32,35] and IGT[33,36] in later years, apparently as a consequence of exposure to an altered metabolic milieu[11,29] during intrauterine life ("fuel-mediated teratogenesis"). Finally, the substantial risk of abnormal carbohydrate metabolism in the mother subsequent to a diagnosis of GDM[28,83–86] makes it mandatory that glucose tolerance be evaluated by early and long-term postpartum follow-up. Thus, comprehensive programs for the detection and diagnosis, as well as aggressive and early treatment, of GDM are clearly justified.

Screening and Diagnosis

Screening for GDM by criteria based on clinical risk factors and past obstetric history is nonspecific and fails to detect one-third to one-half of the subjects with GDM who are identified by universal screening.[44–46,87,88] Three international workshop-conferences on GDM[44–46] have recommended that all pregnant women should be screened for glucose intolerance by measurement of glucose in venous blood performed between the 24th and 28th week of gestation. In our center, venous plasma glucose is measured 1 hour after subjects receive 50 g oral glucose. Those with values ≥140 mg/dL undergo a full diagnostic 100-g oral glucose tolerance test using the criteria of O'Sullivan and Mahan,[28] as adapted by the National Diabetes Data Group[43] for interpretation of results. The screening and diagnostic criteria for GDM are summarized in Exhibit 26-2.

Subclassification

Subjects with GDM are subclassified according to the level of FPG as indicated in Exhibit

Exhibit 26-2 Screening and Diagnostic Criteria for Gestational Diabetes Mellitus

---

Screening for Gestational Diabetes

1. By glucose measurement in plasma

2. 50-g oral glucose load, administered between the 24th and 28th week, and without regard to time of day or time of last meal, to all pregnant women who have not been identified as having glucose intolerance before the 24th week

3. Venous plasma glucose measured 1 hour later

4. A value of ≥140 mg/dL in venous plasma indicates the need for a full diagnostic glucose tolerance test.

Diagnosis of Gestational Diabetes Mellitus

1. 100-g glucose load, administered in the morning after overnight fast for at least 8 hours but not more than 14 hours, and after at least 3 days of unrestricted diet (≥150 g carbohydrate) and physical activity

2. Venous plasma glucose is measured fasting and at 1, 2, and 3 hours. Subject should remain seated and not smoke throughout the test.

3. Two or more of the following venous plasma concentrations must be met or exceeded for positive diagnosis:
   Fasting, 105 mg/dL
   1 hr, 190 mg/dL
   2 hr, 165 mg/dL
   3 hr, 145 mg/dL

Source: Adapted with permission from *Diabetes* (1985;34 [Suppl 2]:123–126), Copyright 1985, American Diabetes Association Inc.

26-1. Such stratification has been used by us and others to guide therapy and has proved to be valuable in predicting maternal and fetal outcomes.

Etiology and Pathogenesis

On the basis of clinical presentations and limited follow-up experiences, GDM has usually been deemed to be a variant of NIDDM. However, much epidemiologic data from our center and others indicate that GDM entails much genotypic as well as phenotypic heterogeneity and that some of the women with GDM may actually have slowly evolving IDDM.[51,89]

Treatment

Goals of treatment are the same for GDM as for PGDM and have been described above. Nutritional management is addressed in a separate section of this chapter.

Insulin. The precise place of insulin treatment of GDM is not fully defined.[3-5] In the small group of patients with overt hyperglycemia (FPG ≥130 to 140 mg/dL), there is little, if any, controversy.[44,46] In the majority, the primary objective of therapy with insulin is the prevention of macrosomia and other perinatal morbidities. The degree of such risks and their specific relationship to the magnitude of maternal hyperglycemia GDM are the major issues of controversy.[45,46] In our center, women with FPG of 130 mg/dL or greater (sometimes designated as GDM class B_1) are started on treatment with insulin immediately after diagnosis.[3-5] The remainder are initially followed on diet alone (see below), and insulin therapy is confined to those whose FPG remains or becomes elevated to ≥105 mg/dL and/or those whose 1-hour postmeal (usually breakfast) plasma glucose concentration is ≥140 mg/dL on two successive determinations (ie, above the upper limit for FPG in normal pregnancy). As indicated in the reports of three international workshop-conferences on GDM,[44-46] many others use a similar approach to insulin therapy in GDM. Some have advocated the use of "prophylactic" insulin routinely in GDM patients older than 25 years of age,[90,91] and others have used very strict treatment criteria that have resulted in the treatment of 50 to 85% of women with class A_1 GDM with insulin.[92,93] We have refrained from using sulfonylureas in GDM because of their known transplacental passage and potentiality for acting on fetal ß-cells.

Monitoring Metabolic Control. All patients with GDM monitor urinary ketones in the first voided morning specimen to facilitate the detection of inadequate dietary carbohydrate intake (accelerated starvation). FPG and 1-hour postbreakfast plasma glucose measurements are obtained at each outpatient visit to help determine the need for insulin therapy. Those receiving treatment with insulin monitor capillary blood sugar before meals (four times a day) at home to assist in making insulin dosage adjustments on a weekly basis in consultation with the physician or nurse practitioner. We also request that patients monitor postprandial blood glucose levels on 2 or more days per week. To validate their accuracy on an ongoing basis, patients doing fingerstick blood sugar testing also have plasma glucose measurements obtained at each outpatient visit to compare with simultaneously obtained fingerstick determinations.

Delivery

Goals for the management of GDM during labor and delivery are the same as those outlined previously for women with PGDM. In our experience, insulin therapy is rarely required to maintain normoglycemia during labor in women with GDM. Furthermore, most of them will not require the resumption of therapy with insulin during the postpartum period.

Postpartum Follow-Up

The diagnosis of GDM bears significant implications for long-term maternal health. During pregnancy, one cannot distinguish, with certainty, between evolving type I or type II diabetes and transitory glucose intolerance, which will subside postpartum. Postpartum reclassification and long-term follow-up are therefore essential. Within the first year postpartum, a significant proportion of our patients with GDM display IGT or diabetes mellitus[83,86] by NDDG criteria.[43] For women in whom FPG during pregnancy is overtly elevated (FPG $\geq$130 mg/dL), the incidence is 75 to 90%.[83,86] It is likely that in many of these, abnormalities in glucose tolerance antedate pregnancy.[83,94] Although their testing procedures differed somewhat, workers from eastern Germany,[95] Australia,[96] and Saudi Arabia[97] have also reported high incidence of abnormal glucose tolerance during the first 1 or 2 years of postpartum follow-up. Many others have shown that GDM, based on a variety of diagnostic criteria, identifies women at high risk

for the later development of diabetes mellitus and that the incidence increases progressively with time from the index pregnancy.[28,83–86, 94–98]

We and others have identified certain characteristics that can be determined during pregnancy that convey a higher risk for postpartum glucose intolerance.[83,86,98–100] These include relative insulinopenia, severity of glucose intolerance at diagnosis, obesity, early gestational age at diagnosis, racial/ethnic origin (increased in Hispanics), and family history of maternal diabetes. Using multiple logistic regression, we found that relative insulin deficiency (lower basal insulin levels and blunted acute-phase insulin response to oral glucose) and the severity of antepartum hyperglycemia (fasting and 2-hour values) were independently associated with the presence of diabetes mellitus in the early postpartum period.[86] Obesity (associated increased insulin resistance) and blunted integrated insulin responses (area under the curve) were independent predictors in those who developed diabetes mellitus up to 5 years postpartum. It is likely that some of, or all, the other prognostic factors (early gestational age at diagnosis, racial/ethnic origin, and family history of maternal diabetes) are mediated through the independent associations noted above.

NUTRITIONAL INTERVENTION

Nutritional intervention in pregnancies complicated by diabetes has typically been based on the nutritional recommendations of the National Research Council for Healthy Pregnancies[101] and the American Diabetes Association.[102] However, several specific questions remain:

- How many calories should be provided?
- How should the carbohydrate or calories be distributed?
- Should the diet differ for women who are obese?

There are insufficient research data available to provide conclusive answers to these questions. The following summarizes what is currently known and accepted and describes how we apply these principles at the Northwestern University Diabetes in Pregnancy Center.

Normal Pregnancy

Basic Principles

Dietary recommendations for pregnancy complicated by diabetes have evolved with the passage of time (see ref. 103 for historical review). In recent years, nutritional recommendations for diabetes in pregnancy have closely paralleled those for normal pregnancy. On the basis of epidemiologic data indicating an apparent optimal weight gain during pregnancy of 22 to 30 lbs[101] and calculations of the caloric requirements thought necessary to effect this (an additional 200 to 300 calories/day above nongestational needs), diets have been devised and prescribed for all pregnant diabetic women, without consideration being given to diabetic class or pregestational maternal weight. For pregnant women with type II diabetes or GDM who are obese, presumed "normal diets" for pregnancy may be excessive and unnecessarily complicate efforts to achieve optimal control of hyperglycemia. The recent report and new recommendations of the Institute of Medicine of the National Academy of Sciences entitled *Nutrition in Pregnancy*[104] would suggest that such is the case. These recognize the inverse relationship between prepregnancy weight and desirable weight gain (varying from 15 to 40 lb). Accordingly, nutrition advice should be individualized on the basis of pregestational maternal weight and other factors including amount of physical activity. Interest in physical fitness and pursuit of physically active life styles are common among women of reproductive age. Data regarding hemodynamic, metabolic, and hormonal responses to physical exercise in pregnant women are still somewhat limited, and the potential use of exercise to augment insulin sensitivity and facilitate the treatment of diabetes in pregnancy remains a subject of continuing inquiry. However, clinical reports suggest that many women continue moderate physical exercise during pregnancy without apparent adverse effects (see

Chapter 6).

The following pattern of weight gain can be anticipated in normal pregnant women who are of average height and at optimal weight before conception: 2 to 4 lb (1 to 2 kg) in the first trimester and approximately 0.8 lb/wk during the second and third trimesters, for a total of 24 to 28 lb (11 to 13 kg). Current recommendations for protein intake call for the addition of 10 g/d above the 0.8 g/kg per day (recommended dietary allowances) for nongravid subjects.[104] Intake of calories must vary at different stages of pregnancy to produce this pattern. The World Health Organization recommends an increase of 150 kcal in the first trimester and 350 kcal during the last two trimesters.[105] However, estimates of substantially lower caloric increments have also been made.[101,104] It is emphasized that the current recommendations are based on achieving the desired pattern of weight gain rather than representing arbitrary formulas for dietary intake. Some women gain excessively due to the misconception that totally unrestricted eating during pregnancy is permissible. In the case of women with diabetes, excessive weight gain may also be attributable to prescribing a large increase in calories too early in the pregnancy or to the administration of excessive amounts of insulin and the development of frequent hypoglycemia early in pregnancy, when insulin needs may actually decrease. The dietitian should be alerted to these possibilities if the patient comments on constantly being hungry with an adequate intake or if the patient has a rapid weight gain.

In Women Who Are Obese

Most dietitians are familiar with modifying caloric intake based on weight changes and feel comfortable using various formulas as guidelines. However, it is more difficult to find such guidelines for pregnant women who are obese. Based on patient-reported prepregnancy weight, women who are obese appear to gain less weight than women who are at or below their IBW before pregnancy. It has also been reported that optimal perinatal outcome in obese women is associated with substantially smaller weight gain than in normal-weight subjects.[106] It should be remembered that a weight-maintaining diet for an obese subject may contain more calories than the 35 to 38 kcal/kg IBW that is recommended for normal pregnancy.

The use of diets that restrict caloric intake below the above levels is more controversial.[107] Although pregnancies in severely obese women are often considered to be at high risk for perinatal complications, the use of caloric restriction has been approached with caution. Much of the concern has been engendered by the reports of impaired childhood IQ of offspring whose mothers (diabetic and nondiabetic) experienced ketonemia during pregnancy.[108–110] Because the propensity for exaggerated ketonemia in pregnancy (ie, accelerated starvation) can be easily unmasked by simply skipping a meal[24,25] or substantially limiting carbohydrate intake, there is general concern that a reduction of total caloric intake will also put obese pregnant women at risk for accelerated starvation. A second reason for caution about the restriction of caloric intake during pregnancy is the apparent association between lowest weight gain and poor pregnancy outcome, regardless of maternal level of prepregnancy weight.[106]

Restriction of calories has long been advised in several centers with no apparent ill effects. Thus, Pedersen[111] reported the use of 1200- to 1500-calorie diets for obese women during pregnancy whether diabetic or nondiabetic, and Garrow[112] advocated restriction of fat and total calories for all obese pregnant women. Coetzee et al[113] reported average daily intake of 1600 calories in normal pregnancy and restriction of calories in obese subjects with diabetes to 1000 calories. However, these were not controlled trials in which detailed assessments of neonatal outcome were obtained. Recent studies concerning the effects of different nutritional regimens on maternal metabolic parameters and neonatal outcome are therefore of importance. It is clear that caloric restriction does restrain maternal weight gain. This was documented most clearly

by Borberg et al.[114] Obese nondiabetic women received diet plans based on 1800- to 2000-calorie diets (with from 150 to 180 g carbohydrate). They were compared with a similar group eating to appetite. From 16 weeks to delivery, the dieted group gained on average 6.2 kg, in contrast to the 12.6 kg gained in those eating ad libitum. Similar findings in women with GDM, most of whom were obese, have been reported from the same institution by Dornhorst et al.[115] Thirty-five subjects with GDM who were prescribed diets ranging from 1200 to 1800 calories/d gained half as much weight as their nondiabetic control group (matched for age, degree of obesity at entry, race, and parity) who were eating as dictated by appetite. The effects of maternal calorie restriction on fetal weight are uncertain. The limited data that are available are discussed in conjunction with the discussion of GDM. Effects on perinatal outcome and long-term development have not been examined in detail or in sufficient numbers to reach conclusions about efficacy or safety.

Pregnancy Complicated by Diabetes Mellitus

Basic Principles

The considerations that form the basis of dietary recommendations in normal pregnancy have generally been used as the foundation for guidelines for the management of diabetes in pregnancy. Implementation varies depending on specific targets for total calories and carbohydrate/protein/fat composition and distribution.[103] As indicated above, most authors do not recommend that exercise be curtailed during pregnancy in women who have been physically active before gestation. The same can be recommended for women with diabetes mellitus, unless obstetric or medical problems supervene. The American Diabetes Association has indicated that the use of various sweeteners is acceptable in the management of diabetes and has made no specific recommendations that their use in pregnancy be curtailed.[102] However, because saccharin[116] does cross the placenta in small concentrations and is cleared slowly from the fetal circulation and aspartame[117] is hydrolyzed rapidly in the gastrointestinal tract to its constituent products (aspartic acid, methanol, and phenylalanine), some patients and professionals are cautious about the ingestion of these substances during pregnancy.

In Women with Diabetes and Obesity

In addition to the general issues regarding dietary recommendations for obese pregnant women that have been discussed above, specific considerations apply to obese women with PGDM or GDM. First, because caloric restriction in obese nongravid subjects with diabetes is often associated with reduction in insulin resistance and improvement in glucose tolerance, a hypocaloric diet would be an attractive therapeutic alternative during pregnancy if the same improvements could be demonstrated.[107] However, concerns arising from the propensity for accelerated starvation[24,25] with hypocaloric diets are perhaps even greater in women with glucose intolerance.

Some results have been reported. We have shown that the magnitude of accelerated starvation in women with GDM is similar to that of normal pregnant women,[25,118] so that any effort to treat GDM must include careful metabolic surveillance. Knopp et al[119] measured 24-hour metabolic profiles in a limited number of obese GDM patients who received 2400 calories/d, 1600 to 1800 calories/d (33% reduction), or 1200 calories/d (50% reduction). When calories were reduced by 33%, fasting and 24-hour mean glucose, basal insulin, and basal triglycerides tended to fall. Unfortunately, circulating ketones were not reported in this group. However, plasma FFAs were not higher, and the women did not develop ketonuria. With a 50% reduction of calories, fasting and 24-hour mean glucose levels declined significantly, as did fasting insulin and triglyceride. However, concentrations of plasma FFAs and ß-hydroxybutyrate increased, the latter by two- to threefold. Maresh et al[120] also obtained 24-hour profiles in subjects with GDM and nondiabetic controls in the third tri-

mester, both before and 4 to 5 weeks after beginning treatment of those with GDM. The GDM patients were allocated to caloric restriction alone or dietary restriction plus subcutaneous insulin. Treatment by diet alone resulted in improved but not normal glucose profiles, whereas those with GDM who also received subcutaneous insulin had glucose profiles identical to nondiabetic controls. Before treatment, plasma ß-hydroxybutyrate concentration was higher in GDM patients than in controls during much of the day. GDM patients treated with diet restriction had ß-hydroxybutyrate levels at the upper normal range throughout the 24-hour period, whereas levels with insulin-treated GDM were not different from controls throughout most of the 24-hour period. Jovanovic-Peterson and Peterson[121] found a reduction in postprandial blood glucose levels with moderate caloric and carbohydrate restriction in GDM, which in their hands could be achieved without a concomitant development of ketonuria. In the studies noted above, ketonuria, when measured, did not appear to be enhanced in diet-restricted patients except in studies of Knopp[119] where calories were reduced by 50%. However, in the study by Dornhorst et al,[115] wherein diets as low as 1200 calories were used, data on ketonuria are not presented.

At the Northwestern University Diabetes in Pregnancy Center

Basic Principles

We follow the general principles for the dietary management of diabetes in pregnancy that have been reviewed in the previous sections. However, actual details of implementation are individualized for each person. As part of the team approach to management, we involve the team dietitian in developing an overall strategy of treatment, including preconceptual planning when possible. In that case, the initial basic dietary approach can be carefully planned to limit the number of future changes. For example, we emphasize the role of regular mealtimes and a bedtime snack whenever the initial plan is developed, even though it is not always necessary to include a snack until the last half of pregnancy. We write specific nutrition prescriptions that are based on an individual's IBW. For those not familiar with meal planning and selection of portion sizes, we initially recommend a total caloric intake of 30 to 32 kcal/kg IBW for the preconception period and first trimester and 36 to 38 kcal/kg IBW in the second and third trimester. Distribution of carbohydrate, protein, and fat is approximately 50, 15, and 35%, respectively. For the "average" woman, who is 5'4" in height and 58 kg IBW, the 38-kcal/kg IBW diet translates into 2200 kcal, 275 g carbohydrate, 80 g protein, and 85 g fat. The distribution of calories and carbohydrates is approximately 2/2, 2/7, 2/7, and 1/7, with full meals spaced at 5-hour intervals and a bedtime snack 4 hours after dinner. Adequate carbohydrate intake at bedtime reduces the likelihood of overnight ketonemia (accelerated starvation) in subjects treated with diet alone and helps prevent nocturnal hypoglycemia in those who are treated with insulin. If either occurs, the insulin regimen may need adjusting or an extra starch or fruit is added to the evening snack.

Modifications of this basic plan are made by the dietitian and patient to meet individual preferences and to achieve optimal metabolic control and appropriate weight gain. These measures will avoid ketonemia and promote good glycemic control in most patients with GDM or NIDDM and many with IDDM. Some professionals advocate much greater restriction of carbohydrate in an effort to minimize postprandial hyperglycemia especially at breakfast as well as advising patients to reduce their carbohydrate intake in an upcoming meal when they encounter premeal hyperglycemia.[121,122] We do not advise our patients to try these more complex techniques to optimize metabolic control until they fully understand all of the basic concepts of nutrition and the use of short- and intermediate-acting insulin for the management of diabetes mellitus.

We encourage that alcohol be avoided throughout pregnancy and recommend that in-gestion of all sweeteners and caffeine be limited. Actual food choices are based on each individual's food preferences. However, a high fiber intake is recommended to those who experience constipation due to the iron supplement or pregnancy itself.

Finally, we try to provide the patient with an adequate understanding of how to modify her diet and other aspects of treatment for sick days or hypoglycemic reactions. Such information is also helpful if she develops nausea and vomiting, although our patients are advised to call any member of the team whenever they are not feeling well or have questions about their management.

Diet Planning before Conception

As indicated above, our goal is to initiate contact between our diabetic patients who are planning a pregnancy and the dietitian who will work with them during pregnancy. The diet plan that is developed (30 to 32 kcal/kg IBW) is used until 14 to 16 weeks of gestation if weight gain is appropriate. When possible, during preconception care, we initiate or maintain the insulin regimen that will be used throughout the pregnancy.

Pregestational Diabetes Mellitus

We act quickly if a subject has not been under our care before conception or has not achieved satisfactory metabolic control. In some cases, this still entails hospitalization for 1 to 3 days to ensure that the patient has the tools needed to achieve these objectives. The initial dietary approaches differ, depending on when in the course of pregnancy the consultation occurs and whether the patient is hospitalized. If the initial diet prescription is for 30 to 32 kcal/kg IBW, the plan is constructed in a way that will easily accommodate an increase to 36 to 38 kcal/kg IBW after 14 weeks of gestation when increased appetite and rapid weight gain supervene. Strict adherence to the schedule for meal and snack times and the intake of accurate portion sizes are stressed. If the patient is hospitalized, having her observe portion sizes of the food she is served provides an ideal teaching tool. Follow-up sessions with the dietitian are important, whether or not a change in total calories is required at a later time. Contacts are mandatory if recurrent problems such as hypoglycemia occur and/or if weight gain is substantially above or below expected ranges.

Gestational Diabetes Mellitus

Diet is the cornerstone of treatment and is implemented as soon as possible after the diagnosis of GDM is established. As in normal pregnancy, the meal plan is based on 36 to 38 kcal/kg IBW for both the normal-weight subjects and the 50 to 60% of our cases who are obese.[51] Although some evidence suggests that hypocaloric diets might be used safely and effectively in the latter group (see discussion above), we believe that widespread use of caloric restriction for GDM should await confirmation of such results in larger populations, with careful neonatal and long-range follow-up of the offspring to assess fully the impact of such therapy.[107] Several points regarding GDM deserve additional emphasis. First, the nutritional consultation often is the patient's first encounter with a dietitian, during which the patient may still be in the initial phase of her reaction to the diagnosis that has only recently been made. Second, the caloric intake represented by the prescription of 36 to 38 kcal/kg IBW may actually impose a significant reduction in food intake for some subjects, in particular those who are severely obese (prepregnancy weight ≥150% IBW) or have already experienced marked weight gain (ie, more than 30 lb) during their pregnancy. Occasionally, calories are increased to promote adherence to a meal plan. Finally, follow-up contact is necessary for all women with GDM, even those who do not receive treatment with insulin, because of the difficulty many subjects have in dealing with the diagnosis of GDM and the complex medical and obstetric treatment plan they must follow.

Postpartum

Contact with the dietitian is continued after delivery for several reasons. First, guidance is needed in making the transition from the diet during pregnancy to the nutritional requirements postpartum. Second, the initial postpartum approach varies depending on whether the mother will breastfeed her baby or immediately begin her efforts to return to her prepregnancy weight and nutritional state. Finally, the dietitian should also be used as a resource for infant nutrition and to support establishment of good eating habits in the child.

During Lactation. Breastfeeding is encouraged for a woman with PGDM or GDM, if that is her preference. Very little information is available about the impact of lactation on metabolic control, but what has been observed is that blood glucoses may be more variable during lactation in women with IDDM.[123] The extent of variability may depend on the amount of milk produced and the frequency and regularity of feeding. There is some evidence that exposure to breast milk rather than cow milk lessens the risk of developing IDDM in offspring.[124] The woman who is breastfeeding requires additional nutrients, and caloric restriction should not be imposed during the period of lactation. However, some women lose weight with breastfeeding because the caloric demands during full lactation are even greater than during gestation.[101] We usually recommend that the mother continue to receive 38 kcal/kg IBW or more during lactation. Adequate education and support of breastfeeding must be provided so that the mother will know the rewards as well as the frustrations of nursing and be prepared to accommodate work, travel, and other activities in her plan for managing her diabetes and breastfeeding her infant.

Restoration of Pregravid Weight. At the end of pregnancy, women are often looking forward to delivery so that they can begin to lose the weight that they gained during gestation. This is an opportune time for the health team to support this behavior and encourage nutritional follow-up. Plans for weight reduction should be presented as part of comprehensive postpartum management. A detailed program should be developed before discharge from the hospital for patients who are not breastfeeding their infants.

However, as noted above, hypocaloric diets should not be initiated in a woman who is breastfeeding until she decides to terminate lactation. It is important to make programs for diet and exercise available to women who have had GDM, particularly those who are obese. Although conclusive evidence is not yet available to show that these measures can forestall the development of overt diabetes mellitus in later years, there have been some reports that suggest that is the case,[125] and such efforts seem prudent in light of the demands that obesity makes on insulin secretion. A National Institutes of Health–supported multicenter clinical trial that will test interventions aimed at preventing the development of NIDDM in high-risk populations, including women with previous GDM, has recently been initiated.

REFERENCES

1. Freinkel N, Dooley SL, Metzger BE. Care of the pregnant woman with insulin-dependent diabetes mellitus. *N Engl J Med.* 1985;313:96–101.

2. Gabbe SG. Medical complications of pregnancy. Management of diabetes in pregnancy: six decades of experience. In: Pitkin RM, Zlatnik FJ, eds. *Yearbook of Obstetrics and Gynecology. Part 1. Obstetrics.* Chicago, Ill: Yearbook Medical Publishers; 1980;37–49.

3. Metzger BE, Phelps RL, Dooley SL. The mother in pregnancies complicated by diabetes mellitus. In: Porte D Jr, Sherwin RS, eds. *Ellenberg & Rifkin's Diabetes Mellitus.* 5th ed. Norwalk, Conn: Appleton & Lange; in press.

4. Buchanan TA, Unterman TG, Metzger BE. The medical management of diabetes in pregnancy. *Clin Perinatol.* 1985;12:625–650.

5. Metzger BE, Purdy LP, Phelps RL. Diabetes mellitus and pregnancy. In: DeGroot LJ, ed. *Endocrinology.* 3rd ed. Philadelphia, Pa: WB Saunders Co; 1994:1464–1481.

6. Mintz DH, Chez RA, Hutchinson DL. Subhuman primate pregnancy complicated by streptozotocin-induced diabetes mellitus. *J Clin Invest.* 1972;51:837–847.

7. Hytten FE, Leitch I. Components of weight gain. In: Hytten FE, Leitch I, eds. *The Physiology of Human Pregnancy.* 2nd ed. Oxford: Blackwell Scientific Publications; 1971:286–387.

8. Goodner CJ, Freinkel N. Carbohydrate metabolism in pregnancy. IV. Studies on the permeability of the rat placenta to 1131 insulin. *Diabetes.* 1961;10:383–392.

9. Pitkin RM, Spellacy WN. Physiologic adjustments in general. In: *Laboratory Indices of Nutritional Status in Pregnancy.* Washington, DC: National Academy of Sciences; 1978:1–8.

10. Shibasaki T, Odagiri E, Shizume K, Ling N. Corticotropin-releasing factor-like activity in human placental extracts. *J Clin Endocrinol Metab.* 1982;55:384–386.

11. Freinkel N. The Banting Lecture 1980: of pregnancy and progeny. *Diabetes.* 1980;29:1023–1035.

12. Freinkel N, Metzger BE. Metabolic changes in pregnancy. In: Foster DW, Wilson JD, eds. *Williams Textbook of Endocrinology.* 8th ed. Philadelphia, Pa: WB Saunders Co; 1992:993–1005.

13. Beck P, Daughaday WH. Human placental lactogen: studies of its acute metabolic effects and disposition in normal man. *J Clin Invest.* 1967;46:103–110.

14. Kalkhoff RK, Kim HJ. The influence of hormonal changes of pregnancy on maternal metabolism. In: *Pregnancy Metabolism, Diabetes and the Fetus.* Amsterdam: Excerpta Medica; 1979:29–46. CIBA Foundation Symposium no. 63.

15. Page EW. Human fetal nutrition and growth. *Am J Obstet Gynecol.* 1969;104:378–387.

16. Cahill GG Jr, Owen OE. Some observations on carbohydrate metabolism in man. In: Dickens F, Randle PJ, Whelan WJ, eds. *Carbohydrate Metabolism and Its Disorders.* New York, NY: Academic Press; 1968:497–522.

17. Young M. Placental transfer of glucose and amino acids. In: Camerini-Davalos RA, Cole HS, eds. *Early Diabetes in Early Life.* New York, NY: Academic Press; 1975:237–242.

18. Puavilai G, Drobny EC, Domont L, et al. Insulin receptors and insulin resistance in human pregnancy: evidence for a postreceptor defect in insulin action. *J Clin Endocrinol Metab.* 1982;54:247–253.

19. Freinkel N. Effects of the conceptus on maternal metabolism during pregnancy. In: Leibel BS, Wrenshall GA, eds. *On the Nature and Treatment of Diabetes.* Amsterdam: Excerpta Medica Foundation; 1965:679–691.

20. Herrera E, Knopp RH, Freinkel N. Carbohydrate metabolism in pregnancy. VI. Plasma fuels, insulin, liver composition, gluconeogenesis and nitrogen metabolism during late gestation in the fed and fasted rat. *J Clin Invest.* 1969;48:2260–2272.

21. Felig P, Lynch V. Starvation in human pregnancy: hypoglycemia, hypoinsulinemia, and hyperketonemia. *Science.* 1970;170:990–992.

22. Metzger BE, Freinkel N. Regulation of maternal protein metabolism and gluconeogenesis in the fasted state. In: Camerini-Davalos R, Cole H, eds. *Early Diabetes in Early Life.* New York, NY: Academic Press; 1975:303–311.

23. Metzger BE, Hare JW, Freinkel N. Carbohydrate metabolism in pregnancy. IX. Plasma levels of gluconeogenic fuels during fasting in the rat. *J Clin Endocrinol Metab.*1971;33:869–873.

24. Metgzer BE, Ravnikar V, Velesis R, et al. Accelerated starvation and the skipped breakfast in late normal pregnancy. *Lancet.* 1982;1:588–592.

25. Metzger BE, Freinkel N. Accelerated starvation in pregnancy: implications for dietary treatment of obesity and gestational diabetes mellitus. *Biol Neonate.* 1987;51:78–85.

26. Freinkel N, Metzger BE, Nitzan M, et al. Facilitated anabolism in late pregnancy: some novel maternal compensations for accelerated starvation. In: Malaise WJ, Pirart J, eds. *Proceedings of the VIIIth Congress of the International Diabetes Federation.* Amsterdam: Excerpta Medica; 1974:474–488. International Congress Series no. 312.

27. Phelps RL, Metzger BE, Freinkel N. Carbohydrate metabolism in pregnancy. XVII. Diurnal profiles of plasma glucose, insulin, free fatty acids, triglycerides, cholesterol and individual amino acids in late normal pregnancy. *Am J Obstet Gynecol.* 1981;140:730–736.

28. O'Sullivan JB, Mahan CM. Criteria for the oral glucose tolerance test in pregnancy. *Diabetes.* 1964; 13(27):82–85.

29. Freinkel N, Metzger BE. Pregnancy as a tissue culture experience: the critical implications of maternal metabolism for fetal development. In: *Pregnancy Metabolism, Diabetes and the Fetus.* Amsterdam: Excerpta Medica; 1979:3–23. CIBA Foundation Symposium no. 63.

30. Freinkel N, Lewis NJ, Johnson R, et al. Differential effects of age versus glycemic stimulation on the maturation of insulin stimulus-secretion coupling during culture of fetal rat islets. *Diabetes.* 1984;33:1028–1038.

31. Pedersen J. Weight and length at birth of infants of diabetic mothers. *Acta Endocrinol.* 1954;16:330–343.

32. Pettit DJ, Baird HH, Aleck KA. Excessive obesity in offspring of Pima Indian women with diabetes during pregnancy. *N Engl J Med.* 1983;308:242–245.

33. Pettit DJ, Aleck KA, Baird HA, Carraher MJ, Bennett PH, Knowler WC. Congenital susceptibility to NIDDM. Role of intrauterine environment. *Diabetes.* 1988;37:622–628.

34. Martin AO, Simpson JL, Ober C, et al. Frequency of diabetes mellitus in mothers of probands with gestational diabetes: possible maternal influence on the predisposition to gestational diabetes. *Am J Obstet Gynecol.* 1985;151:471–475.

35. Metzger BE, Silverman B, Freinkel N, Dooley SL, Ogata ES, Green OC. Amniotic fluid insulin concentration as a predictor of obesity. *Arch Dis Child.* 1990;65:1050–1052.

36. Silverman BL, Metzger BE, Cho NH, Loeb CA. Impaired glucose tolerance in adolescent offspring of diabetic mothers: relationship to fetal hyperinsulinism. *Diabetes Care.* 1995;18:611–617.

37. Alcolado JC, Alcolado R. Importance of maternal history of noninsulin dependent diabetic patients. *BMJ.* 1991;302:1178–1180.

38. Thomas F, Balkau B, Vauzelle-Kervrodan F, Papoz L, the CODIAB-INSERM-ZENECA Study Group. Maternal effect and familial aggregation in NIDDM. The CODIAB Study. *Diabetes.* 1994;43:63–66.

39. Gauguier D, Nelson I, Bernard C, et al. Higher maternal than paternal inheritance of diabetes in GK rats. *Diabetes.* 1994;43:220–224.

40. Aerts L, Holemans K, Van Assche FA. Maternal diabetes during pregnancy: consequences for the offspring. *Diabetes Metab Rev.* 1990;6:147–167.

41. Susa JB, Sehgal P, Schwartz R. Rhesus monkeys made exogenously hyperinsulinemic in utero as fetuses, display abnormal glucose homeostasis as pregnant adults and have macrosomic fetuses. *Diabetes.* 1993; 43(suppl 1):86A. Abstract.

42. Connell FA, Vadhiem C, Emmanuel I. Diabetes in pregnancy: a population based study of incidence, referral for care and perinatal mortality. *Am J Obstet Gynecol.* 1985;151:598–603.

43. National Diabetes Data Group. Classification and diagnosis of diabetes mellitus and other categories of glucose intolerance. *Diabetes.* 1979;28:1039–1057.

44. Freinkel N, Josimovich J, Conference Planning Committee. American Diabetes Association Workshop-Conference on Gestational Diabetes. Summary and recommendations. *Diabetes Care.* 1980;3:499–501.

45. Freinkel N. Summary and recommendations of the Second International Workshop-Conference on Gestational Diabetes Mellitus. *Diabetes.* 1985;34(suppl 2):123–126.

46. Metzger BE, the Organizing Committee. Summary and recommendations of the Third International Workshop-Conference on Gestational Diabetes Mellitus. *Diabetes.* 1991;40(suppl 2):197–201.

47. Hare JW. Maternal complications. In: Hare JW, ed. *Diabetes Complicating Pregnancy. The Joslin Clinic Method.* New York, NY: Alan R. Liss, Inc; 1989:81–98.

48. White P. Pregnancy and diabetes. Medical aspects. *Med Clin North Am.* 1965;49:1015–1024.

49. Ogata ES, Freinkel N, Metzger BE, et al. Perinatal islet function in gestational diabetes: assessment by cord

plasma C-peptide and amniotic fluid insulin. *Diabetes Care.* 1980;3:425–429.

50. Metzger BE, Phelps RL, Freinkel N, et al. Effects of gestational diabetes on diurnal profiles of plasma glucose, lipids and individual amino acids. *Diabetes Care.* 1980;3:402–409.

51. Freinkel N, Metzger BE, Phelps RL, et al. Gestational diabetes mellitus: heterogeneity of maternal age, weight, insulin secretion, HLA antigens, and islet cell antibodies and the impact of maternal metabolism on pancreative, ß-cell and somatic development in the offspring. *Diabetes.* 1985;34(suppl 2):1–7.

52. Warram JH, Krolewski AS, Gottlieb MS, et al. Differences in risk of insulin-dependent diabetes in offspring of diabetic mothers and diabetic fathers. *N Engl J Med.* 1984;311:149–152.

53. Hare JW, White P. Pregnancy in diabetes complicated by vascular disease. *Diabetes.* 1977;26:953–955.

54. Reece EA, Coustan DR, Hayslett JP, et al. Diabetic nephropathy: pregnancy performance and fetomaternal outcome. *Am J Obstet Gynecol.* 1988;159:56–66.

55. Phelps RL, Sakol P, Metzger BE, et al. Correlation of changes in diabetic retinopathy during pregnancy with regulation of hyperglycemia. *Arch Ophthalmol.* 1986;104:1806–1810.

56. Chew EY, Mills JL, Metzger BE, et al. Metabolic control and progression of retinopathy: the diabetes in early pregnancy study. *Diabetes Care.* 1995;18:631–637.

57. Diabetes Control and Complications Trial Research Group. The effect of intensive treatment of diabetes on the development and progression of long-term complications in insulin-dependent diabetes mellitus. *N Engl J Med.* 1993;329:977–986.

58. Lauritzen T, Larsen KF, Larsen H, et al. Effect of year of near-normal blood glucose levels on retinopathy in insulin-dependent diabetics. *Lancet.* 1983;1:200–203.

59. Kroc Collaborative Study Group. Blood glucose control and the evolution of diabetic retinopathy and albuminuria. *N Engl J Med.* 1984;311:365–372.

60. Freinkel N, Metzger BE. Emerging challenges in diabetes and pregnancy: diabetic embryopathy and gestational diabetes. In: Alberti KGMM, Krall LP, eds. *The Diabetes Annual/4.* Amsterdam: Elsevier Science Publishers; 1988:179–201.

61. From research to practice. Diabetes and birth defects: insights from the 1980s, prevention in the 1990s. *Diabetes Spectrum.* 1990;3:150–184.

62. Mills JL, Baker L, Goldman AS. Malformations in infants of diabetic mothers occur before the seventh gestational week: Implications for treatment. *Diabetes.* 1979;28:292–293.

63. Cousins L, Rigg L, Hollingsworth D, et al. The 24 hour excursion and diurnal rhythm of glucose, insulin, and C-peptide in normal pregnancy. *Am J Obstet Gynecol.* 1980;136:483–488.

64. Gillmer MDG, Beard RW, Brooke FM, et al. Carbohydrate metabolism in pregnancy. Part I—diurnal plasma glucose profile in normal and diabetic women. *BMJ.* 1975;3:399–404.

65. Persson B, Lunell N-O. Metabolic control in diabetic pregnancy. Variations in plasma concentrations of glucose, free fatty acids, glycerol, ketone bodies, insulin and human chorionic somatomammotropin during the last trimester. *Am J Obstet Gynecol.* 1975;122:737–745.

66. Buchanan TA, Schemmer JK, Frienkel N. Embryotoxic effects of brief maternal insulin-hypoglycemia during organogenesis in the rat. *J Clin Invest.* 1986;78:643–649.

67. Pedersen J. *The Pregnant Diabetic and Her Newborn. Problems and Management.* 2nd. ed. Copenhagen: Munksgaard; 1977.

68. Knight GL, Palomaki GE. Maternal serum alpha-fetoprotein and the detection of open neural tube defects. In: Elias S, Simpson JL, eds. *Maternal Serum Screening for Fetal Genetic Disorders.* New York, NY: Churchill Livingstone; 1992;41–58.

69. Ogata ES, Sabbagha R, Metzger BE, Phelps RL, Depp R, Freinkel N. Serial ultrasonography to assess evolving fetal macrosomia: studies in 23 pregnant diabetic women. *JAMA.* 1980;243:2405–2408.

70. Landon MB, Mintz MC, Gabbe SG. Sonographic evaluation of fetal abdominal growth: predictor of the large-for-gestational-age infant in pregnancies complicated by diabetes mellitus. *Am J Obstet Gynecol.* 1990;163:115–121.

71. Keller JD, Metzger BE, Dooley SL, Tamura RK, Sabbagha RE, Freinkel N. Infants of diabetic mothers with accelerated fetal growth by ultrasonography: are they all alike? *Am J Obstet Gynecol.* 1990;163:893–897.

72. Philipps A, Dubin JW, Matti PJ, Raye JR. Arterial hypoxemia and hyperinsulinemia in the chronically hyperglycemic fetal lamb. *Pediatr Res.* 1982;16:653–658.

73. Philipps AF, Porte PJ, Stabinsky S, Rosenkrantz TS, Raye JR. Effects of chronic fetal hyperglycemia upon oxygen consumption in the ovine uterus and conceptus. *J Clin Invest.* 1984;74:279–286.

74. Philipps AF, Rosenkrantz TS, Porte PJ, Raye JR. The effects of chronic fetal hyperglycemia on substrate uptake by the ovine fetus and conceptus. *Pediatr Res.* 1985;19:659–666.

75. Oats JN. Obstetrical management of patients with diabetes in pregnancy. *Baillieres Clin Obstet Gynaecol.* 1991;5:395–411.

76. Amankwah KS, Prentice RL, Fleury FJ. The incidence of gestational diabetes. *Obstet Gynecol.* 1977;49:497–498.

77. Coustan DR, Nelson C, Carpenter MW, Carr SR, Rotondo L, Widness JA. Maternal age and screening for gestational diabetes: a population-based suvey. *Obstet Gynecol.* 1989;73:557–561.

78. Dooley SL, Metzger BE, Cho NH. Gestational diabetes mellitus: the influence of race on disease prevalence and perinatal outcome in a U.S. population. *Diabetes.* 1991;40(suppl 2):25–29.

79. Beischer Na, Oats JN, Henry OA, Sheedy MT, Walstab JE. Incidence and severity of gestational diabetes mellitus according to country of birth in women living in Australia. *Diabetes.* 1991;40(suppl 2):35–38.

80. Hod M, Merlob P, Friedman S, Schoenfeld A, Ovadia J. Gestational diabetes mellitus: a survey of perinatal complications in the 1980s. *Diabetes.* 1991;40(suppl 2):74–78.

81. Philipson EH, Kalhan SC, Rosen MG, et al. Gestational diabetes mellitus. Is further improvement necessary? *Diabetes.* 1985;34(suppl 2):55–60.

82. Widness JA, Cowett RM, Coustan DR, et al. Neonatal morbidities in infants of mothers with glucose intolerance in pregnancy. *Diabetes.* 1985;34(suppl 2):61–65.

83. Metzger BE, Bybee DE, Freinkel N, et al. Gestational diabetes mellitus: correlations between the phenotypic and genotypic characteristics of the mother and abnormal glucose tolerance during the first year postpartum. *Diabetes.* 1985;34(suppl 2):111–115.

84. O'Sullivan JB. Long term follow up of gestational diabetes. In: Camerini-Davalos RA, Cole HS, eds. *Early Diabetes in Early Life.* New York, NY: Academic Press; 1975:503–518.

85. Mestman JH, Anderson GV, Guadalupe V. Follow-up study of 360 subjects with abnormal carbohydrate metabolism during pregnancy. *Obstet Gynecol.* 1972;39:421–425.

86. Metzger BE, Cho NH, Roston SM, Radvany R. Prepregnancy weight and antepartum insulin secretion predict glucose tolerance five years after gestational diabetes mellitus. *Diabetes Care.* 1993;16:1598–1605.

87. Merkatz IR, Duchon MA, Yamashita TS, et al. A pilot community-based screening program for gestational diabetes. *Diabetes Care.* 1980;3:453–457.

88. O'Sullivan JB, Mahan CM, Charles D, et al. Screening criteria for high-risk gestational diabetic patients. *Am J Obstet Gynecol.* 1973;116:895–900.

89. Buschard K, Buch I, Molsted-Pedersen L, Hougaard P, Kühl C. Increased incidence of true type I diabetes acquired during pregnancy. *BMJ.* 1987;294:275–279.

90. Felig P. Body fuel metabolism and diabetes mellitus in pregnancy. *Med Clin North Am.* 1977;61:43–66.

91. Coustan DR, Imarah J. Prophylactic insulin treatment of gestational diabetes reduces the incidence of macrosomia, operative delivery and birth trauma. *Am J Obstet Gynecol.* 1984;150:836–842.

92. Drexel H, Bichler A, Sailer S, et al. Prevention of perinatal morbidity by tight control in gestational diabetes mellitus. *Diabetes Care.* 1988;11:761–768.

93. Mazze RS, Langer O. Primary, secondary, and tertiary prevention: program for diabetes in pregnancy. *Diabetes Care.* 1988;11:263–268.

94. Harris MI. Gestational diabetes may represent discovery of preexisting glucose intolerance. *Diabetes Care.* 1988;11:402–411.

95. Wollf C, Verlohren H-J, Arlt P, Mechmedowa F, Kripylo C, Wetzler C. Development of metabolic disturbances in patients with gestational diabetes—postgestational classification of carbohydrate tolerance. *Zentralbl Gynakol.* 1987;109:88–97.

96. Farrell J, Forrest JM, Storey GNB, Yue DK, Shearman RP, Turtle JR. Gestational diabetes—infant malformations and subsequent maternal glucose tolerance. *Aust NZ J Obstet Gynaecol.* 1986;26:11–16.

97. Al-Shawaf T, Moghraby S, Akiel A. Does impaired glucose tolerance imply a risk in pregnancy? *Br J Obstet Gynecol.* 1988;95:1036–1041.

98. O'Sullivan JB. The interaction between pregnancy, diabetes, and long-term maternal outcome. In: Reece EA, Coustan DR, eds. *Diabetes Mellitus in Pregnancy: Principles and Practice.* New York, NY: Churchill Livingstone; 1988:575–585.

99. Catalano PM, Vargo KM, Bernstein IM, Amini SB. Incidence and risk factors associated with abnormal postpartum glucose tolerance in women with gestational diabetes. *Am J Obstet Gynecol.* 1991;165:914–919.

100. Damon P, Kühl C, Bertelsen A, Molsted-Pedersen L. Predictive factors for the development of diabetes in women with previous gestational diabetes mellitus. *Am J Obstet Gynecol.* 1992;167:607–616.

101. Food and Nutrition Board. *Recommended Dietary Allowances.* 10th ed. Washington, DC: National Academy Press; 1989:1–38.

102. American Diabetes Association. Nutrition principles for the management of diabetes and related complications (techinical review). *Diabetes Care.* 1994;17:490–518.

103. Ney D, Hollingsworth DR. Nutritional management of pregnancy complicated by diabetes: historical perspective. *Diabetes Care.* 1981;4:647–655.

104. National Academy of Sciences. *Nutrition in Pregnancy, Part I: Weight Gain.* Washington, DC: National Academy Press; 1990:10–13.

105. WHO (World Health Organization). *Handbook on Human Nutritional Requirements.* Report of R Passmore, BM Nicol, M Narayana Rao, GH Beaton, and EM Demayer. Geneva: WHO; 1974.

106. Naeye RL. Weight gain and the outcome of pregnancy. *Am J Obstet Gynecol.* 1979;135:3–9.

107. Phelps RL, Metzger BE. Caloric restriction in gestational diabetes mellitus: when and how much? (Editorial). *J Am Coll Nutr.* 1992;11:259–262.

108. Churchill JA, Berendes HW. Intelligence of children whose mothers had acetonuria during pregnancy. In: *Perinatal Factors Affecting Human Development.* Washington, DC: Pan American Health Organization; 1969:30. Science Publication no. 185.

109. Stehbens JA, Baker GL, Kitchell M. Outcome at ages 1, 3, and 5 years of children born to diabetic women. *Am J Obstet Gynecol.* 1977;127:408–413.

110. Rizzo T, Metzger BE, Burns WJ, Burns KC. Correlations between antepartum maternal metabolism and child intelligence. *N Engl J Med.* 1991;325:911–916.

111. Pedersen J. Management of diabetic pregnancy and the newborn infant. In: Pedersen J, ed. *The Pregnant Diabetic and Her Newborn.* Copenhagen: Williams & Wilkins; 1977:223.

112. Garrow JS. Underfeeding and overfeeding and their clinical consequences. *Proc Nutr Soc.* 1976;35:363–368.

113. Coetzee EJ, Jackson WPU, Bemman PA. Ketonuria in pregnancy—with special reference to calorie-restricted food intake in obese diabetics. *Diabetes.* 1980;29:177–181.

114. Borberg C, Gillmer MW, Brunner EJ, et al. Obesity in pregnancy: the effect of dietary advice. *Diabetes Care.* 1980;3:476–481.

115. Dornhorst A, Nichols JSD, Probst F, et al. Caloric restriction for the treatment of gestational diabetes. *Diabetes.* 1991;40(suppl 2):161–164.

116. Pitkin RN, Reynolds WA, Filer LJJ, et al. Placental transmission and fetal distribution of saccharin. *Am J Obstet Gynecol.* 1971;111:280–286.

117. Sturtevant FM. Use of aspartame in pregnancy. *Int J Fertil.* 1985;30:85–87.

118. Buchanan TA, Metzger BE, Freinkel N. Accelerated starvation in late pregnancy: a comparison between obese women with and without gestational diabetes mellitus. *Am J Obstet Gynecol.* 1990;162:1015–1020.

119. Knopp RH, Mages MS, Rassys V, Benedetti T, Bonet B. Hypocaloric diets and ketogenesis in the management of obese gestational diabetic women. *J Am Coll Nutr.* 1991;10:649–667.

120. Maresh M, Gillmer MDG, Beard RW, Alderson CS, Bloxham BA, Elkeles RS. The effect of diet and insulin on metabolic profiles of women with gestational diabetes mellitus. *Diabetes.* 1985;34(suppl 2):89–93.

121. Jovanovic-Peterson L, Peterson CM. Dietary manipulation as a primary treatment strategy for pregnancy complicated by diabetes. *J Am Coll Nutr.* 1990;9:320–325.

122. Nutritional Management during Pregnancy in Preexisting Diabetes. In: *Medical Management of Pregnancy Complicated by Diabetes.* Alexandria, VA: American Diabetes Association; 1993.

123. Whichelow MJ, Doddridge MC. Lactation in diabetic women. *BMJ.* 1983;287:649–650.

124. Kostraba JN, Cruickshanks KJ, Lawler-Heavners J, et al. Early exposure to cow's milk and solid foods in infancy, genetic predisposition and risk of IDDM. *Diabetes.* 1993;42:288–295.

125. Stowers JM, Sutherland HW, Kerridge DF. Long-range implications for the mother. *Diabetes.* 1985;34(suppl 2):106–110.

Chapter 27

Considerations in Caring for Older Persons with Diabetes

Sue McLaughlin

EFFECT OF AN AGING POPULATION ON THE PREVALENCE AND INCIDENCE OF DIABETES

Advancements in medical technology and the institution of preventive health practices have enabled Americans to live longer. The percentage of individuals older than the age of 65 has increased tenfold in the past 90 years, from 3.1 million in 1900 to 31.2 million in 1990. By the year 2030, there will be about 66 million older adults, representing nearly 22% of the population of this country.[1]

As we age, there is an increased prevalence and incidence of impaired glucose tolerance and diabetes, as illustrated in Figure 27-1. Approximately 18% of the individuals older than age 65 have diabetes, and this percentage increases to 40% for those older than age 80.[2] This makes it one of the most common medical problems for this subgroup of our population. Prevalence is higher in blacks, Hispanics, and some native American populations.[3,4]

FACTORS PREDISPOSING THE OLDER PERSON TO DEVELOP DIABETES

Most older people with diabetes have type II or non–insulin-dependent diabetes mellitus (NIDDM). Factors believed to predispose the older person to develop type II diabetes are shown in Figure 27-2. Of these factors, most researchers in this area agree that the main reason for the glucose intolerance of aging is due to a decreased response to insulin, or insulin resistance. Whether the insulin resistance is itself a primary change or is due to the more inactive status of many older people is controversial. Broughton and associates[5] in the United Kingdom demonstrated that when young people were carefully selected to be as inactive as older subjects, there was no difference in insulin action between the two groups. This suggests that inactivity, rather than age, is the cause of insulin resistance in older people.

DETECTION AND DIAGNOSIS

Type II diabetes is often difficult to detect in the older person. Symptoms of weight loss and fatigue or one of the complications of diabetes are more commonly presented than complaints of classic symptoms of polyuria, polyphagia, and polydipsia.[6,7]

Unfortunately, the cumulative effects of unrecognized hyperglycemia may have caused considerable damage by the time diagnosis is made. Diabetes may be detected during an ophthalmologic examination (when diabetic retinopathy is identified) or during an office visit (when a woman's chief complaint is burning on urination or vaginal discomfort, associated with a urinary tract or vaginal infection, exacerbated by hyperglycemia). Gale and associates[8] found that in adult patients who were hospitalized with severe uncontrolled diabetes, 35% of the patients were older than 50, 38% had previously undiagnosed diabetes, and 43% of cases were fatal.

Diagnosis of diabetes in the older person is based on the same criteria as is used for younger individuals[9] (see Chapter 1).

ESTABLISHING BLOOD GLUCOSE TREATMENT GOALS

It is known that blood glucose increases by about 1 to 2 mg/dL per decade after 30 to 40 years of age. As well, postprandial blood glucose may increase by as much as 8 to 20 mg/dL per decade.[7] Due to this seemingly "normal" rise in blood glucose as we age, some clinicians have suggested that treatment goals be age-adjusted.[10] At this time, however, the recommendations for blood glucose goals, set forth by the American Diabetes Association (ADA), are no different for older adults than for younger individuals.[11]

As is true for other age groups, establishment of individual goals for blood glucose should be developed by the patient and his or her family or caregiver in consultation with the health care team.

FACTORS TO CONSIDER FOR MANAGING DIABETES IN THE OLDER PERSON

The factors that should be considered when determining a management plan for the older person with diabetes are shown in Exhibit 27-1. Several of these factors are discussed at greater length.

Effects of the Physiologic Changes of Aging

The physiologic changes of aging present additional challenges for the older person with diabetes. Changes that have the potential to directly affect nutritional status or that may be slowed by nutrition intervention are discussed further.

Changes in Dentition and Swallowing Ability

Available data suggest that 50% of the persons older than age 65 are edentulous.[12] Tooth loss, poorly fitting dentures, and sensitive teeth and gums can make chewing food difficult. If any of these problems exist, nutritious foods such as meat and fresh fruit and vegetables may be avoided, and nutritional deficiencies may result.

Many older persons also have difficulty swallowing due to decreases in saliva secretion and esophageal motility. Food may seem drier and,

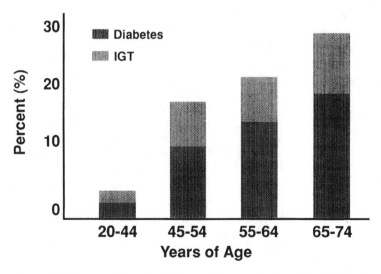

Figure 27-1 Prevalence of Diabetes and Impaired Glucose Tolerance in the United States. *Source:* Reprinted from Halter JB. Geriatric patients, in *Therapy for Diabetes Mellitus and Related Disorders,* Lebovitz HE (Ed), with permission of the American Diabetes Association; Copyright © 1991: 156.

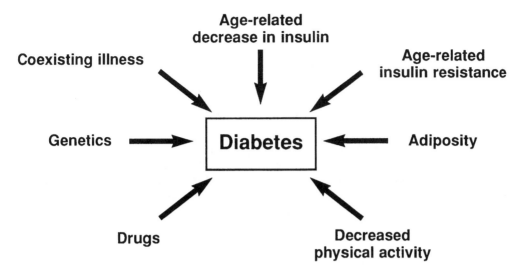

Figure 27-2 Factors Predisposing the Elderly to Diabetes. *Source:* Adapted from Halter JB. *Diabetes Update: Elderly Patients with Non–Insulin-Dependent Diabetes Mellitus.* Kalamazoo, MI: The Upjohn Company; 1990. Copyright © 1994, American Diabetes Association.

therefore, less appealing. Swallowing may also be more difficult, because of decreased mastication and ability to form an adequate bolus of food. The decrease in saliva secretion can also effect the digestive process because the initial digestion of starches, which begins in the mouth, is slowed.[12]

Exhibit 27-1 Factors To Consider for Managing Diabetes in the Older Person

- Remaining life expectancy
- Effects of the physiologic changes of aging
- Patient commitment
- Availability of support services
- Economic issues
- Presence of multiple medical diagnoses
- Presence of diabetes complications
- Use of multiple medications

Source: Adapted from Halter JB, Geriatric patients, in *Therapy for Diabetes Mellitus and Related Disorders*, Lebovitz HE, ed. With permission of the American Diabetes Association, Copyright © 1991: 157.

Poorly controlled diabetes can also lead to gingivitis and periodontitis. Good oral hygiene is particularly important. Texture modification of foods and use of oral supplements may be necessary, in some cases, for nutritional needs to be met.

Changes in Gastrointestinal Function

Age-related decreases in hydrochloric acid, pepsin, and gastric mucous secretion may cause poorer digestion and absorption of nutrients (eg, calcium, iron, and vitamin B_{12}), contributing to gastrointestinal distress (bloating and flatulence) and nutritional deficiencies.[13]

Constipation is a common and chronic problem among older persons, reported to occur in 96% of those older than the age of 65.[14] Contributing causes of this problem include limited dietary fiber intake, use of certain medications (eg, narcotic analgesics) for pain relief, laxative abuse, hypothyroidism, decreased muscle tone in colonic walls, and inadequate fluid intake.

A liberal fluid intake and adequate intake of dietary fiber should help alleviate problems with constipation. Sugar-free powders made from plant fibers can be mixed with water and used if needed.

Changes in Renal and Bladder Function

Several renal changes occur with age. A decline is seen in the number of nephrons, total blood flow, glomerular filtration rate, urinary creatinine excretion, renal concentration ability, sodium conservation, and the glucose resorption rate. As a result of these changes, the older person's ability to handle sodium and protein in the diet is affected.

Bladder function also decreases with age. It is more difficult for the bladder to secrete a small volume of concentrated urine than a larger volume at a lower concentration. This contributes to the increased incidence of urinary tract infections in older people with diabetes. A liberal fluid intake (ie, 8 to 10 cups/d) is recommended to help prevent or alleviate problems.

Changes in the Nervous System

Loss of memory is often associated with the aging process. However, many older persons who are socially and intellectually stimulated show little or no memory loss. Unfortunately, older persons who do suffer from dementia or Alzheimer's disease are at a significant risk for malnutrition, as they may forget to eat. Also, omission or overdosing of medication (diabetes and others) may occur. The importance of having adequate caregivers available is obvious if needs are to be met.

Other nervous system changes include loss of taste, smell, vision, hearing, and touch.

Loss of Taste. It has been estimated that at age 70, a person has 70% fewer taste buds than at age 30. This is due to an inability of taste cells to regenerate.[15] Deficiencies of vitamin A or zinc are also believed to be partially responsible for this decline in function. Various medications and renal failure have also been shown to cause deterioration in the sense of taste.

As a result of the decreased taste sensation, older adults may desire to increase their use of salt and sugar to improve taste satisfaction. This promotes a particular challenge for the older person for whom a restricted diet has been prescribed.

Loss of Smell. The threshold for detecting odors has been shown to be 12 times higher in older adults than their younger counterparts.[16] This is particularly significant, because most food flavor is detected by olfactory perception.[17] Diminished smell acuity may have a large impact on an individual's interest in food and his or her resultant intake.

For these reasons, it may be important to focus on the nonolfactory attributes of a meal (ie, color, texture variations, plate presentation, ambiance) to maintain quality of eating and adequate intake for the older person.

Loss of Vision. Several visual changes occur due to the aging process: a decrease in acuity and the ability to focus on nearby objects, and an increased likelihood for senile cataracts. Older individuals may have difficulty reading educational materials, food labels, or drawing up insulin dosages accurately.

Loss of Hearing. Hearing loss occurs in 40 to 60% of people aged 65 or older and affects more men than women.[18] It is important to assess a patient's hearing level at the beginning of a teaching session and to never make assumptions about what the older person has heard.

Loss of Touch. Older individuals with crippled hands may have trouble preparing food, as well as difficulty feeding themselves. This, in turn, may affect food intake and nutritional status and result in wide fluctuations in blood glucose levels.

Evaluation of supportive services is necessary, and a visit with the occupational therapist often proves helpful.

Changes in the Skeletal System

Many older persons suffer from osteoporosis. This is due in part to decreased intestinal calcium absorption, as well as inadequate dietary intake, and several other factors.[19] In addition to the discomfort and pain caused by the resultant shift in normal bone structure, these individuals are at increased risk for suffering a fracture. In addition to a calcium-rich diet and the use of calcium supplements, a regular exercise routine that is weight-bearing can help to maintain bone density and will enhance glycemic control as well.

Changes in Immune Function

A decline in immune system function often occurs with age. Adequate dietary intakes of protein and zinc will help prevent recurrent illness and promote adequate wound healing. The current recommended daily allowance (RDA) for zinc is 15 mg/d for men and 12 mg/d for women. Zinc is found in meat, liver, eggs, and seafood.[20,21]

Presence of Multiple Medical Diagnoses

Between 80 and 86% of people aged 65 years and older have one or more chronic health conditions, which may include osteoarthritis, hypertension, cardiovascular disease, coronary artery disease, and emphysema.[22]

Coronary artery disease is the most prevalent illness and leading cause of death in persons older than age 65. Individuals with diabetes who have a myocardial infarction have a lower rate of survival at 1 and 5 years postincident than their nondiabetic counterparts.[23]

The incidence of hypertension also increases with age, particularly in the black population.[23] The combination of diabetes and hypertension significantly increases the incidence of renal disease or a cardiovascular or cerebrovascular accident in the person with diabetes.

Presence of Diabetes Complications

In addition to coexisting medical disorders, many older persons with diabetes experience the acute and long-term complications of the disease. These potential problems threaten the safety and quality of life for the older person.

Acute Complications

Hypoglycemia. Hypoglycemia is the most commonly occurring diabetic complication in older people and is associated with improved glycemic control. It may occur in the older person taking either insulin or oral hypoglycemic agents (OHAs).

For those with insulin-dependent diabetes mellitus (IDDM), it has been reported to induce electrocardiographic changes that are identical to ischemia and has also been shown to mimic cardiovascular disease.

A 20 to 31% incidence of hypoglycemia has been reported in older persons treated with OHAs.[10] It is observed most often during the first few years of OHA therapy and in patients taking medications known to potentiate the action of OHAs.

Another potential complication associated with hypoglycemia is the increased likelihood that falls may occur, resulting in injury and the chance of a bone fracture.

Medical nutrition therapy for the older person with diabetes must include information regarding potential causes, signs and symptoms, treatment, and prevention of recurrence for this acute complication, with emphasis on consistent eating patterns including meals and between-meal snacks as needed.

Hyperglycemia. Uncontrolled hyperglycemia is not a benign condition for individuals of any age. Table 27-1 lists some of the problems and discomforts caused by hyperglycemia that adversely affects the quality of life for the older person with diabetes.[24]

Hyperosmolar Hyperglycemic Nonketonic Syndrome. Left unchecked, uncontrolled hyperglycemia may progress to an even more severe condition known as hyperosmolar hyperglycemic nonketonic syndrome (HHNS). It is found more commonly in the older person than diabetic ketoacidosis (due to fewer older persons with IDDM) and is a condition of equal severity.

The four major clinical features of HHNS are (1) severe hyperglycemia (blood glucose greater than 600 mg/dL), (2) absence of or slight ketosis, (3) plasma or serum hyperosmolality (340 mOsm), and (4) profound dehydration.[25] Precipitating causes of this condition include the use of medications (ie, diuretics, phenytoins, ß-blockers, and glucocorticoids), surgical stress, infections, loss of thirst, and renal disease.

When initially seen, most patients have had polyuria and polydipsia for days to weeks and are therefore markedly dehydrated, with dry mucous membranes and doughy skin. The mentally alert patients usually complain of extreme thirst, weakness, and fatigue. For others, mental status may range from mild confusion to hallucinations to coma.

Treatment of HHNS includes hospitalization with insulin administration and fluid replacement. Therapy should be tailored to the needs of the individual. The amount of fluid lost usually contains about 60 mEq/L of sodium and potassium. To prevent the occurrence of cerebral edema, the blood glucose level should be lowered cautiously and the hyperosmolarity should be reversed slowly as well. To avoid hypo-glycemia, initial insulin dosages should be small, because some of these patients will be extremely sensitive to insulin. The mortality rate for HHNS is high, occurring in about 12 to 50% of patients.[26]

Chronic Complications

In addition to the acute complications just discussed, the older person with diabetes may develop long-term complications. This may occur if asymptomatic, undetected hyperglycemia was present for several years before diagnosis.

Macrovascular Complications. There is a twofold increased risk for myocardial infarction, stroke, and renal insufficiency compared with others of the same age who do not have diabetes. Also, the risk for amputation is increased almost tenfold.[2]

Table 27-1 Effects of Uncontrolled Hyperglycemia on the Older Person with Diabetes

Effect of Hyperglycemia	Resultant Problem
1. Altered ability of endogenous opioids to bind to their receptors	Diminished pain threshold
2. Osmotic diuresis	Incontinence Insomnia and nocturia; blurred vision; possible cognitive impairments; weight loss; loss of muscle mass, strength, mobility, and stability; hyperosmolar hyperglycemic nonketotic syndrome Sodium depletion and dehydration, with possible hypotension in some people Trace mineral deficiency (ie, zinc, chromium, magnesium)
3. Increased platelet adhesiveness	Increased atherosclerosis with increased chance for myocardial infarction (MI) or cardiovascular accident (CVA) and poorer recovery post-accident
4. Impaired granulocyte and macrophage function	Increased incidence of infection and poor wound healing
5. Increased red blood cell reformability	Aggravated peripheral vascular disease
6. Altered ability to aid tissue repair/restoration due to decreased nutrients available to tissues	Accelerated aging

Microvascular Complications. Microvascular complications such as retinopathy or nephropathy may also be present. Macular edema is the major cause of visual loss in older persons with diabetes. Cataracts, glaucoma, and third nerve palsies also appear to be more prevalent in these individuals than their nondiabetic counterparts. There is an increased risk of developing end-stage renal disease, as well as the age-related decline in kidney function and increased prevalence of hypertension, as mentioned earlier.

Neuropathy. Sensorimotor neuropathy (ie, loss of sensation in the hands and feet) may cause an older person to burn him- or herself on the stove or to have an injury to a foot or toe go unnoticed until infection sets in.

Autonomic neuropathy may cause bladder dysfunction, resulting in urinary incontinence and/or recurrent urinary tract infections. It may also contribute to constipation problems. Blood pressure regulation may also be affected, resulting in orthostatic or postprandial hypotension, which may increase the risk for falls and subsequent injuries.[23]

Use of Multiple Medications

The presence of multiple medical diagnoses in the older population is accompanied by an increased usage of prescription and over-the-counter (OTC) medications. Individuals older than age 65 take an average of 5.6 prescribed medications per day,[27] as well as a wide variety of OTC drugs.

Many of these medications have the potential to have an effect on nutritional status in several ways. They may suppress or stimulate the appetite or alter digestion, absorption, metabolism, utilization, or excretion of a nutrient. Table 27-2 lists the effects that various medications have on the nutritional status of the older person. Table 27-3 identifies some of the medications that commonly interfere with blood glucose control.[28–30]

As an integral part of the diabetes management team, the registered dietitian should become familiar with the effects of these medications, so that potential problems, as well as management solutions, may be identified.

COMPONENTS OF MEDICAL TREATMENT FOR THE OLDER PERSON WITH DIABETES

Components of treatment for the older person with diabetes include medical nutrition therapy, exercise, diabetes medications, if needed, and blood glucose monitoring.

Medical Nutrition Therapy

The goals of medical nutrition therapy for the older person with diabetes include:

- Assist in meeting goals for glycemic control
- Provide adequate calories to promote weight maintenance, loss, or gain, as appropriate
- Provide adequate calories and nutrients to prevent nutrition deficiencies and malnutrition
- Assist in meeting goals for control of hypertension, lipid disorders, and other medical problems
- Identify diabetes management goals that promote safety, quality of life, and health

Although the importance of glycemic control for the older individual with diabetes should be underscored, it must be balanced with an equal concern for preventing nutritional deficiencies. The meal plan must incorporate individual preferences, as well as ethnic influences and customs. It must also include modifications that will promote positive outcomes for accompanying medical conditions.

Calorie Requirements and Body Weight

Calorie needs are known to decrease by 20 to 30% during the 40 to 70 years that pass between young adulthood and old age.[31] This is believed

Table 27-2 Effects of Drugs on Nutritional Status of the Elderly

Mechanism	Drug	Nutritional Implication
Intake of food		
Increased appetite	Lithium carbonate	Possible weight gain
Decreased appetite	Amphetamines	Decreased caloric intake
Taste sensitivity	Cocaine	Dehydration; decreased taste sensitivity
	Lidocaine	Decreased salt and sweet sensitivity
Absorption of nutrients	Mineral oil	↓ Carotene, vitamins A, D, K absorption
	Neomycin	↓ Absorption of fat, carbohydrate, protein, fat-soluble vitamins, vitamin B_{12}, calcium, iron
	Colchicine	↑ Loss of fat, carotene, Na, K, vitamin B_{12}, and lactose
	Tetracyclines	↓ Absorption of calcium, iron, magnesium, xylose, amino acids, and fat
		↓ Synthesis of vitamin K by intestinal bacteria Can cause steatorrhea
	Cathartics	Intestinal calcium and potassium loss; glucose absorption
	Phenolphthalein	↓ Absorption of vitamin D and calcium
	Potassium chloride	↓ Absorption of vitamin B_{12}
	Antacids	↓ Absorption of iron and calcium
Metabolism affect	Methotrexate	Folate antagonist
	Phenytoin	↓ Serum levels of folate, vitamin B_{12}, pyridoxine, 25–)H vitamin D_3, and calcium; possible osteomalacia
	Corticosteroids	↓ Absorption of calcium and phosphorous
		↑ Urinary excretion of vitamin C, calcium, potassium, zinc, and nitrogen
		↓ Serum zinc
		↑ Blood glucose, serum triglycerides, serum cholesterol
Increased excretion	Aspirin	↑ Urinary folate excretion
	D Penicillamine	↑ Urinary excretion of pyridoxine, zinc, and copper
	Penicillin	↑ Urinary excretion of potassium
	Tetracyclines	↑ Urinary excretion of vitamin C, riboflavin, nitrogen, folic acid, and niacin
	Thiazides	↑ Urinary excretion of potassium, magnesium, zinc, and riboflavin
		↓ Carbohydrate tolerance
		Possible potassium and magnesium depletion

Source: Reprinted with permission from *The Female Patient* (1982;7:PC32/21), Copyright © 1982, PW Communications Inc.

to be due to the reduction in lean body mass, with resultant reduction in basal metabolic rate. Failure to exercise regularly or limit portion sizes of food may result in a net weight gain over the years. Evidence has shown that there is a strong association between body weight and the prevalence of diabetes, with an increase in body weight promoting insulin resistance and hyperinsulinemia. For every 20% increase over an individual's ideal body weight, the risk of diabetes increases more than twofold.[7]

Although obesity is uncommon in the older population as a whole, it is more prominent in both women and men older than 65 who have diabetes than their nondiabetic counterparts, occurring in 25% of women aged 65 to 74 with diabetes, compared with 15% without diabetes, and in 6% of men this age with diabetes compared with 1.5% of those without diabetes.[32]

Because older individuals are at risk for nutritional deficiencies and malnutrition, weight loss to improve glycemic control and associated medical conditions such as hypertension and hyperlipidemias should be gradual (ie, 0.5 to 1 lb/wk). A modest weight reduction of as little as 10 to 20 pounds has been shown to improve glycemic control.[33]

Of course, not all older persons with diabetes are obese. It has been suggested that weight reduction not be implemented for those older than 70 years of age unless they are at least 20% overweight.[29]

Nutrient Composition of the Diet

As the ADA's 1994 Nutrition Recommendations suggest, the ideal composition of the diabetic diet is unknown at this time.[34] Guidelines should be based on the individual needs of the older person, with consideration of blood glucose goals and the presence of associated medical conditions that will respond favorably to changes in dietary habits.[30] Long-established eating patterns (ie, where, when, and with whom a person eats), as well as food preferences and

Table 27-3 Medications That Commonly Interfere with Blood Glucose Control

Potentiate Hypoglycemia	*Potentiate Hyperglycemia*
• Alcohol	• Corticosteroids (Prednisone)
• Allopurinol (Lopurin)	• Some diuretics, such as furosemide (Lasix) and all thiazide diuretics
• Anticholinergics, such as dicyclomine (Bentyl)	
• ß-adrenergic antagonists, such as atenolol (Tenormin) and metoprolol (Lopressor)	• Epinephrine (Primatene Mist)
	• Estrogens
• Clofibrate (Novofibrate)	• Niacin (vitamin B_3)
• Haloperidol (Haldol)	• Phenothiazines, such as chlorpromazine (Thorazine)
• H_2-receptor antagonists, such as cimetidine (Tagamet) and ranitidine (Zantac)	
	• Phenytoin (Dilantin)
• Monoamine oxidase inhibitors, such as phenelzine sulfate (Nardil)	• Rifampin (Rifadin)
• Phenylbutazone (Azolid)	• Sympathomimetics, such as theophylline (Duraphyl)
• Salicylates, such as aspirin	• Nonsteroidal anti-inflammatory drugs (NSAIDs)
• Sulfonamides, such as trimethoprim/ sulfamethoxazole (TMP/SMX; Bactrim)	

Source: Adapted with permission from Deakins D. Teaching Elderly Patients about Diabetes. *American Journal of Nursing* (1994;94[4]:38–42), Copyright © 1994, American Journal of Nursing.

intolerances, and financial limitations combine to have an effect on the likelihood that dietary recommendations will be implemented.

The percentage of calories provided by carbohydrate will vary, depending on the individual's eating habits and glucose and lipid goals. Higher carbohydrate percentages have been found to cause hypertriglyceridemia and suboptimal blood glucose control in some individuals with type II diabetes.

Many older individuals will be pleasantly surprised to learn that current scientific evidence does not support restriction of sucrose in the diet for reasons of glycemic control.[34] Teaching should include a discussion of how to incorporate sweets in the diet to prevent misunderstandings and overuse of foods that are also high in fat content or low in nutrient density.

Protein. The 1989 RDA for protein is set at a minimum of 63 g/d for males and 50 g/d for women, age 51 and older.[20] The ADA 1994 Nutrition Recommendations suggest that protein be provided in amounts similar to 0.8 g/kg body weight per day, which is approximately 10% of calories.

Debate exists among gerontologists regarding whether this amount is adequate to meet the needs of the older person. Those advocating higher intakes argue that (1) protein digestion and metabolism is reduced with age and (2) protein foods contain much-needed iron and minerals. Those in favor of lower intakes point out (1) the resultant reduction in stress on the kidneys and (2) that with a reduced lean body mass, less is needed for tissue repair.[35]

At the present time, recommendations of the ADA seem prudent and may be adjusted for individual needs during periods of stress, infection, etc.

Fat. The U.S. Dietary Guidelines recommend a fat intake of 30% of total calories, cholesterol intake limited to 300 mg/d, and a limitation of saturated fats to one-third of the total fat intake or 10% of total calories. Because of the increased risk for cardiovascular disease, which accompanies diabetes, the ADA underscores the recommendations for cholesterol and saturated fat. However, current ADA guidelines do not include a recommended percentage of total calories to be supplied by fat. Although a lower-fat diet seems prudent for many, the accompanying increase in the percentage of calories from carbohydrate may be detrimental to glycemic control and triglyceride levels. Also considering the risk for malnutrition and lower body weights in the very old, a low-fat, low-cholesterol diet may not be appropriate for some individuals.

Fiber. Although fiber in normal dietary amounts is not believed to affect blood glucose, it should still be encouraged, along with adequate fluids, to promote bowel regularity. Although daily consumption of 20 to 35 g of fiber is recommended, older individuals may not tolerate this amount. Goals regarding fiber intake should be determined on an individual basis.

Micronutrients. Although both aging and diabetes have been shown to be independently associated with alterations in micronutrient status, at present, routine supplementation of vitamins and minerals is not recommended for older individuals. However, certain conditions may warrant a trial supplementation of specific nutrients, as indicated below.

Zinc. Zinc supplementation has been found to facilitate wound healing in several uncontrolled studies with elderly subjects.[36,37] Hallbook and Lanner[37] found that venous leg ulcers healed faster in patients with serum zinc levels greater than 110 mg/dL (either at baseline or after supplementation) than in patients with lower serum zinc levels. Some gerontologists have suggested a 3-month trial of zinc supplementation (70 mg elemental zinc, three times daily) for this patient population.[38]

Additional research is needed to quantify whether zinc supplementation is truly beneficial for these individuals, and if so, in what dosage and for what duration.[39]

Vitamin C. Vitamin C is known to aid wound healing by promoting collagen formation and increasing the tensile strength of the wound. Because many elderly patients have problems with vascular fragility and are thereby at increased risk for skin breakdown and decubitus ulcers, some physicians have prescribed a trial dosage of vitamin C as a preventive measure.[40]

If the decision is made to institute a trial of supplemental vitamin C (ie, 500 to 1000 mg/d), it is important to recognize these potential problems: inaccuracies in blood glucose monitoring results, possible precipitation of oxalate stones, and rebound scurvy in the occasional patient.[39,41]

Again, more research is needed in this area to determine whether supplementation with vitamin C is beneficial.

Calcium. As people age, they often decrease their use of dairy products and, as a result, reduce their intake of calcium. Also, lack of exposure to sunlight, of particular concern for those home-bound or confined to bed, may result in a vitamin D deficiency. Insufficient vitamin D affects the body's ability to use and retain calcium. These factors and others combine to increase the older person's risk for osteoporosis.

The National Institutes of Health Osteoporosis Consensus Conference has recommended that older individuals, including those with diabetes, be encouraged to take 1000 mg of elemental calcium per day.[42] Guidelines for supplementation include[35] (1) calcium carbonate is the best-absorbed preferred form, (2) test: 75% of a calcium tablet should dissolve in 6 oz vinegar within 30 minutes if it is of desirable absorbability, (3) avoid use of dolomite, bone meal, and aluminum-based antacids as supplements, (4) combine calcium with a small amount of vitamin D or lactose to enhance absorption, and (5) avoid concurrent supplementation with iron.

Sodium. Many older individuals with diabetes are also hypertensive. Current ADA recommendation suggest a daily sodium intake of 2400 mg/d for individuals with mild-to-moderate hypertension and no more than 3000 mg/d for others, as is recommended for the general population.[34]

As mentioned earlier, as the sense of taste declines with age, many older persons compensate by adding extra salt to their food. Adherence to a sodium-restricted diet will be particularly difficult for these individuals.

If, after a 3-month trial with the sodium-restricted diet, no changes are seen in blood pressure, it may be best to discontinue the sodium restriction. Older persons with diabetes have multiple challenges and are given multiple management recommendations. If recommendations are not effective in producing the desired outcomes, they should be discontinued.

Exercise

Exercise is an important component of treatment for the older person with diabetes. In addition to its beneficial effects on glucose metabolism,[7,43] serum cholesterol levels, and cardiovascular fitness,[44] it has been shown to increase bone density, muscle strength, and flexibility. One study by Fiatarone and associates[45] found that exercise increased stability and decreased the chances of falling, even for individuals in their nineties. Older persons may also benefit from an enhanced psychological well-being and improvement in appetite when exercise has been incorporated into their normal routine.[38]

Despite these benefits, the use of exercise in the older person as a treatment modality is considered controversial. Individuals with cardiovascular disease, poor vision, arthritis, or Parkinson's disease or who are at increased risk for falls or injury may not be candidates for an exercise regimen.

For those individuals in whom exercise is recommended, the regimen should begin with stretching and flexibility exercises, followed by 20 to 30 minutes of low-impact aerobic exercise at a pace that maintains the pulse rate between 100 and 120 beats per minute.[29,46] Swimming or water aerobics may be appropriate for the older person with arthritis or when weight-bearing exercises are not recommended.

The above obviates the need for an exercise program that is tailored to fit the individual needs and capabilities of the older person. Older patients need to be closely evaluated before an exercise program is instituted and monitored carefully thereafter.

Diabetes Medications

If a trial of dietary modifications and exercise is insufficient to maintain blood glucose levels within the goal range, diabetes medication must be initiated. Drug therapy may consist of an OHA, insulin, or a combination of both.

Oral Hypoglycemic Agents and Metformin

Oral hypoglycemic agents and/or metformin may be used to treat the older person. Use should be instituted at the lowest possible dose and gradually increased. It is recommended that chlorpropamide (Diabinese) be avoided in persons older than 60 years of age because it reduces free water clearance and produces an unacceptably high risk for hyponatremia. Due to its route of excretion via the kidney and its half-life of 35 hours, a higher incidence of hypoglycemia has occurred in the past with chlorpropamide.[47]

The following dietary implications should be recognized when counseling the older person who takes an OHA: (1) note whether the OHA is to be taken before or with a meal to enhance absorption. (2) As discussed previously, the OHAs can potentially cause hypoglycemia, particularly among older persons who tend to skip meals.

If the fasting blood glucose is extremely elevated on diagnosis (ie, >250 mg/dL), administration of OHAs is unlikely to be sufficient for managing glycemic control, and insulin therapy is indicated.

Insulin

The primary goal of insulin therapy for the older person should be to achieve the best glycemic control, with the least risk of hypoglycemic, while using the simplest regimen.

Several insulin regimens are currently being used to treat diabetes in the older person. In addition to the multiple regimens used for those with type I, individuals with type II may receive a single shot of intermediate-acting insulin before bedtime, a split mixed dose of intermediate-acting and regular insulin given one to two times per day, intermediate-acting insulin given with OHAs, or a premixed solution of intermediate- and short-acting insulin.[48]

The dosage and time of insulin administration should be patterned around the person's usual eating habits, rather than the reverse.

Monitoring

Blood glucose monitoring is a vital component of diabetes management and can assist the older person by providing a "black and white" evaluation of glycemic control, including identification of hypoglycemic episodes. Through advances in technology, monitoring devices have become much simpler to read and operate, enhancing use for older persons with dexterity and vision problems.

Recommendations regarding how frequently the older person should perform blood glucose monitoring depend on several factors, including the relative stability of diabetes control, whether diabetes medication (either insulin or OHA) has been prescribed, patient ability or willingness to perform the testing procedure, availability of support systems, and financial resources.

Blood glucose monitoring results are often an effective tool for reinforcing meal-planning principles and identifying potential areas where dietary or medication adjustments may be needed.

SPECIAL CONSIDERATIONS FOR THE OLDER PERSON WITH DIABETES RESIDING IN A LONG-TERM CARE FACILITY

Five percent of older Americans (approximately 1.5 million) live in long-term care (LTC) facilities. More than half of them are at least 80 years old, and nearly 12% have diabetes, which represents both diagnosed and undiagnosed cases.[49]

Exhibit 27-2 Outcomes of Malnutrition in Older Persons

Physical

- Increased risk of infection
- Respiratory difficulties (diaphragm atrophy; decreased hypoxic drive, vital capacity, tidal volume, and respiratory rate)
- Skin breakdown with ulceration
- Poor wound healing (delayed collagen synthesis; fibroblastic proliferation; neovascularization)
- Prolonged postoperative complications
- Increased morbidity and mortality
- Musculoskeletal difficulties (weakness; poor mobility, work capacity, and potential for rehabilitation)
- Cardiac difficulties (decreased cardiac reserve; altered electrocardiogram; decreased myocardial contractility)

Social-Psychological

- Apathy
- Irritability
- Memory loss
- Confusion

Economic

- Increased medical costs

Source: Reprinted with permission from *Journal of the American Dietetic Association* (1992;92:1109–1116), Copyright © 1992, The American Dietetic Association.

Statistics indicate that compared with their nondiabetic counterparts, individuals with diabetes are more likely to require placement in these institutions. In a study of LTC residents by Mooradian and associates,[50] it was discovered that individuals with diabetes had a higher incidence of renal failure, proteinuria, retinopathy, and infections of the urinary tract and skin, compared with their nondiabetic counterparts. They were also more likely to have peripheral vascular disease.[50] Also, these individuals typically

suffer from multiple diseases,[51] thereby compounding the effect on overall health status.

Medical nutrition therapy plays a vital role in diabetes management for residents of these facilities. Two nutrition-specific problems (malnutrition and dehydration) that pose a particular challenge for these individuals are discussed further.

Malnutrition

Individuals residing in LTC facilities are at significantly higher risk for malnutrition than those living at home.[52] Incidence in institutionalized adults has been reported to range from 10 to 85%.[53] Malnutrition often goes unrecognized in the elderly, because its manifestations (excessive loss of lean body mass) resemble the signs and symptoms of the aging process. It is associated with negative physical, psychosocial, and economic outcomes as illustrated in Exhibit 27-2.[53] These outcomes, combined with the detrimental effects of hyperglycemia, cause residents of the LTC facility to be prime targets for poor health and diminished quality of life. It is the responsibility of the registered dietitian, dietary staff, and other members of the health care team to ensure that the nutrition needs of these individuals are being met.

Nutrient Needs

In general, nutrient needs of the older LTC resident with diabetes do not differ from those for his or her non-LTC counterpart. However, an increase in calories and protein is usually required when infection, skin breakdown, or some other type of catabolic or debilitating process is present (eg, cancer, cardiovascular accident [CVA], etc). Vitamin-mineral supplementation (eg, vitamin C, zinc, calcium) may also be recommended in certain cases, as discussed earlier.

Modifications to the usual diet can be made by altering the nutrient density and content of foods (ie, fortification), increasing the frequency of feedings, and/or using medical nutritionals. Enteral or parenteral nutrition may also be needed in some cases. Refer to Chapter 32 for more information on enteral and parenteral feedings for the individual with diabetes.

Provision of Meals and Snacks in the LTC Facility

The first step in meeting a resident's nutrition needs is to ensure that meals and snacks are provided as intended. It is the resident's right to be served attractive, nutritious food of good quality in a timely manner. The facility's dietary staff must also be knowledgeable regarding portion sizes and appropriate menu substitutions. Alternative foods must be available should the resident have a dislike for the regular menu item.

The Omnibus Reconciliation Act (1987) requires that LTC facilities routinely offer three meals and a bedtime snack to residents. Also, not more than 14 hours should pass between a substantial evening meal and breakfast the following day, except on weekends and holidays. On these days, 16 hours may elapse between a substantial evening meal and breakfast, provided a "nourishing snack" is given at bedtime.

Provision of between-meal snacks is particularly important for the elderly resident who has diabetes. They can be vital in preventing hypoglycemic episodes for those who require insulin or OHAs to manage their diabetes. Mid-morning and evening snacks are not typically offered; therefore, a physician's order will be needed if these are to be provided. The composition of the standard bedtime snack may also need to be altered, as some facilities offer only one food item. Again, individualization is the key.

Calorie Needs and Weight Goals

Calories should be prescribed to assist the LTC resident in attaining and maintaining a reasonable body weight. One study conducted by Mooradian and associates[50] found body weight of LTC residents to fall midway between non-LTC residents with diabetes (higher weights) and LTC residents without diabetes (lower weights). Almost 21% of LTC residents with type II diabetes were 20% or more under average body weight, when compared with the 1960 table of average weight and height of Americans aged 65 to 94 years. Only 8.5% were considered overweight.

Most gerontologists and registered dietitians suggest use of a range of normal or calculation of body mass index (BMI) when determining desirable weights for LTC residents, as opposed to using a height/weight table. Healthy older adults should have a BMI between 22 and 27.[54]

Low body weights are epidemiologically associated with a greater morbidity and mortality in the elderly as a whole. Therefore, weight loss for the older LTC resident should not be a goal in and of itself but rather a method for improving serum glucose and lipid levels and the severity of hypertension, as applicable, after considering the risk/benefit ratio for each individual.

Do Residents of a LTC Facility Need a Special Diet for Diabetes?

Rather than prescribing set calorie levels (eg, 1200, 1500, 1800), some LTC facilities have opted to use a "liberalized geriatric diet," which still follows the basic principles of a diabetic diet (ie, consistency, balanced nutrients, low saturated fat) but incorporates regular canned fruit, a small portion of regular dessert, etc, within the pattern of the approved menu cycle.

As the ADA 1994 Nutrition Recommendations indicate, these practices are in agreement with current research findings. In 1987, Coulston and associates[55] investigated whether significant changes occurred in glycemic control when a diabetic versus a regular diet was provided to 18 NIDDM residents over a 16-week period. As Figure 27-3 illustrates, no significant differences were noted.[55]

Dehydration

Dehydration is considered by many gerontologists to be the most common fluid and electrolyte disturbance in older persons. Reports of its incidence in LTC residents range from 12 to 25%.[56] The etiologies for its occurrence are listed in Exhibit 27-3.

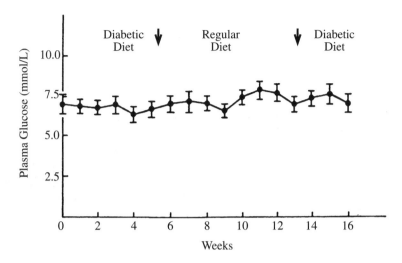

Figure 27-3 Weekly Fasting Plasma Glucose Concentrations from All 18 Patients ($\bar{x} \pm$ SEM). *Source:* Reprinted with permission from Coulston AM, Mandelbaum D, Reaven GM. Dietary management of nursing home residents with non–insulin-dependent diabetes mellitus. *American Journal of Clinical Nutrition* (1990;51:67–71), Copyright © 1990, American Society for Clinical Nutrition.

Exhibit 27-3 Etiologies of Dehydration in the Older Person

Physiologic
- Diminished thirst perception
- Inability of aging kidneys to concentrate urine in response to a fluid deficit

Medical
- Medications, especially diuretics and sedatives
- Fever and infection
- Diarrhea and vomiting
- High solute feedings (particularly high protein)
- Cardiovascular and renal disease
- Diminished level of consciousness
- Poorly controlled diabetes

Environmental
- Elevated environmental temperature
- Use of air-fluidized beds

Situational
- Purposeful fluid restriction to prevent urinary incontinence
- Lack of caregiver assistance to provide fluids

Source: Reprinted with permission from Campbell SM. Maintaining hydration status in elderly persons: problems and solutions. In: *DNS Support Line* (1992;14(3):7–10), Copyright © 1992, The American Dietetic Association.

As with malnutrition, identifying individuals who are clinically dehydrated is particularly complicated because clinical signs of dehydration (reduced skin turgor, confusion, lethargy, and falling) are often assumed to be normal signs of aging.[57]

For the older person with diabetes the osmotic diuresis and dehydration that results from hyperglycemia may cause hypernatremia, resulting in the potentially fatal condition described previously, HHNS.

Glycemic control and provision of adequate fluids are two obvious, yet sometimes elusive, methods of preventing dehydration in the older individual with diabetes. Residents of the LTC facility should be encouraged to drink the water and other fluids provided them not only at mealtime but between meals as well.

A general guide for ensuring adequate fluid intake is to provide 1 mL fluid per calorie consumed. Daily fluid needs can also be calculated based on 30 mL water per kilogram body weight. Additional fluids will be needed if any of these conditions are exhibited: infection, mild vomiting (≥500 mL/d), diarrhea (≥1000 mL/d),

Exhibit 27-4 Factors for Consideration When Conducting a Home Health Care Assessment of Nutritional Needs

---

Financial Status
- Is the individual able to afford the variety of foods comprising a well-balanced diet?
- Is the individual eligible to receive food stamps, home-delivered meals (ie, Meals on Wheels), or interested in participating in a congregate feeding program (ie, senior nutrition site)?

Food Procurement and Preparation
- Who does the shopping and cooking?
- Is obtaining transportation to the store a problem?
- Do physical disabilities prevent the individual from preparing food?
- What kind of cooking facilities are available?

Living Situation and Support Systems
- Does the individual live alone?
- Are family members or friends available to provide assistance?

Behavior Disorder
- Does the individual have problems with substance abuse, mental illness, depression, or will to live?

Education Needs
- Does the client have a clear understanding of his or her diet and how to put it into practice?
- Are there vision or literacy problems that prevent the client from purchasing foods that are appropriate or reading educational materials?

---

elevated environmental temperature, diuretic or multiple medication use, high-protein feedings, history of dehydration, or diabetes out of control.[57]

DIABETES MEDICAL NUTRITION THERAPY IN THE HOME HEALTH CARE SETTING

According to the 1990 report of the American Association of Retired Persons, 95% of older adults live in our communities. Many of them lack adequate social support services to assist them in adequately managing their diabetes and other medical conditions. If diabetes was diag-

nosed during hospitalization, very limited teaching may have occurred before discharge, leaving the older person with feelings of helplessness and inadequacy. Although the outpatient clinic is an excellent option for continuance of teaching, some older people will have a difficult time returning for scheduled classes or appointments, due to financial constraints, lack of transportation, etc. Individuals who are truly home-bound may qualify for home health care services, which will make it possible for much-needed care and teaching to continue.

Advantages of the Home Visit

Clients are often much more comfortable and receptive to learning in the familiar surroundings of their own home. Ramsdell and associates[58] found that a home assessment yields valuable information that often is not obtainable during a routine clinic visit. Results of their study showed that the home visit identified up to four new problems and yielded one to eight new recommendations, in comparison with information obtained during the office-based assessment by a general internist. Twenty-three percent of the problems recognized in the home could have resulted in death or significant morbidity.[58]

Use of the Nutrition Screening Initiative's Determine Checklist or Level I or II screen by home health nursing staff on the initial visit with the client will help identify those at nutritional risk who would benefit from a registered dietitian's intervention (see Appendix 4-C in Chapter 4).[54]

In addition to completing a thorough nutritional assessment, Exhibit 27-4 lists some questions to be asked by the registered dietitian when interviewing the home care client. After completing the assessment, the plan of care should be developed and implemented. Mutually determined goals for diabetes management and medical nutrition therapy should be established at the first visit if possible. Observations and recommendations regarding nutritional needs of the client and related concerns must be communicated to the client, physician, family, and/or significant others, as well as to other members of the home health care agency staff who care for the client, to ensure continuity of care.

NUTRITION EDUCATION FOR THE OLDER PERSON WITH DIABETES

Teaching the older person with diabetes about nutrition and diabetes self-care presents both challenges and rewards for the nutrition educator. Many older individuals have one or more chronic conditions in addition to diabetes that may be positively affected by dietary intervention. To be effective, nutrition education (self-management training) must be provided that is multifaceted, yet easy to follow and understand.

Aspects of Aging That Have an Effect on the Learning Process

It is important that the nutrition educator understand the aspects of aging that may have an effect on the learning process. Three areas of change that often affect the older person have been identified: physical health, mental health, and social resources.[59,60] Each of these changes will impact the effectiveness of medical nutrition therapy and should be considered before determining the type of nutrition intervention and educational tools to be used.

Physical Health

Changes in physical health associated with aging were discussed previously in this chapter. In particular, hearing and vision losses, as well as cognitive changes, will affect how well instructions are received and understood by the learner, which has an effect on the rate of adherence overall.

Mental Health

A person's life experiences and perceptions have an impact on readiness and motivation to learn new information at any age. Loss, in many forms (spouse and friends, job, financial security, health and physical function) may make it difficult for the older person to adjust and find new purpose in life.[61,62] Feelings of depression, loneliness, and inability to cope, with resultant denial of illness, may block the learning process. If teaching is to occur, the learner must acknowledge and accept the diagnosis of diabetes and believe that learning to manage the disease will improve the quality of life. Also, it is important to remember that older people are "problem-oriented" learners (ie, they want to be able to apply the information they have learned and are not likely to be motivated to follow instructions or perform tasks well that have little meaning for them).[61]

Social Resources

Social support has been shown to reduce morbidity, lessen exposure to psychosocial stress, and buffer the impact of stress on health.[63] It has also been shown to help motivate and reinforce positive behaviors.[64,65] Families of older persons generally comprise the bulk of their social support.[66] However, a growing number of the older population live alone and may not have a consistent support system, as discussed earlier.

Registered dietitians and other health care professionals can provide vital information and encouragement to these individuals, as well as connecting them with other resources in the community.[67,68]

Strategies for Teaching Older Persons Effectively

Some recommended strategies for teaching older adults are noted in Exhibit 27-5.

Evaluating Teaching Tools

Weinrich and Boyd[69] have identified several key points or questions to be asked when evaluating teaching tools for the older person (see Exhibit 27-6). Choosing effective teaching tools will significantly enhance learning for the older individual with diabetes and can make the difference between short-term learning and long-term success in diabetes nutrition management.

Exhibit 27-5 Strategies for Teaching Older Adults Effectively

1. Teach in a quiet setting that is free of background noise, distractions, and interruptions.

2. Keep teaching sessions short.

3. Present information at a slow pace.

4. Focus your message, using only a few major points per teaching session.

5. Provide concrete, real-life examples that the learner can relate to.

6. Recognize visual, auditory, and cognitive handicaps and disabilities and adapt teaching materials/teaching style to accommodate the learner (large-print materials with limited text, written at a 5th grade reading level; inclusion of simple drawings; face and speak directly to the learner, etc).

7. Use a variety of teaching approaches (eg, visual, auditory) and encourage active participation (return demonstrations, etc.) throughout the learning process.

8. Reinforce verbal teaching with written information.

9. Repeat key concepts frequently and allow plenty of time for questions.

10. Include family or other support persons in the teaching sessions.

Exhibit 27-6 Evaluating Teaching Tools for the Older Person

Is the teaching tool accurate?

Is the teaching tool appropriate for the intended audience?

Are visuals and written materials easy to read (overheads, charts, slides, etc)?

Is the teaching tool appropriate for the type of instructional methods chosen?

Can the teaching tool help the learner meet the behavioral objectives?

Is the psychological tone optimistic, positive, honest, and nonthreatening?

Is the material presented socially acceptable to older adults?

Do the materials speak to the developmental needs of the older person?

Source: Adapted from Weinrich SP, Boyd, M. Education in the elderly: adapting and evaluating teaching tools. *Journal of Gerontological Nursing* (1992;18[1]:15–20), Copyright © 1992, Slack, Inc.

CONCLUSION

Diabetes affects a disproportionate number of older Americans. In addition to managing their diabetes, these individuals are faced with multiple challenges: loss of social support systems, physiologic changes of aging, multiple medical diagnoses, diabetes complications, and declining financial resources. As an integral member of the diabetes management team, the registered dietitian must recognize these challenges and individualize medical nutrition therapy to meet the unique needs of each older person.

REFERENCES

1. American Association of Retired Persons. *A Profile of Older Americans.* Washington, DC: AARP; 1991.

2. Halter JB. Geriatric patients. In: Lebovitz HE, ed. *Therapy for Diabetes Mellitus and Related Disorders.* Alexandria, Va: American Diabetes Association; 1991.

3. Harris MI. Epidemiology of diabetes mellitus among the elderly in the United States. *Clin Geriat Med.* 1990;6:703–729.

4. Bennett PH. Diabetes in the elderly: diagnosis and epidemiology. *Geriatrics.* 1984;39:37–41.

5. Broughton DL, Alberti KGMM, Taylor JR. Peripheral tissue insulin sensitivity in healthy elderly subjects. *Gerontology.* 1987;33:357–362.

6. Goldberg AP, Coon PJ. Non–insulin-dependent diabetes mellitus in the elderly—influence of obesity and physical inactivity. *Endocrinol Metab Clin.* 1987;16:843–865.

7. Lipson LG. Diabetes in the elderly: diagnosis, pathogenesis, and therapy. *Am J Med.* 1986;80(suppl 5A):10–21.

8. Gale EAM, Dornan TL, Tattersal RB. Severely uncontrolled diabetes in the over-fifties. *Diabetologia.* 1981;21:25–28.

9. National Diabetes Data Group. Classification and diagnosis of diabetes mellitus and other categories of glucose intolerance. *Diabetes.* 1979;28:1039–1057.

10. Shuman CR. Optimal insulin use in older diabetics. *Geriatrics.* 1984;39(10):71–89.

11. American Diabetes Association. Position statement: standards of medical care for patients with diabetes mellitus. *Diabetes Care.* 1994;17:616–624.

12. Albanese AA. *Nutrition for the Elderly.* New York, NY: Alan R Liss; 1980.

13. Gastineau CF. Aging and factors influencing the nutritional status of the elderly. In: Haller EW, Cotton GE, eds. *Nutrition in the Young and the Elderly.* Lexington, Mass: DC Heath; 1983.

14. Powers MA, Raimondi MP, Kohrs MB. Diabetes nutrition managment for the elderly. *Diabetes Educ* (special issue: Diabetes in the Elderly). 1983;9:26.

15. Kamath SV. Taste acuity and aging. *Am J Clin Nutr.* 1982;36:766.

16. Clydesdale FM. Meeting the needs of the elderly with the foods of today and tomorrow. *Nutr Today.* 1991;Sept/Oct:13–20.

17. Gerontological Nutritionists Practice Group. Study assesses nutritional risk of olfactory dysfunction. *Gerontol Nutr Newslett.* Winter 1994. Chicago, Ill: American Dietetic Association.

18. Ryan WJ, Hutchinson JM, Hull RH. Conversation: the aging speaker. *ASHA.* 1980;22:423.

19. National Dairy Council. Nutrition and the elderly. *Dairy Council Dig.* 1983;54:19.

20. Committee on Dietary Allowances, Food and Nutrition Board. *Recommended Dietary Allowances.* 10th ed. Washington, DC: National Academy of Sciences; 1989.

21. Wagner PA. Zinc nutriture in the elderly. *Geriatrics.* 1985;40:111.

22. O'Hara NM, White D. Drugs and the elderly. In: Lewis CB, ed. *Aging: The Health Care Challenge.* Philadelphia, Pa: FA Davis Co; 1985.

23. Matz R. Diabetes mellitus in the elderly. *Hosp Pract.* 1986;21(3):195–218.

24. Henry RR, Edelman SV. Advances in treatment of type II diabetes mellitus in the elderly. *Geriatrics.* 1992; 47(4):24–30.

25. American Diabetes Association. *Clinical Education Series: Medical Management of Non–Insulin-Dependent (Type II) Diabetes.* Alexandria, Va. ADA; 1994.

26. Morley JE, Mooradian AD, Rosenthal MJ, et al. Diabetes mellitus in elderly patients. Is it different? *Am J Med.* 1987;83:533–544.

27. Miller LV. Managing the elderly patient with diabetes. *Clin Diabetes.* 1985;4:76–90.

28. Roe DA. Drug–nutrient interactions in the elderly. *Geriatrics.* 1986;41:57.

29. Morley, JE, Perry HM. The management of diabetes mellitus in older individuals. *Drugs.* 1991;41:548–565.

30. Deakins D. Teaching elderly patients about diabetes. *Am J Nurs.* 1994;94(4):38–42.

31. McGandy RB, Barrows CH, Spanias A, et al. Nutrient intakes and energy expenditure in men of different ages. *J Gerontol.* 1966;21:581–587.

32. Peters AL, Davidson MB. Use of sulfonylurea agents in older diabetic patients. *Clin Geriatr Med.* 1990;6:903–921.

33. Wing RR, Koeske R, Epstein LH, et al. Long term effects of modest weight loss in type II diabetic patients. *Arch Intern Med.* 1987;147:1748–1753.

34. American Diabetes Association. Position statement: nurtition recommendations and principles for people with diabetes mellitus. *Diabetes Care.* 1994;17:519–522.

35. McCool A. Nutritional needs for the healthy elderly. In: Kline DA, Kline R, Hulbert G, eds. *Nutrition for the Elderly.* San Marcos, Calif: Nutrition Dimension; 1991.

36. Haegar K, Lanner E, Magnusson PO. Oral zinc sulfate in the treatment of venous leg ulcers. In: Pories WJ, Strain WH, Hsu JM, Woosley RL, eds. *Clinical Applications of Zinc Metabolism.* Springfield, Ill: Thomas; 1974:158–167.

37. Hallbook T, Lanner E. Serum zinc and healing of venous leg ulcers. *Lancet.* 1972;2:780–782.

38. Rosenthal MJ, Hartnell JM, Morley JE, et al. UCLA geriatric grand rounds: diabetes in the elderly. *J Am Geriatr Soc.* 1987;35:435–447.

39. American Diabetes Association. Technical review: selected vitamins and minerals in diabetes. *Diabetes Care.* 1994;17(5):464–479.

40. Reed RL, Mooradian AD. Nutritional status and dietary management of elderly diabetic patients. *Clin Geriatr Med.* 1990;6:883–901.

41. Alhadeff L, Guaitieri CT, Lipton M. Toxic effects of water-soluble vitamins. *Nutr Rev.* 1984;42:33–40.

42. National Institutes of Health Consensus Conference. Osteoporosis. *JAMA.* 1984;252:799–802.

43. Coopan R. Determining the most appropriate treatment for patients with non–insulin-dependent diabetes mellitus. *Metabolism.* 1987;36(suppl 1):17–21.

44. Shephard RJ. The scientific basis of exercise prescribing for the very old. *Am Geriatr Soc.* 1990;38:62–70.

45. Fiatarone MA, Marks EC, Ryan ND, et al. High intensity strength training in nonagenarians. *JAMA.* 1990;263:3029–3034.

46. Ruoff G. The management of non–insulin-dependent mellitus in the elderly. *J Fam Pract.* 1993;36(3):329–335.

47. Melander A, Bitzen PO, Faber O, et al. Sulphonylurea anti-diabetic drugs: an update of their clinical pharmacology and rational therapeutic use. *Drugs.* 1989;37:58–72.

48. Henry RR, Edelman SV. Advances in treatment of type II diabetes mellitus in the elderly. *Geriatrics.* 1992;47(4):24–30.

49. National Center for Health Statistics. *The National Nursing Home Survey.* Hyattsville, Md: NCHS; 1985. Stock no. 017-022-010-658.

50. Mooradian AD, Osterweil D, Petrasek D, et al. Diabetes mellitus in elderly nursing home patients: a survey of clinical characteristics and management. *J Am Geriatr Soc.* 1988;36:391–396.

51. Besdine RW. The date base of geriatric medicine. In: Rowe JW, Besdine RW, eds. *Health and Disease in Old Age.* Boston, Mass: Little, Brown; 1982:1–14.

52. Goodwin JS. Social, psychological and physical factors affecting the nutritional status of elderly subjects: separating cause and effect. *Am J Clin Nutr.* 1989;50:1201–1209.

53. Kerstetter JE, Holthausen BA, Fitz PA. Malnutrition in the institutionalized older adult. *J Am Diet Assoc.* 1992;92:1109–1116.

54. Nutrition Screening Initiative. *Nutrition Interventions Manual for Professionals Caring for Older Americans.* Washington, DC: Nutrition Screening Initiative; 1992.

55. Coulston AM, Mandelbaum D, Reaven GM. Dietary management of nursing home residents with non–insulin-dependent diabetes mellitus. *Am J Clin Nutr.* 1990;51;67–71.

56. Ross Laboratories Medical Department Research, Columbus, OH, conducted with Consulting Dietitians at the 73rd Annual Meeting of the American Diabetes Association, October 1990.

57. Cambell SM. Maintaining hydration status in elderly persons: problems and solutions. In: *DNS Support Line.* Vol. XIV(3). Chicago, Ill: American Dietetic Association, Dietitians in Nutrition Support Practice Group; 1992:7–10.

58. Ramsdell JW, Swart JA, Jackson E, et al. The yield of a home visit in the assessment of geriatric patients. *J Am Geriatr Soc.* 1989;37:17–24.

59. Whitman NI, Graham BA, Gleit CJ, et al. *Teaching in Nursing Practice: A Professional Model.* Norwalk, Conn: Appleton-Century-Crofts; 1986.

60. Weinrich SP, Boyd M, Nussbaum J. Continuing education: adapting strategies to teach the elderly. *J Geriatr Nurs.* 1989;15(11):17–21.

61. Kicklighter JR. Characteristics of older adult learners: a guide for dietetics practitioners. *J Am Diet Assoc.* 1991;91:1418–1422.

62. Alywahby NF. Principles of teaching for individual learning of older adults. *Rehab Nurs.* 1989;14:330–333.

63. Chiriboga D. Social supports. In: Maddox GL, ed. *The Encyclopedia of Aging.* New York, NY: Springer; 1987.

64. Given BA, Given CW. Creating a climate for compliance. *Cancer Nurs.* 1984;7:139–147.

65. Culbert PA, Kos BA. Aging: considerations for health teaching. *Nurs Clin North Am.* 1971;6:605–614.

66. Zarit S, Orr NK, Zarit JM. *The Hidden Victims of Alzheimer's Disease.* New York, NY: New York University Press; 1985.

67. Smiciklas-Wright H, Taylor-Davis S. Educating the geriatric client. In: *DNS Support Line.* Vol. XV(2). Chicago, Ill: American Dietetic Association, Dietitians in Nutrition Support Practice Group; 1993:5–9.

68. Insititute of Medicine, Division of Health Promotion and Disease Prevention. *The Second Fifty Years: Promoting Health and Preventing Disability.* Washington, DC: National Academy Press; 1990.

69. Weinrich SP, Boyd M. Education in the elderly: adapting and evaluating teaching tools. *J Geriatr Nurs.* 1992;18(1):15–20.

Part VII

Nutrition and Specific Clinical Conditions

Chapter 28

Renal Disease and Diabetes

Linda G. Snetselaar

STATISTICS

Overt clinical nephropathy is defined as the presence of persistent proteinuria greater than 500 mg per 24 hours with concomitant retinopathy and elevated blood pressure. Approximately 35% of patients with type I diabetes and 20% with type II diabetes develop nephropathy. Although a higher percentage with type I diabetes get nephropathy, there are many more individuals with type II diabetes with clinically defined nephropathy. Diabetic nephropathy is the single leading cause of end-stage renal disease (ESRD) in the United States. The disease has been the primary cause of more than 50,000 cases of ESRD from 1987 to 1990. ESRD costs the nation more than $7.3 billion annually to treat.[1] Statistics indicate that 35% of new cases of ESRD each year are attributed to diabetes.[2]

Two new studies have shed light on the importance of glycemic and blood pressure control in preventing glomerular changes and preserving renal mass. The Diabetes Control and Complications Trial (DCCT) provided statistically significant evidence that improved glycemic control reduces risk of renal complications.[3] The role that blood pressure control plays in preventing glomerular changes and preserving renal mass was shown through a study funded by the National Institute of Diabetes and Digestive and Kidney Diseases and Bristol-Myers Squibb Pharmaceutical Research Institute.[4] Researchers in this study found that captopril, an angiotensin-converting enzyme inhibitor, reduced the risk of death or ESRD by 50% in persons with insulin-dependent diabetes mellitus (IDDM). The study showed that regardless of the degree of kidney damage, captopril slowed down renal disease and delayed the development of ESRD for all study subjects. The DCCT results are discussed in further detail later in this chapter.

OVERVIEW OF RENAL INSUFFICIENCY

The following reviews the basic functions of the kidney and changes seen in renal insufficiency. Glomerular filtration rate (GFR) represents the kidney's ability to remove wastes effectively from the blood; in a person with normal renal function, GFR averages 100 to 120 mL/min. *Renal insufficiency* is the term applied when the creatinine clearance, a laboratory test used to estimate the GFR, falls between 50 and 20 mL/min.[5]

Protein filtered by the normal kidney is almost completely absorbed by the body. One of the first signs of glomerular damage is proteinuria. However, persons with type I diabetes who have normal kidney function may experience episodes of proteinuria when metabolic control is poor. Newly diagnosed persons with type II diabetes with years of carbohydrate intolerance often have some degree of proteinuria related to nephrosclerosis. This proteinuria does not necessarily lead to kidney failure.[6]

After 20 years of insulin therapy, approximately half of all individuals with IDDM develop persistent proteinuria of variable amounts, with protein losses as high as 20 g/d reported.[6,7]

This clinical symptom marks a steady decline in renal function. In the early stages of nephropathy, persons with type I diabetes may develop a nephrotic syndrome characterized by significant protein losses (>3 g/d) with concomitant hypoalbuminemia, edema, and hyperlipidemia.[7]

The major component of urinary protein is albumin. Depression of serum albumin concentration is anticipated if the liver is unable to synthesize this visceral protein at a rate commensurate with the body's losses. Normal hepatic synthesis of albumin is between 8 to 14 g/d. Protein urinary losses above this level will result in hypoalbuminemia.[8] However, in patients with malnutrition, systemic illness, or liver impairment, moderate proteinuria (3 to 5 g/d) may be associated with a more severe hypoalbuminemia (<2.5 g/dL).

Decreased plasma oncotic pressure may result from low serum albumin levels. Water transudes from the plasma into the interstitial compartment, causing edema. The loss of plasma fluid results in hypovolemia, which triggers renal retention of water and sodium and exacerbates the edema.[9,10]

Potassium excretion mainly occurs in the kidney. Despite renal damage, the normal serum concentration of potassium is maintained because circulating aldosterone stimulates enhanced potassium secretion by the remaining nephrons.[11] Usually, only when renal function is diminished to less than 15% of normal (GFR = 15 mL/min per 1.73 m^2) does hyperkalemia develop. However, diabetic individuals with mild renal insufficiency may develop hyporeninemic hypoaldosteronism, a syndrome characterized by depressed levels of plasma aldosterone.[7,11] Because aldosterone stimulates secretion of potassium with depressed levels, the hypoaldosteronism results in less potassium being secreted, yet increases in circulating potassium occur due to the diminished renal function. This elevation in potassium is not typically seen with mild renal impairment. Mineralocorticoid replacement therapy usually corrects this hyperkalemia. Some individuals may also require a dietary restriction of potassium (2 g/d).[7]

During the 4 to 6 years that elapse from the onset of proteinuria to the development of chronic uremia (creatine clearances <20 mL/min), the diabetic patient develops azotemia, anemia, hypertension, renal bone disease, retinopathy, and neuropathy.[6,7] Diminished erthyropoeitin (EPO) production and shortened red blood cell life span contribute to the anemia of chronic renal failure. In the past, therapy for this anemia included periodic red blood cell transfusions when hematocrit levels are dangerously low. Today, androgen steroid replacement may be prescribed. If a specific deficiency is documented, then supplementation of either iron, pyridoxine, folate, or vitamin B_{12} is warranted.[7] Currently, it is common practice to give patients EPO even before dialysis.

The kidney is the site of activation of vitamin D to either 1,25-dihydroxycholecalciferol (1,25[OH]$_2$D$_3$) or 24,25-hydroxyvitamin D (24,25[OH$_2$]D$_3$).[12] As the GFR falls to less than 25 mL/min, inadequate quantities of these vitamin D$_3$ metabolites are produced, resulting in diminished calcium absorption from the gastrointestinal tract, hypocalcemia, and osteomalacia.[9,13] Compounding this inadequate production, studies have demonstrated that renal patients may have increased requirements of vitamin D due to hyperphosphatemia and elevated parathyroid hormone levels.[13]

With diminished kidney function, renal phosphorus excretion becomes impaired. Parathyroid hormone (PTH) levels rise to facilitate phosphorus output; yet as glomerular function diminishes to less than 25% of normal, this compensatory response becomes less effective, resulting in elevated serum phosphorus levels.[14,15] Thus, renal diabetic patients have secondary hyperparathyroidism, hyperphosphatemia, and vitamin D deficiency that contribute to bone disease. Phosphate-binding antacids are administered in renal insufficiency to prevent hyperphosphatemia. Aluminum hydroxide antacids have been linked to aluminum toxicity. This intoxication may cause dementia and a form of vitamin D-resistant osteomalacia.[16] Many nephrologists recommend calcium acetate or calcium carbonate as the phosphate-binding agent rather than aluminum hydroxide gels. A variety of vitamin D supplements, including $1,25(OH)_2D_3$, $25(OH)D_3$, and dihydrotachysterol, have proved effective in the treatment of renal osteo-dystrophy. Careful regulation of vitamin dosage may prevent the development of hypercalcemia.

Because the kidney plays a role in insulin deg-radation, the diabetic patient with renal dysfunc-tion maintains higher serum insulin levels for a given dose of insulin and is therefore more prone to hypoglycemic reactions. Diabetes control, al-ready complicated by renal insufficiency, is also adversely affected by the widely fluctuating food intakes caused by the anorexia and nausea that may occur in renal failure. Peripheral and autonomic neuropathies associated with long-term diabetes are aggravated by the pres-ence of uremic toxins. One such neuropathy, gastroparesis diabeticorum, is manifested by epigastric discomfort, early satiety, nausea, vomiting, and weight loss.[17] Constipation or di-arrhea may occur from altered peristalsis and from phosphate binders. These complications, coupled with difficulty in achieving good blood glucose control, place patients at high nutritional risk. Metoclopramide is a medication commonly used for treatment; unfortunately, its success rate is suboptimal.

STAGES OF RENAL DISEASE IN PERSONS WITH DIABETES

Hypertrophy/Hyperfunction

This stage is seen as an acute stage at diagno-sis of diabetic nephropathy and appears to be re-lated to elevated blood glucose levels. It is char-acterized by hypertrophy, glomerular hyper-filtration, or an abnormally increased GFR.

Silent

Although the urinary albumin excretion (UAE) is normal, an increased basal membrane thickening may be present. This is the stage when prevention by normalizing glycemic con-trol can be very important. Because it is the si-lent stage, few biologic measures may alert one to this stage. Early slightly elevated levels of se-rum creatinine may be an indicator of needed in-tervention. Serum creatine values beginning at 1.4 for males and 1.2 for females may indicate the need to focus on normalizing blood glucose levels.

Microalbuminuria

This stage describes the at-risk patient. Microalbuminuria is diagnosed when the UAE rate reaches 20 to 200 μg/min in two to three urine samples collected within a 6-month period.

Proteinuria/Overt Clinical Nephropathy

This stage is characterized by persistent proteinuria (>200 μg/min or >500 mg per 24 hours total protein excretion). An increase in UAE may be the earliest manifestation or a marker of overt clinical nephropathy.[3] Table 28-1 provides normal, increased, and clinically significant levels. Renal status can be evaluated by looking at microalbumin, 24-hour urine pro-tein, or the albumin/creatinine ratio. Micro-

Table 28-1 Urinary Albumin Excretion (UAE)

	Normal UAE	Increased UAE	Clinical Nephropathy
Random albumin (μg/mL)	<10	20–200	>200
24-hour protein (mg/24 h)	<15	30–300	>300
Albumin/creatinine ratio	<20	20–300	>300

Source: Data from American Diabetes Association, 1994.

albuminuria is defined as a UAE rate between 20 and 200 mg in an overnight period or 24-hour sample on at least two of three occasions within a 6-month period. Less than 10 µg/min would be considered normal. If the level of albumin falls between 10 and 20, it should be repeated. Levels indicated under the clinical nephropathy category are those at which a protein restriction of approximately 0.8 g/kg per ideal body weight (IBW) per day is recommended.

Nephrotic Syndrome—ESRD

When the disease progresses to this final stage, treatment options include hemodialysis, continuous ambulatory peritoneal dialysis (CAPD), or transplantation. In persons with diabetes who progress to this stage, nearly 100% also present with hypertension and retinopathy, 75% have peripheral neuropathy, and nearly one-third have had a previous myocardial infarction.[18]

URINARY ALBUMIN EXCRETION

Table 28-1 shows clinically significant levels of UAE. The DCCT analyzed UAE in persons with diabetes over a 10-year period. The results, which are presented below highlight the importance of glycemic control in persons with diabetes.

Diabetes Control and Complications Trial

The DCCT included two intervention groups: primary and secondary (see Figure 28-1). These two cohorts of IDDM patients were recruited and studied to answer two separate questions. First, would intensive treatment prevent or delay the development of complications in subjects who had no complications at baseline (primary prevention trial)? Second, would intensive treatment prevent or slow progression of complications in subjects who had early complications at baseline (secondary intervention trial)? The DCCT results indicate that intensive diabetes therapy delays the onset and slows progression of retinopathy and delays the development of microalbuminuria ($\geq$40 mg/24 h) in both cohorts

and the development of overt nephropathy (albuminuria >30 mg/24 h) in the secondary intervention cohort.[3]

In the Primary Prevention Cohort, the cumulative incidence of microalbuminuria ($\geq$28 µg/min) reached 16% after 9 years in the intensively treated group and 27% in the conventionally treated group. Intensive therapy reduced the mean adjusted risk of microalbuminuria by 34% (95% confidence interval [CI] 2, 56; $p = .04$). In the Secondary Intervention Cohort intensively treated group, the baseline UAE rate was less than 28 µg/min, and the cumulative incidence of microalbuminuria was 26% after 9 years. In the conventionally treated group, it was 42%. Intensive therapy reduced the mean absolute risk by 43% (95% CI 21, 58; $p < .001$).

The development of a more advanced level of microalbuminuria ($\geq$70 µg/min) among those who had a baseline UAE of less than 28 µg/min was also noted. In the Primary Prevention Cohort, the cumulative incidence of UAE of 70 µg/min or greater was 3.3% after 9 years in the intensively treated group and 7.0% in the conventionally treated group. In the Secondary Intervention Cohort, the cumulative incidence of this level was 10.0% after 9 years in the intensively treated group and 20.2% in the conventionally treated group. Intensive therapy reduced the mean absolute risk by 56% (95% CI 26, 74; $p = .002$).

In the Primary Prevention Cohort, only three intensively treated subjects and six conventionally treated subjects developed clinical albuminuria ($\geq$208 µg/min). In the Secondary Intervention Cohort, the cumulative incidence of clinical albuminuria was 5.2% after 9 years in the intensively treated group and 11.3% in the conventionally treated group. Intensive therapy reduced the mean absolute risk by 56% (95% CI 18, 76; $p < .01$). In the secondary cohort, 73 subjects (38 assigned to intensive treatment, 35 assigned to conventional treatment) had UAE levels of 28 µg/min or greater at the time of entry into the study. In each treatment group, eight subjects developed levels of 208 µg/min or greater during the course of the study.

Two DCCT Intervention Groups

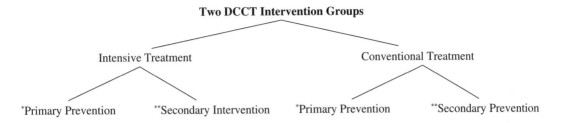

* **Primary**—Prevention cohort patients were required to have IDDM for 1 to 5 years without retinopathy as detected by seven-field stereoscopic fundus photography and to have urinary albumin excretion of less than 40 mg per 24 hours.

** **Secondary**—Prevention cohort patients were required to have IDDM for 1 to 15 years, to have very mild-to-moderate nonproliferative retinopathy, and to have urinary albumin excretion of less than 200 mg per 24 hours.

Figure 28-1 DCCT Intervention Groups. *Source:* Reprinted with permission from The Diabetes Control and Complications Trial Research Group, The Effects of Intensive Treatment of Diabetes on the Development and Progression of Long-Term Complications in Insulin-Dependent Diabetes Mellitus, *New England Journal of Medicine*, 1993;329:977–986, Copyright © 1993, Massachusetts Medical Society.

For the primary, secondary, and combined cohorts, there were no significant differences in creatinine between treatment groups during the study. Only seven subjects in the entire study (two intensive, five conventional) developed urinary UAE of 208 µg/min or more coupled with a creatinine clearance of less than 70 mL/min per 1.73 m². The appearance of hypertension (blood pressure >140/90 mm Hg) did not differ significantly between treatment groups in the primary, secondary, or combined cohorts.

The beneficial effect of intensive therapy on the development of microalbuminuria was consistent in subgroups defined by baseline variables including age, diabetes duration, baseline HbA_{1c}, level of retinopathy, neuropathy, the presence or absence of hyperfiltration (<130 or ≥130 ml/min per 1.73 m²).

In summary, intensive therapy reduced the cumulative incidence and overall hazard rates for the development of microalbuminuria and clinical albuminuria in both the primary prevention and secondary intervention DCCT cohorts. The consistent beneficial effect of intensive therapy at all levels of nephropathy examined suggests that intensive therapy will at least delay progression of nephropathy and may prevent the development of advanced renal disease in IDDM patients.

GENERAL NUTRITIONAL CONSIDERATIONS

Prevention of wide variations in blood glucose levels is key to the medical management of diabetes mellitus. To achieve this goal, matching insulin, dietary intake, and exercise is crucial. Dietary intake must be consistent with insulin levels. Amounts of insulin to cover usual intake must be individualized for each major meal and evening snack.

The American Diabetes Association recommends that with the onset of nephropathy, dietary protein restriction of not less than the adult recommended daily allowance is required—0.8 g of protein per kilogram IBW per day.[18,19] Table 28-2 shows general diet recommendations for hemodialysis and peritoneal dialysis. The Modification of Diet in Renal Disease (MDRD) study showed that it is possible to achieve between 0.6 and 0.8 g/kg of protein per day.

In the early stages of renal insufficiency, dietary intervention may be used to treat symptoms.[20] Hypertensive patients may be prescribed a combination of antihypertensive medication and a low-sodium diet, which may be the only dietary manipulation of the diabetic diet until renal failure develops.

Individuals experiencing ESRD require a 2-g/d sodium restriction in conjunction with diuretic therapy. When edema is severe and medications prove ineffective, the physician may prescribe a severely restricted sodium diet (250 to 500 mg/d) for a period of less than 1 week to promote diuresis.

Cholesterol and fat-restricted diets can be effective in normalizing the hyperlipidemia associated with nephrotic syndrome[6] (see Table 18-5). If diet alone is not effective, drug therapy may be necessary.

In general, optimal protein synthesis is facilitated by provision of adequate energy intake (25 to 35 kcal/kg IBW per day). Table 28-3 provides specific data on activity level and weight status. Positive nitrogen balance in most nephrotic patients can be maintained by provision of protein at levels of 1.5 to 3.0 g/kg IBW per day.[10] High-quantity protein ingestion is contraindicated in azotemic patients; diets providing approximately 1.0 g/kg per day protein with additional replacement of urinary protein losses on a gram-for-gram basis have been recommended for these individuals. (If the patient is obese, protein needs are based on ideal weight; otherwise, these are based on present weight.)

Table 28-2 General Diet Recommendations for Renal Patients[a]

Treatment	Pre-ESRD	Hemodialysis	Peritoneal Dialysis
Protein (g/kg IBW)	0.6–0.8[b]	1.1–1.4	1.2–1.5
Nephrotic syndrome	0.8–1.0		
Energy (kcal/kg IBW)[c]	35–40	30–35	25–35
Phosphorus (mg/kg IBW)	8–12[d]	<17[e]	<17[e]
Sodium (mg/d)	1000–3000 if necessary	2000–3000	2000–4000
Potassium (mg/kg IBW)	Typically unrestricted	Approximately 40	Typically unrestricted
Fluid (mL/d)	Typically unrestricted	500–750 + daily urine output or 1000 mL if anuric	2000+
Calcium (mg/d)	1200–1600	Depends on serum level	Depends on serum level

[a] See specific guidelines for each treatment modality.

[b] The upper end of this range is preferred for diabetes and malnourished patients.

[c] See guidelines (Table 28-3) for estimating energy needs based on weight and activity level.

[d] Whereas 5 to 10 mg/kg IBW is frequently cited in the scientific literature, 5 mg/kg IBW is practical only when used in conjunction with a very low-protein diet supplemented with amino acids or ketoacid analogs.

[e] A diet that is higher in protein may make it impossible to meet the optimum phosphorus prescription.

Source: Reprinted with permission from *National Renal Diet: Professional Guide* (p 6), Copyright © 1993, The American Dietetic Association.

Table 28-3 Estimated Energy Requirements Based on Both Weight Status and Activity Level

Weight	Sedentary (kcal/kg)	Moderate (kcal/kg)	Active (kcal/kg)
≥10% IBW	20–25	30	35
IBW	30	35	40
≤10% IBW	30	40	45–50

Source: Reprinted with permission from *National Renal Diet: Professional Guide* (p 6), Copyright © 1993, The American Dietetic Association.

To maintain adequate calories when reduced-protein diets are used, the American Diabetes Association recommends concentrated carbohydrates, reduced protein foods, and increased total fat with saturated fat intake reduced.[19]

Dietary protein restriction is a long-standing component of the management of kidney failure diseases. Stringent reduction of dietary protein delays the onset of uremic symptoms, such as diarrhea, pruritis, nausea, vomiting, and lethargy, and when dialysis is unavailable, can help prolong life.[20–24] However, strict protein restrictions (0.6 g protein per kilogram IBW) were not shown to change the progression of renal insufficiency in the MDRD study.[25]

Many trials have incorporated keto acids into the dietary protocols. The α-keto analogs of the essential amino acids, except for lysine and threonine, undergo transmission in vitro.[26] Recent MDRD data show that the FDA-approved keto acids do not delay progression of renal disease.[25]

Diets providing a minimum of 30 to 35 calories/kg body weight and 0.8 protein per kilogram have been safely provided to medically stable patients with diabetic nephropathy. During illness or catabolic stress, the diet is liberalized to provide 1.0 to 1.5 g protein per kilogram IBW. Patients on these dietary regimens were closely monitored (bimonthly) to ensure that there was no deterioration in nutritional status. Table 28-2 summarizes nutritional recommendations. Low-protein products are available to assist the patient in following a reduced-protein diet. Exhibit 28-1 provides examples. As stated previously, patients with diabetic nephropathy maintain higher serum insulin levels for a given dose of insulin. Increases in the incidents of hypoglycemia are the result if the dose is not adjusted.

END-STAGE RENAL DISEASE: THE DIALYSIS PATIENT

The individual with ESRD and diabetes mellitus is a prime candidate for malnutrition. In one study, 43 chronic dialysis patients with type I diabetes were evaluated to determine overall nutritional status.[27] Twenty-six percent of those studied were significantly below IBW, 44% were markedly depleted in muscle mass, and 35% had depressed serum albumin levels.

There are many causes of malnutrition. The dialysis process removes small amounts of iron, water-soluble vitamins and minerals, peptides, and amino acids.[22] Significant protein losses occur during peritoneal dialysis.[28] Endocrine disorders reported in chronic renal failure, elevated PTH, and glucagon and peripheral tissue insensitivity to insulin may disrupt nutrient utilization.[29] Renal patients are more prone to catabolic episodes caused by bone disease or gastrointestinal bleeding. People with diabetes have the added insult caused by poor glucose control and diabetic gastropathy. Furthermore, appetite is diminished due to overly stringent dietary restrictions, a metallic taste in the mouth, psychological depression, or the nausea associated with end-stage renal failure.[20] These factors precipi-

Exhibit 28-1 Special Low-Protein Products

	Amount	Weight (g)	Protein (g)	Sodium (mg)	Calories	Phosphorus (mg)
Anellini, low protein, Aproten	1 cup cooked	190	0.3	15	180	10
Baking Mix, low protein, Wel-Plan	1/4 cup	28	0.1	3	90	14
Bread, Unimix, low protein, Kingsmill, prep without milk or egg	1 slice	41	0.1	0	99	19
Chocolate Chip Cookie, low protein, Med Diet	1 cookie	11	0.1	2	56	7
Crackers, low protein, Wel-Plan	1 cracker	8	0.0	32	32	1
Creamy Lemon Herb Sauce, low protein, R&D Labs	1/4 of package, dry	6	0.6	32	21	15
Cut Spaghetti, low protein, Wel-Plan (makes 1 cup cooked)	1/2 cup, dry	50	0.2	30	171	15
Ditalini, low protein, Aproten	1 cup cooked	130	0.3	10	180	10
Garlic Herb Sauce, low protein, R&D Labs	1/4 of package, dry	6	0.8	32	22	27
Gelled Dessert Mix, cherry, low protein, Prono	1/3 cup prepared	55	0.0	8	55	0
Gelled Dessert Mix, lime, low protein, Prono	1/3 cup prepared	55	0.0	6	55	0
Gelled Dessert Mix, orange, low protein, Prono	1/3 cup prepared	55	0.0	8	55	0
Gelled Dessert Mix, strawberry, low protein, Prono	1/3 cup prepared	55	0.0	8	55	0
Imitation Dairy Drink, prepared, low protein, Med Diet	8 fl oz	246	2.4	91	89	97
Macaroni, low protein, Wel-Plan (makes 1 1/4 cup cooked)	1/2 cup, dry	50	0.2	30	171	15
Ratatouille, low protein, R&D Labs	1 package	283	4.0	240	140	76
Rice Starch Bread, low protein, Med Diet (12 slices/loaf)	1 slice	47	0.1	25	155	5
Rigatini, low protein, Aproten	1 cup cooked	130	0.3	10	200	10
Rusks, low protein, Aproten	1 slice	10	0.1	3	42	5
Spaghetti Rings, low protein, Wel-Plan (makes 1 cup cooked)	1/2 cup, dry	70	0.4	48	238	21
Spice Cookie, low protein, Med Diet	1 cookie	11	0.1	2	54	4
Sugar Cookie from Cookie Base, low protein, Kingsmill	2 cookies	28	0.3	83	130	—
Sweet Cookies, low protein, Wel-Plan	1 cookie	10	0.0	2	49	1
Tagliatelle, low protein, Aproten	1 1/3 cup cooked	200	0.4	10	275	15
Tomato Sauce, low protein, R&D Labs	1/4 of package, dry	10	0.3	17	36	8
Vanilla Cream-Filled Wafers, low protein, Med Diet, Aglutella	3 wafers	19	0.1	6	100	4
Vanilla/Chocolate Wafers, low protein, Wel-Plan	3 wafers	25	0.1	4	132	45
Wheat Starch, low protein, dp	1 Tbsp	7	0.0	2	25	3
Wheat Starch, low protein, dp	1/2 cup	56	0.2	20	198	26
Unimix, low protein, Kingsmill, dry mix	1 cup	115	0.3	0	278	53

Source: Reprinted with permission from *Protein Wise Counter*, Nutrition Coordinating Center, Modification of Diet in Renal Disease (MDRD) Study, University of Pittsburgh, Copyright © 1989.

tate clinical malnutrition and jeopardize the quality of life.

Nutritional Assessment Parameters

Accurate assessment of nutritional status enables identification of existing nutritional deficiencies and facilitates planning of corrective measures. Objective data are interpreted to evaluate nutriture in patients with diabetes and chronic renal failure.

Body Composition

Adult dialysis patients generally present above 90% IBW using standard reference tables.[30] However, these patients may have an increase in total body water without evidence of edema, thus diminishing the reliability of body weight.[30,31] Some dialysis patients may tolerate a gradual retention of up to 12 lb fluid with no signs of circulatory overload.[32] Arm circumference (AC) and triceps skinfold (TSF) measurements are used to determine midarm muscle circumference (MAMC), an estimate of muscle mass [MAMC = AC − (0.314 × TSF)]. Low MAMC in dialysis patients correlates with nutritional wasting.[32] Because overhydration may decrease the precision of these anthropometric arm measurements, they should be taken when patients are at or close to estimated *dry weight* (the term used to identify the lowest weight achievable without hypotensive episodes). These parameters are recorded on the arm without vascular access. However, repeatedly administered insulin injections at the midarm site may cause hypertrophy of the tissue, making accurate estimates impossible to obtain.[21] Doing serial measurements in each patient enables early detection of changes in body composition. This information can also be compared with a healthy population using standard reference tables, such as those published by Frisancho.[30] When values fall below the 5th percentiles of these tables, depletion of arm muscle or fat is potentially a problem.

Serum Proteins

An excellent indicator of malnutrition is low serum albumin.[32,33] Serum transferrin, the iron-binding protein, is also a sensitive indicator of protein status, despite small losses during hemodialysis and peritoneal dialysis therapy.[29,34] Depressed serum levels of this visceral protein are reported with iron overload, a condition associated with excessive supplement of iron used to treat the anemia of renal failure.[32,35] Prealbumin and retinol-binding protein are not valid nutritional indices in renal failure due to the impaired degradation of these visceral proteins by the kidney.[32]

Laboratory Parameters

Elevated serum concentrations of numerous nutrients in renal failure are caused by impaired clearance. Creatinine is a by-product of normal muscle turnover routinely excreted by the kidney. A rise in serum creatinine to levels greater than 2.0 mg/dL indicates altered renal function.[33] Creatinine serum concentration is influenced by the total body muscle mass, so a serum creatinine of 6 mg/dL in a small frame-size woman may represent a GFR of 10 mL/min, whereas for a muscular male, it may indicate a GFR of 30 mL/min. Creatinine clearance, derived from serum concentration in relation to 24-hour urinary creatinine excretion, gives a more precise estimation of GFR than does serum creatinine alone. Urine output becomes marginal as renal status diminishes to 10 or 15% of normal function, and serum creatinine is often used as an indicator of kidney function. Serum creatinine levels vary markedly among dialysis patients. However, they typically remain stable for each individual if consistent dialysis is provided.

Serum urea nitrogen concentration, or blood urea nitrogen (BUN), gradually rises throughout the course of chronic renal failure and remains elevated despite initiation of dialysis. If no clinical signs of uremia exist, generally, BUN levels between 60 to 100 mg/dL are acceptable.[33] Diabetic patients develop uremic symptoms at lower BUN levels than other renal patients.[10] BUN, a measure of nitrogen accumulation from protein breakdown, is directly influenced by dietary protein consumption. Catabolic stress, internal bleeding, dehydration, inadequate dialysis, and very high protein intake cause an unexpectedly high rise of BUN in dialysis patients.

Serum potassium values significantly greater than or less than normal are hazardous because of the role that potassium plays in nerve and muscle contraction. Arrhythmias and cardiac arrest may suddenly develop in severely hyperkalemic or hypokalemic patients. Elevated blood glucose levels may lead to life-threatening hyperkalemia in diabetes.[7,20] A 2-g daily restriction of dietary potassium should normalize serum levels despite kidney impairment.[35]

Serum sodium measurements reflect water balance. Elevated levels indicate dehydration with water loss, and depressed levels, water overload. Normalization of serum sodium is implemented by fluid and sodium restriction.

With impaired excretion, phosphorus blood concentration rises as GFR falls below 25 mL/min.[6] In the presence of hyperphosphatemia, serum calcium levels decrease and secondary hyperparathyroidism results.

Despite normalization of serum phosphorus, persistent hypocalcemia indicates a need for calcium and/or vitamin D supplementation. Depressed serum calcium levels also occur in the presence of hypoalbuminemia, because a portion of calcium is bound to this blood protein. Maintaining normal phosphorus concentration in the blood and ensuring a normal phosphorus-calcium product prevents risk of metastatic calcification.[13,33,36]

Good blood glucose control is critically important in diabetic renal failure. Hyperglycemic episodes may result in hyperkalemia, fluid overload (due to increased thirst), and elevated serum triglyceride and cholesterol values.[25] Fasting serum glucose concentrations between 120 to 180 mg/dL are considered reasonable. The microchromatographic measurement of HbA_{1c} may be increased in uremic individuals independent of glucose control.[37] Despite the difficulties with the absolute value of this measure, changes upward and downward from a baseline value can be of value. For example, if HbA_{1c} increases from 7.0 to 10.0, careful daily monitoring of blood glucose is vital. Monitor laboratory parameters on a weekly or monthly basis at the dialysis center, with the blood drawn at the beginning of treatment. Variations in the individual's serum values over time may represent alterations in residual kidney function, medical status, dialysis treatment, nutritional status, and/or dietary intake.

Treatment Modalities in End-Stage Renal Disease

ESRD occurs when the person with renal insufficiency requires either hemodialysis, peritoneal dialysis, or kidney transplantation to sustain life. Most diabetic patients in this country receive hemodialysis, which reflects its widespread availability. Peritoneal dialysis, particularly CAPD, is increasing in popularity. Kidney transplantation is an excellent treatment choice but limited to a relatively small percentage of this patient population because donor kidneys are in short supply and may not be immunologically compatible. Also, some patients are not surgical candidates due to their poor medical status. Although all three treatment modalities are available to both diabetic patients and nondiabetic individuals, people with diabetes are at greater risk of complications and have shorter survival rates than other renal patients.

Hemodialysis Therapy

The creation of an arteriovenous shunt in 1960 allowed hemodialysis therapy to be offered on a long-term basis.[38] Dialysis treatments are scheduled two to three times weekly and last commonly from 3 to 4 hours each time.[14] Blood is removed from the body using a surgically created vascular access (the shunt), then exposed to dialysate solution across a semipermeable membrane. Diffusion and ultrafiltration remove toxins, fluids, and nitrogenous wastes from the blood.

People with diabetic nephropathy experience a higher incidence of hypertensive episodes during hemodialysis, higher morbidity, and higher mortality rates than nondiabetic hemodialysis patients.[36] Due to atherosclerosis in limb arteries, these patients cannot maintain a patent vascular access, thus requiring repeated access surgeries or peritoneal dialysis.[7]

Nutritional Considerations in Hemodialysis Therapy. Renal nutrition in hemodialysis ensures sufficient nutrient intake and avoids an excessive accumulation of metabolic wastes. These criteria are derived from the many nutritional considerations of hemodialysis, including losses of amino acids and peptides, iron, water-soluble vitamins and minerals, fluid, and glucose.[21] Prescribed water-soluble vitamins and minerals replace dialysate losses. By the time maintenance dialysis is begun, the diabetic individual is usually oliguric (urine output of less than 400 mL/d) or anuric (urine outputs of less than 100 mL/d) and thus needs to maintain careful volume control. Retention of 1 L water results in an increase in body weight of 1 kg. Interdialytic weight gains of 1.5 to 2.0 kg are acceptable for most individuals. Fluid removal greater than 4 kg during dialysis treatment may cause dangerous hypotensive episodes. Reducing overall fluid intake and restricting dietary sodium are essential.

Diabetic individuals with poor diabetes control present unique medical management problems. Hyperosmolar nonketotic coma resulting from elevated serum glucose is reported in renal insufficiency.[14] Life-threatening episodes of cardiac arrhythmias due to hyperkalemia develop when blood glucose concentration is markedly increased.[7] Polydypsia associated with hyperglycemia may spur increases in fluid consumption of such magnitude that pulmonary edema or congestive heart failure develops.

Although insulin requirements continually decrease with loss of functioning renal tissue, accurately prescribing insulin dosage remains difficult due to fluctuations in appetite and the delayed gastric emptying associated with both diabetic gastropathy and uremic neuropathy. Insulin administration is modified on dialysis days because glucose losses occur with hemodialysis, whereas insulin is not dialyzable. Hypoglycemic reactions may occur during treatment, despite the presence of glucose in the dialysate. If patients complain of light-headedness, some blood is removed from the arterial line and glucose analyzed by self-monitoring blood glucose techniques. Low blood glucoses are treated with administration of hyperosmolar dextrose (50 g/100 mL) into the venous return line of the dialysis apparatus.[7]

Many health care clinicians do not permit food to be consumed during hemodialysis because of the elevated risk of hepatitis, increased incidence of hypotension, delayed gastric emptying during therapy, or the increased perils involved in staff assisting patients with meals while simultaneously monitoring vital life signs. Diminished food intake on dialysis days contributes to poor blood glucose control and malnutrition documented in the diabetic dialysis population.[20]

Daily oral supplementation with commercial supplements is frequently needed to ensure adequate energy and protein ingestion. Dairy products are no longer promoted because of the increase in phosphorus intake. During bouts of nausea, small (60 to 180 mL), frequent feedings are tolerated best because many supplements have a high sugar content. Elevation of blood glucose can be prevented by using small portions. Regrettably, oral supplementation with diet is difficult due to frequent bouts of nausea and anorexia experienced by these catabolic patients.

In some cases, intradialytic infusion of parenteral nutrition solutions are used to prevent nutritional debilitation without disrupting the patient's life style. Hypertonic formulations are administered into the vascular access via the venous tubing during hemodialysis. Piraino and coworkers[39] observed improvement in dry body weight, appetite, energy intake, and muscle strength in catabolic nondiabetic patients who were given a 1-L solution of mixed amino acids and glucose several times weekly for a period of 20 weeks. No clinical improvement was observed in those patients with wasting due to advanced metabolic bone disease and secondary hyperparathyroidism.

Supporters of this method of nutritional support state that the infused amino acids and glucose replace losses that occur during hemodialysis without causing fluid overload. Some of the infusate is lost during the treatment process. Wolfson et al[40] provided a 1-L amino acid and glucose solution to eight male patients. It was administered at a constant rate into the drip chamber of the venous outflow tubing of the dialyzer. Approximately 80% of infused amino acids were retained. Although these trials indicate promise for this technique in nutritional support, further studies are needed to evaluate the true cost benefits of on-line intradialysis hyperalimentation.

Peritoneal Dialysis Therapy

Due to difficulties in maintaining vascular accesses, some diabetic individuals are treated by peritoneal dialysis. Survival is similar for hemodialysis and peritoneal dialysis in diabetic patients.[41] The peritoneum is used as a dialyzing membrane in peritoneal dialysis. A hyperosmolar dialysate solution is infused slowly into the peritoneal cavity using a surgically placed catheter. This fluid remains in the abdominal area while excess water and uremic toxins cross the membrane from the body by osmosis and diffusion. Pump or simple gravity drip remove this fluid and reinfuse clean dialysate. The dialysate compositions are composed of either 1.5, 2.5, or 4.25% dextrose and contain serum electrolytic content.[42] Higher dextrose-content preparations increase fluid removal. Insulin is added to the dialysate in diabetic patients to reduce the hyperglycemia caused by these solutions. There are two basic types of peritoneal dialysis: CAPD and continuous cyclic peritoneal dialysis (CCPD). These techniques vary in the frequency and length of dialysis.

Excellent uremic clearances have been reported with CAPD. Individuals are on dialysis 24 h/d, 7 d/wk, mimicking the kidneys' ongoing filtration of metabolic wastes. Gravity drip infuses 2 L of dialysate into the body. This dialysate remains in the body for 4 to 8 hours. CAPD is a manually administered process that enables great flexibility during travel. The treatment procedure is simple. Even visually impaired patients can perform their dialysis.

CCPD is a combination of intermittent and CAPD. Patients infuse a 2-L exchange into their abdominal cavity in the morning. This dialysate remains in the body for approximately 14 hours during the day and then is drained. During sleep, three to four cycles of peritoneal dialysis are administered by a peritoneal dialysis cycler machine. This technique eliminates the multiple interruptions associated with CAPD created by dialysis exchanges during the day. Because there are fewer exchanges of dialysate than with CAPD, the risk of peritonitis is reduced. Dialysis is performed daily to prevent accumulation of uremic toxins. However, because CCPD involves training in both techniques of peritoneal dialysis, it is not a commonly used treatment modality.

Nutritional Considerations in Peritoneal Dialysis. Individuals undergoing CCPD and CAPD receive continuous dialysis. Protein losses with CAPD are reported to range from 7 to 14 g/d and increase somewhat during episodes of inflammation of the peritoneum.[43] Losses of approximately 15 g/d of protein are estimated during peritonitis. These losses drop back to baseline values after 2 or 3 days of treatment. The average protein loss with CCPD is 10 to 12 g/d.[44]

Glucose absorption averages 182 ± 61 g/d and is directly related to the dextrose concentration of dialysate.[45] The added glucose calories may be of benefit to some individuals because insufficient energy intake is common in renal failure, but for many patients, this glucose absorption contributes to obesity and hypertriglyceridemia.[45–47] Blumberg and coinvestigators[32] documented elevation in plasma vitamins A and E and depressed levels of vitamins B, B_2, B_6, and C and folic acid in the ten CAPD patients studied. A major advantage of CAPD is its removal of PTH and some phosphorus, which may help improve the metabolic abnormalities contributing to renal osteodystrophy and impaired neurologic functions.[48] Fluid intake can be liberalized given the better volume control associated with CAPD. The removal of excess fluid is fairly easily achieved by the more frequent use of the higher dextrose concentration solutions. Sodium and potassium clearances are also very good with this form of peritoneal dialysis. Dietary intervention is less stringent, thus adding to the appeal of CAPD as a dialysis choice.

Renal Transplantation

Kidney transplantation is an effective treatment option for the diabetic individual with ESRD.[49] Mortality and morbidity rates for transplantation are difficult to compare with dialysis, because it is usually the younger, healthier individual who is a candidate for transplantation. Diabetic patients present with a greater occurrence of complications posttransplantation than do nondiabetic individuals. Medical nutrition therapy after kidney transplantation is focused on correction of deficiencies to achieve an overall good nutrition status.

Some people may not have been dialyzed to their dry body weight due to technical difficulties with dialysis. As a result, they may experience a significant weight loss in the weeks after surgery due to diuresis and present substantially below IBW. Energy intake in these cases should be increased by approximately 300 to 500 calories above daily baseline requirements to facilitate gradual weight gain.

Corticosteroid medications (commonly used to suppress rejection) cause increased hunger and appetite of such magnitude that obesity is a major nutrition problem in the transplantation population. Excessive weight gains can be easily prevented by calorie-controlled diets and exercise.[19]

Supraphysiologic doses of steroids also complicate blood glucose control, with insulin requirements often doubling. Maintaining a consistent pattern of food intake is essential because insulin and steroid dosages will both be periodically adjusted after the transplant. Patients are usually stabilized on immunosuppressive medications and insulin within 6 months postsurgery. At that time, they may return to a standard diabetic diet designed to facilitate blood glucose control.

Many nutrients may be modified during medical nutrition therapy for the transplant patient. Protein ingestion in the range of 1.0 to 1.5 g/kg per day is sufficient to maintain nitrogen balance. Blood pressure control is facilitated by a mild dietary sodium restriction of 3 to 4 g/d. Patients accustomed to limiting fluid intake must be encouraged to drink adequate amounts of liquids to prevent dehydration. Dietary potassium and phosphorus are not restricted unless serum levels become elevated.

Miller et al[50] reported a significant improvement in nutrition status after transplantation in 21 nondiabetic and 24 diabetic patients seen in the outpatient clinic at their facility. Nutrition status was evaluated before and after renal transplantation, with reported improvement in body weight, serum albumin, and serum transferrin noted in the months after surgery. By contrast, the diabetic group had a lower weight for height and MAMC than the nondiabetic group, suggesting that the presence of diabetes may adversely affect nutrition status. Periodic nutrition counseling after transplantation is strongly recommended, particularly for diabetic individuals who experience nutrition deficiencies before surgery.

Nutrition Counseling for Pre-ESRD

Counseling people with diabetes who are also faced with the nutrient restrictions of pre-ESRD is a rewarding and enjoyable process. The registered dietitian integrates subjective information ascertained from the patient interview with evaluation of nutrition status and planned medical treatment to establish patient care plans. This practitioner then collaborates with the physician to determine the diet prescription. The dietitian is responsible for translating the complex prescription into a meal plan tailored to meet metabolic needs and accommodate the individual's life style.

The framework of the dietary regimen is a diabetic-style meal plan, giving consideration to the timing, type, and quantity of foods consumed to facilitate blood glucose control. Food exchange lists modified for sodium and potassium content are used to simplify menu planning (Appendix 28-A). Individuals are encouraged to assist in creating the meal plan by providing feedback regarding usual dietary habits. This interaction cultivates trust and rapport between the dietitian and the patient and facilitates dietary adherence. Because the ramifications of dietary noncompliance may be life-threatening, the dietitian stresses the important role that diet plays in overall medical management.

Educating patients on methods of incorporating a wide variety of foods into their diets while staying within the prescribed dietary guidelines is critical (Appendix 28-B). Periodically, patients may desire items listed on the "Foods to Be Avoided" section of the diet booklet. The dietitian then works with them to set up guidelines for incorporation of these foods in quantities that will not cause physical harm. For example, if the individual desires a frankfurter, it may be suggested that one be consumed the night before dialysis, with the provision that interdialytic weight gain up to that time be less than 1 kg and that there be no evidence of fluid overload. Renal dietitians use this technique to facilitate long-term dietary adherence. Consultation with the nephrologist regarding relaxation of any dietary restriction is recommended.

Blood Glucose Control

The American Diabetes Association stresses the importance of normalizing blood glucose levels in patients who are at risk for or show overt clinical signs of diabetic nephropathy.[19] The careful matching of insulin to food intake is a major consideration in achieving good blood glucose control.

To achieve near-normal HbA$_{1c}$ levels in the DCCT, blood glucose levels were monitored before each meal and an evening snack (at least four times a day) and once a week at 3 A.M. With this close monitoring, it was possible to connect causes of high or low blood glucose levels with daily life situations (eg, overeating, undereating, exercise, stress, timing of insulin injection). For

example, if diet is indicated as a cause of high blood glucose, the day of the week and time of day might be pinpointed along with place of food consumption. By determining specifically when and where a behavior occurs, it is possible to problem-solve strategies to overcome future occurrence.

Reduced Levels of Dietary Protein

To achieve 0.6 to 0.8 g of dietary protein, many of the strategies used in the MDRD study may be of value.

Medical Nutrition Therapy in the MDRD Study

The MDRD intervention program emphasized long-term dietary adherence by supporting patient behavior changes toward dietary goals and by teaching 840 patients to self-manage the behavior change process over an average follow-up period of 2.2 years. The intent was for the dietitians to be largely the facilitators and the patients to be the active agents, the ones who set the goals and solved the problems in reaching for their goals. There were five basic types of MDRD nutrition intervention activities: goal-directed therapy, self-management training, knowledge and skills, modeling, and support activities.

Goal Directed Therapy. Goal-directed therapy was related to stepwise goals set by the dietitian and patient. It provided multiple types of information, both biologic and behavioral. It had a positive focus, which was an advantage of including multiple types because the dietitians were able to judge which type might be most effective and motivating for each patient. Goals communicated high expectations. If patients aimed high, they would work harder and feel a greater sense of success in the long run. Goals reinforced the efforts of patients as well as outcomes or overall performance.

Self-Management Training. The primary form of self-management training was self-monitoring. Patients were expected to keep track of the grams of protein they ate each day. Although the emphasis was on protein, some patients also self-monitored other nutrients such as phosphorus, sodium, or calories, depending on their dietary goals. The dietitians reviewed the patients' self-monitoring records informally or used a study-supplied nutrient analysis system on their personal computers.

Knowledge and Skills (Baseline). Knowledge and skills activities teach patients to discriminate the protein content of foods. Patients were given two protein resources, which allowed them to identify grams of protein in certain amounts of food. Math skills were reviewed, and they were taught to weigh and measure foods and self-monitor. Patients were also taught goal-setting skills and problem-solving skills. Throughout the study, knowledge and skills activities were conducted, always in the context of solving specific problems that patients encountered while trying to reach specific goals that they set. This paved the way for eventual self-management.

Knowledge and Skills (Early Intervention). During early intervention, knowledge and skills activities included a review of the intervention plan, each patient's study diet prescription, goal-setting activities (during early intervention, patients set goals for protein and, for many participants, calories), and problem-solving activities.

Knowledge and Skills (Midintervention). During midintervention, knowledge and skills activities included those for fine-tuning protein and calorie intake. For example, some activities helped patients more precisely estimate portion sizes when eating out. Guidelines were given for nutrients other than protein and calories after these goals were well established. For example, guidelines were provided for phosphorus, potassium, sodium, and high biologic value protein. General guidelines were also given for healthy life style, exercise, and so on.

Knowledge and Skills (Later Intervention). During later intervention, knowledge and skills activities included continued problem solving, plus motivational and relapse prevention activities, and tasks that encouraged the application of

behavioral skills to other life goals. For example, some session topics included using goal setting and problem solving to increase well-being, positive thinking, and other life goals of value to the patients.

The time frame for each of these levels of knowledge and skills depended on each patient's mastery. If early intervention was mastered, the next level, "midintervention," was attempted. Individuals moved at different rates and achieved mastery at their own pace.

Modeling. MDRD modeling activities included sample menus. The dietitians used the study-provided nutrient analysis system on their clinic computers to develop menus. The menus were often based on the patients' self-monitoring records. Patients were given special foods, including low-protein pastas, breads, and high-protein beverage powders for the usual protein group. Recipes and cookbooks were distributed. Food tasting and cooking demonstrations were conducted, and visits were held at restaurants and grocery stores.

Support. Support activities included the dietitian cosigning with the patients during baseline a formal commitment to the study goals and reviewing this commitment throughout follow-up (working with the patient's family, giving patients certificates of accomplishment, appreciation gifts such as mugs and subscriptions to cooking magazines). Phone calls were placed to patients between visits, and mailings included newsletters, birthday cards, and notes of appreciation. Group activities included group visits, dinners, and other social events. There were several relapse prevention activities.

All Activity Categories. All activity categories (goal-directed therapy, self-management training, knowledge and skills, modeling, and support) were emphasized early in the intervention and decreased over time for all diet groups ($p = .000$) except support activities, which remained as frequent over time in patients with more advanced renal disease. At the same time, outstanding adherence was achieved and maintained throughout the intervention program. We conclude that patients learned to manage their own behavior change process. By managing their own medical nutrition therapy, patients became self-sufficient and aware of areas in which change was needed.

CONCLUSION

In summary, medical nutrition therapy in diabetic nephropathy involves careful attention to glucose control and protein modification. Medical nutrition therapy in peritoneal and hemodialysis varies, depending on the specific types used. The keys to long-term diet adherence in ESRD are goal-directed therapy, self-management training, knowledge and skills, modeling, and support.

REFERENCES

1. Nathan OM. *Study Shows Intensive Treatment of Diabetes Can Delay Kidney Complications.* Bethesda, Md: National Kidney and Urologic Disease Information Clearinghouse, National Institute of Diabetes and Digestive and Kidney Diseases, National Institutes of Health; 1994.

2. Selby JV, FitzSimmons SC, Newman JM, Katz PP, Sepe S, Showstack J. The natural history and epidemiology of diabetic nephropathy. Implications for prevention and control. *JAMA.* 1990;263:1954–1960.

3. Diabetes Control and Complications Trial Research Group. The effects of intensive treatment of diabetes on the development and progression of long-term complications in insulin-dependent diabetes mellitus. *N Engl J Med.* 1993;329:977–986.

4. Lewis EJ, Hunsicker LG, Bain RP, Rohde RD. The effect of angiotensin-converting-enzyme inhibition on diabetic nephropathy. *N Engl J Med.* 1993;329:1456–1462.

5. Knochel JP. Pathogenesis of the uremic syndrome. *Postgrad Med.* 1978;64:88.

6. Friedman EA. Diabetic nephropathy: strategies in prevention and management. *Kidney Int.* 1982;21:780.

7. D'Elia J, Kaldany A, Miller DG, et al. Diabetic nephropathy. In: Marble A, Krall LP, Bradley RF, et al, eds. *Joslin's Diabetes Mellitus.* 12th ed. Philadelphia, Pa: Lea & Febiger; 1985:635–664.

8. Mogensen CE. Diabetes mellitus and the kidney. *Kidney Int.* 1982;21:673.

9. Nyberg G, Larsson O, Attman P-O, et al. Time as a risk factor in diabetic nephropathy. *Diabetes Care.* 1985;8:590.

10. Kaufman CE. Fluid and electrolyte abnormalities in nephrotic syndrome. *Postgrad Med.* 1984;76:135.

11. Glassock RJ, Goldstein DA, Goldstone R, et al. Diabetes mellitus, moderate renal insufficiency and hyperkalemia. *Am J Nephrol.* 1983;3:233.

12. Kawashima H, Kurokawa K. Metabolism and sites of action of vitamin D in the kidney. *Kidney Int.* 1986;29:98.

13. Massry SG. Requirements of vitamin D metabolites in patients with renal disease. *Am J Clin Nutr.* 1980;33:1530.

14. Avioli LV. Renal osteodystrophy and vitamin D. *Dialysis Transplant.* 1978;7:244.

15. Nortman DF, Coburn JW. Renal osteodystrophy in end-stage renal disease. *Postgrad Med.* 1978;64:123.

16. Heaf JG, Melsen F. Aluminum deposition in bone due to aluminum hydroxide consumption. *Nephron.* 1985;40:246.

17. Taub S, Mariani A, Barkin JS. Gastrointestinal manifestations of diabetes mellitus. *Diabetes Care.* 1979;2:437.

18. Whittier FC, Evans DH, Dutton S, et al. Nutrition in renal transplantation. *Am J Kidney Dis.* 1985;4:405.

19. American Diabetes Association. Nutrition recommendations and principles for people with diabetes mellitus. *Diabetes Care.* 1994;17:519–522.

20. Levine SE. Nutritional care of patients with renal failure and diabetes. *J Am Diet Assoc.* 1982;81:261.

21. Kopple JD. Nutritional management of chronic renal failure. *Postgrad Med.* 1978;64:135.

22. Kolff WJ. Forced high caloric, low protein and the treatment of uremia. *Am J Med.* 1952;12:667.

23. Kempner W. Compensation of renal metabolic dysfunction. *N C Med J.* 1945;6:117.

24. Alvestrand A, Ahlberg M, Furst P, et al. Clinical results of long-term treatment with a low protein diet and a new amino acid preparation in patients with chronic uremia. *Clin Nephrol.* 1983;19:67.

25. Klahr S, Levey AS, Beck GJ, et al. The effects of dietary protein restriction and blood-pressure control on the progression of chronic renal disease. *N Engl J Med.* 1994;330:877–884.

26. Walser M. Rationale and indications for use of α keto analogues. *J Parenter Enteral Nutr.* 1983;8:37.

27. El Nahas AM, Coles GA. Dietary treatment of chronic renal failure: ten unanswered questions. *Lancet.* 1986;1:597.

28. Wardle EN, Kerr DNS, Ellis HA. Serum proteins as indicators of poor dietary intake in patients with chronic renal failure. *Clin Nephrol.* 1975;3:114.

29. Harvey KB, Blumenkrantz MJ, Levine SE, et al. Nutritional assessment and treatment of chronic renal failure. *Am J Clin Nutr*. 1980;33:1586.

30. Frisancho RA. New standards of weight and body composition by frame size and height for assessment of nutritional status of adults and the elderly. *Am J Clin Nutr*. 1984;40:808.

31. Blumenkrantz MJ, Kopple JD, Gutman RA, et al. Methods for assessing nutritional status of patients with renal failure. *Am J Clin Nutr*. 1980;33:1567.

32. Blumberg A, Hanck A, Sander G. Vitamin nutrition in patients on continuous ambulatory peritoneal dialysis (CAPD). *Clin Nephrol*. 1983;20:244.

33. Frederico CB, Martin BR. Practical applications of nutrition assessment in the chronic hemodialysis population. *Am J Intrav Ther Clin Nutr*. 1983;10:10.

34. Bianchi R, Mariani G, Toni, M, et al. The metabolism of human serum albumin in renal failure on conservative and dialysis therapy. *Am J Clin Nutr*. 1978;31:1615.

35. Miller DG, Levine S, Bistrian B, et al. Diagnosis of protein calorie malnutrition in diabetic patients on hemodialysis and peritoneal dialysis. *Nephron*. 1983;33:127.

36. Shideman JR, Buselmeir TJ, Kjellstrand M. Hemodialysis in diabetics. *Arch Intern Med*. 1976;136:1126.

37. Panzetta G, Bassetto MA, Feller P, et al. Microchromatographic measurement of hemoglobin A, in uremia. *Clin Nephrol*. 1985;20:259.

38. Schribner BH, Babb AL. Chronic hemodialysis in Seattle: 1960–1966. *Dialysis Transplant*. 1986;15:33.

39. Piraino AJ, Firpo JJ, Powers DV. Prolonged hyperalimentation in catabolic chronic dialysis therapy patients. *J Parenter Enteral Nutr*. 1981;5:463.

40. Wolfson M, Jones MR, Kopple JD. Amino acid losses during hemodialysis with infusion of amino acids and glucose. *Kidney Int*. 1982;21:500.

41. Kjellstrand CM. Dialysis in diabetics. In: Friedman EA, ed. *Strategy in Renal Failure*. New York, NY: John Wiley Sons; 1978:345–361.

42. Dolan PO, Greene HL. Renal failure and peritoneal dialysis. *Nursing*. 1975;7:41.

43. Rubin J, Nolph KD, Arfania D, et al. Protein losses in continuous ambulatory peritoneal dialysis. *Nephron*. 1981;28:218.

44. Diaz-Buxo JA, Farmer CD, Walker PJ, et al. Continuous cyclic peritoneal dialysis. A preliminary report. *Int Soc Artificial Organs*. 1981;5:157.

45. Grodstein GP, Blumenkrantz MJ, Kopple JD, et al. Glucose absorption during continuous ambulatory peritoneal dialysis. *Kidney Int*. 1981;19:564.

46. Von Baeyer H, Gahl GM, Reidinger H, et al. Adaptation of CAPD patients to the continuous peritoneal energy uptake. *Kidney Int*. 1983;23:29.

47. Bonnar DM. Rationale for nutritional requirements for patients on continuous ambulatory peritoneal dialysis. *J Am Diet Assoc*. 1982;80:247.

48. Delmez JA, Slatopolsky E, Martin KJ, et al. Minerals, vitamin D, and parathyroid hormone in continuous ambulatory peritoneal dialysis. *Kidney Int*. 1982;21:862.

49. Parfrey PS, Hutchinson TA, Harvey C, et al. Transplantation versus dialysis in diabetic patients with renal failure. *Am J Kidney Dis*. 1985;5:112.

50. Miller DG, Levine SE, D'Elia JA, et al. Nutritional status of diabetic and nondiabetic patients after renal transplantation. *Am J Clin Nutr*. 1986;44:66.

Sample of Exchange Lists for Protein, Potassium, Sodium, and Phosphorus Restricted Diets

MILK

Per portion:

CHO— 6 g
PRO— 4 g
FAT— 0–4 g
(varies)
NA+— 60 mg
K+— 175 mg

Daily Servings _____

Food	Portion
Milk: whole/low-fat/ non-fat	1/2 cup
Evaporated Milk	1/4 cup
Powdered Milk	2 Tbsp powder
Yogurt, plain only	1/2 cup
Ice Cream:	1/2 cup of plain flavored ice cream may be substituted for one item on this list **Once per Week Only!** It is **Not** necessary to use dietetic ice cream.

AVOID: Condensed Milk, Buttermilk, Frappes, Cocoa, Fruit-Flavored Yogurts, Ice Cream with Nuts, Syrups, Marshmallows, or Fruit; Milkshakes or Malted Milks.

MEAT

Per portion:

CHO— 0 g
PRO— 7 g
FAT— 5 g
NA+— 25 mg
K+— 100 mg

Daily Servings _____

Food	Portion
*Meats, Poultry, Fish, Seafood	1 oz
Clams, Shrimp, Oysters, Scallops	5 small
**Cheese: Low sodium	1 oz
Cottage cheese: low sodium/regular	1/4 cup
Egg	1 medium
Peanut Butter: salt-free/regular	1 level Tbsp

AVOID: Canned Salted Fish and Meat, Luncheon Meats, Salted and Smoked Meat and Fish, Regular and Diet, Hard or Processed Cheeses, Frozen Entrees (T.V. Dinners).

---

* If you eat only koshered meats, discuss this with your dietitian.

** Diet cheeses are often low in fat, but are not low in sodium. Due to its high phosphorous content, select cheese only once or twice per week.

Source: Reprinted from Diet Manual with permission of New England Deaconess Hospital, Boston, Massachusetts, 1987.

VEGETABLES

Group A
Per portion:
CHO— 5 g
PRO— 2 g
FAT— 0 g
NA+— 10 mg
K+— 110 mg

Daily Servings _____

Vegetables may be fresh, frozen, or canned WITHOUT SALT or SODIUM COMPOUNDS. Cooking vegetables in large amounts of water and draining off the liquid will lower their potassium content.

Portion Size: 1/2 cup unless otherwise indicated.

Bean Sprouts	Lettuces
Cabbage	Mustard Greens
Cauliflower	Onions
Celery (1 stalk)	*Spinach—raw,
Chicory	loosely packed
Cucumbers	Summer Squash
Dandelion Greens	Swiss Chard
Endive	Turnip Greens
Green Beans	Yellow Wax Beans
Green Peas (1/4 cup)	Watercress
Kale	Zucchini

* Please note that 1/2 cup of raw spinach equals 2 Tbsp of cooked spinach.

Group B
Per portion:
CHO— 5 g
PRO— 2 g
FAT— 0 g
NA+— 10 mg
K+— 180 mg

Due to their higher potassium content limit these vegetables to _____ portions *per week instead* of a vegetable listed in Group A.

Portion Size: 1/2 cup unless otherwise indicated.

Asparagus	Green Pepper
Beets	Kohlrabi
Broccoli	Okra
Brussels Sprouts	Mushrooms, whole
Carrots	Radishes, 10 medium
Collard Greens	Rutabaga
Eggplant	Turnip

AVOID: Artichokes, Bamboo Shoots, Baked Beans, Beet Greens, Chick Peas (Garbanzos), Cowpeas, Dried Peas and Beans, Kidney Beans, Lima Beans, Lentils, Parsnips, Plantains, Potatoes, Sauerkraut, Sweet Potatoes, Tomatoes, Tomato Products, V-8 Juice, Winter Squashes (Acorn, Butternut, Hubbard), Water Chestnuts, and Yams.

BREAD

Per portion:
CHO— 15 g
PRO— 3 g
FAT— 0 g
NA+
  Regular— 150 mg
  Low Sodium— 5 mg
K+— 35 mg

Daily Servings _____

Breads & Bread Products	Portion
Bagel	1/2 medium
Biscuits, Muffin	1 (2" diameter)
White, Rye, Italian, *Whole Wheat	1 slice
Pita (Syrian) Pocket Bread	1/2 6" round
Breadcrumbs, unsalted	3 Tbsp
English Muffin	1/2 plain
Hamburger Roll	1/2 plain
Frankfurter Roll	1/2

Breads & Bread Products continued

Food	Portion
Dinner Roll	1 small
Sponge Cake	1 1/2" cube

Cereals

Food	Portion
Dry: flakes	3/4 cup
puffed	1 1/2 cups
Cooked:	1/2 cup

Crackers

Food	Portion
Animal Crackers	8
Arrowroot Biscuits	5
*Gingersnaps	5
*Graham Crackers	3 plain squares
Lorna Doones	3
Matzoh	4" x 6"
Melba-Toast, salt-free	5 thin slices
Pilot Cracker	1 small
Rice Cakes	2
Uneedas	3
Unsalted Top Saltines	6
Vanilla Wafers	6
Zwieback Toast	3

* Potassium content is approximately 75 mg.

Food	Portion
Pasta	
Macaroni, Noodles, Spaghetti, Shells	1/2 cup cooked

Miscellaneous

Food	Portion
Flour, Tapioca, Cornstarch, Arrowroot	2 Tbsp
Popcorn, unsalted	3 cups/popped
Jello, sweetened, (count as 120 mL fluid)	1/2 cup
*Rice	1/2 cup
*Corn	1/2 cup

* Potassium content is approximately 75 mg.

AVOID: *Cereals:* Instant and Quick Cooking, or Any Cereal Containing Sugars or Marshmallows, or Nuts, Bran Flakes.

AVOID: *Snack Foods:* Potato Chips, Cheese Curls, Salted Crackers, Salted Popcorn, Pudding Mixes, Cakes, Pies, Tortilla Chips.

AVOID: *Vegetables:* Potatoes, Sweet Potatoes, Yams, Dried Peas and Beans, Chick Peas.

AVOID: *Miscellaneous:* Lentils, Wheat Germ, Commercially Prepared Soups, Baking Coating Mixes, Flavored Rice, Noodle, or Potato Mixes.

FRUIT

Group A
Per Portion:

CHO—	15 g
PRO—	0.5 g
FAT—	0 g
NA+—	2 mg
K+—	140 mg

Daily Servings _____

Includes fresh fruit, pure fruit juices, canned, dried, cooked, or frozen fruits without additional sugar. Drain the liquid that fruits are packed in! Be sure to accurately measure all fruit.

Food	Portion
Apples	1/2 medium, 1 small
Apple Juice	1/2 cup
Applesauce (unsweetened)	1/2 cup

Food	Portion
Apricot Nectar	1/3 cup
Blueberries	3/4 cup
Boysenberries	3/4 cup
Cherries	12 large
Cherries, canned	1/2 cup
Cranberries, whole	1 1/2 cups
Cranberry Juice	3/4 cup
Cranberry Juice Cocktail (low-calorie)	1 cup
Fruit Cocktail	1/2 cup
Grapes	15
Grape Juice, frozen, diluted	1/3 cup
Kumquats	4 medium
Lemon	1 medium
Lime	2 medium
Lime Juice	3/4 cup
Loganberries	3/4 cup

Food	Portion
Mango	1/2 small
Peaches, canned only	1/2 cup
Peach Nectar	1/2 cup
Pears, canned only	1/2 cup/2 halves
Pear, fresh	1/2 large
Pear Nectar	1/3 cup
Persimmons, native	2 medium
Pineapple, canned	3/4 cup/2 rings
Pineapple, fresh	1/3 cup
Pineapple Juice	1/2 cup
Prunes, dried	3 medium
Raisins	2 Tbsp
Raspberries	1 cup
Tangerine	2 small

Group B
Per Portion:

CHO—	15 g
PRO—	0.5 g
NA+—	2 mg
K+—	230 mg

Drain the liquid that the fruits are packed in. Be sure to accurately measure all fruits. Due to their higher potassium content, limit to _____ total portions *per week instead* of a fruit listed in Group A.

Food	Portion
Apricots, canned	1/2 cup or 4 halves
Blackberries	3/4 cup
Figs, fresh	2 medium
Figs, dried	1 1/2
Gooseberries	1 cup
Grapefruit sections	3/4 cup
Grapefruit, fresh	1/2
Grapefruit juice	1/2 cup
Orange	1 small
Orange juice	1/2 cup
Peach, fresh or frozen	1 small, 1/2 cup
Plums	2 small
Watermelon (count as 180 mL fluid)	1 1/4 cups

AVOID: Apricots (fresh, dried), Avocados, Banana, Cantaloupe, Casaba Melon, Dates, Honeydew Melon, Kiwi Fruit, Muskmelon, Papaya, Persimmons (tropical), Pomegranate, Prune Juice, Strawberries.

FAT

Per Portion

CHO—	0 g
PRO—	0 g
FAT—	5 g
NA+	
Regular—	50 mg
Low Sodium—	5 mg
K+—	0 mg

Daily Servings _____

Your diet was planned for the use of *regular/low sodium* fats.

Food	Portion
Butter, Margarine, regular/unsalted	1 tsp
Diet Margarine	2 tsp
Vegetable Oils, Shortening, Lard	1 tsp
Mayonnaise, regular/low sodium	1 tsp
Coffee Whiteners	2 Tbsp
Nondairy Whipped Toppings	4 Tbsp

*Creams	
Cream Cheese	1 Tbsp
Heavy Whipping Cream	2 tsp
Light Cream	1 Tbsp
Sour Cream	2 Tbsp
Whipped Cream	2 tsp
Salad Dressing, regular/low sodium	1 Tbsp

_____

* LIMIT your intake of cream to a maximum of 3 servings/day. Cream contains some protein; more than 3 servings need to be calculated into your diet.

AVOID: Avocados, Bacon, Bacon Fat, Bacon Bits, Italian and Bleu Cheese Salad Dressings, Nuts (all kinds), Olives, Salt Pork, Cream Sauces and Salted Gravies.

Educational Tools for Diabetic Individuals with Renal Failure

Teaching Meal Plan Guides

"Your Diabetic Renal Diet"
New England Deaconess Hospital
Department of Dietetics
185 Pilgrim Road
Boston, Massachusetts 02215

"Calorie Controlled Renal Diet"
Council on Renal Nutrition
Dallas/Fort Worth Metroplex Chapter
National Kidney Foundation of Texas, Inc.
13500 Midway Road
Suite 213
Dallas, Texas 75234

"Your Diabetic Kidney Diet"
St. Michael Hospital
2400 West Villard Avenue
Milwaukee, Wisconsin 53209

Cookbooks

"The Eclectic Renal Gourmet"
The Council on Renal Nutrition of New England
c/o The Kidney Foundation of Massachusetts
344 Harvard Street
Brookline, Massachusetts 01246

"Creative Cooking for Renal Diabetic Diets"
The Cleveland Clinic Foundation
9500 Euclid Avenue
Cleveland, Ohio 44106
Attn: Department of Nutritional Services

"Cooking the Renal Way"
Carolyn J. Ostergren, R.D.
3932 N.E. 37th
Portland, Oregon 97212

"Carbohydrate and Sodium Controlled Cookbook"
Trudy O'Regan, R.D.
Washington Hospital
2000 Mowry Avenue
Fremont, California 94538

Chapter 29

Hypertension in Persons with Diabetes

Judith Wylie-Rosett
Sylvia Wassertheil-Smoller

Hypertension is associated with increased risk of diabetic complications, and the risk factors for developing diabetes and hypertension overlap considerably. The American Diabetes Association estimates that hypertension is twice as common among individuals with diabetes as in the general population.[1] This chapter examines the relationship between diabetes and hypertension and the related risks, as well as discussing treatment modalities.

EPIDEMIOLOGY AND NATURAL HISTORY OF HYPERTENSION AND DIABETES

Historical Perspective

Before antihypertensive medications became available in the 1950s, there was no satisfactory treatment, and most patients had uncontrolled high blood pressure. Severe sodium restriction was the focus of dietary intervention. Although reports advocating low-salt diets appeared as early as 1904 in France and 1922 in the United States, the best known intervention in this area was the Kempner rice-fruit diet, which was composed of a daily sodium intake of 150 mg but also was reduced calorie and intake was rich in potassium, thus potentially confounding the effects of sodium restriction.[2]

With the advent of drug therapy, the risk of death from stroke related to hypertension began to be reduced. As antihypertensive medications became widely available, vigorous goal-centered, stepped-care pharmacologic treatment of

hypertension, including more mildly elevated blood pressures, reduced mortality substantially.[3] Rates of awareness, treatment, and control of hypertension have risen dramatically since 1972 when the National High Blood Pressure Education Program was developed. National Health and Nutrition Examination Survey (NHANES) data indicated that in 1971 to 1972 only 51% of the hypertensive individuals were aware of their diagnosis compared with 84% in 1988 to 1991.[3] During that 20-year period, the proportion of hypertensive individuals who were treated with antihypertensive medications rose from 36 to 73%, and control rates of those treated (measured as <160/95 mm HG) increased from 16 to 55%. Death rates from coronary heart disease and stroke have fallen by 50 and 57%, respectively.[3] The decline in death rates appears to be in large part due to the intensification in efforts to detect and treat hypertension.

However, questions about undesirable side effects of antihypertensive medication resulted in a renewed interest in dietary intervention. Many studies have been conducted to evaluate the effects of weight control, sodium restriction, and modification of other nutrient intake on blood pressure.[4–8] In the 1990s, clinical trials continue to provide insights to refine the role of nutrition intervention in the prevention and treatment of hypertension.

Blood Pressure Measurement

The pumping of the heart exerts pressure or force on the walls of the arteries, which is mea-

Exhibit 29-1 Classification of Blood Pressure for Adults Age 18 Years and Older[a]

Category	Systolic (mm Hg)	Diastolic (mm Hg)
Normal[b]	<130	<85
High normal	130–139	85–89
Hypertension[c]		
Stage 1 (Mild)	140–159	90–99
Stage 2 (Moderate)	160–179	100–109
Stage 3 (Severe)	180–209	110–119
Stage 4 (Very severe)	≥210	≥120

[a] Not taking antihypertensive drugs and not acutely ill. When systolic (SBP) and diastolic (DBP) pressures fall into different categories, the higher category should be selected to classify the individual's blood pressure status. For instance, 160/92 mm Hg should be classified as stage 2, and 180/120 mm Hg should be classified as stage 4. Isolated systolic hypertension (ISH) is defined as SBP ≥140 mm Hg and DBP <90 mm Hg and staged appropriately (eg, 170/85 mm Hg is defined as stage 2 [ISH]).

[b] Optimal blood pressure with respect to cardiovascular risk is SBP <120 mm Hg and DBP <80 mm Hg. However, unusually low readings should be evaluated for clinical significance.

[c] Based on the average of two or more readings taken at each of two or more visits after an initial screening.

Note: In addition to classifying stages of hypertension based on average blood pressure levels, the clinician should specify presence or absence of target organ disease and additional risk factors. For example, a patient with diabetes and a blood pressure of 142/94 mm Hg plus left ventricular hypertrophy should be classified as "stage 1 hypertension with target organ disease (left ventricular hypertrophy) and with another major risk factor (diabetes)." This specialty is important for risk management.

Source: Reprinted from *The Fifth Report of the Joint National Committee on Detection, Evaluation and Treatment of High Blood Pressure* (p 4) by the National Heart Lung and Blood Institute, NIH Pub No 93-1088, 1993.

sured as blood pressure. Blood pressure varies throughout the body, with the pressure being greater in the legs than in the arms. However, blood pressure standards are based on measurements obtained from the upper arm. These standards are based on a combination of systolic and diastolic blood pressure. The systolic pressure is the peak pressure at the moment when the heart contracts as it pumps blood out of the heart. The diastolic pressure is the pressure at the moment when the heart relaxes to permit the inflow of blood. Blood pressure is measured by constricting blood flow and by inflating the blood pressure cuff with air. As air is released from the cuff, the reading on the sphygmomanometer corresponding to the first sound heard through a stethoscope measures the systolic blood pressure. The pressure that corresponds with the last sound heard measures the diastolic blood pressure. Blood pressure is measured

based on standards in millimeter of mercury because, traditionally, the sphygmomanometer used columns of mercury to determine blood pressure levels.

Today, blood pressure can be measured using automated techniques. Many devices use self-inflated cuffs for the arm or finger cuffs to provide a digital reading and do not require any clinical skills to determine the blood pressure level. The accuracy of automated measurement can vary, as do readings obtained by more traditional methods. The automated methods, especially those available as coin-operated devices, need to be checked against a more standard measurement. Blood pressure determined by medical care providers may be falsely elevated when a patient is nervous, often due to a "white coat" effect if the medical visit is perceived stressful. Care provider bias or measurement error can also affect clinical values obtained for blood pressure. Multiple determinations when an individual is relaxed are needed to determine the level of blood pressure control.

Classification of Hypertension

The terminology used to describe blood pressure elevation partially reflects the understanding of the risk associated with various blood pressure levels. Criteria for classifying elevated blood pressure, like those used to diagnose diabetes, have been developed by several groups. In the United States, the guidelines for classifying and treating elevated blood pressure generally come from the Joint National Committee on the Detection, Evaluation, and Treatment of High Blood Pressure, but criteria from the World Health Organization are often used internationally.[3] The Joint National Committee classifies a blood pressure of 140/90 mm Hg or more as hypertension.[8]

In 1993, the Joint National Committee changed from using the terms *mild*, *moderate*, and *severe hypertension*, which have been traditionally used to describe increasing degrees of blood pressure elevation, to a classification system based on stages of hypertension. The rationale for this change was that terms such as *mild hypertension* or *moderate hypertension* failed to convey the importance of hypertension as a continuous cardiovascular risk factor. Exhibit 29-1 shows the 1993 classifications of elevated blood pressure. The term *high normal blood pressure* has been included in the 1993 classification system because the rate of cardiovascular events is higher than for individuals with lower pressure levels.

Traditionally, guidelines for treating hypertension have been based on diastolic blood pressure levels. More recent studies, especially the Systolic Hypertension in the Elderly Program, have determined that controlling systolic blood pressure is as important as controlling diastolic blood pressure.[9] The classifications are based on both systolic and diastolic levels. However, relatively little is known about how dietary intervention affects systolic blood pressure because most of the intervention literature to date has focused on the levels of diastolic blood pressure.

Risk Factors

Hypertension is a very common condition and is even more common among those with diabetes. According to the American Diabetes Association, about half of the persons with diabetes older than age 18 have hypertension, compared with about one-quarter of those without diabetes.[10] Population groups at risk for diabetes are also at risk for hypertension. Blacks have the highest rate of hypertension in the world.[11] Blacks develop hypertension at a younger age, and their hypertension is more severe, which may partially account for the increased risk of renal complications and peripheral vascular disease among blacks with diabetes.

Prevalence of hypertension rises with age as does diabetes. Both hypertension and diabetes are risk factors for cardiovascular morbidity and mortality.[12] Among hypertensives, as well as among normotensives, the presence of diabetes confers a two- to threefold greater risk of cardiovascular disease.

Diabetes nearly doubles the risk of cardiovascular disease and of ischemic heart disease, after controlling for other risk factors such as elevated blood pressure and total cholesterol. When combined with the high cholesterol and high blood pressure that the presence of diabetes confers on a 50-year-old woman, the risk of developing heart disease within the next 8 years is four times that of a nondiabetic woman of the same age with normal systolic blood pressure and an acceptable cholesterol level of less than 200 mg/dL.

Natural History and Pathophysiology

Approximately 30 to 75% of diabetic complications are thought to be caused by hypertension.[1] Hypertension, independently of diabetes, is a well-established risk factor for micro- and macrovascular disease. However, there seems to be a synergistic effect between diabetes and hypertension with respect to vascular disease.

Elevation of blood pressure is a major predictor of deterioration of renal function, and as renal function deteriorates, blood pressure usually rises. Thus, hypertension plays a key role in the progression of diabetic kidney disease, and renal insufficiency raises blood pressure. Hypertension has also been linked to progression of retinopathy, which, like nephropathy, is a disease associated with a thickening of the capillary basement membrane.

The role of hypertension in the progression of macrovascular disease appears to be related to the excess pressure exerted on artery walls. The risk of coronary, cerebral, and peripheral vascular disease is greatly increased with elevated blood pressure. Exhibit 29-2 lists clinical manifestations of target organ disease associated with hypertension, all of which are considered to be complications of diabetes as well.

Renin, a hormone produced by the kidneys, is important in the autoregulation of blood pressure, through its conversion to angiotensin. There are inconsistencies in the literature as to the etiology and precise nature of how the renin-angiotensin system is related to the development of insulin resistance, hypertension, and diabetes.[13]

Some people are salt-sensitive, meaning that their blood pressure rises excessively with acute sodium-loading. Persons with diabetes are more likely to be salt-sensitive. However, even though they may be salt-sensitive, a chronic low-sodium diet may or may not lower blood pressure in diabetic patients whose blood pressure is sensitive to acute sodium-loading, in which sodium intake is greatly increased over 1 day or a few days. Nevertheless, persons who are hypertensive and sodium-sensitive are more likely to manifest left ventricular hypertrophy, microalbuminuria, and other metabolic abnormalities that are linked to vascular complication.[14] Whether sodium sensitivity plays a major role in determining the risk of diabetes complications independent of blood pressure control remains to be determined. The mean arterial pressure and glomerular filtration rate are similar in sodium-sensitive and -resistant individuals on both a low- and high-sodium intake. However, when sodium intake is high, the effective renal plasma flow increases in sodium-resistant but not in sodium-sensitive indi-

---

Exhibit 29-2 Manifestations of Target Organ Disease Associated with Hypertension

Organ System	Manifestations
Cardiac	Clinical, electrocardiographic, or radiologic evidence of coronary artery disease Left ventricular hypertrophy or "strain" by electrocardiography or left ventricular hypertrophy by echocardiography Left ventricular dysfunction or cardiac failure
Cerebrovascular	Transient ischemic attack or stroke
Peripheral vascular	Absence of one or more major pulses in the extremities (except for dorsalis pedis) with or without intermittent claudication: aneurysm
Renal	Serum creatinine ≤ 130 µmol/L (1.5 mg/dL) Proteinuria (1+ or greater) Microalbuminuria
Retinopathy	Hemorrhages or edudates, with or without papilledema

Source: Reprinted from *The Fifth Report of the Joint National Committee on Detection, Evaluation and Treatment of High Blood Pressure* (p 4) by the National Heart Lung and Blood Institute, NIH Pub No 93-1088, 1993.

viduals. Thus, sodium-resistant individuals are able to compensate for an increase in sodium intake, and those who are sodium-sensitive are not. This occurs because the filtration fraction and glomerular capillary pressure decreases in sodium-resistant and increases in sodium-sensitive individuals when sodium intake is high. Thus, sodium restriction is theoretically more likely to lower blood pressure in sodium-sensitive than in sodium-resistant individuals.

Paradoxically, both low and high renin levels have been associated with sodium sensitivity.[13,15] Low renin levels are often found in persons with diabetes and may be due to increased extracellular volume and impaired synthesis of or release of renin. Hyperglycemia can increase extracellular volume. Other factors that alter volume status include other metabolic abnormalities and autonomic nervous system dysfunction.

Hyperinsulinemia may be linked through stimulation of renal sodium retention and volume overload or through activation of the sympathetic nervous system and increased norepinephrine, which could result in vasoconstriction. However, more than half of patients with insulin-dependent diabetes mellitus (IDDM) and one-third of those with non–insulin-dependent diabetes mellitus (NIDDM) maintain normal blood pressure despite having high circulating insulin levels and presumably insulin resistance.[1]

TREATMENT MODALITIES

The goal of treatment of persons who have both hypertension and diabetes is to prevent death and disability caused by hypertension with the least disturbance to quality of life,[3] but the American Diabetes Association notes that the optimal blood pressure level for individuals with diabetes is unknown. However, both the American Diabetes Association[1] and the Joint National Committee on Detection, Evaluation and Treatment of High Blood Pressure[3] have established goals for blood pressure control for adults with diabetes as 130/85 mm Hg or less.

The American Diabetes Association estimates that the 30 to 75% of diabetic complications attributable to hypertension are responsive to early detection and aggressive treatment to reduce morbidity and mortality. The goal of treatment is total risk factor reduction. Figure 29-1 illustrates the effects of modifying the risk factors of smoking, high cholesterol, and hypertension in a 50-year-old man or woman with or without diabetes. The risk of any cardiovascular event over the next 8 years[12] for a 50-year-old person who smokes, has an elevated cholesterol level of 230 mg/dL, has elevated blood pressure with a systolic pressure of 160 mm Hg, and has diabetes is 29% for a man and 12% for a woman. If the person did not have diabetes, the risk would be 18% for a man and 7% for a woman. Although it is not possible to undo the presence of diabetes, it is possible to decrease the other risk factors. By relatively modest modifications of these risk factors, the risk for a person with diabetes can be reduced to levels below those for a nondiabetic individual who has higher values for other risk factors. For example, by reducing cholesterol to 200 mg/dL and systolic pressure to 140 mm Hg and by not smoking, the risk is reduced to 12% for a man and 8% for a woman.

Life-style changes should be the foundation of diabetes and hypertension management; these interventions may be the sole therapeutic modality or may be adjunctive to pharmacologic therapy. Antihypertensive drugs vary in their effects on glucose metabolism.

Antihypertensive Medications

Before initiating medication therapy in stage 1 and stage 2 hypertension, a 3-month trial of life-style modification is recommended for patients with diabetes.[1] Medication is instituted at the time of diagnosis if the blood pressure elevation is in stage 3 or 4. This stepped approach to the drug management of blood pressure evolved from the protocols used in the hypertension controlled trials, especially the Hypertension Detection and Follow-up Program (HDFP).[16]

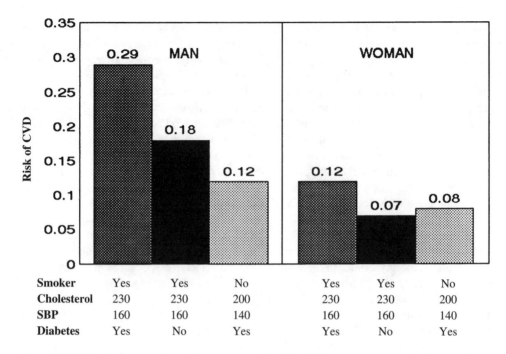

Smoker	Yes	Yes	No	Yes	Yes	No
Cholesterol	230	230	200	230	230	200
SBP	160	160	140	160	160	140
Diabetes	Yes	No	Yes	Yes	No	Yes

Note: CVD includes coronary heart disease, congestive heart failure, cerebrovascular disease, or intermittent claudication.

Figure 29-1 Risk of Cardiovascular Disease within 8 Years Based on Framingham Data. *Source*: Adapted from *The Fifth Report of the Joint National Committee on Detection, Evaluation and Treatment of High Blood Pressure* (p 14) by the National Heart Lung and Blood Institute, NIH Pub No 93-1088, 1993.

Most large-scale hypertension trials have excluded patients with diabetes who were treated with insulin therapy, and relatively few patients with NIDDM participated. To date, there have been no large-scale clinical trials evaluating which antihypertensive agents are the most effective in controlling blood pressure among individuals with diabetes, although some drugs may have deleterious effects on blood lipids and glucose.

Exhibit 29-3 lists various classes of antihypertensive drugs and notes the factors favoring their use and the potential adverse effects related to the management of diabetes. The first level or step of drugs used in controlling hypertension has been diuretics and ß-blockers. Both of these drugs have been shown in large-scale clinical trials, such as HDFP, to reduce mortality

and cardiovascular morbidity.[16] However, both drugs may have certain adverse effects, including deterioration in glucose tolerance. Furthermore, in the Multiple Risk Factor Intervention Trial (MRFIT), diuretic therapy was associated with an increased rate in sudden death in men with resting electrocardiograph abnormalities, and ß-blocker therapy was associated with lipid abnormalities.[17] Diuretics reduce blood volume and thereby reduce the pressure required for the heart to maintain circulation. Thiazide diuretic therapy can cause short-term problems with metabolic control and loss of water-soluble nutrients, especially potassium. Reduction in potassium level is linked to the deterioration in glucose tolerance that is associated with diuretic therapy. Potassium-sparing diuretics can result in elevated potassium levels and are contra-

Exhibit 29-3 Potential Complications of Antihypertensive Drug Classes

Drug	*Potential Complications*
Diuretics	
Potassium losing (thiazides, loop diuretics)	Hypokalemia, hyperglycemia, dyslipidemia, impotence
Potassium sparing	Hyperkalemia, impotence, gynecomastia
Vasodilators	Exacerbation of coronary heart disease, fluid retention
Sympathetic inhibitors	Orthostatic hypotension, impotence, depression
α-**Adrenergic blockers**	Orthostatic hypotension
ß-**Adrenergic blockers**	
Nonselective	Cardiac failure, impaired insulin release with hyperglycemia, hypoglycemia unawareness, delayed recovery from hyperglycemia, impotence
Cardioselective[a]	Blunted symptoms of hypoglycemia, hypertension associated with hypoglycemia, hyperlipidemia, impotence
Angiotensin-converting-enzyme (ACE) inhibitors	Proteinuria, hyperkalemia, leukopenia, agranulocytosis/cough

[a] Cardioselectivity may be lost with high doses.

Source: Adapted with permission from Christieb AR, Treating Hypertension in the Patient with Diabetes. *Medical Clinics of North America* (1982;66:1373–1388), Copyright © 1982, WB Saunders.

indicated for individuals with renal insufficiency or high serum potassium levels. ß-Blockers usually reduce blood pressure by decreasing cardiac output. Unawareness of hypoglycemia is a major adverse side effect that raises concern in using ß-blockers for patients with diabetes.

The effects of ß-blockers and diuretics on blood pressure, quality of life, and other factors differ by race and sex. For example, the Trial of Antihypertensive Intervention and Management (TAIM), as well as other studies, has shown that the ß-blocker atenolol is preferable for white patients and that diuretic therapy is more effective in black patients. The optimum diet–drug combination for black patients was diuretic plus weight loss intervention, whereas for whites, it was atenolol plus weight loss. Quality of life generally remains the same or improves with treatment of hypertension,[18–20] but diuretics may cause impotence, and side effects should be systematically monitored. Weight reduction, interestingly, reduces these side effects. Also, weight loss improves the overall risk profile as well.[21] Although participants in the TAIM study were more successful at losing weight than in reducing sodium intake,[22] the beneficial effect of weight loss on cardiovascular risk, which was mediated though lipid changes, was found in the MRFIT study as well.[17]

Angiotensin-converting-enzyme (ACE) inhibitors decrease angiotensin II-mediated vasoconstriction and synthesis of aldosterone. Blood pressure is decreased as the result of increased vasodilation. The ACE inhibitors reduce microalbuminuria and proteinuria, and these agents may play a role in delaying the progression of diabetic nephropathy that is independent of a blood pressure reduction.[23] Monitoring of potassium and creatinine is important during the first few weeks of ACE inhibitor therapy because hyperkalemia can occur, especially if a patient has renal failure or bilateral renal artery stenosis. ACE inhibitors are contraindicated in pregnancy and should be used with caution in women of childbearing age. Coughing is a common side effect of ACE inhibitors, and angioedema is a rare but serious side effect.[1,3,24,25]

Calcium channel blockers reduce blood pressure through vasodilation.[1,3,25] Some of these calcium antagonists also reduce blood pressure through effects on electrophysiology and hemodynamics. Constipation, diarrhea, and peripheral edema can be side effects of calcium antagonists that may be problematic, especially in patients with neurologic and vascular complications. Elderly patients may have a calcium channel blocker prescribed to control angina.

Weight Reduction

Obesity is linked to both diabetes and hypertension. Weight reduction has been shown to be effective in lowering blood pressure.[4–8] The National High Blood Pressure Education Program Working Group on the Primary Prevention of Hypertension concluded that a weight loss of 4 to 8 kg can improve blood pressure and glycemic control.[26] Data from the TAIM indicate a 4.5-kg (10 lb) weight loss was as effective as step 1 drugs (initial low dose of diuretic or ß-blocker therapy) in lowering blood pressure among overweight hypertensives in stage 1 hypertension.[5,27] When used concomitantly with drugs, weight loss enhanced the effectiveness of diuretics and ß-blockers.

Data from hypertension treatment trials indicate that modest weight loss can reduce the adverse impact of antihypertensive drugs on other cardiovascular risk factors. In the MRFIT, a weight loss of 10 lb (4.5 kg) reduced cholesterol by 10% compared with 7.2% reduction for the weight-stable participants and 3.9% for those who gained weight.[17] Among MRFIT participants, weight loss was less when smoking cessation or antihypertensive drug therapy was implemented.[17] The TAIM demonstrated that weight loss improves overall cardiovascular risk.[20,21]

Data from persons with diabetes also indicate that as the amount of weight loss increases, improvement occurs in lipids (total and subfractions of cholesterol and triglycerides), glucose, and blood pressure.[28]

Sodium Restriction

The American Diabetes Association recommends sodium intake be restricted to 2400 mg or less for individuals with diabetes who have mild-to-moderate (stage 1 or stage 2) hypertension,[29] noting a wide variability to sodium sensitivity.[30] Nevertheless, the general effectiveness of sodium restriction to treat hypertension is still equivocal.

Although traditionally the average sodium intake for Americans was considered to be between 5000 and 10,000 mg, data from NHANES II indicate that the mean intake for males is 3300 mg and for females 2300 mg.[31] The highest level of intake occurs between the teenage years and early adulthood in both sexes. Dietary data from hypertension clinical trials suggest that sodium intake decreases with age and increases with body weight.[4,5,22] Baseline TAIM data obtained in the 1980s suggest that sodium intake of individuals with hypertension who volunteer for clinical trials is lower than in previous clinical trials.[22]

In one small randomized cross-over study of patients with diabetes and hypertension, reducing sodium intake from approximately 4600 to 3150 mg reduced systolic pressure by 11% but did not significantly affect diastolic blood pressure.[32] In the Dietary Intervention Study of Hypertension (DISH), patients who had been previously controlled for more than 5 years with antihypertensive drugs were withdrawn from these drugs and entered into either a weight reduction or sodium restriction program. Sodium restriction (approximately 90 mmol or 2070 mg) was able to retard the relapse to hypertension and the need to restart medication among the lean study participants only. It was not useful in the overweight trial participants.[4]

In the TAIM, a sodium restriction intervention alone (mean level after 6 months of intervention was approximately 110 mmol or 2530 mg) was not effective in lowering blood pressure among mild hypertensives, but subgroup analyses of the data indicated that when individuals lowered their sodium intake to less than 1500 mg/d, blood pressure reduction was comparable with low-dose drug therapy. Only 25% of the study subjects were able to achieve that level of sodium intake despite intensive intervention.[33] Thus, the effort to achieve a long-term sodium restriction diet was not effective. Nevertheless a review by Cutler et al[34] indicates that sodium restriction may be a useful treatment modality.

The question thus is not resolved, but it appears that salt-sensitive individuals will respond to low-salt diets. The problem is that there is no way to identify, a priori, who will be salt-sensitive. Therefore, an empirical approach is necessary. The level of sodium restriction that may be required to achieve a blood pressure effect may also have to be empirically determined. Achieving a sodium level of 1500 mg, as was found to be effective in controlling blood pressure in the TAIM, may be difficult to achieve. The nutritional management of individuals with hypertension and diabetes should consider the interest and willingness to reduce sodium intake.

Few studies have evaluated the effectiveness of sodium restriction in controlling blood pressure in individuals with diabetes. Although sodium sensitivity is common in patients with diabetes and hypertension, in one study investigators did not find a consistent blood pressure response to restricting sodium among individuals with NIDDM. The sodium restriction did not reduce short-term vascular reactivity among patients with diabetes. Relatively little is known to predict how well blood pressure will respond to reduction in sodium intake in a given individual. If the sodium intake appears to be high, it is reasonable to recommend trying to reduce sodium intake to potentially avoid initiating or increasing the dosage of drug therapy. When the interest level and motivation to minimize or avoid drug therapy is high, making a goal of restricting

sodium to a low level (1500 mg) may be warranted.

Some studies have suggested that low renin levels may predict which patients will have a blood pressure response to chronic sodium restriction.[13] Other studies (TAIM and DISH) have indicated that patients with high renin levels have greater blood pressure reduction with salt reduction than those with low renin levels.[15] However, to date renin has not been evaluated as a predictor of which patients with diabetes would be likely to have blood pressure respond to sodium restriction. Furthermore, renin levels are usually obtained only in research studies and require standardized procedures that would be difficult to obtain in clinical practice. Long-term clinical trials are needed to assess how chronic sodium restriction affects the blood pressure elevation that commonly occurs in NIDDM. Studies also need to identify markers for which patients are likely to have blood pressure response to chronic sodium restriction.

Other Dietary and Life-Style Modifications

Excessive alcohol intake can raise blood pressure and reduce responsiveness to antihypertensive medications. Limiting alcohol intake is recommended in the treatment of both diabetes and hypertension.

A high potassium intake may be protective against developing hypertension, and potassium deficiency is associated with an increase in blood pressure. Normal potassium levels should be maintained, preferably from food sources. Most health care providers recommend bananas or orange juice to increase dietary potassium intake. Therefore, other foods rich in potassium such as potato, tomato, legumes, or mango are underused as options to increase intake.

If diuretic therapy results in hypokalemia, an increase in both blood glucose and blood pressure may occur. Potassium supplements, often prescribed as a potassium chloride or a time-released preparation, may be needed to maintain a normal blood potassium level less than 4 mg/dL. Gastrointestinal distress is a side effect of many potassium supplements, especially potassium chloride.

Dietary calcium intake has been shown to be usually inversely related to blood pressure level, and calcium deficiency is associated with increased prevalence of hypertension. A low calcium intake can increase the blood pressure effects of a high-sodium diet. Even though increasing calcium intake may lower blood pressure in some patients with hypertension, there is no way to predict which patients will respond. Therefore, the Joint National Committee recommends following the recommended dietary allowance (RDA) to achieve a calcium intake of 800 to 1200 mg.[3]

A low intake of magnesium has been associated with higher blood pressure. An adequate intake of magnesium consistent with the RDA is needed.[1,3] Unfortunately, nutrient data bases often have inadequate values for magnesium, making assessment intake difficult. At the present time, there is insufficient evidence to warrant supplementation with magnesium to lower blood pressure.

Omega-3 fatty acids in large doses can lower blood pressure. The adverse effects of consuming large quantities of omega-3 fatty acids may include elevation of blood glucose, especially among obese individuals. The Joint National Committee does not recommend the use of omega-3 fatty acid supplements to treat hypertension.[3]

The beneficial effects of regular, moderately intense exercise (40 to 60% VO_{2max}) on blood pressure are well established. When aerobic physical activity is adequate to achieve a moderate level of physical fitness, it appears to reduce the risk of developing hypertension and is helpful in treating hypertension. The Joint National Committee indicates that brisk walking for 30 to 45 minutes three to five times a week appears to be sufficient to achieve the blood pressure effect.[3] Regular aerobic physical activity appears to reduce systolic blood pressure by approximately 10 mm Hg.

Resistance training such as weightlifting can increase blood pressure acutely, which, like the Valsalva maneuver, can precipitate an eye hemorrhage in patients with retinopathy. Therefore, such activities should generally be avoided.

Stress can cause an acute rise in blood pressure. Chronic stress may play some role in hypertension, but the roles of stress management, relaxation therapy, and biofeedback in the management of hypertension are uncertain. Despite short-term demonstration of success, longer-term trials have failed to demonstrate that these techniques are of added benefit in controlling hypertension.

Cigarette smoking can raise blood pressure acutely but does not appear to play a role in developing hypertension. Nevertheless, avoiding tobacco is extremely important in preventing the diabetic complications associated with diabetes and hypertension. An assessment of tobacco exposure and smoking cessation counseling should be integrated into the nutritional management of all patients, especially those with diabetes and hypertension who are at increased risk for complications. Dietitians are increasingly integrating smoking evaluation and counseling into their life-style modification counseling. This integration is needed and may be critical for individuals who may continue to smoke in an effort to control their body weight. Such individuals may need help in the decisional balance between the health risks posed by smoking versus any potential benefit with respect to weight control. Individuals with diabetes and hypertension need to understand how much smoking increases their cardiovascular risk.

INDIVIDUALIZING NUTRITION THERAPY

The nutrition intervention for patients with diabetes and hypertension should be based on a comprehensive evaluation. A careful assessment of the risk profile is needed. Dyslipidemia is common in patients with diabetes and/or hypertension. However, the health status of persons with diabetes and hypertension can vary widely. Some may have hypertension before they develop diabetes. For many of these patients,

Exhibit 29-4 Diabetes and Hypertension Nutrition Recommendations

	American Diabetes Association	*Joint National Committee on Detection, Evaluation, and Treatment of High Blood Pressure*
Calories	Sufficient to attain and/or maintain a reasonable body weight for adults. A mild-to-moderate weight loss of 10 to 20 lb has been shown to improve diabetes control. A moderate calorie restriction of 250–500 calories less than average daily intake is recommended	Lose weight if overweight Reducing fat intake helps reduce calories
Exercise	IDDM—integrate insulin therapy into usual eating and exercise patterns. NIDDM—weight loss is best attempted by a moderate decrease in calorie expenditure. Regular exercise and learning new life-style behaviors are advised	Aerobic regularly
Sodium	For people with mild-to-moderate hypertension, eat 2400 mg or less	Reduce to <100 mmol (2300 mg) or 6 g NaC1
Alcohol	Moderate usage ≤2 alcoholic beverages (1 beverage = 12 oz beer, 5 oz wine, 1 1/2 oz distilled spirits with meals)	Limit 1 oz ethanol (24 oz beer, 8 oz wine, 2 oz 100-proof whiskey)
Fat	Saturated <10% of daily calories, <7% if low-density lipoprotein is elevated. Polyunsaturated fats up to 10% of total calories. Approximate total fat varies with treatment goals: 30%—normal weight and lipids; <30%—obese and elevated lipids; and <40%—evaluated triglycerides unresponsive to fat restriction and weight loss	Stop smoking, reduce dietary saturated fat and cholesterol for overall health
Vitamins/Minerals	If chromium deficient secondary to total parenteral nutrition (TPN), use chromium replacement. Routine evaluation of serum magnesium is recomended in those at high risk for deficiency. Potassium loss may warrant supplementation for patient taking diuretics. Hyperkalemia may warrant potassium restriction in patient with renal insufficiency, hypoaldosteronism, or taking ACE inhibitors	Maintain adequate dietary potassium, calcium, magnesium intake

weight reduction may greatly ameliorate both abnormalities. Nutrition intervention can help reduce some of the adverse effects of antihyper-tensive medication, as well as potentially reduce the dosage needed to control blood pressure. The treatment choice needs to consider the health status and demographic characteristics of the person, which could influence not only the effectiveness but also the impact on quality of life. More research is needed to help guide clinical decision making regarding the treatment of hypertension, especially among black women,[35] who are disproportionately affected by diabetes, hypertension, and the related complications.

Exhibit 29-4 compares the 1994 American Diabetes Association's Nutrition Recommendations[29] and the 1993 Consensus Statement to the guidelines from the 5th Joint National Committee, which were published in 1994. Although there are subtle differences, developing a patient treatment plan can easily be based on both. The American Diabetes Association recommendations tend to provide more guidance for managing patients who have complications. The method for quantifying alcohol equivalents differs slightly, which could potentially cause confusion in using educational materials.

Persons with long-standing diabetes may develop an elevation of blood pressure that is an indication of deterioration in kidney function as a complication of diabetes. For such patients, the primary focus of nutrition therapy should be in managing renal disease and managing cardiovascular risks associated with renal failure. The nutritional management may be assumed by the renal dietitian from the kidney treatment program (see Chapter 28). When a patient develops advanced complications, the nutritional management of the complication may become a higher priority than nutritionally managing the diabetes per se.

When treatment priorities change, patients often become confused. For example, patients are taught to increase potassium intake to prevent hypokalemia related to thiazide diuretic therapy, but restricting potassium intake may be indicated when the antihypertensive medication is changed or when renal deterioration results in hyperkalemia.

Exercise instruction may differ depending on patient status. If a patient has developed a foot ulcer, walking and any weight-bearing exercise is usually contraindicated. Instructions for increasing physical activity may require the expertise of a rehabilitation program. Patients with orthostatic hypotension, which is a common neurologic complication of diabetes, need to stand slowly after reclining.

CONCLUSION

Medical nutritional therapy of diabetes and hypertension overlaps considerably. Weight control is effective in the management of both, and the dietary recommendation for managing diabetes focuses on comprehensive management of cardiovascular risk, which addresses the needs of the high proportion of patients with diabetes who have hypertension. The treatment strategy should be to reduce the risk of micro- and macrovascular complications and to lower overall cardiovascular risk.

REFERENCES

1. American Diabetes Association. Consensus statement: treatment of hypertension in diabetes. *Diabetes Care.* 1993;16:1364–1401.

2. Wassertheil-Smoller S, Langford H, Blaufox MD, Oberman A, Hawkins M. Diuretics and salt restriction in blood pressure control. In: Minick M, ed. *Nutrition and Drugs.* New York, NY: John Wiley & Sons; 1983.

3. Joint National Committee on Detection, Evaluation, and Treatment of High Blood Pressure. *The Fifth Report of the Joint National Committee on Detection, Evaluation and Treatment of High Blood Pressure.* Bethesda, Md: National Institutes of Health, National Heart Lung and Blood Institute; 1993. NIH Publication no. 93-1088.

4. Langford H, Blaufox MD, Oberman A, et al. Dietary therapy slows the return of hypertension after stopping prolonged medication. *JAMA.* 1985;253:657–664.

5. Langford HG, Davis BR, Blaufox MD, et al. Effect of drug and diet treatment of mild hypertension on diastolic blood pressure. *Hypertension.* 1991;17:210–217.

6. Stamler R, Stamler J, Brimm R. Nutrition therapy for high blood pressure: final report of a four-year randomized controlled trial—The Hypertension Control Program. *JAMA.* 1987;257:1484–1491.

7. Trials of Hypertension Prevention Collaborative Research Group. The effects of nonpharmacologic interventions on blood pressure of persons with high normal levels: results of the Trial of Hypertension Prevention, Phase I. *JAMA.* 1992;267:1213–1220.

8. Hypertension Prevention Trial Research Group. The Hypertension Prevention Trial: three-year effects of dietary changes on blood pressure. *Arch Intern Med.* 1990;150:153–162.

9. SHEP Cooperative Research Group. Prevention of stroke by antihypertensive drug treatment in older persons with isolated systolic hypertension. *JAMA.* 1991;265:3255–3264.

10. American Diabetes Association. *Diabetes 1993 Vital Statistics.* Alexandria, Va: ADA; 1993.

11. Intersalt Cooperative Research Group. Intersalt: an international study of electrolyte excretion and blood pressure. *BMJ.* 1988;297:319–328.

12. Anderson KM, Wilson PWF, Odell PM, Kannel WB. An updated coronary risk profile. A statement for health professionals. *Circulation.* 1991;83:356–362.

13. Kaplan NM. The prognostic implications of plasma renin in essential hypertension. *JAMA.* 1975;231:167–170.

14. Campese VM. Salt sensitivity in hypertension: renal and cardiovascular implications. *Hypertension.* 1992;23:531–550.

15. Blaufox MD, Lee HB, Davis B, Oberman A, Wassertheil-Smoller S, Langford H. Renin predicts diastolic blood pressure to nonpharmacological and pharmacological therapy. *JAMA.* 1992;267:1221–1225.

16. Hypertension Detection and Follow-Up Program. Five year findings. I. Reduction in mortality of persons with high blood pressure including mild hypertension. *JAMA.* 1979;242:2562–2571.

17. Caggiula A. A new challenge in antihypertensive therapy: total cardiovascular risk reduction. In: Wassertheil-Smoller S, Wylie-Rosett J, Alderman M, eds. *Cardiovascular Health and Risk Management: The Role of Nutrition and Medication in Clinical Practice.* Littleton, Mass: PSG Publishing Co; 1989.

18. Wassertheil-Smoller S, Blaufox MD, Oberman A, et al. The TAIM Study Group: effect of antihypertensive treatment on sexual function and other quality of life parameters. *Ann Intern Med.* 1991;114:613–620.

19. Croog SH, Levine S, Testa MA, et al. The effects of antihypertensive therapy on the quality of life. *N Engl J Med.* 1986;314:1657–1664.

20. Williams GH, Croog SH, Levine S, Testa MA, Sudilovsky A. Impact of antihypertensive therapy on quality of life: effect of hydrochlorothiazide. *J Hypertens Suppl.* 1987;5:S29–S35.

21. Oberman A, Wassertheil-Smoller S, Langford HG, et al. Pharmacologic and nutritional treatment of mild hypertension: changes in cardiovascular risk status. *Ann Intern Med.* 1990;112:89–95.

22. Wylie-Rosett J, Wassertheil-Smoller S, Blaufox D, et al. Trial of Antihypertensive Intervention and Management: greater attainment of 6 month intervention goals for weight loss than Na/K modification. *J Am Diet Assoc.* 1993;93:408–414.

23. Lewis EJ, Hunsickler LG, Bain RP, Rohde RD, for the Collaborative Study Group. The effects of angiotensin-converting-enzyme inhibition on diabetic nephropathy. *N Engl J Med.* 1993;329:1456–1462.

24. Lam YWF, Sheperd MM. Drug interactions in hypertensive patients: pharmacokinetic, pharmacodynamic and genetic considerations. *Clin Pharmacokinet.* 1990;18:295–317.

25. Cressman MH, Vlasses PH. Recent issues in antihypertensive drug therapy. *Med Clin North Am.* 1988;72:373–397.

26. Working Group on Management of Patients with Hypertension and High Blood Cholesterol Education Programs. Working group report on management of patients with hypertension and high blood cholesterol. *Ann Intern Med.* 1991;114:224–237.

27. Wassertheil-Smoller S, Blaufox MD, Oberman AS, Langford HG, Davis BR, Wylie-Rosett J. The Trial of Antihypertensive Interventions and Management Study: adequate weight loss, alone and combined with drug hypertension. *Arch Inten Med.* 1992;152:131–136.

28. Wing RR, Koeske R, Epstein LH, Nowalk MP, Gooding W, Becker D. Long-term effects of modest weight loss in type II diabetes patients. *Arch Intern Med.* 1987;147:1749–1753.

29. American Diabetes Association. Position statement: nutrition recommendations and principles for people with diabetes mellitus. *Diabetes Care.* 1994;17:519–522.

30. Franz MJ, Horton ES, Bantle JP, et al. Nutrition principles for the management of diabetes and related complications. (American Diabetes Association technical review). *Diabetes Care.* 1994;17:490–518.

31. National Center for Health Statistics. *Vital and Health Statistics: National Health and Nutrition Examination Survey II.* Series 11:231. Washington, DC: U.S. Government Printing Office; 1983.

32. Dodson PM, Beevers M, Hallworth R, Webberley MJ, Fletcher RF, Taylor KG. Sodium restriction and blood pressure in hypertensive type II diabetics: randomized blind controlled and crossover studies of moderate sodium restriction and sodium supplementation. *BMJ.* 1989;298:227–230.

33. Davis BR, Oberman A, Blaufox DM, et al. Trial of Antihypertensive Intervention and Management: lack of effectiveness of low-sodium/high potassium diet in reducing antihypertensive medication requirements in overweight persons with mild hypertension. *Am J Hypertens.* 1994;7:926–932.

34. Cutler JA, Follmann D, Elliott P, Suh I. An overview of randomized trials of sodium reduction and blood pressure. *Hypertension.* 1991;17(suppl 4):I-27–I-33.

35. Anastos K, Charney P, Charon RA, et al. Hypertension in women: what is really known? *Ann Intern Med.* 1993;115:287–293.

Chapter 30

Identifying and Treating Eating Disorders in Persons with Diabetes Mellitus

William H. Polonsky

In this chapter, a decade of research data is reviewed, indicating that eating problems are relatively common in diabetes and that the medical consequences of such behaviors are often grave. Often secretive, ashamed, and/or frustrated, persons with diabetes may describe such problems as uncontrollable binge eating, intense preoccupation with their weight, and/or intentional insulin omission. How can we understand such problems? How widespread and how serious are they? And what are we to do about them?

OVERVIEW OF EATING DISORDERS

Clinical Disorders

Gross disturbances in eating behavior are usually indicative of anorexia nervosa or bulimia nervosa. As presented in Exhibit 30-1, the newly revised fourth edition of the *Diagnostic and Statistical Manual* (DSM-IV)[1] describes anorexia nervosa as a refusal to maintain body weight at or above minimally normal levels for age and height, intense fear of gaining weight or becoming fat, disturbed body image, and (in females) amenorrhea. Bulimia nervosa is characterized by recurrent episodes of binge eating, compensatory behaviors to prevent weight gain (eg, self-induced vomiting, misuse of diuretics or laxatives, and fasting), and preoccupation with body shape and weight. In contrast to earlier editions of the *Diagnostic and Statistical Manual*, DSM-IV has finally recognized insulin omission in patients with diabetes mellitus as a purging behavior that meets the criterion for bulimia nervosa.[1]

Binge eating and compensatory behaviors must have occurred, on average, at least twice weekly for 3 months.

Preoccupation with eating, shape, and weight are common in both disorders. Indeed, bulimic behaviors occur frequently in anorexia (which may explain much of the confusion in earlier classification schemes), although the differences between the disorders are usually clear. Bulimics, for example, are typically of normal weight.[2] In both disorders, females predominate. Males comprise less than 10% of all cases of anorexia nervosa and bulimia nervosa. Among those at greatest risk, women in late adolescence and early adulthood, the prevalence of anorexia nervosa is estimated at 0.5 to 1% and bulimia nervosa at 1 to 3%.[1]

Subclinical Disorders

Less severe disturbances, often referred to as "subclinical" eating disorders, may be even more common than the disorders described above. A subclinical disorder may be considered when the patient meets some of but not all the criteria for bulimia nervosa or anorexia nervosa. There is, however, no commonly accepted definition of subclinical eating disorder, although undue preoccupation with weight and shape would seem to be a necessary feature in all cases.[3] Toward this end, there have been recent efforts[4] to formalize criteria for a newly proposed diagnosis, binge eating disorder, which is characterized by frequent episodes of binge eating (at least twice weekly) and preoccupation

Exhibit 30-1 DSM-IV Diagnostic Criteria for Eating Disorders

---

1. Anorexia Nervosa

A. Refusal to maintain body weight at or above minimally normal levels for age and height (<85% of expected weight)

B. Intense fear of gaining weight or becoming fat, even though underweight

C. Disturbance in the experience of one's body weight, shape, or size (feeling "fat" even though underweight, denying the seriousness of the current low body weight, and/or feeling preoccupied with body weight or shape)

D. In females, amenorrhea (absence of at least three consecutive menstrual cycles)

2. Bulimia Nervosa

A. Recurrent episodes of binge eating, with each episode involving:

  1. consumption of a large amount of food (larger than what most others would eat under similar circumstances)

  2. consumption occurs in a discreet period of time (usually < 2 hours)

  3. feelings of being unable to control one's eating during the event

B. Recurrent compensatory behaviors to prevent weight gain (eg, self-induced vomiting, misuse of laxatives or diuretics, fasting, excessive exercise, and—in diabetes mellitus—insulin omission)

C. Both binge eating and compensatory behaviors must have occurred, on average, at least twice weekly for 3 months

D. Preoccupation with body shape and weight

Source: Reprinted from *Diagnostic and Statistical Manual of Mental Disorders*, 4th ed. With permission of the American Psychiatric Association, Copyright © 1994.

---

with weight and shape, without the use of self-induced vomiting or other compensatory behaviors to prevent weight gain. However, after much debate, binge eating disorder was not accepted as a formal diagnostic category in DSM-IV and thus remains an unofficial subclinical diagnosis. For improved diagnostic purposes, DSM-IV has broadened a third category of eating disorder, known as eating disorder NOS (not otherwise specified), which may include binge eating disorder as well as other subclinical disorders.[1]

Cautions against Overdiagnosis

Extreme care is required when assigning the diagnosis of eating disorder, be it clinical or subclinical. Although an appropriate diagnosis may be overlooked by health care providers, there must be an equal concern with overdiagnosing. For example, overeating is widespread, but such events do not necessarily constitute binge episodes (feeling unable to control one's eating is an essential criterion). Binge eating may be common in populations at great risk, as in female college students,[5] but if bingeing typically occurs, say, only once a month, should this be labeled as a "disorder"? *Disordered eating behaviors, especially when they are infrequent, do not necessarily constitute an eating disorder.*

To guard against overdiagnosing, it must be remembered that obesity is *not* an eating disorder, although binge eating is likely to be a significant contributor in a *subset* of patients (20 to 46%).[6,7] Recent evidence from studies in diabetes supports this viewpoint. In a study of 98 obese non–insulin-dependent diabetes mellitus (NIDDM) patients who were applying to a weight management program, 21% of females and 9% of males met criteria for a serious binge eating problem.[8] In a recent survey of obese women with insulin-dependent diabetes mellitus (IDDM) and insulin-requiring NIDDM, we found that 8 of the 23 IDDM women (35%) reported significant eating problems (5 patients met the screening criteria for bulimia nervosa, and 3 additional patients binged at least twice weekly). Of the 38 NIDDM women, 6 (16%) reported significant eating problems (3 patients met criteria for bulimia nervosa, and 3 additional patients binged at least twice weekly).[9] If obesity were an eating disorder, we would expect that clinically significant eating problems would be apparent in each of these NIDDM and IDDM patients. Instead, disordered eating behavior appeared to be a significant factor in only a few cases.

Similarly, chronic poor adherence to an appropriate diabetic meal plan, although of serious concern, is *not* necessarily an eating disorder. In a recent survey, we found 69 women with IDDM who reported poor adherence to their meal plan (following prescribed recommendations <50% of the time). Only 23 (34%) of these 69 "poor adherers" reported significant eating problems (15 patients met the screening criteria for bulimia nervosa, and 8 additional patients binged at least twice weekly).[9] Again, if poor adherence were equivalent to an eating disorder, we would expect all "poor adherers" to display significant eating problems, and yet only a minority did so.

Etiology

What causes an eating disorder? Biologic, psychological, and social factors are all believed to contribute to the development and maintenance of eating disorders, but in most cases, the actual etiology remains unclear. The pervasive cultural pressures that emphasize unrealistic models of slimness are likely to be an important influence in most cases, although only for those individuals who are psychologically and/or biologically susceptible.[10] For bulimia nervosa in particular, those who are driven to be thin and yet tend to be heavier than their peers may be especially vulnerable.[11,12] Psychological contributors may include affective instability (depressed and rapidly fluctuating mood states, impulsive behaviors), body dissatisfaction, and unreasonably high self-expectations, all contributing to feeling out of control of one's internal life and desiring external means to regain a sense of control. Unfortunately, an unreasonable goal of thinness is often selected as the achievement by which one's sense of control and self-esteem can be regained, although a history of chronic dieting, rigid restraint of one's eating, and belief in "forbidden foods" may commonly lead, for biologic and psychological reasons, to a gross breakdown in cognitive restraints, leading to binge eating and consequent weight *gain*.[13] To cope with this "psychobiologic impasse,"[10] purging strategies may then be used, although, as discussed below, these are commonly ineffective in limiting calories absorbed.[2,14–16]

PREVALENCE OF DISORDERED EATING IN IDDM

Early Research

Although eating disorders were once thought to be rare in diabetes, a growing body of research suggests that such problems may not be so uncommon. The first published case reports began appearing in the early 1980s and soon more and more followed. In a comprehensive review of 57 reported cases of co-occurring IDDM and eating disorders, Marcus and Wing[17] noted that 95% of cases were female (mirroring the prevalence of eating disorders in the general population), the onset of IDDM preceded the eating disorder in 90% of cases, deliberate insulin manipulation to promote weight loss was apparent in the majority (62%) of cases, and poor glycemic control was the norm (noted in 75% of cases).

LaGreca and colleagues[18] examined 30 young women with IDDM, aged 15 to 35, using a structured clinical interview. Based on their glycated hemoglobin (HbA$_1$) level, subjects were divided into three groups of equal size—good, fair, and poor control. Although most of the subjects reported binge eating, those in the poor control group indicated a dramatically higher frequency of bingeing (13 times a month) than those in fair control (7 times a month) and good control (once a month). Also, 70% of those in poor control and 50% of those in fair control reported that they coped with overeating by reducing or omitting their insulin, whereas *none* of those in good control reported insulin manipulation. Although these findings were impressive, they must be interpreted with caution. It was not explained how the subjects were recruited, and thus, we cannot assume that such a sample is a fair representation of the IDDM population.

Dysfunctional Eating Attitudes

Formal investigations have begun to document the actual prevalence, characteristics, and consequences of disordered eating in diabetes. Using standardized psychometric instruments, studies[19–25] have compared the prevalence of dysfunctional eating attitudes in patients with IDDM versus a nondiabetic sample (in all cases, <40 years old).

Eating Attitudes Test

Differences between females with IDDM and nondiabetic females have been consistently found with the Eating Attitudes Test (EAT),[26,27] a self-report scale that measures eating habits and attitudes related to dieting, bulimia, and food preoccupation.[19,23,25] Differences have been most apparent on the dieting subscale, which has led to suggestions that IDDM females are more preoccupied with dieting issues than nondiabetic females. The EAT, however, is replete with diabetes-biased items (eg, "aware of calorie contents of foods I eat," "avoid foods with sugar in them"), to which it would be expected that patients with diabetes would score positively, even when normal eating attitudes are apparent. Thus, the observed IDDM versus nondiabetic differences on the EAT should not be taken too seriously. Attempts to modify the EAT for IDDM patients have been made,[23] but biased items remained (eg, "think about burning calories when I exercise"), suggesting that the EAT, even in modified form, may be inappropriate for use with patients with diabetes.

Eating Disorder Inventory

Significant differences between IDDM and non-IDDM women (aged 16 to 25) have been found on several subscales of the Eating Disorder Inventory (EDI),[28] including drive for thinness and body dissatisfaction,[23] although a re-

cent study examining a younger population (aged 8 to 18), found no such differences.[24]

Eating Disorder Examination

The Eating Disorder Examination (EDE)[29] is a well-respected, standardized clinical interview for the careful quantification of disordered eating behaviors. In comparison to self-report questionnaires, the EDE is much more likely to be a valid and reliable indicator of disordered eating. In several EDE studies with IDDM females, neither young adults[19] nor adolescents[20,24] evidenced more disturbed eating attitudes and behaviors than their non-IDDM counterparts. Also, no differences in eating attitudes and behaviors between males with and without IDDM were found.[19,20,22,23,25]

In total, these data suggest that persons with IDDM are not more likely to have dysfunctional eating attitudes and behaviors than those without IDDM.

Clinical Eating Disorders

The prevalence of diagnosable eating disorders in IDDM has also been examined. Survey studies have reported wildly varying rates of eating disorders, ranging from 2 to 35% of the various samples. These differences are attributable to methodologic problems, including low response rate,[30] age differences in surveyed populations, changes in criteria for eating disorder diagnoses (eg, bulimia nervosa, introduced in DSM-III-R and continued in DSM-IV, makes use of much tighter and more severe criteria than the previously used diagnostic category of bulimia), and the use of different, and often less than appropriate, psychometric measures. Most studies have used a variety of self-report measures for disordered eating, which are appropriate only for screening purposes. Actual diagnoses require a clinical interview.

Nevertheless, careful examination of the available studies reveals that there are important consistencies across many of these studies:

- Rates of anorexia nervosa were generally low (<1%).[31,32]

- Rates of bulimia and bulimia nervosa were generally low in adolescent girls, ranging from 2 to 5%,[9,32,33] and higher in young adult women, ranging from 10 to 12%.[9,31,34]

Although rates for bulimia nervosa in IDDM women appear to peak during late adolescence and early adulthood, rates may remain relatively elevated throughout adulthood. In our recent study, we used the Bulimia Test-Revised (BULIT-R), a self-report questionnaire known to be a sound screening instrument for bulimia nervosa,[35] and found that 11% of those in the 15- to 30-year age group, 6% in the 31- to 45-year age group, and 5% in the 46- to 60-year age group met criteria for bulimia nervosa.[9]

It must be remembered that formal diagnoses were not obtained in these studies. Also, the subject samples were not randomly selected; rather, they were samples of convenience and came mostly from tertiary care centers, which may not accurately represent the general IDDM population.

Recently, several studies have obtained population-based samples and used standardized clinical interviews (the EDE), from which diagnoses were obtained. Similar rates of eating disorders in young adults were observed; specifically, 11% of young IDDM women, aged 17 to 25, met criteria for bulimia nervosa or eating disorder NOS.[19] Unfortunately, in IDDM adolescent girls, the prevalence issue remains unclear, with one study, examining ages 11 to 18, reporting that 9% met criteria for a clinical eating disorder[20] and one study, examining ages 8 to 18, reporting that 0% met criteria.[24] Careful comparisons of young IDDM girls with their non-IDDM counterparts have revealed no differences in the rates of diagnosable eating disorders.[19,20]

Although these data suggest that IDDM patients are no more likely to have clinical eating disorders or disordered eating behaviors and attitudes than the general nondiabetic population, the problem remains a serious one. Among young adult women with IDDM, more than one in ten may be suffering with a diagnosable eat-

ing disorder. Significant though smaller percentages of adolescent and older adult women (perhaps 1 in 20) may be similarly troubled.

Subclinical Eating Disorders

Subclinical disorders are likely to be even more widespread. For example, among Striegel-Moore's[24] subsample of older IDDM adolescents, although no clinical eating disorders were apparent, 71% reported disturbed attitudes regarding their shape and weight and 50% noted excessive weight control efforts. We recently found that, among IDDM females (aged 13 to 60) who did *not* meet screening criteria for bulimia nervosa, 5% reported binge eating at least twice weekly and 12% reported omitting insulin as a means of managing their overeating.[9]

INTENTIONAL OMISSION OF INSULIN

Prevalence

One of the greatest concerns regarding eating disorders in IDDM is the phenomenon of intentional insulin omission. Early in the course of the condition, many young women realize that they can manage their weight through underdosing or omission of insulin (this may often occur at the time of diagnosis, when rapid weight loss occurs despite the consumption of large amounts of calories). By promoting glycosuria, they may eat or overeat without weight gain.[31]

In studies involving standardized clinical interviews, insulin omission in the service of weight control has been found to average 11 to 15% in IDDM women in young adulthood[19] and adolescence.[20,24] As with eating disorders, insulin omission was not apparent in young men.[19,20] Similar findings have been reported from survey research.[31,32,34,36-39] Not surprisingly, binge eating is commonly linked to insulin omission.[18] Even among those who do *not* meet criteria for eating disorders, we found that insulin omission in the service of weight management is significantly more common in those who binge at least twice weekly (42% omitting) than in those who binge less often or not at all (11% omitting).[9]

However, insulin omission does not necessarily indicate the presence of an eating disorder. We found that 31% of a large sample of IDDM women reported insulin omission, but only half of this group indicated that they did so for the purposes of weight management.[38] Insulin omission in the remaining half was more strongly linked to diabetes-specific distress. Among IDDM women with clinical eating disorders, however, intentional omission of insulin is very common and, indeed, appears to be the preferred method for coping with binge eating. Reported rates of omission in this population range from 53 to 86%.[19,32,34,38] In all cases, rates for other compensatory behaviors were markedly lower. In total, these results suggest that insulin omission for weight management may be relatively common among young women with IDDM and that it is strongly associated with disordered eating.

Why Omit?

The popularity of insulin omission lies in the fact that it is a unique form of purging, different from more traditional forms of purging in one very important way—it is an effective form of weight management. Self-induced vomiting, laxative usage, and diuretic use are all inefficient strategies for purging calories, although acute changes in fluid balance may initially disguise this. Because absorption of food begins within minutes in the gastrointestinal tract, vomiting is unable to eliminate all calories consumed and, paradoxically, quite often leads to increased binge eating.[2,16] Similarly, even large doses of laxatives or diuretics do not significantly impair calorie absorption.[14,15] By promoting glycosuria through insulin omission, however, calories are effectively excreted (in concert with fluid depletion).[40] To illustrate, we found that among IDDM women who met screening criteria for bulimia nervosa, those who relied exclusively on traditional forms of purging were significantly heavier (mean body mass index [BMI] = 33.3) than those who reported insulin omission (mean

BMI = 25.1).[9] And yet the consequences of intentional insulin omission, especially in combination with disordered eating, may be severe.

MEDICAL CONSEQUENCES OF DISORDERED EATING IN IDDM

Glycemic Control

Several studies have examined the relationship between eating disorders (mostly bulimia nervosa and eating disorder NOS) and glycemic control in IDDM women.[9,19,20,32,41–43] In almost all cases, those with eating disorders manifested significantly poorer glycemic control than those without eating disorders. For example, we found that the mean HbA_1 for those who met screening criteria for bulimia nervosa was 13.2%, whereas the mean HbA_1 for those not meeting criteria was 10.5%.[9] This was not an uncommon finding; most studies observed a two-point or greater difference in glycated hemoglobin levels between eating disordered and non-eating disordered groups. Given that a similar two-point difference separated the intensive care and standard care groups in the Diabetes Control and Complications Trial (DCCT) (with marked differences in subsequent rates of long-term complications),[44] these findings are likely to be clinically relevant as well as statistically significant.

Long-Term Complications

Several studies have suggested that eating disorders are associated with significantly higher rates of long-term complications.[9,40,42,44]

- Colas et al[41] found that 62% of young IDDM women with eating disorders have retinal lesions versus 20% in a matched non-eating disordered sample.
- We found that retinopathy was apparent in 79% of those IDDM women who met screening criteria for bulimia nervosa versus 52% in those who did not meet criteria. Similarly, neuropathy was apparent in 50% of those with eating disorders versus 20%

in those without. In both cases, these differences remained significant even after controlling for age and duration of illness.[9]

- In a recent prospective study, eating disordered and non-eating disordered patients were reassessed 4 years after initial evaluation. Retinopathy was apparent in eight of nine (89%) young women with a previously suspected eating disorder versus 14 of 56 (25%) without an eating disorder.[44]

In total, these data suggest that eating disorders, especially bulimia nervosa, promote chronically high blood glucose levels and lead inexorably to the early development of long-term complications. In addition to poor glycemic control, inadequate nutrition may also play an important role in the development of such early complications.[42]

Short-Term Complications

Eating disorders, especially bulimia nervosa, have also been linked to more immediate, diabetes-specific complications, especially unstable ("brittle") metabolic control as well as frequent episodes of diabetic ketoacidosis (DKA).[45] In all cases of recurrent DKA, especially among young women, the possibility of dysfunctional eating attitudes and behaviors in combination with intentional insulin omission should be considered. Because it is much rarer, diabetes-specific consequences of anorexia nervosa are less clear, although acute painful neuropathy has been reported in several cases.[42] As noted earlier, the restricting form of anorexia may not present with elevated blood glucose levels. Indeed, with severe limitations on calories, case reports suggest that one of the major consequences may be recurrent severe hypoglycemia.[45]

Importance of Insulin Omission

Intentional insulin omission is likely to be one of the major factors linking eating disorders and the early development of long-term complications. We found that insulin omission in the service of weight management was directly associated with poor glycemic control as well as long-term complications[38]:

- Glycemic control was significantly poorer in omitters (mean HbA_1 = 12.3%) than non-omitters (mean HbA_1 = 10.3%).
- Rates of long-term complications were significantly higher in omitters than non-omitters (for neuropathy, 47 versus 17%; for retinopathy, 72 versus 50%).

Subclinical eating problems may also be associated with significant medical consequences, especially when they are linked to insulin omission.[9] Among those who did *not* meet screening criteria for bulimia nervosa, glycemic control was significantly poorer in omitters (mean HbA_1 = 11.7%) than non-omitters (mean HbA_1 = 10.2%), and rates of neuropathy were significantly higher in omitters (41%) than non-omitters (16%). Similar differences were seen for retinopathy but did not reach significance. Importantly, no significant differences in glycemic control or complication rates were seen between those who reported binge eating at least twice weekly and those who reported less frequent bingeing. Thus, subclinical eating problems in IDDM are not necessarily linked to important medical consequences unless insulin omission is involved.

DISORDERED EATING IN NIDDM

Little data on patients with NIDDM are available. As reported earlier, a recent study of 98 obese NIDDM patients found that 21% of women and 9% of men met criteria for a serious binge eating problem.[8] It is not known whether this is greater than would be found in a matched nondiabetic sample, but it seems unlikely. Surveying a cohort of 71 insulin-requiring NIDDM women, we found that 6% met screening criteria for bulimia nervosa and an additional 7% reported binge eating at least twice weekly. In that same study, 328 IDDM women were also surveyed, and no differences in the prevalence of eating problems between the IDDM and NIDDM samples were observed.[9] As in the IDDM findings presented earlier, it is likely that eating problems are relatively common among NIDDM women as well, but there is nothing to suggest that disordered eating is more common in NIDDM than in the general population. Similarly, it seems likely that disordered eating in NIDDM will contribute to poor glycemic control and higher rates of long-term complications (especially when insulin omission is involved), but there are as yet no data to support these conjectures.

Among insulin-using NIDDM women, insulin omission in the service of weight control appears to be relatively rare. We found that 16% of IDDM women reported insulin omission as a means of managing their weight,[38] yet only 3% of insulin-using NIDDM women reported such behavior.[9] NIDDM patients tend to be older than IDDM patients, so we re-examined these data, limiting the analysis to those women older than 40 years. The findings remained the same—significantly more IDDM women reported omission (10%) than NIDDM women (2%).[9] We suspect that important historical differences may be influential here. For example, those who experience the diagnosis of IDDM are likely to learn, quite directly and powerfully, that insufficient insulin is associated with weight loss. Because the NIDDM diagnosis is not typically linked to weight loss, those with NIDDM are unlikely to learn this lesson.

CONTRIBUTORS TO DISORDERED EATING IN DIABETES

Many researchers suspect that diabetes, especially IDDM, may promote the development of eating disorders, but to date there is little supportive evidence.[46] As noted earlier, the great majority of case reports found that the development of the eating disorder followed the onset of IDDM. However, causal attributions cannot be made, because IDDM typically occurs at a younger age than do eating disorders.[17] Also, the consistent observation that clinical eating disorders are similarly prevalent in those with and without IDDM[19,20,24] argues against an IDDM influence. It remains possible, however, that diabetes may lead to the development of more subclinical eating disorders and/or promote eating disorders that are more intractable to treatment.[47] Although such effects have not yet been substantiated, they seem reasonable, given our understanding of how diabetes education and self-care may influence thoughts and behavior.

Promotion of Chronic Dietary Restraint

As described earlier, a history of chronic dieting, rigid restraint of one's eating, and perception of "forbidden foods" may contribute to the development of eating disorders, especially bulimia nervosa.[13] And in diabetes education, patients are commonly urged to limit and restrain their intake, in terms of food types, amounts, and timing. Also, there is often a strong emphasis on learning to recognize and limit certain foods. Thus, successful diabetes education has tended to promote what may be one of the major risk factors for disordered eating, chronic dietary restraint. As a consequence of such training, patients may become expert at ignoring internal hunger and satiety cues, leading to peculiarly disregulated attitudes toward food. Although preoccupation with food and the consequences of food are strongly encouraged, there may be a markedly decreased enjoyment in eating, with food being increasingly perceived as simple fuel, as another form of medication, or as a tool for merely feeding one's insulin (and/or avoiding hypoglycemia). As internal satisfaction becomes downplayed and the delight and celebration of eating disappears, the potential for more disregulated eating increases, as the individual is more likely to fall prey to other external cues for eating (eg, emotional cues, social situations, and advertisements).

Link between Appropriate Diabetes Self-Care and Weight Gain

Recent evidence suggests that improved glycemic control is associated with consequent weight gain.[43,48-50] In the DCCT, for example, intensively treated patients gained an average of 10 lb *more* than conventionally treated patients.[44] Initiation of insulin treatment for

NIDDM patients after oral agent failure commonly leads to weight gain as well. With improved glycemic control, average weight gains of 5 to 10 lb are not uncommon,[50] although one recent study reported an average weight gain of 17 lb over the first year of insulin treatment.[51]

Also, individuals with IDDM may be significantly heavier than their nondiabetic counterparts, especially among adolescents.[20] No studies have yet examined weight differences between adults with IDDM and nondiabetic adults. For IDDM patients, improved control may lead to weight gain due to a reduction in excreted calories through glycosuria, increased caloric intake secondary to treatment for more frequent hypoglycemia, and/or through the direct, insulin-catalyzed promotion of body fat.[52] For NIDDM patients, the most important factor may be the treatment-induced exacerbation of hyperinsulinemia. Especially for those women sensitive to current cultural pressures for thinness, such weight gain may be viewed as a very significant "complication" of diabetes, although health care providers are often insensitive to the importance of this issue. As reported above, a heavier starting weight, body dissatisfaction, and feelings of loss of control over one's body may be important risk factors for eating disorders, especially bulimia nervosa. Yet each of these factors may be linked with "successful" diabetes care. Not surprisingly, disordered eating behaviors in IDDM and NIDDM women have been found to be strongly linked to weight, with disordered eating more prevalent among heavier women.[9,24]

Greater Prevalence of Depressed and Fluctuating Moods

Depression appears to be more prevalent in IDDM and NIDDM than in the general population, although it is not clear that the prevalence in diabetes is higher than in any other chronic illness.[53] Also, large fluctuations in blood glucose levels, which are naturally more common in diabetes (especially IDDM), are commonly associated with marked shifts in mood.[54] Thus, individuals with IDDM and NIDDM may be more vulnerable to depressed and fluctuating moods and, consequently, a perceived loss of control over one's body. As described earlier, both are believed to be significant contributors to the development of disordered eating.

Promotion of Unreasonably High Self-Expectations

In many cases, coping with diabetes and the frustrations of diabetes self-care may lead to the development of perfectionistic tendencies. Often inadvertently, health care providers as well as family members may categorize blood glucose results as either "good" or "bad." Similarly, poor adherence to one's meal plan is often labeled as "cheating." This may encourage patients to adopt a dichotomous style of thinking in regards to diabetes self-care, presuming that their self-care is satisfactory only when all aspects are rigorously followed (ie, they are being "perfect"). Because the vagaries of insulin therapy and diabetes management commonly lead to blood glucose data that are less than perfect, patients with such unreasonable self-expectations are often deeply disappointed and/or shamed by their "poor" accomplishments. Unreasonably high expectations for self-care may be further encouraged when providers set vague and/or unreasonable treatment goals for their patients. It must be emphasized, however, that no studies have yet examined the prevalence of perfectionism in diabetics. If a higher rate is found, this would suggest that disordered eating behaviors, which are associated with high self-expectations, are encouraged by provider and family communications that regularly promote (albeit inadvertently) unreasonable and/or dichotomous self-care goals.

Uniquely Effective Form of Purging

For those who are frustrated with managing their weight, the intentional omission of insulin can seem an enormously seductive opportunity. As described earlier, insulin omission is a uniquely potent means of purging calories. And despite the catastrophic long-term consequences, a significant number of IDDM women choose to manage their weight by this means. It is not craziness or stupidity that drives such behavior. Rather, given the powerful short-term positive reinforcers that are associated with omission, it is a choice that is intelligible:

- Regular omission leads to *liberation from eating restraints* (because calories are efficiently eliminated) and *less effort expended on the self-care regimen.* For example, because omission promotes higher blood glucose levels, patients may reduce the frequency of blood glucose testing (eg, "Why bother? It's always high anyway"). Indeed, we found that omitters report poorer adherence than non-omitters to providers' recommendations for blood glucose testing as well as meal-planning recommendations.[38]
- With fewer self-care efforts, omitters may find it relieving that they do not need to think about IDDM as often; thus, *"denial" of diabetes is more achievable.*
- With chronically high blood glucose levels, *hypoglycemic episodes are less likely to occur.* This may be of particular importance because omitters report being more fearful of hypoglycemia than non-omitters.[38]

Of interest, we found that the major independent predictors of omission were not disordered eating attitudes and behaviors but fear of normoglycemia (fear that improved glycemic control would lead to weight gain) and diabetes-related distress.[38] In total, significant positive reinforcers for insulin omission are apparent. In exchange for short-term (eg, fatigue and blurred vision) and long-term (microvascular and macrovascular) complications, omitters may be able to manage their weight successfully while freeing themselves from many of the IDDM self-care hassles (although they remain more distressed about their diabetes).

These data suggest that many of the risk factors associated with the development of eating disorders may be pronounced in the diabetic population, suggesting that disordered eating behaviors may be more common in diabetics—especially in IDDM and among those at greatest risk, young women. Further research will be needed to clarify whether this is so. Also, because bulimia nervosa in the general population is commonly an addictive and hard-to-break habit, it is reasonable to suspect that the illness may become significantly more intractable in IDDM in which two additional advantages are obtained, a weight management strategy that actually works and freedom from many of the constraints of diabetes self-care. It is likely that most cases reflect a difficult combination of dysfunctional attitudes toward diabetes as well as dysfunctional eating attitudes.[38]

ASSESSMENT

Common Presentations

Although cases of anorexia nervosa may occasionally occur, disordered eating in diabetes will most commonly present as a variant of bulimia nervosa. The most likely presentations are

- Traditional bulimia nervosa, in which IDDM and NIDDM patients use traditional forms of purging (eg, self-induced vomiting) and, if they are taking insulin, avoid the intentional omission of insulin. Clinical lore suggests that many of these patients may continue to manage their diabetes adequately; thus, glycemic control in such patients may not necessarily be poor.
- Diabetes-specific bulimia nervosa, in which patients (primarily IDDM) use insulin omission as the predominant form of purging. Poor glycemic control and poor regimen adherence are common in this population.[9,46] Recurrent, and unexplained, episodes of DKA may also be apparent. Anecdotal data, however, suggest that many of these patients are successful at administering just enough insulin to avoid DKA.

- "Passive" bulimia, falling in the eating disorder NOS category, in which patients, typically those with IDDM who are on intensive regimens using multiple shots of adjustable regular insulin, have frequent episodes of binge eating or overeating and cope with the potential weight gain by passive purging. Specifically, the patient does not compensate for the increased calorie intake by appropriately increasing the regular insulin dosage. Although dramatic omission of the basal insulin dosage does not typically occur, frequent repetition of such behaviors will lead to chronically elevated blood glucose levels.

- Chronic binge eating (or binge eating disorder), a subclinical disorder in which IDDM and NIDDM patients have frequent episodes of uncontrolled overeating without any subsequent purging behaviors. Elevated blood glucose levels and weight gain are common results.[8]

Identifying Disordered Eating

Given the shame of many patients concerning their disordered eating as well as the common desire to avoid displeasing their health care providers, patients may tend to hide their problematic behaviors; thus, the signs and symptoms of eating disorder pathology are not likely to be obvious in many cases. How then can such problems be identified?

- Medical markers. The possibility of a clinical disorder should be considered when patients present with

  1. chronically poor glycemic control

  2. recurrent DKA

  3. repeated episodes of hypoglycemia

  4. significant fluctuations in weight, especially when such changes cannot be easily explained

- Nonjudgmental questions. To promote an honest discussion/investigation of eating problems, it is vital that the health care provider be as nonjudgmental as possible.

Rather than asking "You don't have any eating problems, do you?" the provider might try a more inclusive open-ended approach, such as "Almost everyone with diabetes struggles with eating; what is that struggle like for you?" Creating an atmosphere of nonjudgmental acceptance is essential.[55]

- Patient self-reports. Even mild self-reports of binge eating, purging, or weight preoccupation should be thoroughly investigated. To begin assessing weight preoccupation, for example, patients may be asked how frequently they think about their weight or shape or how they feel about looking in mirrors or using scales. Details, especially about binges, are essential. Make sure to ask about the specific foods eaten as well as the amounts.

- Self-report screening questionnaires. As described earlier, the EAT includes many diabetes-biased items, which may make interpretation difficult, but there are several other excellent scales with fewer biased items, such as the EDI and the BULIT-R. Administration of such scales may aid in earlier detection of eating problems. Also, these instruments may be useful during an education session as a means to catalyze conversation concerning eating attitudes. The EDI can be obtained from Psychological Assessment Resources (Odessa, FL) and the BULIT-R from its authors (Dr. Mark Thelen, Department of Psychology, University of Missouri—Columbia, MO 65211).

- Young women with IDDM. Careful consideration should be given when evaluating patients in this highest-risk population.

It is important to remember that a clinical interview is required to confirm the diagnosis of an eating disorder. Providers must be conservative when suspecting the presence of an eating disorder. There is no need to stigmatize all obese patients, poor adherers to the self-care regimen, or even insulin omitters (especially those who omit infrequently), because such problems are not necessarily linked to disordered eating.

TREATMENT

A typical case is as follows: Janet, an attractive 27-year-old, single woman with a 14-year history of IDDM, is referred for treatment. She is bright and well educated and is employed full-time as an industrial designer. Despite a mixed-split insulin regimen, her glycated hemoglobin levels (obtained irregularly) over the past several years have been very high, pointing to an average blood glucose level of 350 mg/dL. Mild retinopathy and peripheral neuropathy are apparent. With great shame and many tears, Janet describes a 9-year history of disordered eating, including nightly episodes of binge eating (typically, at least 1 lb of chocolate candy, always eaten in secret) usually followed by the intentional omission of her bedtime NPH insulin. Her eating is chaotic throughout the day and only rarely does she have actual meals, especially not in the morning when she is often too nauseated from high blood glucose levels. She weighs herself at least once each day and, depending on the result, may reduce her morning NPH and regular insulins as well as her suppertime regular insulin. As a teenager, she was hospitalized for DKA on three occasions (secondary to her eating problems) but has not been hospitalized since then. Although Janet has not monitored her blood glucose levels in many months ("Why bother? I know the result will always be high!"), she has become sensitive to the early signs of DKA and has managed to take just enough insulin to avoid hospitalization. She avoids visits with her endocrinologist as much as possible and does her best to "not think about diabetes and the terrible damage I am doing to myself." Janet is relatively content at her current weight but knows that she must stay very vigilant. She is anxious to start exercising, but due to her high glucose levels, she is much too exhausted to begin to do so. She is significantly depressed, angry about diabetes, and frightened about long-term complications, but she feels unable to stop her disordered eating

behaviors. Her weight is the most important thing to her, and the possibility of weight gain is terrifying. Remarkably, she has managed to keep her eating problems secret from her fiance as well as her family.

Interventions for eating disorders in individuals with diabetes, such as Janet, have rarely been studied. To date, only case studies have appeared in the research literature, focusing on treatment for anorexia nervosa[56,57] and bulimia nervosa.[47,58,59] These reports as well as anecdotal data suggest that eating disorders in IDDM may be more difficult to treat than eating disorders in the general population.[47] Principles for treatment include hospitalization, negotiated diabetes management, outpatient psychotherapy, and other intervention.

Hospitalization

Medical crises such as DKA, metabolic abnormalities, and malnutrition (especially in anorexia nervosa) may necessitate acute medical hospitalization. For patients such as Janet, however, the eating disorder often goes unrecognized, and the rapid normalization of blood glucose levels leads to rehydration, likely to be followed by acute edema and/or rapid weight gain. For the weight-conscious patient, such "improvement" can be very frightening and is likely to promote a renewed cycle of insulin omission and bingeing after hospitalization. In these more severe cases, psychiatric hospitalization, especially in an eating disorders unit, is often preferable. Such specialized units can help patients to normalize their eating habits, recognize and address the underlying emotional component to their bingeing, cope with the ensuing weight fluctuations in a structured setting, and face any related psychiatric issues (eg, depression).

Negotiated Diabetes Management

Aggressive attempts to promote appropriate insulin usage, regular blood glucose testing, and reasonable meal planning are likely to be met with significant resistance. If they are initially willing to cooperate, patients who are presented with strict self-care guidelines are likely to gain weight rapidly, which they are unlikely to tolerate for any reasonable length of time, leading to further binge eating, insulin omission, and/or dropping out of treatment. A flexible and gradual approach is imperative, and the perception of self-control (that the patient is in charge of her regimen, body, and fate) should be continually emphasized. Changes in diabetes management should be slow and always negotiated with the patient. At first, negotiated changes may even be of minimal value in promoting glycemic change but still of great importance in establishing a cooperative treatment relationship. As an initial step in treatment, for example, Janet agreed to stabilize her insulin dosages at breakfast and dinner, begin taking 1 U of NPH at bedtime (substantially less than what was prescribed) and testing her blood glucose once each day. In this manner, she retained a sense of control over her fate and body, self-efficacy was promoted, a behavioral habit of bedtime insulin usage was reinitiated, nondichotomous thinking was engendered (as she began to realize that there were reasonable choices for self-care other than "perfect" or "bad"), and intolerably rapid weight changes were avoided. Changes in the prescribed insulin regimen should also be considered. In particular, intensive insulin regimens (involving short-acting insulin before meals as well as long-acting insulins) allow for greater flexibility and modification of eating habits and thus may be preferable in many cases. In a series of case reports, Peveler and Fairburn[47] found that bulimic patients on intensive insulin regimens displayed greater improvement in glycemic control than those patients on one or two injections per day.

Outpatient Psychotherapy

Interdisciplinary treatment for such patients is essential. In most cases, psychotherapy should be a central facet of treatment; thus, referral to a mental health professional, preferably one who is knowledgeable about diabetes, is very important. Recent attention has focused on cognitive-behavioral therapy (CBT), in which significant improvements in bulimia nervosa have been documented.[60] In a modified CBT approach in IDDM, psychotherapy focuses initially on behavioral interventions to achieve a minimally acceptable level of glycemic control, educate about eating disorders in diabetes, assess and stabilize disordered eating behaviors (using food records and initial recommendations for meal timings), and problem-solve toward a gradual reduction in purging and bingeing. Cognitive interventions are soon introduced as well, which focus on modifying dysfunctional beliefs about weight and body shape, examining the cognitive and emotional aspects of bingeing, and exploring negative attitudes about diabetes and diabetes management.

In the nondiabetic population, CBT treatment commonly focuses on helping patients to end their severe dietary restraint through the gradual introduction of forbidden foods into the daily meal plan. In IDDM patients, however, this may seem antithetical to the prescribed treatment regimen. Thus, the therapist must walk a narrow line between encouraging continued restraint and advocating poor self-care adherence.[47] For example, Janet was not encouraged to give up nightly chocolate; rather, she and her therapist worked to end the secretiveness, shame, and "uncontrollability" of her bingeing by staging chocolate "tastings" during their early sessions and also negotiated to find a life-style compromise between no chocolate and too much chocolate. As expected, when given permission to "cheat" in this manner (thus retaining her sense of personal control), her desire for chocolate began to dramatically subside.

Additional Interventions

Family involvement, group interventions, and medication trials should also be considered. It is often helpful to include at least one family member or friend in the treatment process.[46] Whether adolescent or adult, the patient may benefit from acknowledging the eating problems to loved ones, thus ending years of guilt and isolation. It may also be important to openly examine and modify family attitudes and behaviors regarding self-care lapses, given that patients commonly suspect that family members are judging or controlling their eating behaviors. Group psychotherapy treatment for eating disorders has been shown to be helpful[61] and such an approach for young IDDM women with eating disorders may also prove to be of value.[46] Finally, antidepressant medications may be of value as one component of treatment, as it may attenuate the need for eating binges as well as reduce associated depression in some cases.[62] It must be emphasized, however, that the overall value of antidepressants in such complex treatment cases is likely to be relatively limited. Medication should not be considered as the sole intervention for eating disorders in diabetes.

Severe cases, such as Janet's, are likely to be rare in most practices. More commonly seen are cases of chronic binge eating, especially in obese NIDDM patients. In these cases, principles of treatment will be similar. Hospitalization is unlikely to be necessary, but negotiated diabetes management and CBT remain as essential features of treatment. Effective group programs for obese binge eaters have been developed and tested,[63] and adapting these programs for NIDDM patients would be straightforward.

TREATMENT AND PREVENTION TIPS

Dietitians can play an essential role in treating and preventing eating disorders in diabetes. The most important recommendations are as follows:

1. Establish relationships in which patients feel comfortable in being honest about their weight concerns as well as their frustrations with diabetes.

2. In a nonjudgmental and collaborative manner, regularly ask all patients, especially those in the high-risk groups, about insulin omission, episodes of binge eating, and diet behaviors. There should be an emphasis on the normalization of such concerns, that preoccupation with weight, binge episodes, and the temptation to omit insulin are understandable behaviors and are not that unusual.

3. In a proactive fashion, inform all appropriate patients about the basic principles of dieting, including common myths, dangers, and frustrations.

4. All patients on insulin, especially young women with IDDM, should be forewarned about the difficulties of weight management as glycemic control is tightened, and alternative strategies should be discussed and planned (eg, exercise).

5. Recommended eating changes should be respectfully negotiated with the patient. All actions and even the choice of words should convey to the patients that they are in ultimate control of their own eating. For example, be wary of such instructions as "I think we will give you an extra protein exchange for your evening meal." Instead, consider a more respectful intervention, "You might feel better if you ate a little extra protein at your evening meal. How would you feel about trying that?" Above all, avoid becoming a "diet plan dictator."

6. When negotiating eating changes, set individualized goals and tasks that are reasonable, concrete, short-term, and achievable. In this manner, we are helping patients to achieve "success experiences" with meal plan changes, thus engendering greater self-efficacy and reducing the likelihood that patients will become discouraged with treatment. Toward these ends, a generic meal plan should never be presented to the patient. The starting point for all eating change negotiations should be the patient's current eating pattern.

7. As much as possible, avoid eating restraints and forbidden foods. Indeed, negotiate meal plans that include regular opportunities for "imperfect" eating (as in

Janet's nightly chocolate "tastings"), which are likely to reduce the feelings of deprivation that lead to bingeing. Because such episodes are scheduled, diabetes management plans can be modified to minimize blood glucose elevations.

8. When disordered eating behaviors are present, use informal, cognitive-behavioral strategies to identify and overcome the emotional and behavioral factors that may be contributory. Excellent examples of such an approach are seen in Schlundt[55] and Strowig and colleagues.[64]

9. If you suspect a serious eating problem, refer to an appropriate mental health professional.

combination with the unusual pressures of diabetes self-care, fear of normoglycemia in IDDM women (leading to weight gain) may be more widespread than was previously assumed. Among IDDM women, it seems likely that most cases of disordered eating go undetected,[46] potentially indicating a large group of poorly controlled patients who are not receiving appropriate treatment. There are as yet little data available on eating disorders in NIDDM patients. The few studies to date suggest that subclinical eating disorders (especially chronic binge eating) are far from rare. For IDDM and NIDDM patients, appropriate assessment, treatment, and prevention strategies are urgently needed.

CONCLUSION

Eating problems, especially bulimia nervosa and eating disorder NOS, are relatively common in diabetes. It appears that the highest-risk group is young women with IDDM, in which clinical eating disorders are likely to occur in more than 10% of patients. As has been suspected, the consequences of such behaviors are grave. Disordered eating is associated with poor metabolic control and markedly higher rates of long-term complications. Insulin omission is the most common form of purging and may be the major factor in determining serious medical consequences. There do not appear to be more eating disorders in the IDDM population compared with the nondiabetic population, and there is as yet no good evidence that IDDM promotes the development of eating disorders. However, eating disorders in IDDM may be more resistant to treatment than common eating disorders, especially given the seductive and addictive nature of insulin omission in the management of body weight. Subclinical eating disorders, usually related to binge eating, also appear to be common and are linked to poor glycemic control and long-term complications (especially when insulin omission is involved). As a consequence of our cultural preoccupation with slimness in

REFERENCES

1. American Psychiatric Association. *Diagnosis and Statistical Manual of Mental Disorders.* 4th ed. Washington, DC: American Psychiatric Association; 1994.

2. Fairburn CG. Cognitive-behavioral treatment for bulimia. In: Garner DM, Garfinkel PE, eds. *Handbook of Psychotherapy for Anorexia Nervosa and Bulimia.* New York, NY: Guilford Press; 1985:160–192.

3. Fairburn CG. The definition of bulimia nervosa: guidelines for clinicians and research workers. *Ann Behav Med.* 1987;9:3–7.

4. Spitzer RL, Yanovski S, Wadden T, et al. Binge eating disorder: its further validation in a multisite study. *Int J Eating Disorders.* 1993;13:137–153.

5. Gray J, Ford K. The incidence of bulimia in a college sample. *Int J Eating Disorders.* 1985;4:201–210.

6. Marcus MD, Wing RR. Binge eating among the obese. *Ann Behav Med.* 1987;9:23–27.

7. Yanovski SZ, Nelson JE, Dubbert BK, Spitzer RL. Association of binge eating disorder and psychiatric comorbidity in obese subjects. *Am J Psychiatry.* 1993;150:1472–1479.

8. Wing RR, Marcus MD, Epstein LH, Blair EH, Burton LR. Binge eating in obese patients with type II diabetes. *Int J Eating Disorders.* 1989;8:671–679.

9. Polonsky WH, Anderson BJ, Welch G, Lohrer PA, Aponte JE, Jacobson AM. Disordered eating in women with IDDM and insulin-treated NIDDM. In preparation.

10. Johnson C, Connors M. *The Etiology and Treatment of Bulimia Nervosa: A Biopsychosocial Perspective.* New York, NY: Basic Books; 1987.

11. Agras WS, Kirkley BG. Bulimia: theories of etiology. In: Brownell KD, Foreyt JP, eds. *Handbook of Eating Disorders*. New York, NY: Basic Books; 1986:367–368.

12. Fairburn CG, Cooper PJ. Self-induced vomiting and bulimia nervosa: an undetected problem. *BMJ*. 1982;284:1153–1155.

13. Polivy J, Herman CP. Dieting and bingeing: a causal analysis. *Am Psychol*. 1985;40:193–201.

14. Bo-Lynn G, Santa-Ana CA, Morawski SG, Fordtran JS. Purging and calorie absorption in bulimic patients and normal women. *Ann Intern Med*. 1983;99:14–17.

15. Garner DM, Rockert W, Olmsted MP, Johnson C, Coscina DV. Psychoeducational principles in the treatment of bulimia and anorexia nervosa. In: Garner DM, Garfinkel PE, eds. *Handbook of Psychotherapy for Anorexia Nervosa and Bulimia*. New York, NY: Guilford Press; 1985:513–572.

16. Kaye WH, Weltzin TE, Hsu LKG, McConaha CW, Bolton B. Amount of calories retained after binge eating and vomiting. *Am J Psychiatry*. 1993;150:969–971.

17. Marcus MD, Wing RR. Eating disorders and diabetes. In: Holmes CS, ed. *Neuropsychological and Behavioral Aspects of Diabetes*. New York, NY: Springer-Verlag; 1990:102–121.

18. LaGreca AM, Schwarz LT, Satin W. Eating patterns in young women with IDDM: another look. *Diabetes Care*. 1987;10:659–660.

19. Fairburn CG, Peveler RC, Davies B, Mann JI, Mayou RA. Eating disorders in young adults with insulin dependent diabetes mellitus: a controlled study. *BMJ*. 1991;303:17–20.

20. Peveler RC, Fairburn CG, Boller I, Dunger D. Eating disorders in adolescents with IDDM: a controlled study. *Diabetes Care*. 1992;15:1356–1360.

21. Robertson P, Rosenvinge JH. Insulin-dependent diabetes mellitus: a risk factor in anorexia nervosa or bulimia nervosa? An empirical study of 116 women. *J Psychosom Res*. 1990;34:535–541.

22. Rosmark B, Berne C, Holmgren S, Lago C, Renholm G, Sohlberg S. Eating disorders in patients with insulin-dependent diabetes mellitus. *J Clin Psychiatry*. 1986; 47:547–550.

23. Steel JM, Young RJ, Lloyd GG, MacIntyre CCA. Abnormal eating attitudes in young insulin-dependent diabetics. *B J Psychiatry*. 1989;155:515–521.

24. Striegel-Moore RH, Nicholson TJ, Tamborlane WV. Prevalence of eating disorder symptoms in preadolescent and adolescent girls with IDDM. *Diabetes Care*. 1992;15:1361–1368.

25. Wing RR, Norwalk MP, Marcus MD, Koeske R, Finegold D. Subclinical eating disorders and glycemic control in adolescents with type I diabetes. *Diabetes Care*. 1986;9:162–167.

26. Garner DM, Garfinkel PE. The Eating Attitudes Test: an index of the symptoms of anorexia nervosa. *Psychol Med*. 1979;9:273–279.

27. Garner DM, Olmsted MP, Bohr Y, Garfinkel PE. The Eating Attitudes Test: psychometric features and clinical correlates. *Psychol Med*. 1982;12:871–878.

28. Garner DM, Olmsted MP, Polivy J. Development and validation of a multidimensional Eating Disorder Inventory for anorexia nervosa and bulimia. *Int J Eating Disorders*. 1983;2:15–34.

29. Cooper Z, Fairburn C. The Eating Disorder Examination: a semi-structured interview for the assessment of the specific psychopathology of eating disorders. *Int J Eating Disorders*. 1987;6:1–8.

30. Hudson JI, Wentworth SM, Hudson MS, Pope HG. Prevalence of anorexia nervosa and bulimia among young diabetic women. *J Clin Psychiatry*. 1985;46:88–93.

31. Birk R, Spencer, M. The prevalence of anorexia nervosa, bulimia, and induced glycosuria in diabetic females. *Diabetes*. 1987;36(suppl 1):88.

32. Rodin GM, Craven J, Littlefield C, Murray M, Daneman D. Eating disorders and intentional insulin undertreatment in adolescent females with diabetes. *Psychosomatics*. 1991;32:171–176.

33. Powers PS, Malone JI, Coovert DL, Schulman RG. Insulin-dependent diabetes mellitus and eating disorders: A prevalence study. *Compr Psychiatry*. 1990;31:205–210.

34. Stancin T, Link DL, Reuter JM. Binge eating and purging in young women with IDDM. *Diabetes Care*. 1989;12:601–603.

35. Thelen MH, Farmer J, Wonderlich S, Smith M. A revision of the bulimia test: the BULIT-R. *Psychol Assessment*. 1991;3:119–124.

36. Marcus MD, Wing RR, Jawad A, Orchard TJ. Eating disorders symptomatology in a registry-based sample of women with insulin-dependent diabetes mellitus. *Int J Eating Disorders*. 1992;12:425–430.

37. Marcus MD, Wing RR, McDermott MD, Dodge BA. Disordered eating is related to glycemic control in a population-based sample of women with IDDM. *Diabetes*. 1990;39(suppl 1):9A.

38. Polonsky WH, Anderson BJ, Lohrer PA, Aponte JE, Jacobson AM, Cole CF. Insulin omission in women with IDDM. *Diabetes Care*. 1994;17:1178–1185.

39. Biggs MM, Basco MR, Patterson G, Raskin P. Insulin withholding for weight control in women with diabetes. *Diabetes Care*. 1994;17:1186–1189.

40. Widom B, Weakland BS, Friedlander E, Kinsley BT, Simonson DC. Mechanisms of weight gain during intensive insulin therapy. *Diabetes*. 1992;41(suppl 1):59A.

41. Colas C, Mathieu P, Tchobroutsky G. Eating disorders and retinal lesions in type 1 (insulin-dependent) diabetic women. *Diabetologia*. 1991;34:288.

42. Rodin GM, Johnson LE, Garfinkel PE, Daneman D, Kenshole AB. Eating disorders in female adolescents with insulin-dependent diabetes mellitus. *Int J Psychiatry Med*. 1986–1987;16:49–57.

43. Steel JM, Young RJ, Lloyd GG, Clarke BF. Clinically apparent eating disorders in young diabetic women: associations with painful neuropathy and other complications. *BMJ*. 1987;294:859–861.

44. DCCT Research Group. The effect of intensive treatment of diabetes on the development and progression of long-term complications in insulin-dependent diabetes mellitus. *N Engl J Med*. 1993;329:977–986.

45. Rydall A, Rodin G, Olmsted M, Devenyi R, Daneman D. A four year follow-up study of eating disorders and medical costs in young women with IDDM. *Diabetes*. 1994;43:8A.

46. Rodin GM, Daneman D. Eating disorders and IDDM: a problematic association. *Diabetes Care*. 1992;15:1402–1412.

47. Peveler RC, Fairburn CG. The treatment of bulimia nervosa in patients with diabetes mellitus. *Int J Eating Disorders*. 1992;11:45–53.

48. DCCT Research Group. Weight gain associated with intensive therapy in the DCCT. *Diabetes Care*. 1988;11:657–673.

49. Wing RR, Klein R, Moss SE. Weight gain associated with improved glycemic control in population-based sample of subjects with type I diabetes. *Diabetes Care*. 1990;13:1106–1109.

50. Genuth S. Insulin use in NIDDM. *Diabetes Care*. 1990;13:1240–1264.

51. Lindstrom T, Eriksson P, Olsson AG, Arnqvist HJ. Long-term improvement of glycemic control by insulin treatment in NIDDM patients with secondary failure. *Diabetes Care*. 1994;17:719–721.

52. Torbay N, Bracco EF, Geliebter A, Stewart IM, Hashim SA. Insulin increases body fat despite control of food intake and physical activity. *Am J Physiol*. 1985;248:R2120–R2124.

53. Lustman PJ, Griffith LS, Gavard JA, Clouse RE. Depression in adults with diabetes. *Diabetes Care*. 1993;15:1631–1639.

54. Gonder-Frederick LA, Cox DJ, Bobbitt SA, Pennebaker JW. Mood changes associated with blood glucose fluctuations in insulin-dependent diabetes mellitus. *Health Psychol*. 1989;8:45–59.

55. Schlundt D. Emotional eating: Assessment and treatment. *Diabetes Spectrum*. 1993;6:342–343.

56. Peveler RC, Fairburn CG. Anorexia nervosa in association with diabetes mellitus—a cognitive-behavioral approach to treatment. *Behav Res Ther*. 1989;27:95–99.

57. Malone GL, Armstrong, BK. Treatment of anorexia nervosa in a young adult patient with diabetes mellitus. *J Nerv Ment Dis*. 1985;173:509–511.

58. Bubb JA, Pontious SL. Weight loss from inappropriate insulin manipulation: an eating disorder variant in an adolescent with insulin-dependent diabetes mellitus. *Diabetes Educator*. 1991;17:29–32.

59. Featherstone HJ, Beilman BD. Diabetic hyperglycemia and glycosuria as a manifestation of bulimia. *South Med J*. 1984;77:936–937.

60. Fairburn CG. The current status of the psychological treatments for bulimia nervosa. *J Psychosom Res*. 1988;32:635–645.

61. Enright AB, Butterfield P, Berkowitz B. Self-help and support groups in the management of eating disorders. In: Garner DM, Garfinkel PE, eds. *Handbook of Psychotherapy for Anorexia Nervosa and Bulimia*. New York, NY: Guilford Press; 1985:491–512.

62. Walsh BT. Fluoxetine treatment of bulimia nervosa. *J Psychosom Res*. 1991;35:33–40.

63. Smith DE, Marcus MD, Kaye W. Cognitive-behavioral treatment of obese binge eaters. *Int J Eating Disorders*. 1992;12:257–262.

64. Strowig SM, Basco M, Cercone S. A cognitive behavioral approach to diabetes management. *Diabetes Spectrum*. 1994;7:341–342.

Chapter 31

Care for Persons with Diabetes during Surgery

Judith M. Gaare-Porcari
Julie O'Sullivan-Maillet

Patients with diabetes spend more time in the hospital than the general population. In 1983, the incidence of hospitalization was 2.4 times higher and the length of stay was approximately 1.7 days longer for patients with diabetes than for those without the disease.[1] In 1992, hospitalization rates increased 2.87 times higher and length of stay increased to 2.8 days longer than for people without diabetes mellitus. Other health care commodities (ie, nursing homes, home care, medical equipment, prescription drugs, and outpatient medical care) are also used more often by patients with diabetes.[2]

Because of metabolic imbalances resulting from their disease, persons with diabetes have increased risk for degenerative vascular complications that involve the eyes, kidney, heart, and coronary arteries, the extremities, and the nervous and cerebrovascular system; all these complications may be amenable to surgical intervention. Increased operative risk may also be secondary to the risk factor of age. People with diabetes are generally older, and age increases the likelihood of surgery.

Despite these statistics, operative risk is no greater for people with diabetes mellitus than for the general population.[3] Careful preoperative workup, adequate insulin provision, and maintenance of fluid and electrolyte balance lessen operative risk.

The objectives of this chapter are to (1) review the pathophysiology of diabetes, starvation, and injury, (2) relate the metabolic responses to these conditions, and (3) present the rationale and mechanisms of nutritional support

in the patient with diabetes who may experience major physical stress due to accidental trauma, injury, or surgery.

METABOLIC DEMANDS OF SURGERY AND INJURY

Metabolic Response

Four hormonal responses to injury/stress in normal humans cause the four stages of surgical convalescence. The initial hormonal response is salt and water conservation mediated by aldosterone and antidiuretic hormone, which supports circulating volume. Sufficient fluid is retained so that "third spacing" can occur, and the wound naturally becomes edematous. This fluid retention also leads to weight gain and an increased circulating volume and consequent decrease in serum parameters (ie, albumin) used to evaluate nutritional status. Changes in insulin and counterregulatory hormone (eg, glucagon, catecholamines, growth hormone, glucocorticoids, thyroid hormone) secretion and sensitivity mediate the other three stages. Augmented hepatic gluconeogenesis provides adequate glucose for the nervous system, red and white blood cells, the renal medulla, and the healing wound. Skeletal muscle proteolysis provides amino acid precursors for gluconeogenesis and hepatic protein synthesis. Lipolysis provides free fatty acids as an energy source for the non–glucose-dependent tissues.

These responses are linked to the four stages of surgical convalescence, each influencing nutrient requirements. The first phase is marked by nitrogen losses that generally cannot be reduced by provision of exogenous nitrogen sources (ie, protein). The beginning of the second stage, marked by spontaneous diuresis, signals anabolism and a reduction in nitrogen excretion. As long as adequate energy and nitrogen are provided, the third stage of positive nitrogen balance and weight gain can occur. When nitrogen equilibrium rather than positive nitrogen balance occurs, the patient is said to be in "late anabolism," the fourth stage of convalescence.

The diabetic state has been likened to a fasted or starved state in that energy requirements are met by the mobilization of tissue stores so that fatty acids and ketones become the fuel. Catabolic (or counterregulatory) hormone levels are elevated relative to insulin similar to the profile in the stressed nondiabetic person.

The relative insulin deficiency caused by the increased catabolic hormones is augmented by the relative or absolute insulin deficiency of the diabetic state. Therefore, the catabolic state of surgery or trauma may be more severe (or enhanced) in the patient with diabetes. Hyperglycemia and consequent dehydration are the net risks from hormonal changes.

This brief discussion can be summarized in five points. (1) Protein catabolism occurs secondary to both the stress response and diabetes mellitus. This protein (nitrogen) loss may not be attenuated by energy and protein intake. (2) Gluconeogenesis, secondary to an imbalance between insulin and the counterregulatory hormones, occurs as a consequence of both the stress response and diabetes mellitus. (3) Lipolysis occurs for the reasons identified in (2). (4) Fluid retention and fluid shifts secondary to the stress response are an important clue to the stage of surgical convalescence. (5) Nutritional parameters, namely, weight and laboratory data, are influenced by the fluid shifts.

SURGICAL RISKS AND COMPLICATIONS IN THE PATIENT WITH DIABETES MELLITUS

Any surgical procedure carries a degree of risk. Each patient must be evaluated for underlying system dysfunction: cardiovascular, respiratory, immune, renal, and neurologic. Marginal function of any system will increase surgical risk and the possibility of postoperative complications. The following discussion is restricted to issues pertinent to the patient with diabetes mellitus. The reader is referred to surgical textbooks for a broader discussion of the pathophysiology of complications.

Infection

The risk of infection is relative to the capacity of the immune system. Nutritional status, medications, and concurrent disease influence immune function. Impaired immune status is associated with increased susceptibility to infection. Systemic infection influences all other systems, whereas local infection influences wound healing. The patient with poorly controlled diabetes may be more susceptible to systemic infection/sepsis. When hyperglycemia exceeds 200 mg/dL, leukocyte and granulocyte function is impaired. Poorly controlled diabetes is likened to a starved state, and malnutrition is closely linked to depressed immune function.[4] Infections of particular concern for persons with diabetes include candidiasis, gram-negative infections, and unusual infections such as mucormycosis.

Wound Complications

Delayed wound healing is a grave operative morbidity and is especially impaired in the patient with diabetes mellitus and a history of chronic hyperglycemia.[5] Healing is influenced by poor nutritional status (especially protein depletion, ascorbic acid status [collagen synthesis], vitamin A status [epithelialization], zinc status), marked dehydration or edema, severe anemia, medications such as corticosteroids and cytotoxic agents, and irradiation. Poor peripheral circulation and sensory neuropathy delay wound healing and encourage opportunistic infection. Wound dehiscence (separation of the surgical wound), secondary to microangiopathy, uremia, immunosuppression, sepsis, hypoalbuminemia, and obesity, is more prevalent in patients with diabetes mellitus.

Cardiac Complications

Atherosclerosis and coronary artery disease with and without symptoms are more prevalent in patients with diabetes mellitus. Autonomic neuropathy, a complication in 20 to 40%[6] of long-standing cases of diabetes mellitus, is associated with an increased risk of arrhythmia and sudden death.[7] Diabetes complicated by autonomic neuropathy is associated with the lack of hyperdynamic reactions and an increased risk of hypotensive reaction unrelated to blood loss during surgery.[8,9]

Gastrointestinal Complications

Anesthesia and surgical manipulation decrease the normal propulsive activity of the gut. The increased gastric volume (secondary to gastroparesis) in patients with diabetes mellitus increases the likelihood of pneumonitis during anesthesia.[10] The additive effects of medications (opiates in particular), inflammatory conditions, and pain may result in postoperative ileus. Diabetic gastroparesis is often asymptomatic, and the patient may experience increased incidence and duration of ileus. Symptomatic gastroparesis may present as nausea and vomiting. These conditions delay the resumption of oral intake postoperatively.

Renal Complications

Nephropathy complicates fluid and electrolyte management and alters insulin pharmacokinetics. Diabetic nephropathy predisposes patients to renal injury and/or acute renal failure. Neurogenic bladder may result in catheterization and increased risk of infection. Uncontrolled osmotic diuresis may lead to hypotension and acute tubular necrosis.

Age

Older patients (ie, those older than age 55) may be expected to have some generalized arte-riosclerosis and potential limitation of myocardial, renal, and pulmonary reserve. A large percentage of patients with non–insulin-dependent diabetes mellitus (NIDDM) fall into this age category[11] and it seems that the independent operative risk factors of age and diabetes mellitus might have a synergistic effect.

Obesity

The prevalence of NIDDM is greater in the person who weighs greater than 140% of ideal body weight. Obese patients characteristically have higher incidences of postoperative wound complications, thromboembolism, and pulmonary dysfunction (atelectasis).

ASSESSMENT AND EVALUATION OF NUTRITIONAL CARE

Medical nutrition therapy is one of the keys to successful diabetes care and postoperative management.[12] A registered dietitian should be an involved member of the treatment team.[13] Surgical patients with diabetes should be considered at high nutritional risk, especially if the need for surgery (ie, amputation) is related to long-term poor control. Prior illness, disease, or surgical intervention may have caused the patient to restrict food intake for days or weeks, predisposing the patient to nutrient depletion and weight loss. Excessive nutrient losses from vomiting, diarrhea, bleeding, and/or malabsorption may also contribute to nutrient depletion. The physiologic effects of nutritional depletion are well described and depress the function of every organ system.

Parameters to be considered in the perioperative nutritional care plan of a person with diabetes include those identified in Exhibit 31-1. Monitoring and intervention can begin as soon as surgery is anticipated. Additional considerations include energy and nitrogen requirements, special micronutrient needs, and response to nutrition intervention.

Energy Requirements

The energy needs of patients with diabetes in the perioperative period are considered the same as those of a stressed nondiabetic person. Energy requirements are a function of the metabolically active tissue, specifically the lean body mass fraction. Energy expenditure and therefore requirements can be determined by indirect calorimetry or estimated by using a formula. Indirect calorimetry data specific to patients with diabetes undergoing surgery are not available.

Metabolic rate is calculated as either the basal metabolic rate (BMR) or the resting energy expenditure (REE). The major difference between the measurements is that the basal value is measured during the postabsorptive state and the REE is not. This difference in measurement technique accounts for the approximately 10% difference in values obtained. This 10% difference is the thermic effect of food (TEF), also known as the specific dynamic action of food and diet-induced thermogenesis. The energy expenditure formulas of both Harris-Benedict[14] and Boothby et al[15] estimate REE, although the Harris-Benedict formula (Exhibit 31-2) is by far the most widely used by practitioners.

Exhibit 31-1 Parameters To Consider When Planning Perioperative Nutrition Therapy

- Type of surgery and ramifications to gastrointestinal tract
- Medications
- Degree of diabetic gastroparesis
- History of ketoacidosis or nonketotic hyperosmolar coma
- Weight loss despite normal or increased intake (>10% usual body weight is significant)
- Recent polydipsia, polyuria, polyphagia
- Dietary adherence
- Serial glycated hemoglobin values
- Glycosuria/ketonuria
- Serial blood glucose values
- Intraoperative or postoperative complications

These solutions to mathematical models may not represent the patient's actual needs. Elderly and sick patients may have altered body composition (lean body mass deficits), which decreases energy requirements as compared with needs estimated by formulas. Furthermore, factorial corrections for stress, disease, activity, and food use (which may be additive or offsetting) may cause the practitioner to provide more calories than the patient requires. This becomes an issue when caring for a starved patient who may be at risk for the "refeeding syndrome." Overfeeding may exacerbate or create poor glycemic control. Clinical monitoring should include daily weights, strict intake/output, and an initial and then twice weekly complete laboratory panel until a relationship between weight, overall fluid balance, serum albumin, and phosphorus can be established.[16,17]

The refeeding syndrome as an entity is well described in patients who have been fed calories in excess of requirements. It may occur whether the calories are administered orally, enterally, or parenterally. The syndrome is associated with precipitous falls in serum phosphorus and rises in blood glucose. If unchecked, it can lead to death from respiratory compromise. Solomon and Kirby[18] authored an excellent review of the literature and condition.

Nitrogen Requirements

A goal of nutrition management is to attain positive nitrogen balance. This is a function of both nitrogen or protein intake and energy provision. Patients who have been injured, undergone surgery, or have systemic infection retain less of

---

Exhibit 31-2 Harris-Benedict Equation

Men: $66.473 + 13.752W + 5.003H - 6.755A$
Women: $66.096 + 9.563W + 1.85H - 4.676A$

where **W** is weight in kilograms;
H is standing height in centimeters; and
A is age in years.

Table 31-1 Selected Micronutrients: Reference Ranges and Supplementation Guidelines

	Adult Reference Range	Critical Value	Supplementation
Magnesium[a]	1.3–2.1 mEq/L 0.65–1.05 mmol/L	<0.5 mEq/L <0.5 mmol/L	PO: 400–1200 mg/d divided in doses bid to qid IM/IV: 1 g q6h for 4 doses
Zinc[b]	83–96 µg/dL 12.7–14.7 µmol/dL	<70 µg/dL <10.7 µmol/L	PO: 60 mg elemental zinc; 220 mg zinc sulfate
Chromium[b]	0.10–0.20 ng/mL	Not identified	PO: 200 µg chromium chloride
Phosphorous[a]	2.7–4.5 mg/dL 0.87–1.45 mmol/L		IV: 1–1.5 mmol/kg
Vitamin K	Not available	Not identified	PO: 10–20 mg

[a] Reference values from Fischbach.[19]

[b] Reference values from Gibson.[26]

the nitrogen provided than does a healthy or nutritionally depleted person. Positive nitrogen balance or equilibrium may be difficult to attain until the stress response wanes.

The goal is to provide adequate protein in the range of 1.2 to 1.7 g protein per kg actual dry body weight per day to counteract the effects of obligatory nitrogen losses (related, as described earlier, to surgical convalescence) and maximize the amount of nitrogen retained. An empirical guideline when nephropathy exists is closer to the range of 1.0 to 1.5 g protein per kg actual dry body weight per day. Nitrogen retention may not be as great, because the provision is less, but the kidney will not be as taxed.

Special Micronutrient Needs

It is accepted, although not unequivocally established, that vitamin and mineral needs are increased during healing and the recovery process and that micronutrient deficiencies have an adverse effect on the healing and the recovery process. That requirements and use of vitamins and minerals provided in enteral and parenteral formulas are different from those administered orally is not clearly established by accurate bal-

ance studies. Reliable, static markers of micronutrient status are not readily available, and this hampers diagnosis of marginal and sometimes overt deficiencies. Serial measurements are a more reliable, although less practical, index. Dose-related resolution of symptoms is the best marker of depleted stores and subsequent replenishment. Certain vitamins and minerals deserve special mention, and guidelines are offered in Table 31-1, although at least the recommended daily intake for all known essential vitamins and minerals should be provided.

Surgical drains often present at operative sites to prevent or drain fluid accumulations and/or excessive diarrhea or urination are avenues for excessive magnesium and zinc loss. Generally, deficiency may be primary (ie, prolonged state of nothing by mouth [NPO] or use of dextrose 5% in water), or secondary (ie, malabsorption, renal disease involving tubular dysfunction, or enhanced urinary excretion especially with chronic diuretic use or glycosuria). People with diabetes commonly have increased urinary excretion of magnesium,[20,21] although serum concentrations may be normal or lower.[22] The same pattern of increased urinary excretion[23,24] and normal or lower[25] blood concentrations of zinc has been found. Serum mineral concentration is the most frequently used index of mineral status. Static serum measurements have limited usefulness as parameters in the stressed patient.[26] Serial measurements are recommended to monitor the response to supplementation.

Chromium deficiency has been associated with impaired glucose tolerance; however, most patients with diabetes are not chromium-deficient. Supplementation of patients with impaired glucose tolerance is associated with improved blood lipid profiles.[27,28] Marginal status may be a risk if there are excessive losses of body fluids. It is reasonable to assess serum chromium levels if deficiency is suspected.

Although phosphorus plays a role in many body functions, phosphorylation is a central process in energy metabolism. Phosphate depletion has been associated with the administration of intravenous glucose without sufficient phosphorus, the treatment of diabetic acidosis, and excessive use of aluminum hydroxide antacids. Patients with diabetes may be at risk for hyperphosphaturia. The serum phosphorus level should be carefully monitored and kept within normal limits.

Particular attention should be given to vitamin K status in surgical patients because of its important role in blood clotting. Supplementation after a prolonged antibiotic course may be necessary as antibiotics destroy the normal intestinal flora that synthesize vitamin K. Supplementation may also be considered with concurrent long-term anticoagulant therapy.

Response to Nutrition Intervention

It must be recognized that malnutrition and surgical stress alter body composition. Despite the careful estimation and provision of energy, protein, and micronutrients, there are patients who will lose weight postoperatively, and increased calories do not always curtail this weight loss. Spontaneous diuresis and consequent weight loss occur as an encouraging response to adequate nutrient provision[29] as well as herald the second and third phases of convalescence.

Note that the patient will have fluid input less than output (I<O) and that the weight change is a reflection of this loss of body water.

Monitoring weight, fluid balance, and serum albumin assesses progress. During early surgical convalescence, weight gain (fluid intake greater than output [I>O]) may occur with a concurrent decrease in serum albumin as body water compartments shift. If the patient is euvolemic (fluid intake equals output [I=O]), weight gain is likely a positive sign, and the serum albumin is expected to rise accordingly. If the patient retains fluid, the normal course of surgical convalescence (first phase), deteriorating renal function (marked by changes in laboratory parameters), or malnutrition may be the cause. The latter cause is often identified by default.

The response to nutrition intervention can also be gauged by the complication rate. It is expected that poorly nourished patients have a higher complication rate than well-nourished patients.

NUTRIENT PROVISION

Oral Feedings

The patient with diabetes who undergoes an uncomplicated surgical procedure should resume adequate oral feedings within 2 to 3 days once gastrointestinal tract function has resumed. During the period before adequate oral feedings resume, obligatory carbohydrate needs must be met orally, enterally, or intravenously. These calories are necessary to prevent unnecessary fat and protein catabolism. If the oral route is chosen, the traditional progression of a fluid diet to a diet of regular consistency may be initiated. The value of this tiered progression should be argued against.

It is acceptable, but not optimal, for semi-starvation (ie, provision of only maintenance fluids) to remain unchecked in the well-nourished patient for up to 7 days postoperatively.[30] Once this deadline is met, consideration must be given to alternate methods of nutrition support. Nutrition support should be considered earlier if the patient has a history of weight loss greater than 10% usual body weight or other signs of malnutrition or if the length of time before oral feedings can be expected to resume is greater than 7 days.[31]

Liquid Diets

Liquid diets may be unavoidable as preparation for diagnostic tests. For these situations, the emphasis is the provision of obligatory glucose (150 g/d). Both the clear liquid and full liquid diets provided to the patient with diabetes mellitus should contain sucrose and/or other simple carbohydrates. A clear fluid diet contains items that are clear fluids at room temperature (eg, gelatin, broth, tea, ginger ale); a full liquid diet contains all items that are liquid at room temperature (eg, custard, pudding, milk, cream of wheat or rice cereal, cream soup). Liquid diets containing noncaloric foodstuffs are equivalent to semistarvation. Unsupplemented liquid diets will not meet all nutrient needs and should be advanced to solid food as quickly as possible.

If foods of a liquid consistency are all that can be tolerated and supplemental tube feeding is not considered, then the practitioner may choose to supplement the diet with modular macronutrient components, polymeric, monomeric, and/or micronutrient supplements.

Solid Food Diet

The principles of a solid food diet in diabetes mellitus should be followed by the postoperative patient who can manage oral intake. Patients often have a depressed appetite after surgery. Because erratic oral intake disrupts blood glucose control based on intermediate- or long-acting insulin or oral hypoglycemic agents, steady caloric intake is a primary goal. A notation of any uneaten carbohydrate should be made and replacement carbohydrate provided according to the total available glucose (TAG) (Exhibit 31-3). This is especially important for the patient with insulin-dependent diabetes mellitus (IDDM). A minimum of 150 g carbohydrate per 24 hours is essential to prevent ketosis.

Oral Supplements

Commercial nutrient supplements enable the practitioner to offer an adequate diet when swallowing is unimpaired and oral intake is insufficient. Supplements should be calculated as part of a calorie-controlled plan, and therefore carbohydrate must be replaced when the products are not eaten. The carbohydrate base of these products differs. Which product to offer is decided by the patient's acceptance or refusal of the particular sample offered.

The hospitalized patient may have altered taste due to age, disease, or medication. It may be difficult for a patient to consume three or four servings of the same product every day. It may be more successful to vary the products and account for the macronutrient content in the diet calculation. The supplements of choice have a normal macronutrient distribution (ie, carbohydrate 50%, protein 20%, fat 30%). First consideration may be given to a product that is artificially sweetened. If possible, the carbohydrate component of the product should be predominately complex carbohydrate. Soy polysaccharide products have been used in patients with NIDDM, and blood glucose management was improved as compared with other formulas.[32]

Exhibit 31-3 Total Available Glucose

TAG = (1.0 × g carbohydrate) + (0.58 × g protein) + (0.10 × g fat)

Common foods used as carbohydrate substitutes:
- 1/2 cup gelatin, regular = 15 g glucose
- 1/2 cup orange juice = 15 g glucose
- 3/4 cup ginger ale = 15 g glucose
- 1/2 cup ice cream = 15 g glucose

For example, if a patient did not consume 1 cup skim milk and 1 cup cooked carrots from the tray, use of the formula would determine that 29 g glucose would need to be replaced and that 12 oz of ginger ale would be a suitable substitute.

TAG = {(1.0 × 12) + (0.58 × 8) + (0.10 × 0)} + {(1.0 × 10) + (0.58 × 4) + (0.10 × 0)} = 28.96

For any oral regimen, blood glucose can be managed with split doses of intermediate-acting insulin, intermediate-acting insulin with supplemental regular insulin before meals or supplements, or oral hypoglycemic agents as appropriate. It is reasonable to expect the patient to resume blood glucose self-management as soon as possible.

Enteral Nutrition Support

Enteral nutrition support is provided to those patients who cannot manage an adequate oral intake and who have a functional digestive system. The risks of enteral nutrition should not be considered less serious than those of parenteral nutrition.

Commercially prepared formulas should be chosen over blenderized mixtures because they are less likely to be contaminated and are of a known composition. If contamination and composition conditions can be met, formulas made from modular components or whole food can be acceptable. The choice of formula depends on the calculated nutrient needs and consideration of specific metabolic and clinical conditions.

The risk of hyperosmolar nonketotic coma should be considered when a high (ie, >45% total calories) carbohydrate formula is selected. Fluid requirements need to be met, and insulin needs to be carefully managed.

There are data to support the use of soy polysaccharide-enriched formulas in patients with diabetes.[33-35] The product studied differs from conventional formulas in four ways: (1) the addition of soy polysaccharide, (2) the substitution of fructose for sucrose, (3) the lower total carbohydrate content, and (4) the substitution of fat calories for carbohydrate calories. Each of these modifications alone may favorably influence blood glucose values.

Peters and Davidson[33] concluded that the postprandial glycemic response was a function of the total carbohydrate load rather than the type of carbohydrate. In this report, no significant difference was found between the glycemic response of patients with IDDM who received soy polysaccharide-enriched formulas versus a product containing hydrolyzed cereal solids, vegetables, and fruits. Significant differences were established when "fat-enriched" formulas were compared with formulas of usual composition.[33,35]

Micronutrient status must be monitored in patients receiving fiber-enriched formulas because of the chance that the fiber will bind micronutrients. Gastrointestinal transit time is influenced by the addition of fiber and a high-fat content of the diet. This is an important consideration in patients with diabetes who may have asymptomatic gastroparesis.

Aspiration pneumonia can be a complication. The risk of aspiration may be exaggerated in diabetic patients secondary to diabetic gastroparesis. Metoclopromide and cisapride have been used to enhance gastric emptying in patients with diabetes, although it has been suggested that the patients may become refractory to the drugs.[36,37] Hyperosmolar enteral feedings and rapid infusion into the stomach can exacerbate gastroparesis.[38]

Diarrhea, which is often associated with improper formula administration or formula intolerance, may also be secondary to massive antibiotic therapy. If diarrhea develops, cause should be determined by ruling out impaction, side effects of medication, bacterial overgrowth, the use of enemas, previously undiagnosed maldigestion or malabsorption, or diabetic diarrhea. In an extreme situation, dehydration as a result of diarrhea may precipitate hyperosmolar nonketonic coma. Reduction of the rate or strength of enteral feeding will not influence diarrhea caused by any of these factors; manipulation will likely cause inadequate energy and essential nutrient provision to the patient and thereby induce a semistarved state.

Blood Glucose Management

Blood glucose control is a balance between gluconeogenesis of the stress response and the hyperglycemia characteristic of diabetes mellitus and exogenous carbohydrate administration. A program in which enterally fed patients receive four or more bolus feedings per day mimics the traditional diabetic meal pattern and helps ensure optimal blood glucose control. Bolus feedings are often discouraged though because (1) they may increase the risk of aspiration, (2) there is an inherent problem of maintaining accuracy under gravity drip conditions, and (3) it is thought that gastrointestinal tolerance to an enteral formula may be improved by a constant infusion rate.

There is little support in the literature for the latter premise, and research and practice have not ascribed better tolerance of an enteral formula to the use of feeding pumps and a constant infusion rate. Some practitioners maintain that the usefulness of enteral feeding pumps lies in ensuring that the patient receives the prescribed volume.

Patients being fed by the constant infusion of enteral formula may initially be given subcutaneous regular insulin coverage every 6 hours, with the goal of maintaining blood glucose levels in the 200- to 250-mg/dL range. Additional insulin as sliding scale coverage based on capillary blood glucose monitoring may decrease the blood glucose to the goal of 150 to 200 mg/dL. After 2 days, approximately 100% of the necessary subcutaneous regular insulin dose should be given as subcutaneous intermediate-acting insulin in the morning, supplemented with sliding scale insulin coverage, and the patient's blood glucose levels should be monitored every 4 to 6 hours. It has been suggested that two or three doses of intermediate-acting insulin given every 12 or 8 hours should ensure reasonable blood glucose levels when the patient is receiving a continuous-drip enteral formula. Rarely, regular insulin every 6 hours can be continued if unsatisfactory results are obtained with other regimens. The tube feeding should not be abruptly discontinued. When this occurs, an alternate source of carbohydrate is mandatory.

If the enteral feeding drip rate can be ensured and the patient can maintain a peripheral intravenous line, an insulin drip can be provided. However, there is a risk of hypoglycemia if the enteral feeding stops and the insulin drip continues. This practice may be more practical in an intensive care unit setting where constant monitoring is possible.

It is recommended that blood and urine glucose and acetone be monitored every 6 hours in patients with diabetes receiving enteral nutrition. Accurate intake and output records (with parenteral and enteral fluids differentiated) are mandatory for successful monitoring. The evaluation of blood glucose levels permits proper insulin coverage, and the urine readings give the practitioner information regarding glycosuria and substrate use. Fluid balance indicates the presence of polyuria or impending dehydration. Serial weight measurements should be correlated with fluid balance.

Parenteral Nutritional Support

Parenteral nutrition is necessary when the postoperative patient cannot adequately digest or absorb sufficient amounts of nutrients via the gastrointestinal tract. Pre-existing malnutrition secondary to diminished oral (per os) intake, maldigestion, or malabsorption warrants postoperative parenteral nutrition in an effort to reduce the risk of surgical complications. The distinction between peripheral and central (or total) parenteral nutrition is the access site.

Obligatory glucose needs must be met daily. However, glucose-based parenteral nutrition is not recommended. The unbalanced metabolism of the person with diabetes favors the use of mixed fuel solutions. Mixed fuel (equicaloric lipid and glucose) solutions are best tolerated and associated with the fewest metabolic side effects. Exceptions to this recommendation are patients who have impaired fat clearance and/or fat intolerance. Carbohydrate intolerance is exacerbated by a high-glucose provision, and insulin requirements are increased correspondingly. The postoperative[39,40] patient can metabolize up to approximately 5 to 7 mg glucose per kg actual body weight per minute[-1]. Providing amounts greater than this may result in conversion of glucose to fat and exceed ventilatory reserve and cause respiratory decompensation. Lipids should be provided at no greater than 2.5 g per kg actual body weight per day.

An alternative to dextrose-containing solutions is available. Glycerol moieties serve as the carbohydrate substrate in this solution. Patients receiving this solution and additional fat emulsion as a peripheral parenteral nutrition solution required less insulin to maintain blood glucose in the range of 150 to 200 mg/dL than did other patients with diabetes randomized to an isocaloric and isonitrogenous dextrose-amino acid solution.[41]

Nutrition support research in the past decade has created amino acid solutions enriched with particular amino acids. The advantage of branched-chain-enriched solutions has not been established despite more than 10 years of active investigation. It is probable that advantages exist in isolated cases. Evidence to date strongly suggests that provision of glutamine benefits the stressed postoperative patient as obligatory nitrogen losses are attenuated.

Blood Glucose Management

The principles of blood glucose management for peripheral parenteral nutrition (PPN) and total parenteral nutrition (TPN) are identical, although less insulin is required with PPN due to lower glucose delivery. Insulin-dependent patients as well as patients previously maintained on oral hypoglycemic agents can be managed in the same manner. Use of human insulin is the standard, particularly if the patient has had no previous experience with insulin or when the need can be considered temporary (as with an NIDDM patient with a serious infection or with a postoperative stress response) because antibodies may form to beef or pork insulin, resulting in insulin resistance. This resistance may present in a matter of weeks or years.

The methods of maintaining blood glucose in the 150- to 200-mg/dL range are straightforward. Insulin may either be added to the parenteral solution or provided as a separate insulin drip. Only regular insulin may be added to the parenteral formula and is the method of choice. Adsorption occurs to both glass and polyvinyl chloride bags and intravenous tubing, but investigators have found consistent insulin delivery. To compensate for the adsorption problem, an additional 1 to 3 U of regular insulin can be added. Alternatively, an insulin drip can be set up through a separate intravenous line. This method has a greater risk of inducing hypoglycemia if there is substrate interruption and the insulin drip is not discontinued.

The practitioner may feel justified in "weaning" or "tapering" the patient with diabetes who receives solutions containing greater than 10% final dextrose concentration. Weaning or tapering means that a reduced rate of infusion is given for the first and last 2 to 4 hours of infusion. This period gives the body time to equilibrate to the changes in carbohydrate provision.

It is recommended that both blood and urine glucose and acetone be monitored every 4 hours in patients with diabetes receiving parenteral nutrition. Accurate intake and output volumes should be documented. Blood glucose monitoring permits adequate insulin coverage, urine readings give the practitioner information concerning glycosuria and substrate use, and fluid balance demonstrates incidence of polyuria or impending dehydration. Serial weight values should be correlated with fluid balance.

PERIOPERATIVE CARE OF THE PATIENT WITH DIABETES

Evaluation

Historical records of glucose control, coexisting disease, complexity of the surgical procedure planned, and method of insulin administration during surgery all influence the level of control achieved during the perioperative period. Preoperative evaluation should ideally be performed in an outpatient setting. Data reviewed should include the history of insulin or oral hypoglycemic agent use; history of ketosis or hyperosmolar nonketotic coma; diet pattern and compliance; recent polyuria, polydipsia, or polyphagia; recent weight loss; demonstrated glucosuria; blood glucose response to previous surgery; and serial glycated hemoglobin values. A complete history and physical examination should be included in the admission workup. Recommended tests generally include an electrocardiograph to rule out pre-existing myocardial infarction, autonomic screening (ie, respiratory sinus arrhythmia, Valsalva's maneuver, head-up tilt, cold pressor test), a chest x-ray to identify pneumonia or pulmonary edema, a urinalysis to rule out urinary tract infection and identify proteinuria, a full panel of electrolytes and pH to provide baseline serum parameters and to identify any anion gap, and actual height and weight measurements. Diabetic ketoacidosis (DKA) and euglycemic DKA must be recognized and treated before surgery is attempted. Under usual circumstances, all efforts are made to hydrate the patient appropriately and control hyperglycemia before surgery. Many of the complications of diabetes place the surgical patient at increased risk. Many of the potential risks for postsurgical complications can be identified preoperatively and prevented.

Cardiac status, as assessed by a variety of measures, is less stable in the patient with diabetes undergoing an operation and is the leading cause of mortality. Atypical hemodynamic behavior[42] is typical in the group, and the patients are at special risk for hypotension unrelated to blood loss. The patients with diabetes are more likely to require vasopressors to maintain intraoperative blood pressure. There is a higher risk of cardiac lability among those diabetic patients with confirmed autonomic deficits.

Gastroparesis complicates preoperative care and may be compounded by the perioperative use of opiates. The practice of keeping a patient "NPO past midnight" might not be adequate to ensure an empty stomach in the patient with diabetes.[43] A longer fast may decrease the risk, but this is not common practice. Gastric emptying may be enhanced and thus the risk of aspiration during and after anesthesia may be decreased by use of metaclopromide. It is unaffected by cisapride given in the immediate preoperative period.[44]

The patient with diabetes requires close monitoring intraoperatively. General anesthesia can increase levels of growth hormone (increased levels of which are seen in uncontrolled diabetes) and glucocorticoids, and increase sensitivity to various drugs, which may lead to respiratory depression. Intraoperative acidosis due to carbon-dioxide retention or hypoxia or as a direct effect of the anesthetic agent can occur. Emergency surgery may pose special problems for the surgical team if metabolic control is unsteady or nonexistent.

Routine postoperative care will help identify common postoperative complications (see Exhibit 31-4). Complications are more threatening to the person with diabetes than the nondiabetic person, but they need not be more severe. Often, a precipitous rise in blood glucose signals the acute onset of a complication. If this is not recognized quickly, metabolic decompensation may ensue. Alternatively, blood glucose may quickly drop after an abscess is drained, during a severe gram-negative bacterial infection, or when the stress response wanes.

Exhibit 31-4 Postoperative Complications

- Intensive Care Unit syndrome, delirium tremors
- Phlebitis, fever
- Hematoma, seroma, wound dehiscence
- Atelectasis, pulmonary aspiration, pneumonia, postoperative pleural effusion, pneumothorax
- Fat embolism
- Dysrhythmia, myocardial infarction, left ventricle failure
- Pulmonary edema
- Hemoperitoneum
- Gastric dilation, bowel obstruction, fecal impaction
- Prehepatic jaundice, hepatocellular insufficiency, posthepatic obstruction
- Cholecystitis
- Urinary retention, urinary tract infection, oliguria, renal failure
- CVA, convulsions

Fluid Management

Fluid management in the euvolemic state should be a dextrose-saline solution with added potassium. Regular insulin may be added to the fluid or infused separately. A fluid infusion rate of 100 mL/h (5 g of dextrose per hour) should be matched with a minimum of 1 to 2 U of insulin. Blood glucose values should be carefully monitored and the solution rate(s) titrated as necessary to maintain glycemic control.

The patient with diabetes is prone to volume depletion during periods of uncontrolled glycosuria and concomitant polyuria. Postoperative use of loop diuretics may increase the risk of dehydration. This condition can present as poor skin turgor and/or postural hypotension. The resulting decreased blood volume causes decreased renal perfusion and may precipitate prerenal azotemia.

To treat markedly contracted vascular volume, saline with added potassium in an amount adequate to maintain vital signs and central venous pressure is usually given. Ringer's lactate, a glycogenic precursor, was associated with higher blood glucose values in at least one study in patients with diabetes[45] and is thus not recommended. It is necessary to replace blood bicarbonate if the blood pH is 7.0 or less or the blood bicarbonate is less than 9 mEq/L. The provision of 40 to 90 mEq of bicarbonate per liter of hypotonic saline should cause the blood pH to rise to within normal limits. At this point, further bicarbonate should not be given as it potentiates rebound metabolic alkalosis as ketones are metabolized. This alkalosis can cause potassium shifts that may induce cardiac arrhythmias. Replacement of potassium (20 to 30 mEq/h) and phosphorus (3 mmol/h) will probably be necessary.

Blood Glucose Management

Patients receiving oral hypoglycemic agents should receive them until the day of surgery, except for those receiving chlorpropamide, glyburide, or metformin, which, because of their long half-life, should be changed to a short-acting sulfonylurea several days before surgery. Similarly, patients taking long-acting insulin should be managed with an intermediate-acting insulin preparation several days before surgery.

Published recommendations for insulin provisions on the day of surgery and during the procedure vary greatly. Patients may be managed by subcutaneous injection, continuous intravenous infusion (0.25 to 0.35 U of insulin per gram of glucose) or continuous subcutaneous insulin infusion. Recommendations vary from the usual dose of insulin to a slightly reduced dose to a significantly reduced dose on the morning of surgery. A continuous intravenous infusion is generally recommended for all patients except patients with well-controlled NIDDM.[46] The chosen regimen should begin the night before surgery or, at the latest, 7:00 A.M. the morning of surgery.[47] For all methods, frequent and reliable blood glucose determinations should be made to avoid hypoglycemia. A tendency toward low blood glucose values after surgery is common.

Perioperative control of blood glucose to within physiologic limits is associated with lower morbidity in the patient with diabetes. Regular insulin subcutaneously every 4 to 6 hours may be used in patients with NIDDM who have acceptable control (fasting plasma glucose of 180 mg/dL, glycated hemoglobin of 10%), surgery duration less than 2 hours, noninvasive procedures of the body cavity, and food intake anticipated postoperatively. When blood glucose exceeds 250 mg/dL in the perioperative period, patients with NIDDM should be managed with insulin. Some surgeons and anesthesiologists prefer the addition of short-acting insulin to an intravenous solution (continuous intravenous infusion of 1.0 to 2.0 U/h) as it avoids potential hypoglycemia. Insulin injected subcutaneously does not act as quickly and is therefore not recommended.

The pregnant patient undergoing delivery should be managed the same way, as insulin needs decrease dramatically during labor and after delivery, and blood glucose can be more accurately manipulated. Long-standing steroid use, as in patients who have had an organ transplant, causes insulin resistance and therefore increases requirements during surgery. Hypothermia (cardiac bypass graft, open heart, and transplantation types of surgery) also increases insulin requirements.[48]

Insulin requirements that may have greatly increased in the intraoperative period will gradually diminish to preoperative levels. Sharp increases or decreases in blood glucose can signal postoperative complications such as infection or abscess. Blood glucose should be checked every 4 to 6 hours and sliding scale regular insulin provided. Urine glucose and acetone should be checked on the same schedule to monitor for glucosuria or impending ketosis. The blood glucose may be higher than usual the first few mornings after surgery due to the surgery and reduced exercise.[49]

Outpatient surgical procedures generally warrant use of modified subcutaneous insulin regimens. Hirsch and McGill[50] identified two regimens for administration of insulin to patients accustomed to taking split doses of intermediate-acting and regular insulin: (1) one-third to one-half the usual dose of each type on the morning of surgery; or (2) one-half to two-thirds the intermediate-acting dose and little or no regular insulin the morning of surgery. These authors also noted that no change should be made for patients receiving long-acting insulin because the patient should have adequate insulin levels from that given the previous day.

Glucose infusions should be provided, and intraoperative blood glucose values should be assessed. The physician may choose to use a continuous intravenous infusion regimen, and based on the results of one study,[51] better metabolic control may be achieved with the method.

Patient Education

The type of surgery, risks, implications, and potential complications should be explained and discussed with the patient by the health care team. If enteral or parenteral nutritional support is anticipated postoperatively, the physician should make this clear. The registered dietitian should meet the patient to discuss past dietary habits, food preferences, tolerances, and allergies and to identify pre-existing nutrient deficiencies so that the nutritional status of the patient can be assessed. Nutrient needs should be explained to the patient. This education may later facilitate the patient's cooperation with the nutritional care plan.

The operative placement of any type of feeding tube should be discussed with the patient preoperatively, as should the anticipated placement of a nasoenteric feeding tube postoperatively. The patient should understand that this tube is necessary to ensure optimal nutrition during the recovery period and may not be permanent. The enteral nutrient formula should be discussed with the patient by either the physician or registered dietitian. The patient should understand that (1) the formula contains all known essential nutrients, (2) the body recognizes the nutrients the same as those in food taken orally, (3) it is a safe way to provide nutrition, and (4) provided that the patient does not suffer from maldigestion or malabsorption, the formula should be tolerated well. The patient should understand that the care of the feeding tube requires clean technique and that the tube must be flushed before and after medications, after the feeding is stopped for any reason, and before the feeding is resumed. This step is taken in an effort to prevent residue buildup. If an enteral pump is used, the patient should know how to operate it and be aware of trouble-shooting techniques.

The risks and benefits of placing a central catheter for parenteral nutrition should be explained to the patient by the physician. The physician or registered dietitian should discuss the parenteral solution with the patient, particularly explaining that (1) the body recognizes and uses the parenteral solution similarly to food ingested normally, (2) all known essential nutrients can be provided by this route, (3) parenteral nutrition may be a temporary mode of maintaining nourishment until the gastrointestinal tract is functioning again and the patient is able to maintain adequate intake, (4) it is a safe way of providing nutrients for as long as is necessary, (5) when oral feedings are resumed, the dietitian will be available to help the patient choose foods wisely, and (6) when oral intake is established, the parenteral nutrition will be tapered and later stopped when intake is adequate. Basic principles of nutritional monitoring should be explained to the patient. It is advisable to tell the patient that the staff will be monitoring blood levels of electrolytes and weighing the patient daily. It is prudent to explain that initial weight loss is not uncommon and is usually a good prognostic indicator as extra fluid, not body mass, is lost.

The patient should be advised that the site of the catheter has to remain sterile. An insecure dressing should be reported to the nurse so that it can be changed. The patient should know not to touch the port(s) of the catheter at any time.

CONCLUSION

Management of the increased risk factors a patient with diabetes undergoing surgery faces is critical to the operation. Metabolic decompensation and microvascular disease compromise the patient. Efforts should center around (1) preoperative identification of compromised organ function, (2) resolution of factors influencing compromised function as can be done, (3) assurance of adequate nutrition in the postoperative period, and (4) attainment of physiologic blood glucose values through manipulation of the insulin regimen.

REFERENCES

1. Harris MH, Hamman RH, eds. *Diabetes in America, National Diabetes Data Group.* NIH Publication no. 851468. 1985.

2. American Diabetes Association. *Direct and Indirect Costs of Diabetes in the United States in 1992.* Alexandria, Va: American Diabetes Association; 1993.

3. Palmisano JJ. Surgery and diabetes. In: Kahn CR, Weir GC, eds. *Joslin's Diabetes Mellitus.* 13th ed. Philadelphia, Pa: Lea & Febiger; 1994:955–961.

4. Myrvik QN. Immunology and nutrition. In: Shils ME, Olson JA, Shike M, eds. *Modern Nutrition in Health and Disease.* 8th ed. Philadelphia, Pa: Lea & Febiger; 1994;623–662.

5. Goodson WH, Hunt TK. Wound healing with diabetes mellitus. *Surg Clin North Am.* 1984;64:762.

6. Burgos LG, Ebert TJ, Assidao C, et al. Increased intraoperative cardiovascular morbidity in diabetics with autonomic neuropathy. *Anesthesiology.* 1989;70: 591–597.

7. Page MM, Watkins PJ. Cardiopulmonary arrest and diabetic autonomic neuropathy. *Lancet.* 1978;1:14–16.

8. Knüttgen D, Weidemann D, Doehn M. Diabetic autonomic neuropathy: abnormal cardiovascular reactions under general anesthesia. *Klin Wochenschr.* 1990; 68:1168–1172.

9. Pfeifer MA. Conclusions. *Diabetes Spectrum.* 1990;3: 45–48.

10. Olsson GL, Hallen B, Hambraeus-Jonzon K. Aspiration during anaesthesia: a computer aided study of 185,358 anaesthetics. *Acta Anaesthesiol Scand.* 1986;30:84–92.

11. Task Force on Diabetes Data Collection and Analysis of the American Diabetes Association Council on Epidemiology and Statistics. *Diabetes 1993 Vital Statistics.* Alexandria, Va: American Diabetes Association; 1993.

12. American Dietetic Association. Position statement: nutrition recommendations and principles for people with diabetes mellitus. *J Am Diet Assoc.* 1994;94(5):504–506.

13. Daly A, Arky RA. Nutritional management. In: Lebovitz HE, DeFronzo RA, Genuth S, Kreisberg RA, Pfeifer MA, Tamborlane WV, eds. *Therapy for Diabetes Mellitus and Related Disorders.* Alexandria, Va: American Diabetes Association; 1991;92–99.

14. Harris JA, Benedict TG. *Biometric Studies of Basal Metabolism in Man.* Washington, DC: Carnegie Institute of Washington; 1919. Publication no. 279.

15. Boothby WM, Berson J, Dunn HL. Studies on the energy of metabolism of normal individuals: a standard for basal metabolism with a nomogram for clinical application. *Am J Physiol.* 1936;116:468–484.

16. Starker PM, LaSala PA, Askanazi J, et al. The influence of preoperative total parenteral nutrition upon morbidity and mortality. *Surg Gyn Obstet.* 1986;162:569–574.

17. Starker PM, LaSala PA, Forse A, Askanazi J, Elwyn DH, Kinney JM. Response to total parenteral nutrition in the extremely malnourished patient. *J Parenter Enter Nutr.* 1985;9:300–302.

18. Solomon SM, Kirby DF. The refeeding syndrome: a review. *J Parenter Enter Nutr.* 1990;14:90–97.

19. Fischbach F. *A Manual of Laboratory & Diagnostic Tests.* 4th ed. Philadelphia, Pa: JB Lippincott; 1992.

20. Walter RM Jr, Uriu-Hare JY, Olin KL, et al. Copper, zinc, manganese, and magnesium status and complications of diabetes mellitus. *Diabetes Care.* 1991;14:1050–1056.

21. Ponder SW, Brouchard BH, Travis LB. Hyperphosphaturia and hypermagnesuria in children with IDDM. *Diabetes Care.* 1990;13:437–441.

22. Saggese G, Federico G, Bertelloni S, Baroncelli GI, Calisti L. Hypomagnesemia and the parathyroid hormone-vitamin D endocrine system in children with insulin-dependent diabetes mellitus: effects of magnesium administration. *J Pediatr.* 1991;119:677–678.

23. Honnorat J, Accominotti M, Broussole C, Fleuret AC, Vallon JJ, Orgiazzi J. Effects of diabetes type and treatment on zinc status in diabetes mellitus. *Biol Trace Elem Res.* 1992;32:311–316.

24. Golik A, Ramot Y, Maor J, et al. Type II diabetes mellitus, congestive heart failure, and zinc metabolism. *Biol Trace Elem Res.* 1993;39:171–175.

25. Rohn RD, Pleban P, Jenkins LL. Magnesium, zinc and copper in plasma and blood cellular components in children with IDDM. *Clin Chem Acta.* 1993;215:21–28.

26. Gibson RS. *Principles of Nutritional Assessment.* New York: Oxford University Press; 1990:543–544.

27. Mertz W. Chromium in human nutrition: a review. *J Nutr.* 1993;123(4):626–633.

28. Abraham AS, Brooks BA, Eylath U. The effects of chromium supplementation on serum glucose and lipids in patients with and without non–insulin-dependent diabetes. *Metabolism.* 1992;41(7):768–771.

29. Keys A, Brozek J, Henschel A, et al. *The Biology of Human Starvation.* Minneapolis, Minn: University of Minneapolis Press; 1950.

30. Queen PM, Caldwell M, Balogun L. Clinical indicators for oncology, cardiovascular, and surgical patients: report of the ADA Council on Practice Quality Assurance Committee. *J Am Diet Assoc.* 1993;93(3):338–344.

31. Shils ME. Parenteral nutrition. In Shils ME, Olson JA, Shike M, eds. *Modern Nutrition in Health and Disease.* 8th ed. Philadelphia, Pa: Lea & Febiger; 1994:1430–1458.

32. Galkowski J, Silverstone FA, Brod M, Issac RM. Use of low carbohydrate enteral formula as a snack for elderly patients with type 2 diabetes. *Clin Res.* 1989;37:89A.

33. Peters AL, Davidson MD. Effects of various enteral feeding products on postprandial blood glucose response in patients with type I diabetes. *J Parenter Enter Nutr.* 1992;16:69–74.

34. Peters AL, Davidson MD, Issac RM. Lack of glucose elevation after simulated tube feeding with a low-carbohydrate, high-fat enteral formula in patients with type I diabetes. *Am J Med.* 1989;87:178–182.

35. Harley JR, Pohl SL, Issac RM. Low carbohydrate with fiber versus high carbohydrate without fiber enteral formulas: effect on blood glucose excursion in patients with type II diabetes. *Clin Res.* 1989;37:141A.

36. *USP DI, Vol. I: Information for the Health Care Professional.* Tauton, Mass: Rand McNally; 1994:1894–1898, 2896–2898.

37. Nompleggi D, Bell SJ, Blackburn GL, et al. Overview of gastrointestinal disorders due to diabetes mellitus: emphasis on nutritional support. *J Parenter Enter Nutr.* 1989;13:84–91.

38. Champagne MT, Ashley ML. Nutritional support in the critically ill elderly patient. *Crit Care Nurs Q.* 1989;12(1):15–25.

39. Wolfe RR, Allsop JR, Burke JF. Glucose metabolism in man: responses to intravenous glucose infusion. *Metabolism.* 1979;28:210–220.

40. Wolfe RR, O'Donnell TF Jr, Stone MD, et al. Investigation of factors determining the optimal glucose infusion rate in total parenteral nutrition. *Metabolism.* 1980;29:892–900.

41. Lev-Ran A, Johnson M, Hwang DL, Askanazi J, Weissman C, Gersovitz M. Double-blind study of glycerol vs. glucose in parenteral nutrition of postsurgical insulin-treated diabetic patients. *J Parenter Enter Nutr.* 1987;11:271–274.

42. Tseuda K, Huang KC, Dumont SW, Wieman TJ, Thomas MH, Heine MF. Cardiac sympathetic tone in anaesthetized diabetics. *Can J Anaesth.* 1991;38(1):20–23.

43. Radioo DM, Rocke DA, Brock-Utne JG, Marszalek A, Englebreck HE. Critical volume for pulmonary acid aspiration: reappraisal in a primate model. *Br J Anaesth.* 1990;65:248–250.

44. Reissell E, Taskinen MR, Orko R, Lindgren L. Increased volume of gastric contents in diabetic patients undergoing renal transplantation: lack of effect with cisapride. *Acta Anaesth Scand.* 1992;36:736–740.

45. Thomas DJB, Alberti KGMM. The hyperglycemic effects of Hartmann's solution in maturity-onset diabetics during surgery. *Br J Anaesth.* 1978;50:185–188.

46. Arauz-Pacheco C, Raskin P. Surgery and anesthesia. In: Lebovitz HE, DeFronzo RA, Genuth S, Kreisberg RA, Pfeifer MA, Tamborlane WV, eds. *Therapy for Diabetes Mellitus and Related Disorders.* Alexandria, Va: American Diabetes Association; 1991:147–154.

47. Hirsch IB, McGill JB, Cryer IE, White PF. Perioperative management of patients with diabetes mellitus. *Anesthesiology.* 1991;74:346–359.

48. Stephens JW, Krause AH, Peterson CA, et al. The effect of glucose priming solutions in diabetic patients undergoing coronary artery bypass grafting. *Ann Thorac Surg.* 1988;45(5):544–547.

49. Karhunen U, Summanen P, Laatikainen L. Concomitant problems to the anaesthesia of diabetic vitrectomy patients. *Acta Ohpthalmol.* 1987;65:190–196.

50. Hirsch IB, McGill JB. Role of insulin management of surgical patients with diabetes mellitus. *Diabetes Care.* 1990;13:980–991.

51. Christiansen CL, Schurizek BA, Mailing B, Knudsen L, Alberti KGMM, Hermansen K. Insulin treatment of the insulin-dependent diabetic patient undergoing minor surgery. *Anaesthesia.* 1988;43:533–537.

Chapter 32

Gastrointestinal Issues in Persons with Diabetes

Carol Rees Parrish

Seventy-five percent of all patients with diabetes have recurrent gastrointestinal (GI) symptoms. These include abdominal discomfort, nausea, vomiting, constipation, diarrhea, fecal incontinence, and dysphagia (see Table 32-1). Diabetic autonomic neuropathy is present in about 20 to 40% of patients with diabetes mellitus. Clinical symptoms of enteric diabetic autonomic neuropathy are associated with long-standing insulin-dependent diabetes mellitus (IDDM), history of poor glycemic control, and advanced age, as well as pre-existing autonomic neuropathies such as bladder dysfunction, sweat disorder, orthostatic hypotension, and impotence. Nephropathy and retinopathy may also accompany this disorder. It is also worth noting that pancreatic insufficiency, celiac sprue, and pernicious anemia (PA) occur at a higher incidence in this patient population.

This chapter reviews what is known about diabetes and its effect on the GI tract clinical symptoms, as well as medical therapy and nutrition intervention. Special emphasis is given to gastroparesis, as the nutritional ramifications can be significant.

GI POINTS OF INTEREST

The GI tract[1] (Figure 32-1) is a magnificent example of cooperation and coordination, achieving its primary function of providing nutrients to the rest of the body in an effortless manner under most circumstances. It is approximately 20 ft in its entirety and has a surface area rivaling that of a football field. The GI tract also serves as an important immune barrier.

Oral Cavity

Beginning with the oral cavity, food is initially prepared for digestion by mastication and lubrication before delivery to the stomach. Salivary amylase is released in the mouth to initiate the breakdown of complex carbohydrates to simple sugars.

Esophagus

The esophagus is about 45 cm long and has the capability to distend up to 2 in. in diameter. The esophagus propels food by means of peristaltic action and allows passage of the food through the lower esophageal sphincter (cardiac sphincter or gastroesophageal [GE] junction) into the stomach. The lower esophageal sphincter is responsible for preventing reflux of gastric (stomach) contents back into the esophagus; also, by remaining closed, it allows pressure to build up in the stomach to aid in gastric emptying.

Stomach

The fully distended stomach is roughly the size of a football and can hold up to 2 quarts of food or fluids. The role of the stomach is fourfold.[2,3] First, it stores food and controls gastric emptying so that food is delivered to the small bowel at rates at which it can be assimilated. Second, it breaks food up into tiny particles by

Table 32-1 Effect on GI System of Diabetes Mellitus

Disease	Target Organ	Pathology or Abnormality	Symptoms/ Signs	Pathophysiology
Diabetic autonomic neuropathy	Esophagus	Candidiasis Esophagitis	Dysphagia	↓ E-G sphincter pressure; impaired peristalsis Delayed emptying
	Stomach	Gastritis; gastric atrophy	Epigastric discomfort	Autoimmune polyglandular disease
			Macrocytic anemia (occasional pernicious anemia)	Intrinsic factor deficit
			Fullness, nausea, vomiting	Delayed emptying
			Obstructive second-degree bezoar	
	Small intestines		Diarrhea, often nocturnal	Motility disturbance
			Steatorrhea	
		Villous atrophy	Malabsorption	Gluten sensitivity (celiac sprue)
		Mild mucosal inflammation	Malabsorption	Bacterial overgrowth
	Upper abdomen	Radiculopathy	Pain	Nerve-muscle overactivity
	Pancreas	Chronic pancreatitis	Malabsorption Abdominal pain	Unknown (if alcohol and gallstones clearly not responsible)
	Gallbladder	Cholelithiasis; cholecystitis Globally— uncertain	Abdominal pain	?Lithogenic bile Impaired contractility gallbladder
	Colon		Constipation Obstipation	Motor disturbance
	Rectum		Fecal incontinence	Impaired internal sphincter
Insulin-dependent diabetes	Liver	Steatosis; steatonecrosis ↑ glycogen; fibrosis	Hepatomegaly; possible Sx liver disease w/icterus ↑ AST, ALT, GGT	Obesity ?insulin effect or deficit
Ketoacidosis	Stomach	Gastritis, occ. hemorrhagic	Bleeding, mild	Probable effects of severe acidosis, hypotension, ?infection
	Pancreas		Abdominal pain; ↑ amylase (nonpancreatic); occ. ↑ serum triglycerides;	Unknown
	Liver		↑ AST, ALT	
	Abdomen		Pain	Gastric atony; ileus, gastritis

Note: Sx, symptoms; AST, aspartate aminotransferase; ALT, alanine aminotransferase; GGT, gamma-glutamyl transferase.

Source: Reprinted from Ryan JC, and Sleisenger MH. Effects of Systemic and Extraintestinal Disease on the Gut. In: Sleisenger MH, Fordtran JS. *Gastrointestinal Disease—Pathophysiology, Diagnosis, Management.* 5th ed (p 201), with permission of WB Saunders, © 1993.

the process of trituration (antral contraction/ grinding or "gastric mastication") making them susceptible to pancreatic enzyme attack; it also selectively inhibits passage of larger food particles through the pylorus. Third, hydrochloric acid secretion aids in initiation of protein digestion. It is also a potent bacteriocidal agent (destroys bacteria). Fourth, the parietal cells of the stomach synthesize intrinsic factor, which is essential for B_{12} absorption.

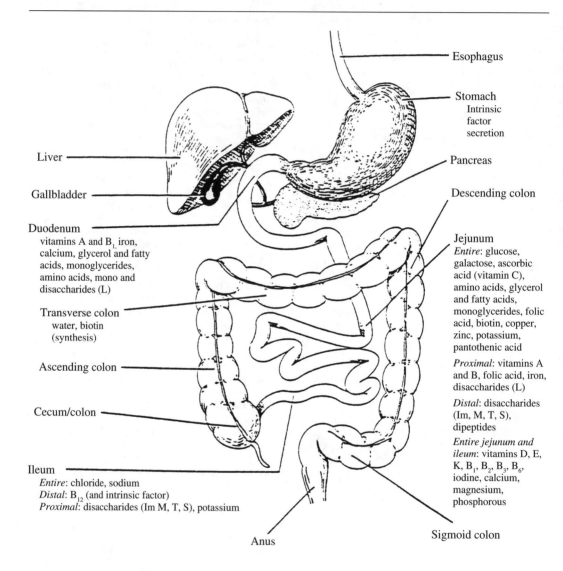

The exact sites for absorption of manganese, cobalt, selenium, chromium, molybdenum, and cadmium are unknown. L = lactose; Im = isomaltose; M = maltose; T = trehalose; S = sucrose.

Figure 32-1 Sites of Absorption. *Source*: Reprinted with permission from Caldwell MD, Kennedy-Caldwell C: Normal nutritional requirements. *Surgical Clinics of North America.* 1981;61(3):491. Copyright © 1981, WB Saunders.

The vagus nerve is intimately involved in gastric motility and secretion which is mediated through sight, smell, taste, and the act of eating. The vagus nerve stimulates acid and pepsin secretion, both important for digestion. Peristaltic activity is also triggered by gastric distension.

Functionally, the stomach is divided into two compartments, the fundus and the antrum (Figure 32-2). The fundus, or first portion of the stomach, does not contract but primarily serves as a receptacle for storage and empties through pressure gradient changes. Because of their fluidity, liquids tend to flow by gravity into the dependent antrum easier than solids. Correspond-ingly, liquid nutrients tend to empty from the stomach sooner than solids, often beginning only minutes after eating. Liquid emptying is generally preserved in persons with gastroparesis.

The antrum is responsible for reducing the particle size of food to less than 1 mm. Integration of gastric and duodenal motor function and receptive relaxation before coordinated release into the duodenum must also occur for normal gastric emptying. Three essential functions are required for gastric emptying of solids: the grinding action of the antrum; the mechanism that senses and allows finely suspended particles

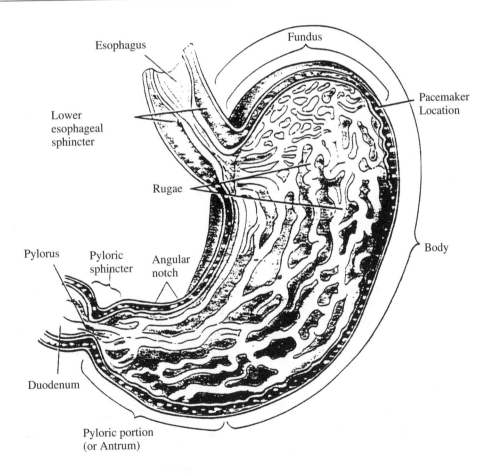

Figure 32-2 Anatomy of the Stomach. *Source:* Reprinted from *Advanced Nutrition and Human Metabolism* (p 35) by SM Hunt and JL Groff with permission of West Publishing Co., © 1990.

to pass through the pylorus, retaining larger particles for further mixing and grinding; and the propulsive mechanism, primarily fundic, that propels fluids and fine particles into the duodenum.

In addition to the above functions, the stomach is also the origin of the migrating motor complex (MMC). The MMC (also known as the "intestinal housekeeper") is bursts of muscle contractions originating in the stomach and propagating throughout the gut every 90 to 120 minutes in the interdigestive period. The MMC operates between meals to clear undigested material and debris from the stomach and along the entire GI tract until expelled. Functionally, it is similar to cilia in the respiratory tract. Motility disorders affecting the distal stomach (antrum and pylorus) are often associated with alterations in the MMC and result in retention of indigestible material with potential bezoar formation.

Small Bowel: Duodenum, Jejunum, Ileum

The first portion of the small bowel, or duodenum, is about 10 in. in length and has a tremendous absorptive capacity. Bile salts and pancreatic secretions enter here. The demarcation between duodenum to jejunum is called the duodenojejunal flexure or, more commonly, the ligament of Treitz. The jejunum is approximately 8 ft long. Most food is digested and absorbed in the first 5 ft of small bowel, underscoring the tremendous efficiency of this segment. The ileum, or terminal portion of the small bowel, is about 4 ft in length. This segment plays an integral role not only in B_{12} absorption but also in the recycling of bile salts (enterohepatic circulation).

Large Bowel: Colon

The colon is about 5 ft in length. The ileocecal valve separates the ileum from the colon, preventing bacterial colonization and reflux of stool back into the ileum. The colon provides the last opportunity to retrieve fluid and electrolytes before expulsion from the body. Dietary fiber (in-

digestible) can be used by colonic flora for fuel, and in the process, short-chain fatty acids (SCFAs) are produced. It is now known that SCFAs are the preferred substrate of colonocytes, aid in fluid and electrolyte absorption, and help to maintain the overall health of the colon. Also, up to 10% of a person's resting energy expenditure can be met by SCFAs produced by colonic flora.[4,5]

PATHOPHYSIOLOGY

The pathophysiology[6-8] of diabetes mellitus in the GI tract is not clearly understood. Many of the signs and symptoms are believed to be related to disruption in the neuronal innervation along the GI tract.

Esophagus and Dysphagia

Motility alterations in the esophagus are often responsible for the dysphagia that is seen in patients with diabetes mellitus.[9,10] Impaired peristalsis, absence of coordinated motor activity, and decreased resting lower esophageal sphincter pressure can be seen in 75% of persons with diabetes, especially those who have concurrent gastroparesis.

Manometry is the procedure used to determine esophageal motility. A probe is placed through the nose or mouth into the lower esophagus, and pressure recordings, reflective of the strength of muscular contractions within the body of the esophagus, are obtained, as are recordings from both the upper and lower esophageal sphincters.

One study[11] suggested reflux esophagitis and candidiases may be more common in IDDM, and although motility is not affected, dysphagia can result.

A word about dysphagia in general—dysphagia, or difficulty swallowing, can occur as a result of injury anywhere from the oropharynx to the GE junction. Oropharyngeal dysphagia can occur as a direct or indirect effect of diabetes. Thirty percent of patients with diabetes have cerebrovascular accidents that may affect their ability to swallow normally.

Clinically, it is not uncommon to hear that a "patient does not have a gag reflex." Although the gag reflex may be a crude response to impending aspiration of food or fluids, it is not responsible for one's ability to protect the airway and prevent aspiration. Coughing is the response necessary to prevent aspiration into the lungs. Another way to help understand the difference is to put a toothbrush too far back in the mouth and experience the response (gagging) versus remembering the last time one had food or fluid "go down the wrong tube" and the violent coughing and eye tearing that ensued. It is clinically incorrect to report that a patient does or does not have a gag reflex and presume this correlates with one's ability to prevent aspiration.

GASTROPARESIS

Gastroparesis,[12–14] or "stomach paralysis" (also known as gastroparesis diabeticorum, diabetic enteropathy, gastric stasis, diabetic gastropathy, or delayed gastric emptying) is one of the most disquieting complications of diabetes mellitus. Although other etiologies exist for gastroparesis, approximately 30% of persons with diabetes are plagued with this disorder. Gastric stasis can also be transient as a result of medications or acute conditions such as infections or ischemia (see Exhibit 32-1). Correction of the underlying disturbance or adjustment in medications should be pursued. It is important to note that gastroparesis waxes and wanes and that patients can have lengthy quiescent periods.

Next to diabetes mellitus, postvagotomy syndrome is the most common etiology for gastroparesis. As noted above, the vagus nerve is the primary stimulus for antral contraction. In patients with partial gastrectomy or vagotomy, as many as 5% of patients will develop abnormalities in gastric emptying.

Motility disorders isolated to the distal stomach (antrum, pylorus) manifest as delayed solid emptying with normal liquid emptying. Fundic, or proximal, disorder may delay both solids and liquids. In most cases of diabetic gastroparesis, liquid emptying is preserved over that of solids.

The basic defect in gastric stasis of diabetes is thought to be neuropathic in origin rather than myopathic. The correlation with autonomic neuropathy is fairly consistent. The mechanism involved is believed to be related to cholinergic dysfunction in the upper GI tract.

Signs and Symptoms

Clinical symptoms associated with gastroparesis are early satiety, persistent postprandial fullness, anorexia, nausea, vomiting (especially food ingested hours earlier), abdominal pain, halitosis, and fluctuating glycemic control. Because gastroparesis is often found in persons with nephropathy, it can be difficult to sort out in the setting of uremia. Also, hyperglycemia (>200 mg%) has been shown to impair gastric emptying and thus contribute to gastric stasis.[15–17] To further confuse the issue, alterations in gastric emptying can cause variations in glycemic control, making tight control difficult.

Diagnosis

Diagnosis of gastroparesis[3] is primarily a clinical assessment, usually after upper endoscopy has ruled out mechanical or functional obstruction of the stomach or upper intestine. However, a radionuclide gastric emptying study[18] is sometimes used to aid in the diagnosis, although one study[19] showed delayed gastric emptying in 27% of patients who also had visceral autonomic neuropathy, but not all patients were symptomatic. The patient is required to consume a solid meal that is tagged with a radioactive label (technitium). In a supine position, gastric emptying is measured with nuclear imaging. In the event a patient cannot take solids, a liquid can be used (eg, Ensure). Each item has an expected rate of emptying based on controls at the particular facility.

NUTRITION ASSESSMENT

Nutrition assessment in a patient with diabetes begins with a severity of nutrition risk assess-

Exhibit 32-1 Factors That May Affect Gastric Emptying

Mechanical Obstruction
duodenal ulcer
prepyloric ulcer
pyloric channel ulcer
idiopathic pyloric stenosis
gastric carcinoma
duodenal carcinoma
pancreatic carcinoma or pseudocyst
duodenal Crohn's disease
superior mesenteric artery syndrome

Acid-Peptic Diseases
gastric ulcer
gastroesophageal reflux disease

Diabetes Mellitus

Post-Gastric Surgery
vagotomy
gastric resection
Roux-en-Y gastrojejunostomy
fundoplication

Disorders of Gastric Smooth Muscle
hollow viscus myopathy
scleroderma
polymyositis
dermatomysitis
muscular dystrophy
amyloidosis
systemic mastocytosis

Neuropathic Disorders
hollow viscus neuropathy
Shy-Drager syndrome
Parkinson's disease
paraneoplastic syndrome
central nervous system or labyrinthine disorders
scleroderma
abdominal epilepsy
abdominal migraine
high cervical cord lesions

Gastritis
atrophic gastritis
viral gastroenteritis

Metabolic/Endocrine Disorders
hypothyroidism
hyperthyroidism
hyperparathyroidism
hypokalemia
hypomagnesemia
hyperglycemia (glucose >200 mg%)
hypo- and hypercalcemia

Medications
anticholinergics
narcotic analgesics
L-Dopa
tricyclic antidepressants
aluminum-containing antacids
sulcralfate
alcohol
beta-agonists
progesterone

Ischemia
atherosclerosis
vasculitis?

Idiopathic Disorders
non-ulcer dyspepsia
gastric dysrhythmias
gastroduodenal dissynchrony
idiopathic pseudo-obstruction
irritable bowel syndrome

Psychogenic Disorders
anorexia nervosa
bulimia
depression

ment (see condensed version in Exhibit 32-2). This will determine whether nutrition intervention should begin immediately or whether a delay is safe while medication adjustment is being made.

Anthropometrics

The most basic and noninvasive criterion in determining nutrition risk is percentage of weight change over time[20] (Table 32-2). Weight loss can be reported as spuriously high in persons with significant dehydration (not uncommon in a patient admitted with nausea, vomiting, and hyperglycemia). Before assessing total weight loss, be sure the client is fully rehydrated to the point of euvolemia (blood urea nitrogen/creatinine ratio should normalize to baseline for that person, and weight should stabilize within

Exhibit 32-2 Nutrition Assessment (Condensed Version)

A. Anthropometrics
1. Height
2. Weight
   a. actual
   b. usual body weight
   c. % weight change
   d. preferred weight

B. Medical/Surgical History
GI anatomy

C. Symptoms
1. Early satiety
2. Morning fullness
3. Aversion to meats and high-fat foods

D. Diet History
1. Prior restrictions
   a. prescribed by physician (fat, fiber, etc.)
   b. self-imposed
2. Vitamin/mineral supplements, etc.
3. Typical intake prior to admission
4. Food allergies/intolerances
   milk/milk products
5. Prior total parenteral nutrition/tube feeding
   length of time, problems; formula, route

E. Dentition
Own teeth, dentures/do they fit?, dental care

F. Laboratory Data
1. Chem 7: Magnesium, phosphorous, calcium, albumin, cholesterol, triglyceride
2. CBC: Hemoglobin/hematocrit, mean corpuscular volume, red cell size distribution width, iron, ferritin
3. B_{12}
4. 25-OH vitamin D
5. HbA_{1c} (glycosylated Hb)
6. 24-hour urinary protein

G. Stooling
Diarrhea/constipation

H. Medication
1. Insulin versus oral hypoglycemic agent
2. Prokinetics
3. H_2 blockers, prilosec
4. Pancreatic enzymes
5. Laxatives
6. Metamucil

Source: Copyright © 1994 CR Parrish, RD, CDE, CNSD.

24 to 28 hours). Distinguishing true weight loss versus fluid loss helps not only to identify clients who are significantly compromised, but will guide therapy as well.

Anyone with significant weight loss is at risk for refeeding syndrome[21] and should be fed judiciously, starting with basal needs until potassium, magnesium, and phosphorus are repleted if serum levels fall.

Determining a client's preferred weight in the initial interview may also unmask potential underlying eating disorders in this population.

Nutrition History

In working with persons with gastroparesis, a detailed diet history is an important guide in determining what, if any, nutrition intervention is needed. Clearly, the patient who cannot keep down water has much less chance of success with nutrition therapy than a patient who can keep most foods down. It is not uncommon that patients, often by trial and error, will arrive at a diet fairly low in fiber and fat due to a perceptible decrease in their symptoms.

Particular attention should be paid to dentition. If a patient cannot adequately masticate solids, solid foods may have to be finely ground or pureed. Even in patients with good dentition but severe gastroparesis, increasing the surface area of the food might be of benefit. Good dental hygiene is especially important in patients with chronic vomiting, as the enamel around the teeth

Table 32-2 Evaluation of Weight Change[a]

Time	Significant Weight Loss	Severe Weight Loss
1 week	1–2%	>2%
1 month	5%	>5%
3 months	7.5%	>7.5%
6 months	10%	>10%

[a] % weight change = severity and significance of weight loss.

$$\% \text{ weight change} = \frac{\text{usual weight} - \text{actual weight} \times 100}{\text{usual weight}}$$

may be compromised from chronic acid exposure, thereby increasing risk of caries and halitosis.

LABORATORY PARAMETERS

Laboratory assessment requires careful scrutiny. Given confounding factors of renal disease, and possible poor glycemic control, especially in a hospital setting with superimposed infections, laboratory values may reflect an acute process versus the patient's actual nutritional status. Nutritional assessment is, after all, a comparison of objective data and clinical judgment.

Glycemic Control

Glycemic control must be determined before a lengthy workup for gastroparesis begins. As elevated serum glucose has been shown to precipitate gastric stasis, it is important to distinguish between poor glycemic control and its effect on gastric emptying versus true gastroparesis. Glycated hemoglobin is the best tool for determining glycemic control over time. Clearly, any nutritional therapy specific for gastroparesis is moot without good glycemic control. Nutrition therapy should always be aimed at optimal control.

Visceral Proteins

Albumin, prealbumin, and transferrin may all be low in the setting of nephrotic syndrome (defined as 3 g or more of protein lost per 24 hours). Proteins in the range of 40 to 150 kd are lost in the urine. The above-mentioned proteins are 69, 61, and 76 kd, respectively.[22] It is important to determine renal function in these patients for the purposes of monitoring the effects of nutritional intervention. A 24-hour urine collection for protein is essential for unexplained low serum albumin in the setting of adequate intake. Serum levels of the aforementioned proteins should not be altered if microalbuminemia is present.

Albumin, prealbumin, and cholesterol are negative acute-phase reactants and therefore can appear quite low in stressed states. Prealbumin is degraded by the kidney and as a result can appear falsely elevated in patients with acute failure. However, once dialysis is initiated, prealbumin will often return below normal limits.[20]

Lastly, prealbumin is affected by serum glucose levels. Hyperglycemia is a catabolic state, and given the short half-life of prealbumin, it will reflect catabolism as a function of poor glucose control and return below normal limits.[23]

Iron

Iron status[24] should be assessed in patients with severe gastroparesis. The best indicator of iron stores and impending iron deficiency is serum ferritin. The caveat is that ferritin is an acute-phase reactant and therefore should not be obtained in inflammatory or septic conditions.[25] The following factors may account for iron deficiency in patients with gastroparesis:

1. decreased intake, especially red meats (it is not uncommon to hear anecdotal reports of red meat aversion)

2. decreased availability in hypo- or achlorhydric states

3. defective digestion of meat secondary to altered trituration

Gastric acidity is required to dissociate and dissolve iron salts from food. Ferric iron (Fe^{3+}) is reduced to ferrous iron (Fe^{2+}) in the stomach, with the Fe^{2+} being 100 times more soluble at intestinal pH (5.5 to 6.5). Approximately two-thirds of iron in food is bound in the form of iron salts. The remaining one-third is heme iron in the form of red meat (if red meat is consumed). Because heme iron is chelated by the heme porphyrin, it does not require gastric acidity for absorption. Pancreatic proteases digest heme proteins liberating soluble heme iron complexes, which are absorbed directly by a carrier for heme on the intestinal absorptive cell.[26]

Cyanocobalamin (B12)

Pernicious anemia has a reported incidence ranging from 2 to 30/1,000 in persons with diabetes.[27] However, these studies include only those patients with evidence of megaloblastic anemia. In a more recent study, latent PA was found to have a prevalence of 11% based on serum B_{12} levels, and parietal cell and intrinsic factor antibodies.[28] The authors concluded that PA has a long preclinical course and that it would be worthwhile to screen this patient population.

Magnesium

Low magnesium has been found in up to 30% of patients with diabetes mellitus.[29–31] Hypomagnesemia has been associated with gastroparesis and therefore should be addressed in the overall workup.[32] As it is an intracellular cation, low serum levels reflect a total body deficit. However, total body deficit can occur with normal serum levels (normal range, 1.5 to 2.4 mEq/L).

Magnesium plays an important role in many enzyme functions and is required for all enzymatic reactions involving adenosine triphosphate. Clinical manifestations of magnesium deficiency are:

1. hypocalcemia—thought to be secondary to impaired secretion of parathyroid hormone and renal and skeletal resistance
2. hypokalemia—42% of patients will also have low serum potassium. Refractory potassium repletion in the setting of potassium supplementation will often correct with magnesium supplementation
3. neuromuscular hyperexcitability, cardiac arrhythmias, hypertension, myocardial infarction, and altered glucose homeostasis

Potential causes for magnesium deficiency in diabetes might include diuretics, renal wasting secondary to glucosuria-induced osmotic diuresis, diarrhea, and malabsorption.

In addition to being aware of the effects of low serum magnesium, one needs to look for it.

It is often not part of the standard hospital chemistry panel, and replacement is often slow and inadequate (see Exhibit 32-3). The standard dose of intravenous 2 g $MgSO_4$ contains 16 mEq of Mg, the U.S. recommended dietary allowance, which is meant to maintain levels, not replace pre-existing deficiencies. *Note:* As magnesium is excreted by the kidney, caution must be taken in patients with renal insufficiency (<30 mL/min).

NUTRITION AND GASTRIC EMPTYING

Gastric emptying is influenced by a number of factors, including volume, composition, consistency, and caloric content of the meal as well as by body position.[2,3,33] Liquids leave the stomach faster than solids; however, as caloric density increases, emptying rates decrease.[34] Fats, sugars, certain amino acids (especially L-tryptophan), and titratable acids of high osmolarity trigger sensory mechanisms in the intestine, which in turn inhibit gastric emptying. Of these nutrients, the most potent inhibitor of gastric emptying is fat.

Fat has a number of inhibitory effects on stomach emptying, stimulation of cholecystokinin release by fat being one of the more powerful. Cholecystokinin acts to slow gastric emptying via relaxation of the fundus and pyloric contraction. Medium-chain *fatty acids,* especially those with chain lengths of 10 to 14 carbons, are more potent inhibitors than long-chain *fatty acids.* However, medium-chain *triglycerides* do not inhibit gastric emptying to any great extent.[35] The emptying time of long-chain *triglycerides* is similar to that of solids.[36]

Elemental diets take longer to empty from the stomach than blended "whole" food of comparable caloric composition, probably due to the amino acid content and the hypertonicity of formulas.[37] However, it is important to note that this may not be of clinical importance.

Soluble fiber also has an inhibitory effect on gastric emptying, although fiber of any type may be met with intolerance in these patients.[38]

Exhibit 32-3 Guidelines for Intravenous Magnesium Replacement Therapy

Category	Magnesium Dose
Daily requirements	0.4 mEq/kg/24 h 2 mEq/g N/24 h
Serum magnesium = 1–1.4 mEq/L	Initial: 1 mEq/kg over 24 h Follow: 0.5 mEq/kg over 24 h × 5 d
Electrolyte depletions	Initial: 6 g over 3 h Follow: 5 g over 6 h Follow: 5 g q 12 h × 5 d
Serious reactions	Initial: 2 g over 2 min Follow: 5 g over 6 h Follow: 5 g q 12 h × 5 d

Note: 50 percent $MgSO_4$ = 0.5 g/mL or 4 mEq/mL, 10 percent $MgSO_4$ = 0.1 g/mL or 0.8 mEq/mL.

Source: Data from Oster JR, Epstein M, *American Journal of Nephrology*. 1988;8:34, S Karger AG; and from *Critical Care Medicine*. 1991;12(6):32–46, Williams & Wilkins.

Fiber-containing stool softeners should also be avoided.

Nutrition Intervention

Glycemic control is sometimes difficult to achieve in patients with gastroparesis. Because the patient cannot reliably keep food down, insulin dosing is a problem (majority of patients with gastroparesis are type I); hypoglycemia or hyperglycemia may result. The primary aim, then, is to get the nausea and vomiting controlled enough so that the patient can tolerate food and fluids with some regularity. At the same time, glucose must be controlled to remove the potential contribution of hyperglycemia to delayed emptying. In terms of patient comfort, small frequent meals with an emphasis on liquids are most successful during acute exacerbation of gastroparesis. Walking or remaining upright after meals can also be of benefit. Some patients also complain that foods begin to "back up as the day goes on." Limiting solids to breakfast and lunch and then switching to liquid nourishment the rest of the day may be the solution. There is no single way to do this.

Fat

Fat restriction is one of the first dietary restrictions placed on patients with gastroparesis, and although fat clearly can slow gastric emptying, relief of symptoms varies with each patient. Personal experience suggests that fat in association with solid foods is more problematic than liquid fat (ie, whole milk does not seem to make much difference compared with skim; some patients tolerate milkshakes and ice cream very well).

Fiber

It is common in patients with gastroparesis to have alterations in the MMC. During the interdigestive period, the MMC normally sweeps residual food, fiber, and other stomach contents from the stomach and small intestine. Retention of indigestible solids can lead to bezoar formation, particularly in the presence of hypo- and achlorhydria, which may accompany diabetes.

A gastric bezoar[39,40] is a mass of indigestible material found in the stomach and is made up of a variety of substances (similar to a hair ball in a cat). Phytobezoars, the most common, are made up of plant and vegetable fibers; however, persimmons (disopyrobezoar) and hair (trichobezoar) are also found. More recently, there have been case reports of medication bezoars including sucralfate and hygroscopic gum laxatives.[41,42] Predisposing factors in the formation of bezoars are hypochlorhydria, large particle size, indigestibility, poor mastication, gastric outlet obstruction, and altered antral motility, all of which can be present in a patient with diabetes mellitus. Bezoars themselves can cause gastric outlet obstruction and hence are one of the differential diagnoses in the workup of a patient for gastroparesis.[43] Once a bezoar has been found, treatment may be removal at the time of endoscopy or by use of a Teledyne Water Pik that breaks up the bezoar and allows it to pass on through the GI tract.[44]

Because of the potential for bezoar formation, high-fiber foods should be limited or avoided altogether, especially in patients who have presented with a bezoar in the past. High-fiber foods associated with bezoar formation include the following: oranges, persimmons, coconuts, berries, green beans, figs, apples, sauerkraut, Brussels sprouts, potato peels, and legumes.[45] Because the diet is low in fiber, constipation can be an unwanted side effect. Appropriate laxatives such as docusate sodium or sorbitol with adequate fluids will help.[46]

Dentition

Patients who have poor dentition may benefit from finely ground or pureed food, not only because of their inability to masticate but also to improve gastric emptying.

Body Positioning

Body positioning is an important consideration, as lying flat will not enhance gastric emptying. In fact, it may encourage reflux in patients with hiatal hernia or a history of reflux disease. In the hospital setting, it is important to have patients sit up during and for at least 30 minutes after their meal.

Iron

As discussed earlier, iron can be a chronic problem in this patient population, especially if hypo- or achlorhydria is present. Because red meats are often not well tolerated, heme iron intake may be limited to nonexistent.

Intolerance to iron supplementation is not uncommon, especially in patients with underlying gastric discomfort. On questioning, patients have generally tried only one formulation (usually $FeSO_4$ 325 mg TID or a total of 180 mg iron per day). Side effects of iron supplementation are usually dose-related; therefore, lowering the dose or even switching from a tablet to an elixir may increase tolerance and compliance. Remember, some iron is better than none. Examples of common iron supplements used can be found in Table 32-3.

Calcium

Bone health is another area of concern, and unfortunately, milk intolerance is not uncommon. One of the possible reasons for this can be due to coexisting small bowel dysmotility with subsequent bacterial overgrowth. Although calcium absorption primarily occurs in the duodenum, it can be absorbed throughout the entire small bowel; therefore, some "protection" is afforded. Patients with coexisting celiac sprue are at much greater risk of osteopenia due to marked decrease in calcium absorption and warrant special attention to calcium intake and bone health.

Cyanocobalamin (B_{12})

Due to the higher incidence of pernicious anemia in this patient population, any patient with known achlorhydria, elevated mean corpuscular volume, gastrectomy, or terminal ileal resection should have serum B_{12} checked. Vitamin B_{12} can be given intramuscularly as 100 µg or 1,000 µg every 1 to 3 months, respectively.

Nutrition Support

In refractory cases of diabetic gastroparesis, enteral tube feeding may be the only answer. Total parenteral nutrition is *rarely* necessary. Because liquid emptying is generally preserved, theoretically gastric feedings may be successful. However, even if a patient tolerates this form of feeding for a time, long-term tolerance is very doubtful. In the event this is the only option, a gastric feeding trial should be undertaken to determine the potential for success. Goal flow should be reached and sustained for at least 24 hours before consideration of percutaneous endoscopic gastrostomy (PEG) placement or possibly a nasogastric tube. Bolus feedings are contraindicated due to volume sensitivity of the gastroparetic stomach.

Nasoduodenal or nasojejunal feedings may work for short-term feeding; however, if patients experience any regularity to their vomiting, the risk of tube dislodgement is very high. Similarly, long-term percutaneous endoscopic jejunostomy or PEJ (small bowel access through a PEG tube with a "jejunal arm") feeding can also be problematic. This is because the J arm is threaded through a PEG and is "free floating" and therefore can migrate back into the stomach. The most common PEG tube used is a 20-French, which may only allow a tube with a 6-French internal diameter to be passed through, depending on which one is used. Tube clogging as a result of medications can be a problem when the smaller bore (6,8-French) tubes are used. If a PEG-J must be used, insert a PEG tube that can accommodate a 9- or 10-French tube to be used in conjunction.

A surgically placed jejunostomy (J-tube) is the best route for long-term enteral feeding in a patient with gastroparesis.[47] This route of feeding guarantees consistent nutrient and fluid delivery even in the setting of continued nausea and vomiting. Patients with increasing hospital admissions due to chronic nausea and vomiting are good candidates for this intervention, even if their nutritional status is only somewhat compromised. Quality of life is an important consideration, and keeping patients home with a means to infuse nutrients, fluids, and medications during acute exacerbations is a worthwhile goal.

Table 32-3 Commonly Used Iron Supplements

Product	Dosage [a] Form/Strength	Elemental Iron (mg)
Ferrous sulfate		
Tablet	325 mg	60
Solution	300 mg/5 ml	60
Feosol	220 mg/5 ml	44
Fer-In-Sol	15 mg/0.6 ml	15
Ferrous gluconate		
Fergon[R]	320-mg tablet	37
Ferrous fumarate		
Vitron C	1 tablet	66 (w/125 mg vit C)
Polysaccharide iron complex		
Nu-Iron	1 capsule	150 mg

[a] Usually given BID or TID.

Source: Copyright © 1994, CR Parrish, RD, CDE, CNSD.

Once a J-tube is in place and the stomach is bypassed, any polymeric enteral formula can be used. A fiber-containing formula is preferable for maintenance of colonic flora whenever possible. Although data are lacking, patients with dysmotility along the entire GI tract or with known bacterial overgrowth may not tolerate fiber-containing formulas due to fermentation by gut flora. There are no special formulas that have proven efficacy in terms of glycemic control. If a patient requires insulin before enteral feedings, they will require insulin regardless. If a patient is volume-sensitive or wants to infuse the least number of hours at night, a more calorically dense formula will allow this. Because the jejunum is volume-sensitive, continuous feedings, usually overnight so the patient is not burdened during the day, is ideal. Bolus feeding the small bowel is not well tolerated. Although a pump is generally recommended, gravity drip is possible. Flow rate tolerance is unique to the individual and can be quite high (one of our patients feeds at 160 mL/h overnight without problems).

Water flushes are key in this patient population, unless fluid restriction is necessary. With the added concern of osmotic diuresis when the renal threshold for glucose is exceeded (180 mg%), more water is probably better than less. This can be provided as water flushes every 4 to 6 hours over the course of the day. Some patients are able to take fluids by mouth and may only require additional water through their tube during exacerbations. Another alternative patients may choose is to dilute their formula and run higher flow rates to infuse water concurrent with their feeding. Most patients can assess their changing fluid needs by responding to thirst or a noticeable decrease or darkening of their urine output.

One last consideration, especially in patients with lower caloric requirements but perhaps higher micronutrient needs, is to determine the amount of the U.S. RDA delivered in the volume of formula they will be discharged on. Vitamin/mineral elixirs can be given via the J-tube if necessary. There are very little data on long-term jejunostomy feeding and potential micronutrient deficiencies as a result of bypassing the duodenum.

If a patient is relying almost exclusively on J-tube feedings, iron status should be monitored routinely. The rationale is that the preferred brush border for iron absorption is in the duodenum, which is bypassed with J-tube feedings. In patients who get very little to no heme iron, especially in low acid-producing states, deficiency may develop. In a retrospective chart review, 67% of jejunostomy-fed patients were found to have poor iron stores.[48]

PROKINETIC AGENTS

Treatment for diabetic gastroparesis is based on a combination of pharmacotherapy and nutrition intervention. Prokinetic or promotility means forward motion. Prokinetic agents (see Table 32-4) have important therapeutic benefits in disorders of GI smooth muscle. Four currently used prokinetic agents are reviewed here.[49,50]

There is a vomiting center in the brain, located in the lateral reticular formation. Also, there is a chemoreceptor trigger zone located on the floor of the fourth ventricle. Nausea and vomiting can result from a number of factors; in gastroparesis, the mechanism is still unknown. Metoclopropamide (Reglan) is one of the most commonly used prokinetic agents on the market. It has central antiemetic action as well as peripheral actions on GI motility. It can be given enterally, subcutaneously (SC), and intravenously (IV). Delayed absorption may occur in patients with gastroparesis who receive metoclopropamide orally. It may be necessary to give these patients a "loading" dose SC or IV to initiate gastric and small bowel motility and then follow with oral dosing. The main side effects of Reglan are drowsiness, restlessness, and anxiety. Tardive dyskinesia is a more serious potential side effect at higher doses and can be permanent. Furthermore, Reglan should not be used in patients who are being treated for Parkinson's disease as it may counter the effects of L-Dopa.

Cisapride (Propulsid) was recently made available in the United States. It has very similar

Table 32-4 Prokinetic Agents

Agent	Activity Site	Mechanism of Action	Receptor Affinity	Available Routes/Doses	Side Effects	Drug Antagonists
Metoclopramide (Reglan)	Esophagus, stomach, and small bowel	Antiemetic. Increases gastric/duodenal contractions and improves gastroduodenal coordination. Increases lower esophageal sphincter pressure	Central dopamine antagonist (D_2 receptor) 5HT-4 receptor agonist	IV / PO (tab, elixir) / SC — 5 mg / 10 mg TID QID	Drowsiness. Dystonic reactions/tardive dyskinesia. Restlessness/anxiety. Hyperprolactinemia: amenorrhea, impotence, galactorrhea	Alcohol, barbiturates, benzo diazepenes, should not be used in Parkinson's patients, or with anticholinergics
Domperidone (Motilium) (experimental)	Stomach and proximal small bowel	Antiemetic. Increases gastric/duodenal contractions and improves gastroduodenal coordination	Peripheral dopamine antagonist (does not cross blood-brain barrier)	PO 10–30 mg QID	Hyperprolactinemia: amenorrhea, impotence, galactorrhea	Hypoacidity can decrease bioavailability
Cisapride (Propulsid)	Esophagus, stomach, small bowel, colon, gallbladder	Increases gastric/duodenal contractions and improves gastroduodenal coordination. Increases small bowel and colonic motility	Facilitates acetylcholine release from myenteric plexus 5HT-4 agonist	PO 10–20 mg QID	Rare headaches. Slight loose stool or increased frequency	Should not be used with anticholinergics
Erythromycin	Esophagus, stomach, and small bowel	Increases gastric antral contractions and phase III MMC activity in small bowel ("pharmacologic antrectomy")	Motilin agonist	PO 250 mg q d TID IV 100–200 mg QID	Abdominal cramps, diarrhea, transient nausea	Promotes cardiovascular side effects of seldane
Sandostatin (Octreotide)	Stomach, small bowel, gallbladder, sphincter of Oddi	Stimulates fasting motility (phase III MMC) in small bowel. Inhibits fed pattern in stomach and small bowel, stimulates rapidity of sphincter of Oddi phasic activity (Tachyodea), inhibits gallbladder motility		SC 50–100 µg at night	Transient nausea, loose stool, gallstones possible after 6 months of treatment, slight weight loss	
Misoprostol (Cytotec)	Small bowel, colon	Stimulates secretion in small bowel and increases colonic motility		PO 400–1600 µg/d	Abdominal cramping, diarrhea, can induce abortion in 1st trimester	

Source: Copyright © 1994 CR Parrish, RD, CDE, CNSD, and RW McCallum, MD.

effects to Reglan; however, it also enhances colonic motility. Cisapride does not cross the blood-brain barrier and therefore does not have the same side effects as Reglan. Nor does it have the same potent antiemetic properties.

Erythromycin, in addition to its antibiotic effects, has been found to accelerate solid emptying in smaller doses. By impairing gastric sieving, it allows larger food particles to leave the stomach, an action described as "pharmacologic antrectomy."

Domperidone (Motilium) is currently available in 58 countries but has not yet been cleared for use in the United States. It acts peripherally like cisapride; however, it has a potent central antiemetic effect because its site of action on the chemoreceptor trigger zone lies outside the blood-brain barrier. It has a unique pharmacologic niche in patients with Parkinson's disease who also have gastroparesis.

SMALL BOWEL AND COLON

Diarrhea and Malabsorption

Diabetic diarrhea is primarily diagnosed by exclusion.[51–53] It occurs in approximately 10 to 20% of patients with long-standing poorly controlled diabetes.[7] The diarrhea is intermittent, although it can be persistent and associated with nocturnal incontinence. Malabsorption is uncommon, but if present, conditions such as pancreatic insufficiency, bacterial overgrowth, and celiac sprue should be excluded. Possible mechanisms of diarrhea in patients with diabetes mellitus include

- abnormal motility of the small bowel or colon
- bacterial overgrowth in the small bowel
- anorectal dysfunction
- exocrine pancreatic insufficiency
- intestinal secretion
- celiac sprue
- bile acid catharsis
- foods containing polyols (sugar alcohols)

- lactose intolerance
- medications

Diarrhea does not necessarily mean malabsorption; therefore, before an expensive, lengthy workup is embarked on, it is important to determine whether diarrhea is actually present. Loose stools, increased frequency, and increased volume can all be labeled as diarrhea; most patients define it by the first two criteria.[54] Distinguishing low-volume from high-volume diarrhea will help to determine the underlying etiology; therefore, collecting stool for weight is the first step toward diagnosis. Diarrhea is usually defined as greater than 250 mL of stool per day or greater than three stools per day. Once diarrhea is documented, workup should include medications and infectious agents as possible etiologic factors. Making a patient "NPO" or "resting the GI tract" is unnecessary and may cause atrophy of an already injured intestine (unless, of course, enteral stimulation causes an aggravation of the diarrhea).

Before malabsorption should be suspected in patients with diarrhea, actual intake needs to be documented. Weight loss in the setting of *adequate intake* and diarrhea (and good glycemic control in a patient with diabetes) is a cardinal sign for malabsorption. However, malabsorption *can* occur without diarrhea. The first step is to obtain a qualitative fecal fat (a spot check for fat in the stool). Qualitative and quantitative fecal fat (72 hour) requires the patient to *take in* fat. All too often, fecal fat studies are interpreted as negative while the patient has been NPO, on clear liquids, or off the floor for procedures. Less than 6 g of fat per day in the stool is considered normal.[55] Clinical pearl—if a fecal fat (qualitative or quantitative) is ordered on a patient,

1. Make sure a diet of 100 g fat per day is ordered.

2. Inform the patient! Many of these patients have been told to restrict fat or have found that it makes them sick and they do not

know that they need to consume all the fat on their tray for diagnostic purposes.

3. Do a calorie count for grams of fat ingested *concurrent* with the stool collection.

Pancreatic Insufficiency

Pancreatic insufficiency can be seen in patients with diabetes[56,57] and is the most common cause of malabsorption in this population. Nutrition intervention in the past was aimed at restricting fat in the diet. Although fat restriction will decrease malabsorption, it is unnecessary with *adequate* pancreatic enzyme supplementation. Gastric acid suppressing agents such as histamine 2 receptor antagonists (famotidine, ranitidine) are necessary to prevent degradation of oral pancreatic enzymes in the stomach, unless sustained release formulations are used or the patient has achlorhydria. If enteral tube feeding is required in these patients, *noncoated* enzymes such as viokase can be added to the formula (1/2 tsp/120 mL) or given every 4 hours via the tube in 10 to 20 mL of water or normal saline. Elemental diets are expensive and unnecessary.[58] It has been shown that even in patients with total pancreatectomy, 60% of intact proteins will be absorbed.[59] In another study,[60] fat digestion was not impaired until lipase outputs were decreased to approximately 10% of normal.

Pancreatitis

A word about pancreatitis[8]:

1. Severe pancreatitis with destruction of the pancreas can lead to diabetes. Usually 90% of pancreatic function must be lost before clinical signs are apparent.

2. Pancreatitis can also exacerbate diabetes.

3. Chronic alcoholic pancreatitis will cause diabetes in up to 70% of patients, especially those with calcification of the pancreas.

4. Adenocarcinoma of the pancreas is two to four times more frequent in patients with established diabetes mellitus and alcohol-

ism. It is difficult to determine at times whether the cancer caused the diabetes or vice versa. In 80% of patients presenting with pancreatic cancer and diabetes, the diabetes is discovered within a year of the time the cancer is clinically apparent. For a recent review of pancreatic cancer and diabetes, see McLaughlin[61]; however, the need for elemental or hydrolyzed formulas via gastric or jejunal tube is not consistent with this author's clinical experience.

Bacterial Overgrowth

Bacterial overgrowth[62] is another potential cause of malabsorption in patients with diabetes. Intestinal stasis and hypo- or achlorhydria predispose these patients to overgrowth of their normal intestinal flora. Diarrhea is thought to result from deconjugation of bile salts in the small bowel, with resultant interference in micelle formation and fat malabsorption. Bacterial metabolism of dietary protein can result in protein malnutrition similar to kwashiorkor in severity. Proteins may be partially degraded, followed by deamination, producing fatty acids and ammonia. The ammonia may then be absorbed and incorporated into urea synthesis. Therefore, despite adequate dietary protein intake, a significant proportion may be lost to bacterial degradation. Treatment with antibiotics will eliminate the problem. In patients with recurrences of bacterial overgrowth, rotating antibiotics are often used to avoid antibiotic resistance (10 days each month, alternating three different antibiotics).[63]

Celiac Sprue

Celiac sprue,[64] also known as gluten-sensitive enteropathy or nontropical sprue, is receiving increased attention in the diabetic population. Reportedly, it occurs in 1.5 to 11% of persons with diabetes mellitus.[65,66] Diagnosis is confirmed by small bowel biopsy, where the intestinal mucosa is found to be flat with loss of absorptive intestinal villi. Antigliadin antibody testing as a newer diagnostic tool is gaining recognition before overt signs of malabsorption arise. A gluten-free (gliadin-free) diet, in addition to whatever diabetic regimen the patient is on, will attenuate the problem. Regeneration of the normal intestinal architecture can take up to 6 to 8 months, depending on dietary compliance. Because the diet is so complex, it is not enough to provide patients written materials without careful personal instruction. Many gluten-free diets used by hospitals are incorrect and should be updated annually to reflect the continuing changes and new additives in our food supply. An excellent resource for the most up-to-date- information is the Gluten Intolerance Group of North America in Seattle, Washington (206/325-6980).

Lactose intolerance is not uncommon in patients with celiac sprue. The lactase enzyme is found in the tips of the villi, which is the last to regenerate on a gluten-free diet. Although lactose in this setting is not harmful, patients may be more comfortable on a lower-lactose diet initially. After 1 month or so, this can be liberalized as tolerated.

Diabetic Diarrhea

After all the above-mentioned etiologies for diarrhea are ruled out, diabetic diarrhea is diagnosed by exclusion. Normal intestinal motility and electrolyte transport are regulated by enteric and autonomic neurons. Intestinal fluid and electrolyte secretion and absorption are determined by a balance of these two processes. In diabetic patients, there may be impaired absorption capability and an up-regulation of luminal secretion, causing the homeostatic balance to shift to net secretion and altered motility. Efforts to treat this disorder are empiric with the aim of reducing symptoms. Diet modification, bulking agents, cholestyramine, opiates, Reglan, and various antidiarrheals have been tried without consistent results. Fedorak et al[67] reported a significant reduction in stool output in a few patients given clonidine, which reduces diarrhea by enhancing mucosal absorption of fluid and electrolytes and by inhibiting anion secretion.

Constipation

Constipation[46,68] is the most common GI complaint in patients with diabetes mellitus. It is most likely related to an underlying autonomic neuropathy. Medical therapy is the mainstay of treatment; high-fiber diets have not been proven to be efficacious.

Fecal Incontinence

Rectal-anal incontinence[7,8,57] is one of the more distressing of the GI symptoms. The internal sphincter is solely innervated by the autonomic nervous system; therefore, autonomic dysfunction is thought to be the cause. Normal sphincter resting tone and reflexive internal sphincter relaxation triggered by rectal distention are impaired. Management is empiric with biofeedback and antidiarrheal agents.

RESEARCH

One interesting area of research in gastroparesis includes placement of pacing wires in the stomach. This is usually done at the time of jejunostomy tube placement. The hope is to stimulate the "gastric pacemaker" and perhaps "jump start" the stomach into normal contractions.

Medications, especially promotility agents, are currently being investigated, and new ones are coming out on the market routinely.

In terms of nutrition, little has been done in the area of controlled trials in patients on long-term jejunostomy feeding. As this is an ever-increasing feeding option, long-term effects of nutrient delivery beyond the duodenum need to be investigated. It is possible that certain nutrients will need to be "uploaded" to meet the needs of these patients, particularly in low-acid states. This is an area wide open to clinical nutritionists and is definitely wanting.

REFERENCES

1. Yamada T. *Textbook of Gastroenterology*. Philadelphia, Pa: JB Lippincott; 1991.
2. Meyer JH. Physiology of the stomach. In: Champion MC, McCallum RW, eds. *Physiology, Diagnosis and Therapy in GI Motility Disorders*. Toronto: Medicine Publishing Foundation; 1988:15–22. Symposium Series 22.

3. McCallum RW. Diagnosis of gastric motility disorders. In: Champion MC, McCallum RW, eds. *Physiology, Diagnosis and Therapy in GI Motility Disorders*. Toronto: Medicine Publishing Foundation; 1988:61–80. Symposium Series 22.

4. Nordgaard I, Hansen BS, Mortensen PB. Colon as a digestive organ in patients with short bowel. *Lancet*. 1994;343:373–376.

5. McNeil NI. The contribution of the large intestine to energy supplies in man. *Am J Clin Nutr*. 1984;39:338–342.

6. Atkinson M, Hosking DJ. Gastrointestinal complications of diabetes mellitus. *Clin Gastroenterol*. 1983;12(3):633–650.

7. Feldman M, Schiller LR. Disorders of gastrointestinal motility associated with diabetes mellitus. *Ann Intern Med*. 1983;98:378.

8. Ryan JC, Sleisenger MH. Effects of systemic and extraintestinal disease on the gut. In: Sleisenger MH, Fordtran JS, eds. *Gastrointestinal Disease—Pathophysiology, Diagnosis, Management*. 5th Ed. Philadelphia, Pa: WB Saunders; 1993:200–206.

9. Vantrappen G. Diagnostic methodology of esophageal problems. In: Champion MC, McCallum RW, eds. *Physiology, Diagnosis and Therapy in GI Motility Disorders*. Toronto: Medicine Publishing Foundation; 1988:51–60. Symposium Series 22.

10. Bernstein G, Rifkin H. Diabetes mellitus: gastrointestinal complications. *Compr Ther*. 1986;12(11):8–12.

11. Parkman HP, Schwartz SS. Esophagitis and gastroduodenal disorders associated with diabetic gastroparesis. *Arch Intern Med*. 1987;147:1477–1480.

12. Read NW, Houghton LA. Physiology of gastric emptying and pathophysiology of gastroparesis. *Gastroenterol Clin North Am*. 1989;18(2):359.

13. Minami H, McCallum RW. The physiology and pathophysiology of gastric emptying in humans. *Gastroenterology*. 1984;86:1592.

14. Kelly D, Camillerio M. Gastrointestinal motility. *Supportline Newslett Diet Nutr Support DPG Am Diet Assoc*. 1991:13(1).

15. Barnett JL, Owyang C. Serum glucose concentration as a modulator of interdigestive gastric motility. *Gastroenterology*. 1988;94:739–744.

16. MacGregor IL, Gueller R, Watts HD, Meyer JH. The effect of acute hyperglycemia on gastric emptying in man. *Gastroenterology*. 1976;70:190–197.

17. Horowitz M, Harding PE, Maddox AF, et al. Gastric and esophageal emptying in patients with type II (non-insulin dependent) diabetes mellitus. *Diabetologia*. 1989;32(3):151–159.

18. Malmud LS, Fisher RS. Scintigraphic evaluation of esophageal transit, gastroesophageal reflux, and gastric emptying. In: Gottschalk A, ed. *Diagnostic Nuclear Medicine*. Vol. 2. Baltimore, Md: William & Wilkins; 1988:663–686.

19. Keshavarzian A, Iber FL, Vaeth J. Gastric emptying in patients with insulin-requiring diabetes mellitus. *Am J Gastroenterol*. 1987;82(1):29–35.

20. Hopkins B. Assessment of nutritional status. In: Gottschlich MM, Matarese LE, Shronts EP, eds. *Nutrition Support Dietetics; Core Curriculum*. Silver Spring, Md: American Society for Parenteral and Enteral Nutrition; 1993:15–70.

21. Solomon SM, Kirby DK. The refeeding syndrome: a review. *JPEN*. 1990;14:90–97.

22. Kaysen DA. Nutritional management of nephrotic syndrome. *J Nutr*. 1992;2(2):50–58.

23. Jain SK, McVie R, Duett J, Herbst JJ. The effect of glycemic control on plasma prealbumin levels in type-I diabetic children. *Horm Metab Res*. 1993;25:102–104.

24. Meyer JH. Chronic morbidity after ulcer surgery. In: Sleisenger MH, Fordtran JS, eds. *Gastrointestinal Disease—Pathophysiology, Diagnosis, Management*. 5th Ed. Philadelphia, Pa: WB Saunders; 1993:731–744.

25. Gibson R.S. Assessment of iron status. *Principles of Nutritional Assessment*. New York, NY: Oxford University Press; 1990:349–376.

26. Conrad ME, Weintraub LR, Sears DA, Crosby WH. Absorption of hemoglobin iron. *Am J Physiol*. 1966; 211:1123.

27. Munichoodappa C, Kozak GP. Diabetes mellitus and pernicious anemia. *Diabetes*. 1979;19:719–723.

28. Davis RE, McCann VJ, Stanton KG. Type I diabetes and latent pernicious anaemia. *Med J Aust*. 1992;156(3): 160–162.

29. Campbell RK, Nadler JN. Magnesium deficiency and diabetes. *Diabetes Educ*. 1992;18(1):17–19.

30. Rude RK. Magnesium deficiency and diabetes mellitus: causes and effects. *Postgrad Med*. 1992;92(5):217–224.

31. Whang R, Whang DD, Ryan MP. Refractory potassium repletion: a consequence of magnesium deficiency. *Arch Intern Med*. 1992;152:40–45.

32. Fisher RS. Gastroduodenal motility disturbances in man. *Scand J Gastroenterol*. 1985;109(suppl):59.

33. Meyer JH. Motility of the stomach and gastroduodenal junction. In: Johnson LR, ed. *Physiology of the Gastrointestinal Tract*. 2nd ed. New York, NY: Raven Press; 1987:613–629.

34. Moore JG, Christian PE, Coleman RE. Gastric emptying of varying meal weights and composition in man—evaluation by dual liquid and solid phase isotopic method. *Dig Dis Sci*. 1981;83:1306.

35. Becker EJ, Jeukendrup AE, Brouns F, Wagenmakers AJM, Saris WHM. Gastric emptying of carbohydrate—medium chain triglyceride suspensions at rest. *Int J Sports Med*. 1992;13 (8):581–584.

36. Hunt JN, Stubbs DF. The volume and energy content of meals as determinants of gastric emptying. *J Physiol (Lond).* 1975;245:209–225.

37. Bury KD, Jambunathan G. Effects of elemental diets on gastric emptying and gastric secretion in man. *Am J Surg.* 1974;127:59.

38. Nompleggi D, Bell SJ, Blackburn GL, Bistrain BR. Overview of gastrointestinal disorders due to diabetes mellitus: emphasis on nutrition support. *JPEN.* 1989;13 (1):84.

39. Salena BJ, Hunt RH. Bezoars. In: Sleisenger MH, Fordtran JS, eds. *Gastrointestinal Disease—Pathophysiology, Diagnosis, Management.* 5th Ed. Philadelphia, Pa: WB Saunders; 1993:758–763.

40. Ahn YH, Maturu P, Steinheber FU, Goldman JM. Association of diabetes mellitus with gastric bezoar formation. *Arch Intern Med.* 1987;147:527–528.

41. Algozzine GJ, Hill G, Scoggins WG, Marr MA. Sucralfate bezoar (letter). *N Engl J Med.* 1983;309:1387.

42. Anderson W, Weatherstone G, Veal C. Esophageal medication bezoar in a patient receiving enteral feedings and sucralfate. *Am J Gastroenterol.* 1989;84(2):205–206.

43. Goldstein S, Lewis JH, Rothstein R. Intestinal obstruction due to bezoars. 1984;79(4):313–318.

44. Rider JA, Foresti-Lorente RF, Garrido J, et al. Gastric bezoars: treatment and prevention. *Am J Gastroenterol.* 1984;79:357–359.

45. Emerson AP. Foods high in fiber and phytobezoar formation. *J Am Diet Assoc.* 1987;87(12):1675–1677.

46. Schiller LR. Gastrointestinal problems in diabetes. *Clin Diabetes.* 1987;5:128.

47. Jacober SJ, Narayan A, Strodel WE, Vinik AI. Jejunostomy feeding in the management of gastroparesis diabeticorum. *Diabetes Care.* 1986;9(2):217–219.

48. Parrish C, Sanfilippo N, Krenitsky J, McCallum R. Nutritional and global assessment of long-term jejunostomy feeding. In: *ASPEN 18th Clinical Congress Manual.* San Antonio, Tex: American Society for Parenteral and Enteral Nutrition; 1994:589. Abstract.

49. Lin HC, Meyer JH. Disorders of gastric emptying. In: Yamada T, ed. *Textbook of Gastroenterology.* Philadelphia, Pa: JB Lippincott; 1991:1213–1240.

50. McCallum RW. Review of the current status of prokinetic agents in gastroenterology. *Am J Gastroenterol.* 1985;80(12):1008–1016.

51. Chang EB. Diabetes and the small intestine. In: *American Gastroenterological Association Postgraduate Course.* Boston, Mass: American Gastroenterological Association; 1993:211–219

52. Ogbonnaya KI, Arem R. Diabetic diarrhea: pathophysiology, diagnosis, and management. *Arch Intern Med.* 1990;150:262.

53. Valdovinos MA, Camilleri M, Zimmerman BR. Chronic diarrhea in diabetes mellitus: mechanisms and an approach to diagnosis and treatment. *Mayo Clin Proc.* 1993;68:691–702.

54. Benya R, Layden TJ, Mobarhan S. Diarrhea associated with tube feeding: the importance of using objective criteria. *J Clin Gastroenterol.* 1991;13(2):167–172.

55. Romano TJ, Dobbins JW. Evaluation of the patient with suspected malabsorption. *Gastroenterol Clin North Am.* 1989;18(3):467–483.

56. Newihi HE, Dooley CP, Saad CS, Staples JS, Zeidler A, Valenzuela JE. Impaired exocrine pancreatic function in diabetics with diarrhea and peripheral neuropathy. *Dig Dis Sci.* 1988;33(6):705–710.

57. Freston JW, Moore JR. Approach to gastrointestinal problems associated with common clinical conditions. In: Yamada T, ed. *Textbook of Gastroenterology.* Philadelphia, Pa: JB Lippincott; 1991:928–931.

58. Silk DB, Grimble GK. Relevance of physiology of nutrient absorption to formulation of enteral diets. *Nutrition.* 1992;8:1–12.

59. Steinhardt HJ, Wolf A, Jakober B, et al. Nitrogen absorption in pancreatectomized patients; protein vs. protein hydrolysate as substrate. *J Lab Clin Med.* 1989;113: 162–167.

60. DiMagno EP, Go VLW, Summerskill WHJ. Relations between pancreatic enzyme outputs and malabsorption in severe pancreatic insufficiency. *N Engl J Med.* 1973;288(16):813–815.

61. McLaughlin S. Pancreatic cancer and diabetes. *Diabetes Educ.* 1994;20(1):20.

62. Bjorneklett A, Hoverstad T, Hoviq T. Bacterial overgrowth. *Scand J Gastroenterol.* 1985;20(suppl 109): 123–132.

63. Colemont LJ, Camilleri M. Chronic intestinal pseudo-obstruction: diagnosis and treatment. *Mayo Clin Proc.* 1989;64:60–70.

64. Hartsook E. Celiac sprue and insulin dependent diabetes mellitus. *Gluten Intolerance Group Newslett.* 1987;13 (2):2–8.

65. Barera G, Bianchi C, Calisti L, et al. Screening of diabetic children for coeliac disease with antigliadin antibodies and HLA typing. *Arch Dis Child.* 1991; 66(4):491–494.

66. Collin P, Salmi J, Hällström O, et al. High frequency of coeliac disease in adult patients with type I diabetes. *Scand J Gastroenterol.* 1989;24:81–84.

67. Fedorak RN, Field M, Chang EB. Treatment of diabetic diarrhea with clonidine. *Ann Intern Med.* 1985;102:197.

68. Kim CH. Managing GI complications of diabetes. *Cont Int Med.* 1992:77–86.

Chapter 33

Dental Care and Persons with Diabetes

Riva Touger-Decker
David A. Sirois

Ongoing and planned reform in health care systems will continue to result in significant changes in practice settings and in the spectrum of services provided by primary and specialty care providers. Most notably, primary care providers must expand their recognition of disease in multiple organ systems and play a central role in the multidisciplinary management of their patient. The dietetic and dental professions have already begun this transdisciplinary practice by recognizing the essential link between diet, nutrition, and oral health. This chapter describes specific diet, nutritional, and oral health factors related to diabetes and the manner in which these factors influence one another and the patient's overall well-being. The final section describes guidelines for prevention and treatment of dental diseases.

Systemic disease influences oral health, and conversely, oral health can influence the natural history of systemic disease. Simply stated, the oral cavity is an organ system that influences, and is influenced by, other organ systems. Specifically in diabetes, in which meal timing and composition is critical, both the dental and dietetic professional must be aware of the oral complications of diabetes and the relationship between these complications, nutritional health, and diabetes control. Improved interdisciplinary communication and comprehensive patient care will be achieved through (1) greater recognition of diabetes- and nutrition-related oral disease; (2) identification of nutrition and diet risk factors that contribute to oral disease; (3) profes-

sional and patient education; and (4) appropriate counseling and treatment of patients with diabetes, often requiring consultation between dietetic and dental professionals.

EFFECTS OF DIABETES ON THE ORAL CAVITY

Diabetes can lead to a variety of oral complaints or abnormalities, mostly as a direct result of hyperglycemia (Exhibit 33-1). Alterations in oral cellular metabolism, immune surveillance, and vascular integrity as well as altered salivary chemistry all may occur in patients with diabetes.[1]

Periodontitis and gingivitis are well-recognized oral complications of diabetes mellitus[2-4] (Exhibit 33-1). *Periodontitis* refers to inflammation and destruction of the attachment apparatus of the teeth, including the ligamentous attachment of the tooth to the surrounding alveolar bone (Figure 33-1). The gingiva represents the soft tissue component of the periodontium, comprised of the oral mucosa that covers a small portion of the tooth root and crown. Inflammation of only the soft tissue component of the periodontium is termed *gingivitis*. Both forms of periodontal disease (gingivitis and periodontitis) result from infection by pathologic oral bacterial flora, which are present in dental plaque. The progression of periodontitis is influenced significantly by local and systemic health, particularly conditions that impair or alter the local or systemic immune response. Periodontitis can lead to extensive local bone loss, resulting in tooth loss and, in severely immunocompromised individuals, to serious bacteremia.

It is well established that diabetes, particularly when poorly controlled, is associated with a higher prevalence of gingivitis and destructive periodontitis.[2–4] The susceptibility to periodontal disease in diabetes, although primarily related to the presence of common dental bacterial plaque, is likely directly related to several diabetes-related pathologic events. Impaired neutrophil chemotaxis and macrophage function are well-known events in diabetes.[5,6] These immune defects diminish the host's capacity to identify and destroy periodontal bacterial pathogens. Pathologic tissue destruction due to diabetes-related altered collagenase and ß-glucuronidase activity, as well as a host of cellular immune mediators, contribute to the periodontal tissue destruction.[7–9]

One recent study demonstrated that ß-glucuronidase, an enzyme associated with connective tissue destruction, levels were significantly higher in poorly controlled diabetics and good metabolic control was the only predicting variable for enzyme levels when considered with

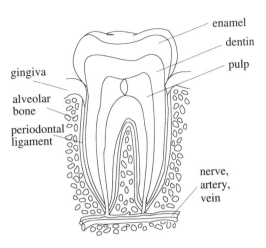

Figure 33-1 Normal Tooth Anatomy

microbes, plaque, age, duration, and type of diabetes.[10] Increased salivary glucose results in additional bacterial substrate and plaque formation.[11–13] Increased salivary calcium contributes to plaque calcification (calculus formation), which results in local periodontal irritation and inflammation. Finally, diabetes-related microangiopathies and vascular permeability abnormalities can lead to altered tissue metabolism and immune surveillance, which favor periodontal disease progression.[5,14–16]

Preventive periodontal therapy must be included in the comprehensive care of the diabetic patient, particularly poorly controlled diabetes (see Exhibit 33-2). Therapy includes explicit hygiene instruction for the patient and frequent periodic examinations and prophylactic dental

Exhibit 33-1 Common Oral Complications of Diabetes

Symptom	Contributing Factor(s)
Periodontal disease	Impaired immune surveillance Salivary hypercalcemia and hyperglycemia Microangiopathy Altered cellular metabolism and enzyme activity
Xerostomia	Hyperglycemia
Candidiasis	Hyperglycemia Impaired immune surveillance
Altered taste	Altered salivary chemistry Microangiopathy
Burning mouth or tongue	Microangiopathy and neuropathy

Exhibit 33-2 Periodontal Preventive Maintenance Program

1. Dental checkup and periodontal prophylaxis (cleaning) every 3–6 months.
2. Explicit oral hygiene instructions:
   - brush at least twice daily (preferably after meals)
   - instruction in proper tooth brushing technique
   - rinse after meals when brushing is not possible
   - floss daily or at least twice weekly
   - comply with regular checkups

Exhibit 33-3 Xerostomia

Contributing Factors:

Medications:
anticonvulsants
antidepressants
antihistamines
narcotics
diuretics
hypotensive agents
muscle relaxants
minor tranquilizers

Illnesses:
diabetes
AIDS
Sjogren's syndrome
rheumatoid arthritis

Complications:
oral candidiasis
rampant dental caries
burning mouth
dysphagia
altered taste

Management:
1. prescription topical fluoride in custom mouthpiece
2. limit fermentable carbohydrates
3. artificial saliva
4. salivary stimulation (pilocarpine, bethanechol)
5. dental recall visits, cleaning, hygiene instruction

cleaning. Many diabetic patients will benefit from the use of topical or systemic antimicrobial medications during the treatment of active periodontal disease or as part of a preventive maintenance program. When periodontal surgery is planned, additional perioperative considerations become critical, such as adjustments in diet and medication usage.

Xerostomia, or dryness of the mouth, is a side effect of many medications and a common complication of diabetes mellitus[17–22] (see Exhibit 33-3). Decreased salivary flow contributes to a variety of oral infections and sensory disorders, including oral candidiasis, rampant dental caries, periodontal disease, altered taste, and burning mouth. Subjective complaints of oral dryness should always be verified by evaluation of

salivary flow, volume, and consistency because there is often poor correlation between the perception of dryness and actual decreased salivary flow. Interestingly, although complaints of oral dryness are common among patients with diabetes, the evidence for decreased flow is controversial, and there are conflicting reports of salivary flow rates among patients with diabetes.[13,23]

Oral candidiasis is an opportunistic fungal infection commonly associated with hyperglycemia and is a frequent complication of diabetes. *Candida albicans* is a constituent of the normal oral microflora but rarely colonizes and infects the oral mucosa. Common predisposing factors for oral candidiasis include immunosuppression, individuals who wear dentures and practice poor oral prosthesis hygiene, and chronic use of broad-spectrum antibiotics.[24] The combination of xerostomia, compromised immune function, and increased salivary glucose as a substrate for fungal growth are the major contributing factors to candidiasis in diabetes.[25–28] Although typically appearing as superficial white patches that are easily removed to reveal the underlying red mucosa, candidiasis may also appear as a purely erythematous area and may be overlooked or misdiagnosed. Although often asymptomatic, candidiasis can cause painful oral burning and, particularly when the oropharynx or esophagus is involved, limit eating and drinking. Initial treatment may require systemic antifungal medications followed by daily maintenance therapy using topical antifungal rinses. Management of oral candidiasis is summarized in Exhibit 33-4.

Altered taste in patients with diabetes is often due to altered salivary chemistry, xerostomia, and/or candidiasis. The person with diabetes who complains of altered or bad taste should be evaluated for each of these likely causes. Salivary flow rates and a cytology smear for *Candida* are simple, inexpensive tests whereas sialochemistry requires more sophisticated and costly analyses. Diabetic microangiopathy and autoimmune neuropathy have also been suggested as a cause for altered sensations as well as *burning mouth or tongue*.[15,29] Less commonly,

Exhibit 33-4 Oral Candidiasis

Presentation:
white or red patches on buccal mucosa or tongue that can be rubbed off, leaving a red or bleeding surface

Complications:
dysphagia
burning mouth or tongue
altered or bad taste
secondary infection

Management:
1. gentle debridement
2. topical oral antifungal*
3. systemic antifungal followed by topical maintenance therapy

* Avoid topical antifungal medications with sweeteners, which can contribute to rampant dental caries when xerostomia is present.

nutritional deficiencies of iron and several B vitamins including folate can lead to burning mouth.[30] Hematologic and nutritional evaluation can identify these deficiencies that respond to diet therapy. When there is no associated, treatable physical or biochemical abnormality, burning mouth can be improved using a variety of tricyclic antidepressant medications. Unfortunately, a nearly universal side effect of the tricyclic antidepressants is xerostomia, which may compound candidiasis and dental caries.

DENTAL DIET/NUTRITION ASSESSMENT

The close relationship between the sequelae of diabetes and oral manifestations that have an effect on diet detailed in the previous section support the need for nutrition risk evaluation in the dental office. It is incumbent on the dentist to inquire as to the patient's problems with chewing or swallowing or other changes in the oral cavity that affect the ability to eat as well as questions about oral hygiene techniques. The dentist's role is to provide diet counseling as it relates to oral health (ie, oral conditions wherein

the ability to eat a regular diet is altered or when diet may play a role in oral diseases such as tooth decay). Before counseling, dentists must first evaluate nutrition risk as well as diet in their patients.

A nutrition risk evaluation can be quickly obtained by the dentist during initial and periodic examinations using a simple evaluation form shown in Exhibit 33-5. The risk factors listed in Exhibit 33-6 include data already collected by the dentist but, when examined from a different perspective, that of nutrition risk. This form may be completed by the dentist or dental auxiliary personnel during initial and periodic patient visits. Elements of the medical/dental history of particular concern in patients with diabetes are listed in Exhibit 33-7.[31] These questions can be addressed by the dentist on initial and periodic patient visits as a component of comprehensive patient care. The number and type of risk factors present in conjunction with oral examination findings and dental treatment plans provide the dentist with a determination of patient needs for nutrition education or diet intervention.

Significant weight gain or loss as a risk factor provides clues as to the impact of changes in masticatory function on eating ability. Medication and health histories provide clues to possible risk factors in the patient's dental picture. For example, xerostomia may be related to medications independent of the diabetes[22] (see Exhibit 33-3).

Biting and chewing are difficult when occlusion, the pattern in which opposing teeth come together, is altered. When teeth are missing or severely decayed, occlusion of the anterior (front) or posterior (back) teeth may be altered, causing difficulty biting and chewing, respectively. Ill-fitting dentures can also limit variety in food selection, reducing intake of fresh fruits and vegetables and whole grains due to altered mastication.[32,33] Treatment focuses on dental restoration and modification in diet consistency to maximize eating ability.

Preoperative diet evaluation is imperative for oral surgery patients to ensure appropriate postoperative diet composition and medication tim-

Exhibit 33-5 Nutrition Risk Evaluation of the Individual with Diabetes

Note: This screening form is completed on all patients by the dentist during the initial visit and then at periodic checkups.

MEDICAL HISTORY:

Ht: ___ft ___inches   **Wt:** ____lbs
 Wt 6 months ago: ____lbs
 (>10% wt change in <6 months indicates
  nutrition risk)

No	Yes	
____	____	Medications with drug-nutrient reactions
____	____	Hypertension
____	____	Immunosuppressive disorder(s)
____	____	Risk factors relative to diabetes:_____
____	____	Physical disability having an effect on ability to eat
____	____	Substance abuse
____	____	Eating disorder (anorexia/bulimia)
____	____	Pregnancy/nursing (circle one)
____	____	Age >65 years old
____	____	Diabetic sequelae: _____
____	____	Diabetic management plan: _____

DENTAL EXAM:

No	Yes	
____	____	Pocket depths _____
____	____	Gingival index _____
____	____	Extensive caries
____	____	Lack of occlusion: anterior posterior (circle which apply)
____	____	Edentulism
____	____	Full/partial dentures
____	____	Soft tissue lesions suggestive of nutrition risk
____	____	Planned dental procedures requiring diet modification

PERSONAL HISTORY: (These risk factors combined with one or more of the above indicates the need for further diet evaluation.)

No	Yes	
____	____	Smoker
____	____	Receiving public assistance for food
____	____	Runs out of money during the month for food
____	____	Special diet modifications:_____ _____
		Vitamin/mineral/nutrition supplements:_____
____	____	Recent (<6 months) loss of significant other

Exhibit 33-6 Dental Nutrition Risk Factors Indicating Need for Diet Intervention

Dentures (new or replacement)

Edentulism (partial or complete tooth loss)

Oral surgery planned

Extensive caries

Extensive dental restorative work affecting occlusion

Periodontal disease

Xerostomia

Altered taste

Burning tongue/mouth

Eating disorder

Exhibit 33-7 Elements of the Medical/Dental History for Individuals with Diabetes

- Symptoms and laboratory test results (glycated hemoglobin, blood glucose) related to diabetes

- Current diabetes management program, including medications, diet, and glucose monitoring

- Frequency, severity, and cause of acute complications such as hypoglycemia and ketoacidosis

- Symptoms and extent of chronic complications associated with diabetes: micro/macroangiopathies, peripheral neuropathy

- Psychosocial and economic factors that may influence diabetes and dental care management

- Prior or current infections

- Weight, weight change (comparison with growth charts in children), % desirable weight, % usual weight

- Blood pressure

- Other medications; vitamin/mineral/nutrition supplements

- Problems chewing, biting, or swallowing foods, xerostomia, mouth pain

Source: Wray D, Dagg JH. Diseases of the blood and blood-forming organs. In: Jones JH, Mason DK, eds. *Oral Manifestations of Systemic Disease.* 2nd ed. London: Bailliere Tindall; 1990:660–713.

ing and dose (ie, oral hypoglycemic agents and insulin). Individuals with periodontal disease, xerostomia, candidiasis, or burning mouth can benefit from diet evaluation to determine presence of risk factors such as frequency of consumption of fermentable carbohydrates, frequency and types of liquids consumed, and diet adequacy.

The three possible outcomes of dental nutrition risk evaluation the dentist may reach are (1) reinforcement of the current diet along with oral hygiene techniques to minimize tooth decay and plaque buildup; (2) completion of a diet recall or food diary and dental-nutrition counseling in the dental office; or (3) referral to a registered dietitian (RD) for comprehensive nutrition therapy. All individuals should receive diet education on prevention of caries, periodontal disease, and candidiasis.

DIET EVALUATION

Diet evaluation and counseling should be considered for individuals with any of the risk factors listed in Exhibit 33-6. Diet data collected includes a typical day's recall or multiday (three-day) food diary to get a "snapshot" of the individual's eating pattern, showing sequence, frequency, and types of foods selected daily. Also, a food frequency questionnaire evaluating meal and snack foods, as well as daily and weekly consumption, helps the health provider to evaluate the overall adequacy of the diet and provides information on types of foods consumed at meals and snacks. Diet evaluation includes diet adequacy based on the food guide pyramid, individual eating plan for diabetes, and decay-promoting potential.

Diet risk factors associated with dental disease go beyond intake of sugar and other fermentable carbohydrates. The primary factors are

- food form: liquid, solid and sticky, long-lasting
- frequency of consumption of fermentable carbohydrates
- nutrient composition

- sequence of food intake
- combinations of foods

These factors determine the decay-promoting potential of the diet. Figure 33-2 lists common sources of fermentable carbohydrates on the food guide pyramid. A scoring system for determining the level of decay-promoting risk is noted in Exhibit 33-8.

The counseling plan focuses on individual diet quality based on the food guide pyramid, diabetic meal plan, and counseling needs along with presence of any additional risk factors such as weight loss or psychosocial problems. Examples include modification of consistency of decay-promoting foods and/or frequency of eating/drinking or guidelines for xerostomia or postoperative diet. Monitoring and follow-up should include periodic diet recalls to evaluate counseling outcome.

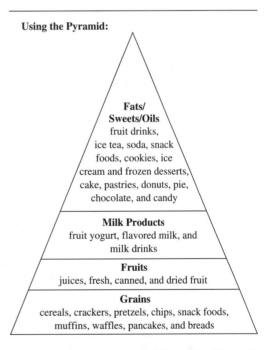

Using the Pyramid:

Fats/ Sweets/Oils
fruit drinks, ice tea, soda, snack foods, cookies, ice cream and frozen desserts, cake, pastries, donuts, pie, chocolate, and candy

Milk Products
fruit yogurt, flavored milk, and milk drinks

Fruits
juices, fresh, canned, and dried fruit

Grains
cereals, crackers, pretzels, chips, snack foods, muffins, waffles, pancakes, and breads

Note: "Diet" or sugar-free cakes, cookies, and muffins are also sources of fermentable carbohydrate.

Figure 33-2 Fermentable Carbohydrate Sources

Exhibit 33-8 Decay-Promoting Potential

Scoring the Sweets	Decay-Promoting Potential		

Scoring the Sweets

Using the dietary recall of an ordinary weekday...
- Classify each sweet as liquid, solid and sticky, or slowly dissolving.
- For each time a sweet was eaten, either at the end of a meal or between meals (at least 20 minutes apart), place a check in the frequency column.
- In each group, add up the number of sweets eaten and multiply by the number provided. Write down the number of points.
- Add up all the points for the total score.

Example:
10:00 A.M. 1 jelly donut
12:00 NOON ham and cheese sandwich
    1 c milk
    1 cupcake
3:00 P.M. 1 coke
5:00 P.M. 1 cough drop

Form	Frequency	Points
Liquid	✓ x 5 =	5
Solid and Sticky	✓ ✓ x 10 =	20
Slowly dissolving	✓ x 15 =	15

TOTAL SCORE = <u>35</u>

Sweet Score:
5 or less	Excellent
10	Good
15 or more	"Watch Out" Zone

Decay-Promoting Potential

Form	Frequency	Points
Liquid soft drinks, fruit drinks, cocoa, sugar and honey in beverages, nondairy creamers, ice cream, sherbet, gelatin dessert, flavored yogurt, pudding, custard, popsicles	____ x 5 =	
Solid and Sticky cake, cupcakes, donuts, sweet rolls, pastry, canned fruit in syrup, bananas, cookies, chocolate candy, caramel, toffee, jelly beans, other chewy candy, chewing gum, dried fruit, marshmallows, jelly, jam	____ x 10 =	
Slowly Dissolving hard candies, breath mints, antacid tablets, cough drops	____ x 15 =	

TOTAL SCORE = _____

Note: If your score is in the watch out zone, nutrition counseling is warranted.

Source: Reprinted from Nizel A and Papas A. *Nutrition in Clinical Dentistry* (p283) with permission of WB Saunders, Copyright © 1989.

DIET AND DENTAL HEALTH EDUCATION

The previous sections of this chapter detail several oral manifestations of diabetes in the teeth and oral mucosa, which are affected by diet. The purpose of this section is to highlight counseling strategies for dental and dietetic professionals to use when treating individuals with diabetes.

Prevention of Decay and Periodontal Disease

Diet and oral hygiene are the cornerstones of prevention of tooth decay and plaque buildup, which can lead to periodontal disease. Exhibit 33-8 lists only simple sugar examples of liquid, solid and sticky, and slowly dissolving foods. However, all fermentable carbohydrates including those listed in Exhibit 33-8 can be reclassified into these three categories. Fermentable car-

Exhibit 33-9 Dental Health Guidelines

- Eat cariostatic foods for snacks: nuts, cheese, popcorn, vegetables
- Limit between-meal eating and drinking of fermentable carbohydrates
- Brush, rinse, or chew sugarless gum after eating sticky foods (crackers, chips, pretzels, dry cereal, fruit, bananas)
- Pair cariogenic foods with cariostatic foods based on nutrient composition
- Avoid regular (sugared) hard candies, lozenges, gum, and other sweets
- Choose sugar-free alternatives, if desired

bohydrate foods (Figure 33-2) are considered "cariogenic" or decay-promoting. The presence of any of these six carbon sugars in the mouth provides substrate for cariogenic bacteria, such as *Streptococcus mutans* to flourish. The *form* of the food is indicative of the length of exposure of the oral cavity to the sugar. Liquids are rapidly cleared by the mouth and have low adherence potential to teeth. Solid foods such as pretzels, crackers, and dry cereals take longer to leave the mouth and tend to adhere to teeth or in the interproximal spaces between teeth. Slowly dissolving foods, such as regular hard candy or gum, take the longest to clear the mouth, therefore result in a prolonged exposure time of the sugar in the oral cavity. *Frequency* is an important variable because each consumption of a fermentable carbohydrate results in a 20- to 30-minute exposure time for bacteria and bacterial acid production.[33] *Nutrient composition* also influences cariogenic risk.[34] Nuts and peanut butter, which are primarily fat, are cariostatic (they do not promote decay). They "coat" tooth enamel, producing a protective coating.[35-37] Cheese is also a cariostatic food, stimulating an alkaline saliva (or buffer), reducing plaque-forming bacteria, and increasing the clearance rate of fermentable carbohydrates.[38,39] Casein and whey proteins found in milk, yogurt, and cheese help reduce enamel demineralization by increasing calcium and phosphate in plaque.

Although many individuals with diabetes avoid concentrated sweets and many simple sugars, fermentable carbohydrate foods[34] are still common in the diabetic diet.[35] Important variables to consider are the frequency of consumption of such foods and oral hygiene practices used after meals and snacks. Food *sequence and combination* can also influence cariogenic risk. Crackers alone are cariogenic; however, combining them with cheese, a cariostatic food, lowers the cariogenic potential. Adding milk to dry cereal reduces its adherence capabilities, thus lowering the associated cariogenic risk.[40]

Exhibit 33-9 provides guidelines on prevention of dental diseases for individuals with diabetes. Coordination of diet guidelines with proper oral hygiene is critical.

Modification for Dental Procedures

Individuals with diabetes scheduled for surgery should consult with their physician regarding possible adjustment of insulin or oral hypoglycemic agent doses, particularly when the diabetes is poorly controlled. Dentists need to inform patients of the anticipated length of

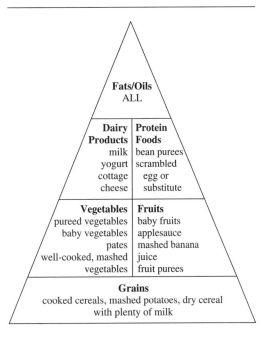

Figure 33-3 Dental Semisolid Diabetes Diet Guidelines

treatment time and remind them to eat their normal meal before the appointment. Compliance with these preoperative recommendations should be confirmed before the surgical procedure begins.

Postoperative diet counseling should include a soft or liquid diet consistent with the composition and timing of the patient's normal diabetic diet. Guidelines on modified foods to select in each food group of the food guide pyramid should be provided. An example of a semisolid diet is shown in Figure 33-3. RDs are encouraged to consult with dentists in the design of a series of modified diabetes diet guidelines for such situations.

RESTORATIVE DENTAL WORK

Restorative dental work refers to dentures (removable prostheses), bridgework (fixed prostheses), and simple tooth fillings. Studies have documented that chewing and biting difficulties pre- and postdenture placement can reduce intake of fresh fruits and vegetables and whole grains.[32] Counseling strategies focus on consistency modification to ensure intake of a nutritionally adequate diet. A soft diet that minimizes the need for biting into or chewing foods and avoids nuts and seeds that can get caught in the dentures is needed initially. Patients should be encouraged to reintroduce other foods on an as-tolerated basis.

XEROSTOMIA, BURNING TONGUE, AND CANDIDIASIS

Diet management focuses on (1) reducing pain before meals to stimulate appetite, (2) providing very moist, temperate, mildly seasoned foods, and (3) proper oral hygiene after all meals and snacks to reduce risk of tooth decay. The dentist may also prescribe artificial saliva or medication that increases saliva secretion. Extremes in temperature should be avoided. Simi-

---

Exhibit 33-10 Dental Questions for the RD To Use in Patient Care

1. Do you have any tooth or mouth problems that make it difficult for you to eat?   _____Yes _____No

2. Do you wear dentures?   _____Yes _____No
   If yes, do you use them for eating?   _____Yes _____No
   If you DO NOT use your dentures for eating, why? _____

3. Do you ever experience any of the following:
   dry mouth   _____Yes _____No
   burning tongue   _____Yes _____No
   bleeding gums   _____Yes _____No
   infections in your mouth   _____Yes _____No

4. Do you have periodontal disease?   _____Yes _____No

5. Do you have trouble biting any foods?   _____Yes _____No
   If yes, please indicate what foods: _____

6. Do you have trouble chewing any foods?   _____Yes _____No
   If yes, please indicate what foods: _____

7. How many times a day do you:
   brush your teeth   _____
   floss your teeth   _____
   rinse your mouth after meals or snacks   _____

larly, strong seasonings, citrus fruits/juices, and foods with nuts or seeds should be avoided to minimize discomfort and maximize intake. All foods should be moistened with gravies, broth, or other suitable liquids. Individuals on fat- or sodium-restricted diets should be cautioned to read labels and select products consistent with their diet prescription. Sugar-free gum and mints may increase salivary flow, thereby adding to the patient's comfort level. Patients should be cautioned to avoid sugared (regular) hard candies, throat lozenges, and gum because in the presence of reduced saliva they increase the risk for tooth decay. Likewise, most oral topical antifungal medications used to treat oral candidiasis contain carbohydrate sweeteners, which promote dental caries. An alternative to cariogenic topical preparations is systemic antifungal therapy or the use of a vaginal troche (clotrimazole) that contains no sweetener.

CONCLUSION

Overall health management of the individual with diabetes requires a multidisciplinary effort. We have long recognized the impact of diet on cardiovascular health, serum glucose, and renal function and readily collaborate with specialists in cardiology, endocrinology, and nephrology. Dentists are specialists in the oral cavity, where diet can have a significant impact on oral health.

Dentists are responsible for counseling patients on diet as it relates to oral health. The RD is responsible for reinforcing that counseling and incorporating oral health guidelines into diet counseling sessions as well as incorporating questions about oral health problems into nutrition assessment protocols. The materials provided in this chapter can be individualized and provided to patients by an RD or dentist. Incorporation of this material into a diabetes management program ensures comprehensive management of individuals with diabetes by a multidisciplinary team of health experts.

The role of the RD is constantly expanding. In regards to the oral health of individuals with diabetes, the RD is responsible for

- asking questions about known dental sequelae of diabetes such as periodontal disease, xerostomia, and oral infections
- incorporating guidelines to promote optimal oral health and prevent disease into counseling plans
- referring patients to dentists when they present with untreated dental problems that interfere with their ability to consume an adequate diet

Dental health questions (Exhibit 33-10) can be incorporated into routine nutrition screening and assessment forms that already include the health questions covered in Exhibit 33-7. The RD and dentist can collaborate in patient management to maximize patient well-being, health, and comfort. Diet health is critical for oral health in individuals with diabetes. Dentists and RDs together must reinforce the importance of balanced diet and proper oral hygiene practices to promote optimal health and prevent disease complications.

REFERENCES

1. Lamey PJ, Darwazeh AM, Frier BM. Oral disorders associated with diabetes mellitus. *Diabetes Med.* 1992;9:410–416.

2. Emrich LJ, Shlossman M, Genco RJ. Periodontal disease in non-insulin diabetes mellitus. *J Periodontol.* 1991;62:123–131.

3. Tervonent T, Oliver RC. Long-term control of diabetes mellitus and periodontitis. *J Clin Periodontol.* 1993;20:431–435.

4. Glavind L, Lund B, Loe H. The relationship between periodontal status and diabetes duration, insulin dosage, and retinal changes. *J Periodontol.* 1968;39:341–347.

5. Genco R, VanDyke TE, Levine MJ, Nelson RD, Wilson ME. Molecular factors influencing neutrophil defects in periodontal disease. *J Dent Res.* 1986;65:1379–1391.

6. Drell DW, Notkins AL. Multiple immunological abnormalities in patients with type-I (insulin-dependent) diabetes mellitus. *Diabetologica.* 1987;30:132–143.

7. Rifkin BR, Vernillo AT, Golub LM. Blocking periodontal disease progression by inhibiting tissue-destructive enzymes: a potential therapeutic role for tetracyclines and their chemically-modified analogues. *J Periodontol.* 1993;64:819–827.

8. Johnson RB. Morphological characteristics of depository surface of alveolar bone of diabetic mice. *J Periodont Res.* 1992;27:40–47.

9. Ramamurphy NS, Golub LM. Diabetes increases collagenase activity in extracts of rat gingiva and skin. *J Periodont Res.* 1983;18:23–30.

10. Oliver RE, Tervonent T, Flynn DG, Keenen KM. Enzyme activity in cervicular fluid in relation to metabolic control of diabetes and other periodontal risk factors. *J Periodontol.* 1993;64:358–362.

11. Ferguson MM, Silverman S. Endocrine disorders. In: Jones JH, Mason DK, eds. *Oral Manifestations of Systemic Disease.* 2nd ed. London: Bailliere Tindall; 1990:593–615.

12. Feller RP, Shannon IL. The secretion of glucose by the parotid gland. *J Am Assoc Dent Res.* 1975;54:570(abstract).

13. Marder MZ, Mandel ID. Salivary changes in juvenile diabetics. *J Am Assoc Dent Res.* 1976;55:679(abstract).

14. Joseph CE, Farnousch A. Current concepts of periodontitis. *J Calif Dent Assoc.* 1984;12:43–53.

15. Dreizen S, Levy BM, Stern MH, Bernick S. Human lingual atherosclerosis. *J Am Assoc Dent Res.* 1974;53:420(abstract).

16. Russel BG. Gingival changes in diabetes mellitus. *J Am Assoc Dent Res.* 1977;56:411(abstract).

17. Ben-Aryen H, Serouya R, Kanter Y, Szargel R, Laufer D. Oral health and salivary composition in diabetic patients. *J Diabetic Complications.* 1993;7:57–62.

18. Screenby LM, Yu A, Green A, Valdini A. Xerostomia in diabetes mellitus. *Diabetes Care.* 1992;15:900–904.

19. Chinn H, Brody H, Silverman S, DiRaimando V. Glucose tolerance in patients with oral symptoms. *J Oral Therapeutics.* 1966;2:261–269.

20. Brightman VJ, Silvert M, Blasberg B, Peterson D, McWilliams R. Blood sugar, blood lipids and oral sensory disorders. *J Am Assoc Dent Res.* 1976;55:929(abstract).

21. Conner S, Iranpour B, Mills J. Alterations in parotid salivary flow in diabetes mellitus. *Oral Surg.* 1970;30:55–59.

22. Navazesh M, Ship I. Xerostomia: diagnosis and treatment. *Am J Otolaryngol.* 1983;4(4):283–292.

23. Marder MZ, Abelson DC, Mandel ID. Salivary alterations in diabetes mellitus. *J Am Assoc Dent Res.* 1975;54:391(abstract).

24. Mooney M, Thomas I, Sirois D. Oral candidiasis. *Int J Dermatol.* In press (1995).

25. Aly FZ, Blackwell CC, Mackenzie DA, Weir DM, Clarke BF. Factors influencing oral carriage of yeasts among individuals with diabetes mellitus. *Epidemiol Infect.* 1992;109:507–518.

26. Ueta E, Osaki T, Yoneda K, Yamamato T. Prevalence of diabetes mellitus in odontogenic infections and oral candidiasis: an analysis of neutrophil suppression. *J Oral Pathol Med.* 1993;22:168–174.

27. Mosci P, Vecchiarelli A, Cenci E, Puliti M, Bistoni F. Low-dose streptozotocin-induced diabetes mellitus in mice. I: Course of *Candida albicans* infection. *Cell Immunol.* 1993;150:27–35.

28. Mencacci A, Romani L, Mosci P, Cenci E. Low-dose streptozotocin-induced diabetes mellitus in mice. II: Susceptibility to *Candida albicans* infection correlates with the induction of a biased Th2-like antifungal response. *Cell Immunol.* 1993;150:36–44.

29. Keene JJ. Arteriosclerotic changes within the diabetic oral vasculature. *J Dent Res.* 1075;54:77-82.

30. Wray D, Dagg JH. Diseases of the blood and blood-forming organs. In: Jones JH, Mason DK, eds. *Oral Manifestations of Systemic Disease.* 2nd ed. London: Bailliere Tindall; 1990:660–713.

31. American Diabetes Association. Standards of medical care for patients with diabetes mellitus. *Diabetes Care.* 1991;14(suppl 2):10–13.

32. Meehan K, Touger-Decker R, Vogel R. The relationship between oral health and nutrition status in denture patients. *J Dent Res.* 1995;74(SI):79.

33. Hollister MK, Weintraub JA. The association of oral status with systemic health, quality of life and economic productivity. *J Dent Educ.* 1993;57(12):901–912.

34. Krasse B. The cariogenic potential of foods—a critical review of current methods. *Int Dent J.* 1985;35:36–42.

35. American Diabetes Association. Nutrition recommendations and principles for people with diabetes mellitus. *J Am Diet Assoc.* 1994;94(5):504–511.

36. Anderson M, Bales D, Karl-Ake O. Modern management of dental caries: the cutting edge is not the dental bur. *J Am Dent Assoc.* 1993;124:37–44.

37. Nizel A, Papas A. Dietary counseling for the prevention and control of dental caries. In: Nizel A, Papas A, eds. *Nutrition in Clinical Dentistry.* Philadelphia, Pa: WB Saunders; 1989:277–308.

38. Nizel A, Papas A. The role of nutrition in prevention and management of periodontal disease. In: Nizel A, Papas A, eds. *Nutrition in Clinical Dentistry.* Philadelphia, Pa: WB Saunders; 1989:309–338.

39. Krobicka A, Bowen WH, Pearson S, et al. The effects of cheese snacks on caries in desalivated rats. *J Dent Res.* 1987;66(6):1116–1119.

40. Bowen WH, Pearson SK. Effect of milk on cariogenesis. *Caries Res.* 1993;27:461–465.

Chapter 34

Persons with Diabetes and HIV/AIDS

Cade Fields-Gardner

Infection with the human immunodeficiency virus (HIV) and the condition of acquired immunodeficiency syndrome (AIDS) has historically been treated as a terminal disease. Today, much like diabetes, HIV and AIDS is evolving into a chronic manageable disease. Therefore, with optimal management we will expect patients to realize a normal life expectancy. This change in philosophy has challenged clinicians and researchers to develop and implement new strategies to preserve nutritional status and quality of life. Optimal management will depend on the ability of the clinician and patient to address successfully the multitude of factors that characterize the complications, including diabetes, of HIV disease.

Currently, more than 500,000 cases of AIDS have been reported to the Centers for Disease Control (CDC). These numbers do not include all the estimated 1 million or more persons who may be infected with HIV. CDC forecasts growing numbers of HIV-infected women, children, homeless, and injection drug users (IDU). HIV is transmitted from person to person through infected bodily fluids. Because the virus is so fragile and easily destroyed by exposure to air or common household bleach, high-risk exposures are primarily through injection of contaminated blood (eg, shared needles of IDU), sexual transmission through vaginal or anal intercourse, and perinatal transmission. Universal precautions (Exhibit 34-1), recommended regardless of a person's HIV status, is appropriate in all patient care and can protect against transmission of HIV as well as transmission of other infections to the immunocompromised person. Documentation on this and more detailed information on transmission, incidence by geographic location and risk group, infection control, forecasts, and other HIV-related issues are available through CDC Information Services.[1]

The CDC defines HIV disease progression to a diagnosis of AIDS according to symptoms, infections and neoplasms, and decreasing clinical markers of immune function (CD4 count). Up to 20% of reported AIDS cases qualify for the diagnosis with "wasting syndrome," defined by the CDC as an unintentional loss of body weight and presence of diarrhea that is not explained by other AIDS-related diagnoses. It has been estimated that 80 to 90% or more of patients with HIV disease will experience the consequences of malnutrition. It has also been suggested that malnutrition may be preventable and treatable in HIV disease.

The time from exposure to the virus, enough to convert to a positive test for its presence, to a diagnosis of AIDS may range from months to years. A patient is considered a long-term survivor when surviving more than 18 to 24 months beyond their first AIDS-defining diagnosis (ie, *Pneumocystis carinii* pneumonia, Kaposi's sarcoma). Many AIDS patients have survived with their CDC case-defining diagnosis for more than a decade. Prognosis for survival is best determined by body cell mass (protein stores) and other markers of nutritional well-being. Longer-term survival means that patients live to experience many of the complications of chronic disease and drug therapies.

Exhibit 34-1 Infection Control

Item	Comments
Handwashing	Hands should be washed with soap and water before and after each procedure
Gloves	Gloves should be worn when caring for open lesions or wounds, handling secretions or excretions (emesis, urine, stool, blood, wound secretions), handling body-fluid soiled linens or other items, providing oral care if contact with oral lesions or blood is likely, or other situations in which contact with bodily fluids is likely
Lab coats or smocks	Lab coats or protective smocks should be worn when soiling of caregiver or clothing is likely
"Sharps" and needles	Needles should not be recapped but disposed of in puncture-resistant container
Disposable supplies	Nonsharp soiled disposable items should be packaged in heavy plastic bags or double bags for disposal according to community solid waste disposal regulations
Environmental safety	Counter or other surfaces and nondisposable supplies soiled by secretions or excretions should be disinfected with a 10% bleach solution or a mycobacteriocidal disinfectant; regular dishwashing and laundry cleaning with soap and water should be sufficient for dishes and laundry; routine household cleansing agents can be used for appliance and other household cleaning; special care should be taken with pet care—it is recommended to have someone other than the HIV/AIDS patient clean cages and litter boxes; durable medical equipment (eg, glucose monitoring machines) are carefully cleaned with a 10% bleach solution before returning to general circulation

Source: Courtesy of the Visiting Nurses Association of San Francisco (*AIDS Home Care and Hospice Manual,* 1987).

DIABETES IN HIV DISEASE

Diabetes has been recognized as a complication of HIV infection and AIDS since the mid-1980s.[2] Diabetes in HIV patients may be temporary (a few weeks to 2 years) or permanent according to the underlying pathophysiology. Some HIV patients may have a personal or family medical history of diabetes. Glucose intolerance and hyperglycemia may also be present during infections, many of which are "opportunistic," occurring in immune-compromised states such as advanced HIV disease. Other mechanisms include pancreatic islet cell destruction and various hormonal imbalances seen in HIV-related complications and associated treatments.

Researchers and clinicians have recorded acute or chronic pancreatitis in conjunction with some of the medications or viral infections commonly seen in HIV/AIDS (Exhibit 34-2). Although the clinical features are similar to those seen in non–HIV-related pancreatitis, effects range from transient to long term. The primary intervention for medication or viral-induced pancreatitis will be the discontinuation of the medication or offending viral treatment. Symptomatic treatment will include blood glucose control through insulin administration and meal timing. In cases of transient pancreatitis, close monitoring will help to determine when it is appropriate to discontinue dietary restrictions and/or insulin administration. In addition to treatment for temporary or permanent diabetes, other medical needs, such as the prevention of malnutrition and wasting, should be addressed concurrently.

Nutrition therapy is of primary importance in the maintenance and restoration of lean body mass, tolerance to therapy, improved quality of life, and the ability to conduct activities of daily

Exhibit 34-2 Examples of Infection- or Medication-Induced Diabetes Mellitus in HIV Patients

Factor	*Mechanism*
Cryptosporidiosis (*Cryptosporidium* sp.)[1]	Opportunistic infection presence associated with incidence of pancreatitis
CMV (cytomegalovirus)[2,3]	Systemic opportunistic infection; suggestions have been made that CMV should be suspected with idiopathic pancreatitis in HIV disease
zalcitabine (ddC, HIVID)[4]	Used in treatment of HIV (antiretroviral); associated with pancreatitis
didanosine (ddI, Videx)[5,6]	Used for treatment of HIV infection (antiretroviral); reports of diabetes-like glucose tolerance curves to frank pancreatitis; estimations of incidence are as high as 70%
Histoplasmosis (*Histoplasma capsulatum*)[7]	Opportunistic infection that may affect the gastrointestinal tract and many organ systems (including lungs)
KS (Kaposi's sarcoma)[7]	Identified as possible cause; may be direct effect of pancreatic KS on pancreas function
Octreotide (Sandostatin)[8]	Used for management of chronic diarrhea in HIV disease; suggested mechanism is the prevention of pancreatic exocrine secretion acting as a "physiologic gallstone" leading to acute pancreatitis
Pentamidine (Pentam 300)[9]	Used for treatment of *Pneumocystis carinii* pneumonia; hypoglycemia during IV treatment is associated with pancreatitis and temporary or long-term insulin-dependent diabetes; possible mechanism is ß-cell dysfunction
TB (*Mycobacterium tuberculosis*)[10]	May affect several organ systems; prophylaxis for previous exposure is recommended

REFERENCES

1. Dowell S, Holt E, Murphy FK. Pancreatitis associated with HIV infection. Paper presented at the V International Conference on AIDS, Montreal, Canada, 1989:250. Abstract MBP233.
2. Joe L, Ansher AF, Gordin FM. Severe pancreatitis in an AIDS patient in association with cytomegalovirus infection. *South Med J.* 1989;82(11):1444–1445.
3. Wilcox CM, Forsmark CE, Grendell JH, Darragh TM, Cello JP. Cytomegalovirus-associated acute pancreatic disease in patients with acquired immunodeficiency syndrome. Report of two patients. *Gastroenterology.* 1990;99(1):263–267.
4. Remick S, Follansbee S, Olson R, Pollard R, Reiter W, Salgo M. Safety and tolerance of zalcitabine (ddC, HIVID) in a double-blind comparative trial (ACTG114;N3300). Paper presented at IX International Conference on AIDS, Berlin, Germany, 1993:488. Abstract POB26-2115.
5. Maxson CJ, Greenfield SM, Turner JL. Acute pancreatitis as a common complication of 2',3'-dideoxyinisine therapy in the acquired immunodeficiency syndrome. *Am J Gastroenterol.* 1992;87(6):708–713.
6. Seidlin M, Lambert JS, Dolin R, Valentine FT. Pancreatitis and pancreatic dysfunction in patients taking dideoxyinosine. *AIDS.* 1992;6(8):831–835.
7. Brandao-Mello CE, Basilio CA, Correa-Lima MB, Valle HA, Silva MA. Pancreatitis and AIDS—a clinicopathological review of 142 cases. Paper presented at 8th International Conference on AIDS, Amsterdam, Netherlands, 1992:B111. Abstract POB-3147.
8. Gradon JD, Schulman RH, Chapnick EK, Sepkowitz DV. Octreotide-induced acute pancreatitis in a patient with acquired immunodeficiency syndrome. *South Med J.* 1991;84(11):1410–1411.
9. Kallas EG, Galvao LL, Rolad RK, Medeiros EA, Levi GC, Mendonca JS. Pentamidine induced ketoacidosis in acquired immunodeficiency syndrome patients. Paper presented at IX International Conference on AIDS, Berlin, Germany, 1993:474. Abstract POB26-2031.
10. Desmond N, Kingdom E, Tanner A, Coker R, Harris JR. Pancreatic tuberculosis: an unusual manifestation of HIV infection. Paper presented at IX International Conference on AIDS, Berlin, Germany, 1993:341. Abstract POB07-1232.

living. Clinical treatment of insulin-dependent diabetes mellitus or non–insulin-dependent diabetes mellitus in HIV/AIDS may be similar to treatment of these conditions found in noninfected individuals. Yet some of the characteristics of the nutritional care plan may be affected by processes unique to HIV/AIDS patients. Both diabetes and HIV disease can predispose a person to increased rates of infection and a delayed healing process. These, combined with the complications of inadequate intake, malabsorption, and altered metabolism of nutrients, can make working with diet and blood glucose control particularly complex. To maximize therapeutic success, nutritional care plans should prioritize and address each of the complications and diagnoses that may affect nutritional status.

GOALS

In addition to, or as a result of, diabetic complications of HIV disease, patients may experience complications of malnutrition and/or wasting of lean tissue that are vital for well-being and survival.[3] Micronutrient deficiencies and alterations continue to confound clinical interventions and have been documented in as much as 60 to 70% of asymptomatic and 80 to 90% of symptomatic HIV patients.[4,5] Because survival is more closely related to nutritional markers (eg, albumin, transferrin, body cell mass) than to immune function,[3] preservation of nutritional stores becomes a clinical priority. Therefore, clinical goals for the diabetic HIV patient include an emphasis on maintaining fluid status, lean body mass, and clinical markers of protein stores along with control of hyperglycemia and related complications.

Patient-clinician partnerships in developing realistic goals and objectives with specific plans and, as much as possible, measurable results will help to ensure optimal medical management. Medical management of the HIV/AIDS patient with diabetes will include the integration of nutritional strategies to match the overall health care plan for patient-generated priorities of care

and medical prognosis. Nonjudgmental evaluation and recommendations are crucial to the development of clinician-patient rapport. As with other patients, sensitivity to sex, age, and cultural factors will be important considerations. Additionally, with HIV/AIDS patients, confidentiality issues are a high priority.

Patients and their health care team should consider feasibility, priority, and benefit versus burden in setting nutritional objectives. Specifically, each proposed intervention discussion should include the purpose, feasibility in accomplishing stated objectives, and the cost in terms of burden to the patient for the type or amount of expected benefit. If the feasibility of achieving the clinical or psychosocial objective is negligible, a time-limited trial of intervention may be instituted. During the course of the intervention, markers of successfully achieving objectives should be weighed against burden in making the decision to continue or discontinue therapy. In cases of life-sustaining support, legal and ethical issues that are generally state-specific (ie, California's laws may differ from those in Illinois) for the withholding or withdrawal of specific therapies may require team discussion, as well.

NUTRITION EVALUATION

General nutrition evaluation criteria apply to the diabetic HIV patient. Common nutritional problems seen in the HIV/AIDS patient are shown in Exhibit 34-3. Although some patients may have a diagnosis of diabetes that is independent of their HIV status, diabetes can also be a "side effect" of infection and many of the HIV/AIDS-associated therapies.[6] Nutritional evaluation of HIV/AIDS patients should include factors that may anticipate the development of pancreatic dysfunction. Family histories of diabetes, medication profiles, and closely monitored laboratory values can help to identify patients at highest risk for developing pancreatitis and diabetes.

Unfortunately, in cases of viral or medication-induced pancreatitis, rising serum levels of li-

Exhibit 34-3 Examples of Nutritional Problems Seen in People with HIV/AIDS

Problem	Etiology	Strategies
Decreased nutrient intake	Anorexia	• Appetite stimulation • Evaluation of offending medications, depression, symptoms • Food-based strategies to improve intake
	Dysphagia/odynophagia	• Treatment of cause: protein-calorie malnutrition, medications (eg, ddC), infections (eg, cytomegalovirus [CMV], *Herpesvirus* sp., *Candida* sp., Kaposi's sarcoma), others • Food-based strategies to increase intake • Nonvolitional feeding (tube or parenteral feeding)
	Alterations in gastrointestinal motility	• Treatment of cause: medications, infections • Food-based strategies to increase intake, reduce symptoms
Decreased absorption	Lactose/gluten intolerance	• Food-based strategies (ie, lactose-reduced products, gluten-free diet)
	Opportunistic infection or neoplasm	• Treatment for cause of malabsorption • Food and supplement strategies for easier absorption (eg, elemental medical nutritional supplements) • Nonvolitional feeding (tube or parenteral feeding)
	Altered gastric pH	• Food-based strategies to improve nutrient digestion/absorption • Supplements (eg, intramuscular injection of vitamin B_{12})
	Severe diarrhea[a]	• Treatment of causes (ie, opportunistic infection, medications) • Treatment of symptoms with medications and food-based strategies
Altered metabolism	Hypermetabolism	• Treatment of offending infection, neoplasm • Metabolic nutrition support to normalize nutrient levels • Medications to reduce presence of hypermetabolic factors (ie, inflammation)
	Endocrine or other organ system alterations	• Treatment of infection or neoplasm affecting organ systems • Treatment of symptoms by medications • Food-based strategies for stabilization and maintenance (eg, diabetic diet in CMV pancreatitis)

[a] Malabsorption does not always accompany diarrhea; conversely diarrhea does not always indicate malabsorption.

pase and amylase (typical markers of pancreatic dysfunction) are not always seen in HIV/AIDS patients.[7-9] Therefore, it will be important to identify multiple risk factors for diabetes and monitor more common signs of pancreatic dysfunction, such as complaints of sustained abdominal pain and hyperglycemia. Higher than normal levels of blood glucose accompanied by increased triglyceride levels may also be indicative of infection. Sustained or very high levels of blood glucose should be monitored for the potential development of diabetes. Special attention should be paid to patients with suspected or diagnosed cytomegalovirus, cryptosporidiosis, histoplasmosis, Kaposi's sarcoma, and their associated medication therapies (Exhibit 34-3).

In addition to hyperglycemia and pancreatic dysfunction, pinpointing other organ dysfunction and risk factors for nutritional compromise will be key in determining appropriate therapies. Like diabetes, HIV disease and its related complications can place a patient at higher risk for vision impairment and renal, hepatic, and/or gastrointestinal dysfunction. Opportunistic infections can compromise lung function, the nervous system, and the circulatory system. Many of the medications prescribed for HIV patients are toxic to the pancreas, liver, kidney, and other systems. These threaten nutritional status maintenance and restoration, which, in turn, compromise overall well-being.

DIABETES EDUCATION

Of primary concern in HIV care is the battle against wasting and its associated detrimental effects. Providing diabetic education for diabetic HIV patients will be crucial to preventing further health problems and decline. Clinicians should address how to best accomplish nutritional goals with individualized recommendations for calorie level, macronutrient distribution, food-based strategies, and oral supplementation. Resources are listed in Exhibit 34-4. Though studies have suggested an increased need for calories and protein, the initial goal of nutritional intervention in HIV disease is to nutritionally and metabolically stabilize the patient. Estimations of calorie requirements will depend on the patient's clinical profile of infection and fevers, weight history, medication therapies, activity level, presence of malabsorption, and health care plan rehabilitation goals. Priorities should be established for both short- and long-term goals for acute and chronic problems. Overall, it will be important to maintain adequate intake, absorption, and normalization of metabolism as much as possible.

The basic educational needs for HIV/AIDS patients who are diabetic are similar to non-HIV diabetic patients. As with many non-HIV diabetic patients, there may be several specific complications to be aware of when planning a counseling session. The cause of diabetes may also influence the need for detailed counseling. In anticipation of eventual resolution of transient diabetes, it may be more appropriate to provide general dietary guidelines that can be easily followed along with a specific insulin administration schedule. In either case, it is particularly important to spell out nutritional priorities. These include, in order of importance, adequate fluids, calories, protein, and micronutrients. Meal guides stress a rounded diet or administration of nutrients to achieve goals of optimal nutritional status. Emphasis is placed on high-calorie, high-protein foods. However, an increased number of fruit and vegetable servings, although not offering as much in the way of calories, does offer some very important micronutrients, nonnutrient antioxidants, and other food substances that promise to play an important role in long-term HIV management.[10]

Blood glucose monitoring is an important factor in therapy adjustment for diabetic HIV patients. There has been some discussion about the safety of blood glucose testing. Concern lies with the risk for additional infection in the HIV patient and the spread of HIV infection itself, emphasizing the need for standardized utilization of universal precautions (Exhibit 34-1) by both the care provider and the client. In an institutional or home setting, recommendations include carefully disposing of lancets and other

Exhibit 34-4 Resources for HIV-Related Nutrition
Information

The American Dietetic Association

1-800-366-1655

Ask for listing of local dietetic associations or
dietitians who specialize in HIV/AIDS-related care.

The Cutting Edge

P.O. Box 922
Cary, IL 60013
1-708-516-2455

Resource for specific questions on nutritional
management in HIV/AIDS.

National AIDS Clearinghouse

1-800-458-5231

Ask for "database search" of professional and
patient information on nutrition and HIV/AIDS.

Ask for information in conference listing service on
HIV/AIDS educational meetings.

National HIV Nutrition Team

Central Office
P.O. Box 922
Cary, IL 60013
1-708-516-1380

West Coast Office
P.O. Box 5874
Berkeley, CA 94705
1-510-655-3702

Nonprofit multidisciplinary resource for nutrition-
related guidelines and information.

Roxane Laboratories

P.O. Box 16532
Columbus, OH 43216

Write for pamphlet from The American Dietetic
Association, "Living Well with HIV and AIDS: A
Guide to Healthy Eating."

Write for "Living Well with HIV and AIDS" video
tape.

Write for "The Golden Apple Recipe Booklet"
(apple-based recipes for HIV/AIDS patients).

Stadtlander's Pharmacy

1-800-238-7828

Ask for HIV Disease Nutrition Guidelines booklets
in English and Spanish.

Ask for reprints of "Wasting Syndrome" foldout
from Lifetimes II publication.

Ask for reprints of "Nutrition Basics" foldout from
Lifetimes II publication.

---

disposable devices that may come into contact
with blood. If possible, patients should be asked
to throw out their own testing materials with
care and to place lancets or other sharp objects
into a puncture-proof container. Mycobacterial
germicides are preferable for cleaning blood-
contaminated areas. Outside the institutional setting, educators are charged with advising patients against sharing glucose monitoring
machines and other safety precautions. Surfaces
may be cleaned with a 1:10 solution of bleach
and water. In general, the same precautions
should be taught to all patients, regardless of
their HIV status.

Polypharmacy is an additional risk factor in
the control of blood glucose as well as the potential for exacerbation of health risks already faced
by the diabetic HIV patient. Individualized
monitoring guidelines for drug–nutrient interactions should be established. These will include
having the patient self-monitor symptoms and
glucose control as well as other parameters that
may be specific to their drug or other related
therapies (Exhibit 34-5).

Metabolic disturbances in lipid metabolism
have been suggested to play a role in an HIV
patient's ability to appropriately rehabilitate nutritional stores. To counter this problem, current
research in nutrition and HIV disease is concen-
trating on the use of medications (anabolics and
growth hormone) that may help restore lean
body mass in preference to fat stores. It has been
suggested that exercise regimens, emphasized in
many diabetic care plans, may also play an important role in nutritional therapy response for
HIV patients.

When indications or strong risk for malnutrition based on inadequate intake have been identified, such as anorexia or other barriers, several
therapeutic avenues may be explored. Appetite-
stimulating medications have been used to support volitional feeding with a variety of results
and side effects. If appetite stimulation is not appropriate, as in patients with severe odyno-
phagia, nonvolitional feeding becomes an appropriate option. Such options for care may be
best discussed before developing a need for en-

Exhibit 34-5 Additional Potential Side Effects of Medications Associated with Pancreatitis

Medication	Purpose	Additional Potential Side Effects
Acyclovir	Prophylaxis/treatment for *Herpesvirus* sp.	Hepatotoxic, increased serum creatinine, liver function tests, nephrotoxic (esp. in IV infusion)
Amphotericin B	Broad-spectrum antibiotic	Decreased serum calcium, sodium, magnesium; nephrotoxic
Didanosine	Antiretroviral; treatment for HIV	Hepatotoxic, abdominal pain, neurotoxic
Fluconozole	Prophylaxis/treatment for candidiasis, cryptococcus	Gastric/duodenal ulcer or inflammation
Foscarnet	Prophylaxis/treatment for cytomegalovirus	Hepatotoxic, abdominal pain, nausea, renal impairment, nephrotoxic, nephrogenic diabetes insipidus, increased serum creatinine, increased urinary protein, decreased serum potassium, calcium, magnesium
Ganciclovir	Prophylaxis/treatment for cytomegalovirus	Hepatotoxic, granulocytopenia
Ketoconazole	Prophylaxis/treatment for candidiasis, coccidioidomycosis	Impaired steroid synthesis, decreased testosterone levels, gastric/duodenal ulcer or inflammation, increased serum potassium, liver function tests, follicle-stimulating hormone; decreased serum calcium; requires gastric acid for absorption
IV pentamidine	Treatment of *P. carinii* pneumonia	Nephrotoxic, hepatitis, granulocytopenia, hypoglycemia (in short term; with hyperglycemia in long term), decreased serum calcium, sodium
Rifampin	Treatment/maintenance for *M. tuberculosis*	Hepatotoxic
Trimethoprim-sulfamethoxazole	Broad-spectrum antibiotic, prophylaxis/treatment for pneumonia	Hepatotoxic, gastric/duodenal ulcer or inflammation, granulocytopenia (esp. in folate deficiency), neurotoxic, nephrotoxic (B_6 supplementation may reduce toxicity but may also reduce drug efficacy), high serum potassium

Sources: Sanford JP, Sande MA, Gilbert DN, Gerberding JL. *The Sanford Guide to HIV/AIDS Therapy.* Dallas, Tex: Antimicrobial Therapy; 1994. Bartlett J. *Medical Management of HIV Infection.* Glenview, Ill: Physicians & Scientists Publishing Co., Inc.; 1994.

teral or parenteral nutrition to allow the patient to make their most rational decision in choosing such a therapy.

ENTERAL NUTRITION SUPPORT IN DIABETIC HIV/AIDS PATIENTS

Although typical standards of care suggest implementation of nonvolitional feeding when anticipating inadequate intake of more than 7 to 10 days, the HIV patient has a much shorter window of time in which to prevent significant decline.[11] It has been suggested that early identification of risk for poor intake of more than 2 days should be a red flag for nutritional compromise. Rather than try to reverse nutritional decline, a difficult task in HIV patients, it may be more appropriate to institute short- or long-term nonvolitional feedings.

Enteral nutrition, as with most other medical conditions, is the preferred route of nonvolitional feeding. Preservation of the gut as a physical barrier to infection and its continued function as an actively defensive (immune functioning) organ are high priorities. Also, absorptive capacity should be preserved to better ensure both nutrient and medication therapy success. In the diabetic HIV patient, similar considerations exist for feeding with special attention to blood glucose control. Although this particular aspect of HIV care has not been well explored, one may be able to borrow from research on enteral feeding in diabetes.

Glycemic control while providing adequate amounts of fluids, calories, protein, and micronutrients will be important to support immune function and reduce the risk of infection. Protocols that apply to diabetic patients for providing sliding scale insulin administration or oral hypoglycemic agents also apply to diabetic HIV patients. Also, isotonic feedings are suggested to help maintain glycemic control and prevent exacerbation of diarrhea. Because the HIV patient may already be immunocompromised, special care to prevent aspiration pneumonia and other sources of infection should be taken. Closed enteral feeding systems have been suggested to reduce the potential contamination and gastrointestinal infection.

PARENTERAL NUTRITION IN DIABETIC HIV/AIDS PATIENTS

Most standard indications for parenteral nutrition and monitoring guidelines apply to the diabetic HIV patient. As in oral and enteral feeding, care should be taken to identify appropriate candidates as early as possible. Calorie and protein needs may be slightly higher in some HIV patients, depending on their clinical status. Because the gut is an important immune-functioning organ and barrier to infection, it will be important to maintain some form of enteral nutrient intake for patients on total parenteral nutri-

tion (TPN) therapy. Special attention for increased risk of infection in diabetic HIV patients should be balanced with the goals for metabolic maintenance and nutritional repletion.

During acute phases of pancreatitis in HIV/AIDS, parenteral nutrition may be recommended as a temporary support. Care should be exercised, as this can place the patient at an even greater risk for catheter sepsis. Glucose control will be an important part of reducing this risk. Dextrose load guidelines and sliding scale insulin protocols for diabetic patients may be followed. For the diabetic HIV patient, insulin administration in the TPN bag may be preferable to long-term use of subcutaneous injections. Catheter draws are preferable to fingersticks in HIV patients to reduce risk of infection. It will be especially important to have clear protocols on catheter draws to prevent glucose-contaminated specimens.

CONCLUSION

In addition to medication and nutrition therapy for diabetes, the nutritional care plan should address needs for fluid, calorie, and protein intake that may be higher than for many other diabetic patients. Although the indications for oral, enteral, and parenteral interventions are similar to those in other nondiabetic or non-HIV/AIDS patients, additional considerations apply. Because the HIV-infected patient may be less able to recover from nutritional compromise, earlier intervention and closer monitoring for complications related to food safety, aspiration, and catheter sepsis will play important roles in balancing the burden of intervention with its benefit.

Malnutrition in HIV disease is multifactoral. Understanding the causes and roles of decreased intake, malabsorption, and metabolic dysfunction should be addressed as much as possible. In this way, the health care plan goals to stabilize metabolically and/or replete nutritional stores can be realized. Physicians, dietitians, nurses, social workers, physical therapists, pharmacists, and other clinicians can expedite the integration of appropriate nutritional care into the health care plan. Contributions from the entire health care team, including the patient, clinicians, and other care providers, will be essential to the successful nutritional management of the diabetic HIV patient.

REFERENCES

1. Centers for Disease Control Voice/Fax Information Services. *Disease Directory.* Document #000004. Call: 1-404-332-4565.

2. Stahl-Bayliss CM, Kalman C, Laskin OL. Pentamidine-induced hypoglycemia in patients with the acquired immunodeficiency syndrome. *Clin Pharmacol Ther.* 1986;39:271–275.

3. Hellerstein MK. HIV-associated metabolic disturbances and body composition abnormalities: therapeutic implications. *AIDSFILE.* 1994;8(1):1–4.

4. Beach RS, Mantero-Atienza E, Shor-Posner G, et al. Specific nutrient abnormalities in asymptomatic HIV-1 infection. *AIDS.* 1992;6:701–708.

5. Bogden JD, Baker H, Frank O, et al. Micronutrient status and human immunodeficiency virus (HIV) infection. *Ann NY Acad Sci.* 1990;587:189–195.

6. Podolsky S, Zimelman A. Diabetes and AIDS. *Clin Diabetes.* 1993;2:29–35.

7. Olson P, Kennedy C, Miller L. Lack of utility of serial amylase determinations in HIV-infected patients receiving didanosine (ddI). Paper presented at IX International Conference on AIDS, Berlin, Germany, 1993:484. Abstract POB26-2095.

8. Silva MA, Silva MC, Lima TS, Lemos O, Correa-Lima MB, Mello CE. Pancreatitis in AIDS patients. Paper presented at VI International Conference on AIDS, San Francisco, Calif., 1990:359. Abstract 2021.

9. Ruhnke M, Kirsch A, Geiseler B. Pancreatitis in patients with HIV infection. Paper presented at IX International Conference on AIDS, Berlin, Germany, 1993:442. Abstract POB19-1842.

10. Fields-Gardner C. Food-based nutrients as therapeutic options in HIV care. *Bulletin for Experimental Treatment in AIDS.* San Francisco, Calif: AIDS Foundation; September 1994. (Contact Ron Baker, Ph.D., at 415-864-5855, ext. 2041.)

11. Macallan DC, Noble C, Baldwin C, Foskett M, McManus T, Griffin GE. Prospective analysis of patterns of weight change in stage IV human immunodeficiency virus infection. *Am J Clin Nutr.* 1993;58:417–424.

Part VIII

Making It All Work

Chapter 35

Reimbursement for Medical Nutrition Therapy of Diabetes

Sandy Gillespie

As nutrition science and its application in health care made tremendous advances in the past decade, the role of the dietitian emerged as one of essential player on the health care team. Likewise, technology has advanced in diabetes management with improved blood glucose monitoring equipment and supplies, oral hypoglycemic agents, insulin, and insulin delivery systems. As demonstrated by the Diabetes Control and Complications Trial (DCCT), these state-of-the-art therapeutic tools make it possible for the diabetes management team to work with patients to achieve levels of self-management resulting in vastly improved health outcomes and optimal quality of life.[1] The DCCT provided an expanded role for the dietitian on the diabetes management team as medical nutrition therapy was recognized as a key element in achieving glycemic control.[2-6] The American Diabetes Association (ADA) standards of care recognize the critical role of nutrition in diabetes management and recommend individualized nutrition therapy and diabetes self-management training as essential elements of the management plan.[7]

COVERAGE AND REIMBURSEMENT PRACTICES HAVE NOT KEPT PACE WITH ADVANCES

Unfortunately, our health care system and coverage and reimbursement practices have not kept pace with the advances in diabetes and nutrition therapy and the established standards of care. Health care financing decision makers—legislators, regulators, insurance companies, employers, and benefits managers—do not fully recognize the value and cost savings of these services. Persons who have health insurance may be told that the medical services covered by their plans do not include medical nutrition therapy and diabetes self-management training. Nonexistent or inadequate coverage and reimbursement of essential services become barriers to quality care.[8] Because of inability to pay, patients may be denied access to the therapies that, if reimbursed today, will prevent costly complications tomorrow.

RISING HEALTH CARE COSTS AND RESEARCH-BASED RECOMMENDATIONS PROMPT ADVOCACY EFFORTS

An increased awareness of the magnitude of the financial, physical, and emotional costs of diabetes and its complications has prompted advocacy groups, health care providers, patients, and their families to become involved in the national debate on health care reform. In 1992, an estimated 13 million people in the United States have diabetes at an annual cost of $92 billion.[9] There was $37 billion spent on inpatient care, with 27% of that amount ($10 billion) spent for hospitalizations related to the chronic complication of diabetes.[9] We know from the DCCT that tight control of blood glucose levels can result in approximately a 60% reduction of risk for costly complications in insulin-dependent diabetes mellitus (IDDM).[1]

Exhibit 35-1 Third-Party Payment Terms Used

A three-party payor arrangement:

First Party—The client/patient (often provides payment)

Second Party—The provider (physician, health care professional, hospital, clinic)

Third Party—The payor (determines services or supplies covered and renders payment to provider or reimbursement to the client/patient)

- Blue Cross Blue Shield Association
- Commercial insurance company
- Health maintenance organization (HMO)
- Preferred provider organization (PPO)
- Self-funded employer plan
- Medicare, Medicaid (public plans)

Coverage—A third-party payor's acknowledgment that it will contribute to payment of a procedure, service, or supplies

Reimbursement—Level of payment allowed for a covered procedure, service, or supplies

The National Institute of Diabetes, Digestive and Kidney Diseases (NIDDK) has translated the DCCT results into recommendations for all persons with diabetes.[10] The NIDDK has advised that health care reform plans include financing for care and education for persons with diabetes and that managed care programs provide access to comprehensive diabetes care and education to prevent diabetic complications. The expanded role of the dietitian and nutrition management emerging from the DCCT[2-6] highlights the need for registered dietitians (RDs) and certified diabetes educators (CDEs) to become advocates for increased recognition and reimbursement of medical nutrition therapy in diabetes management. Although patients must assume responsibility and accountability for diabetes self-management, including nutrition management, they need the assistance of RD/CDEs to develop these skills. This knowledge is influencing diabetes health care professionals to advocate for coverage and reimbursement of the self-care skills training, equipment, supplies, and medications that are necessary for achieving optimal control.[11]

This chapter will guide the diabetes educator to a greater understanding of reimbursement mechanisms and terminology, how the current system operates, and how to maximize reimbursement potential in private and public plans (see Exhibit 35-1 for terms used).

CURRENT STATUS ON REIMBURSEMENT

Coverage and reimbursement for medical nutrition therapy and diabetes self-management training are inconsistent among third-party payers, both public and private. Payment varies among third-party payers and even within individual companies providing a variety of policies or administering policies for self-insured businesses. In federally funded programs, Medicare and Medicaid, interpretation of regulations varies from state to state. (Table 35-1 provides a summary of overall coverage for diabetes care.)

Reimbursement for Outpatient Services

Surveys

Published survey results vary depending on methods used. The various methods include:

- actual tracking of patient claims and explanation of benefits from third-party payers[12,13]
- insurance companies' responses to a written questionnaire or a telephone interview[14]
- payment experience of individual or program providers of diabetes self-management training.[15,16]

Reimbursement for outpatient medical nutrition therapy is estimated at 17 to 71%,[12-14] whereas reimbursement for diabetes self-management training ranges from 28 to 72%.[15,16]

A 1990 survey of the Consulting Nutritionists (Nutrition Entrepreneurs) Dietetic Practice Group of the American Dietetic Association tracked 438 insurance claims in 16 states for nutrition services provided by dietitians in private practice.[12] Licensed dietitians (RD/LD) in private practice received 68.8% reimbursement versus 43.5% for nonlicensed dietitians (RD only).[12] A 1990 American Association of Diabetes Educators (AADE) survey of 120 programs recognized by the ADA from 40 states indicated 19 to 30% received reimbursement only after attaining program recognition.[16] These survey results suggest that third-party payers equate licensure with assurance of provider qualifications and ADA recognition with quality programs.

*The American Dietetic Association
Reimbursement Database*

The American Dietetic Association established a computerized reimbursement data base in 1993 with the following goals[17]:

- provide computer access to the names of third-party payers reimbursing for medical nutrition therapy and the conditions for reimbursement
- establish a member network from every practice setting and geographic area, which includes individuals who are willing to act as resource persons
- provide reimbursement data needed to support the American Dietetic Association health care reform efforts.

The data base provides accurate, reliable information based on tracking actual claims submitted to insurance companies by dietitians all over the United States. The data base provides an opportunity for dietitians in all practice settings and specialty areas to contribute to a valuable project. As the volume of data increases to at least 1,500 records for an individual state, state-specific details can be tracked. For example, the question, "What commercial insurance companies reimburse, at what rate, for medical nutrition therapy for gestational diabetes in hospital outpatient departments in my state?" will be answered when that state provides 1,500 records into the data base.

Table 35-1 Coverage of Services, Equipment, and Supplies for Diabetes Care

Covered	Medicare	Medicaid Programs	Blue Cross Blue Shield	Commercial Insurers
Outpatient visits to physician	Yes	Yes	Most	Most
Annual eye examination	Yes	Yes	Most	Some
Treatment of retinopathy	Yes	Yes	Yes	Most
Routine foot care	Yes	A few	Most	Some
Outpatient education	Yes	A few	A few	Some
Blood glucose meters/strips	Yes	A few	Most	Most
Insulin and supplies	No	Most	A few	Yes
Prescription drugs	No	Yes	A few	Yes
Continuous subcutaneous insulin infusion	No	A few	A few	Most
Therapeutic shoes	Some	A few	A few	A few

Source: Data from *Diabetes: 1993 Vital Statistics* (p 44) by the American Diabetes Association, 1993.

Medicaid

Medicaid is administered by each state under federal guidelines. The program is the primary source of health care coverage for the poor. It is jointly funded by the federal government and the states, with the states defining eligibility, benefits, and payment. According to information obtained by the American Dietetic Association, 36 state Medicaid programs expressly cover nutrition services.[18] A 1990 survey of 114 diabetes education programs recognized by the American Diabetes Association showed that 28% of respondents received Medicaid reimbursement.[16] Some state Medicaid programs are using health maintenance organizations (HMOs) to provide care to Medicaid recipients.[19] As more state departments of medical assistance negotiate contracts with managed care organizations, diabetes advocates must be actively involved in ensuring that established standards of care guide coverage decisions on services, supplies, equipment, and medications for diabetes care. State affiliates of the American Diabetes Association, local chapters of the Juvenile Diabetes Foundation, and the American Association of Diabetes Educators individual members, and their grassroots advocacy networks can influence policy makers. Providing documentation of the necessity, effectiveness, and cost savings of quality diabetes care is the most convincing way to influence health care policy.

Medicare

Coverage and Reimbursement. Medicare, with more than 34 million beneficiaries, is the largest health insurer in the United States. Ninety-six percent of people aged 65 and older who have diabetes are covered by Medicare.[9] The Medicare program is based on legislation (Title XVIII of the Social Security Act of 1965) and regulations at the federal level and is administered by the Health Care Financing Administration (HCFA).[20] Medicare part A covers inpatient care in hospitals, skilled nursing facilities, home care, and hospice care. Medicare part B covers outpatient hospital services, physician services, durable medical equipment, and other

medical services and supplies. Medical nutrition therapy is not specifically included on the statutory list of medical and other health services but is covered in some states as "incident to a physician's professional services." Insurance companies and Blue Cross Blue Shield Associations, acting as *fiscal intermediaries* (part A) or *carriers* (part B), process Medicare claims and make coverage and reimbursement decisions at the state and local levels. Because interpretation of the regulations by the insurance carriers at the state level varies widely, coverage and reimbursement decisions are inconsistent among carriers, diagnoses, and practice settings. The following excerpt from AEtna's Medicare Newsletter for Georgia illustrates how difficult it can be to obtain reimbursement for outpatient services in a physician office practice setting.

From *AEtna Medicare October, 1992 Special Newsletter:*

Issue 2: Counseling/Education Provided by the Physician's Staff

Counseling or education, i.e., diabetic education, by the physician's staff is not considered to be part of the "face-to-face physician/patient encounter time." If no physician encounter occurred on that day, the visit with the nurse or staff for counseling/education should be billed using CPT code 99211*.[21]

In most cases, CPT (current procedural terminology) code 99211*[22] carries the lowest level of reimbursement ($11.00 to $14.00), even if the RD has spent 1 to 1.5 hours with the patient with newly diagnosed non–insulin-dependent diabetes mellitus (NIDDM). This chapter's author has recently received Medicare reimbursement for medical nutrition therapy and diabetes self-management training provided in a physician's of-

---

fice by using CPT codes for self-care skills, 97540* (30 minutes) and 97541* (15 minutes). AEtna, serving as a Medicare carrier in another state, may interpret the regulations differently than AEtna in Georgia. (A more detailed discussion of coding for medical nutrition therapy and diabetes self-management training follows.) According to the *Medicare Coverage Issues Manual*, section 80-1, Medicare may cover diabetes nutrition education for individuals in a hospital outpatient setting, skilled nursing facility, or home health agency under certain conditions.[23] According to Blue Cross Blue Shield, the intermediary for Georgia, these conditions may include a patient with newly diagnosed diabetes or one whose diabetes is out of control and is not able to understand or comply with handouts or medical information from the physician. Diet education may be covered when "the diet prescribed is of such complexity the patient cannot follow a simple brochure."[24]

Diabetes Education Programs. The *Medicare Coverage Issues Manual*, section 80-2, defines an outpatient hospital diabetic education program as a "program which educates patients in the successful self-management of diabetes."[25] Reimbursement may be made under Medicare for education programs that meet the following criteria:

- Services must be furnished under a physician's order by the provider's personnel and under medical staff supervision.

- Eligible patients have newly diagnosed diabetes and/or unstable diabetes (eg, long-term diabetes with current management problems).

- Program participants must be registered patients of that provider.

- Programs should identify themselves as

programs for non–insulin-dependent patients, insulin-dependent patients, or both.

The program includes education about:

- performance of frequent self-monitoring of blood glucose

- diet and exercise

- an insulin treatment plan developed specifically for the patient who is insulin-dependent

- motivation to use the skills learned to enable self-management.

"The overall goal of outpatient hospital diabetic education programs is self-management of the disease, and each program must be sufficiently flexible to meet the individual needs of the patient. (This does not preclude some sessions of the programs to be given on an outpatient group basis.)"[25]

After the intermediary determines that a program may be covered, the intermediary may request additional documentation to make a claims determination. Possible service codes to use when submitting claim forms include the American Hospital Association Revenue codes 942, 510, or 519.

Proposed Medicare Legislation. Recognizing that Medicare sets the precedent for other third-party payers, diabetes advocates have introduced legislation to ensure coverage for diabetes outpatient self-management training in a variety of practice settings. The Medicare Diabetes Outpatient Self-Management Training Acts of 1995 (House version, H.R. 1073, and Senate version, S. 491) introduced in the 104th Congress are intended to increase access to these essential services for the Medicare population and to correct inconsistencies in current reimbursement practices.[26] The legislation defines and expands coverage for diabetes self-management training. A companion bill, H.R. 1074, expands Medicare coverage for blood glucose monitoring strips. The ADA helped draft the legislation and encourages members to contact legislators to re-

---

*CPT codes, descriptions, and two-digit numeric modifiers only are copyright © 1994, American Medical Association. All rights reserved.

quest their support and sponsorship. If this legislation is not passed in the 104th Congress, it will need to be introduced in the next session of Congress unless health care reform precludes the need for it. As with any proposed legislation, grassroots support and lobbying of legislators by coalitions and by individual constituents are essential for passage.

Private Health Insurance Plans

Blue Cross and Blue Shield Associations, commercial insurance companies, self-insured companies, and managed care organizations comprise the remainder of the third-party payment system. As with public or government programs (Medicare and Medicaid), coverage and reimbursement practices vary widely among private third-party payers, depending on the plan, the services provided, and the practice setting. Many commercial carriers determine reimbursement for medical nutrition therapy and diabetes self-management training on a case-by-case basis.

Reimbursement for Inpatient Services

Few data are available on inpatient reimbursement for specific services because of increasing use of two payment systems: capitation and prospective payments. Under capitated rates, hospitals are reimbursed a fixed flat rate (per person per month) to provide services to a given population, usually HMO subscribers. When the HMO subscriber is admitted to the hospital, the hospital must provide the most cost-effective, efficient care possible because it does not receive any additional monies other than the fixed flat monthly rate. Under the prospective payment system, hospitals are reimbursed on a prospective, cost-per-case basis according to the primary or admission diagnosis. Reimbursement is based on predetermined rates using diagnosis-related groups (DRGs) based on admission diagnosis and comorbid conditions or complications (CCs) (secondary diagnoses). Screening and identifying inpatients with the CC (secondary

diagnosis) of, for example, malnutrition can add to the payment received for a DRG (primary diagnosis).[27,28] Payment systems based on the traditional retrospective fee-for-service approach are becoming rare because these payment systems reimburse individual charges for hospital care regardless of length of stay and use of services and are more costly for the third-party payer.

OPERATING WITHIN THE CURRENT REIMBURSEMENT SYSTEM

Charging for Medical Nutrition Therapy and Diabetes Self-Management Training

Even with the fixed payment systems, RD/CDEs must still document charges for their services. Including charges for medical nutrition therapy and diabetes self-management training on the hospital bill will continue to demonstrate the necessity and use of these services. Many institutions do not charge for RD/CDE services. If services are provided but not charged for, they are invisible to third-party payers. When third-party payers, including Medicare, do not see charges for medical nutrition therapy or diabetes self-management training on hospital billing forms, they assume that the services are not needed or are not being used. They will not include unnecessary or underused services in any future payment arrangements or contracts for hospital services. Hospitals providing services, such as medical nutrition therapy and diabetes self-management training, but not receiving compensation for them may find it difficult to justify continuing to pay the salaries of the service providers (RD/CDEs). Institutions whose payer mix includes only a small percentage of fee-for-service payers can often generate enough revenue from medical nutrition therapy charges to justify staff salaries.[29]

Establishing a Charge System

Initiating a charge system for medical nutrition therapy or diabetes self-management training is a time-consuming process requiring cooperation by institutional finance and billing departments. Step-by-step guides for developing a proposal and tips for implementing a charge system are available.[28–31] Patience and persistence are necessary to overcome the obstacles presented by institutional administrators, physicians, and even RD/CDEs themselves.

Codes for Medical Nutrition Therapy and Diabetes Self-Management Training

The question most frequently asked when considering coverage and reimbursement issues is "Which codes do I use?" The absence of unique and uniform codes identifying medical nutrition therapy services and diabetes self-management training adds to the confusion and complexity of how to obtain maximum coverage and reimbursement for these services. Codes are expressed in an alpha-numeric language and are used by health care professionals to communicate with third-party payers[32–34] (see Table 35-2 for definitions and examples).

Need for Uniform and Unique Codes

Specific codes for nutrition services and diabetes self-management training can facilitate the efficient retrieval of clinical and reimbursement information, which could support research efforts in nutrition and diabetes management. For example, unique codes for medical nutrition therapy and diabetes self-management training would allow tracking of these services by third-party payers or researchers interested in health care use trends. Negotiation for capitated rates by managed care organizations are based on service claims history. The ability to track medical nutrition therapy and diabetes self-management training services as services for which charges have been made supports the inclusion of these services in contracts with health care institutions.

Coverage and Reimbursement

Diagnosis (ICD 9-CM) and procedural/service (CPT, HCPCS, and AHA Revenue) codes are the communication link between providers and third-party payers. Codes represent services and supplies on health insurance claims forms, and many health insurers make coverage and payment decisions based on codes used. Although providers try to use codes that accurately describe services rendered, there are no unique codes for nutrition services or diabetes self-management training. Therefore, providers must try to determine which of the existing codes are most appropriate and will achieve the best reimbursement results.

Numerous Codes in Use

The 1991 AADE Third-Party Reimbursement Survey indicated that respondents used 104 different codes for diabetes self-management training services.[15] Information obtained by the American Dietetic Association also shows that several codes are used to describe similar services.[18]

Proposals for Creating Codes for Medical Nutrition Therapy and Diabetes Self-Management Training

CPT codes are the main codes used for services and supplies in outpatient health care services. These codes are published annually by the American Medical Association (AMA).[22] Proposals for new codes are presented to the AMA CPT Editorial Panel.

The American Diabetes Association Coding Proposal. In 1992 the ADA submitted a proposal to the AMA CPT Coding Committee.[35] The proposal explains the need for uniform and unique codes for diabetes self-management training and specifically requests two codes, a *Single Visit Code* and a *Comprehensive Program Code*. No action has been taken by the AMA as of this writing.

The American Dietetic Association Coding Proposal. In 1993 the American Dietetic Association submitted a proposal to the AMA CPT Editorial Panel explaining the need and requesting uniform and unique codes for nutrition services. The two codes requested are for *Nutrition Assessment* and *Nutrition Treatment*.[32] The

Table 35-2 Coding Systems

Codes	Definitions	Examples	Settings
Diagnosis and Procedure			
ICD-9-CM	International Classification of Diseases, 9th Revision Clinical Modification Diagnoses and Hospital Procedures	648.8 Gestational Diabetes V.65.3 Dietary Surveillance and Counseling	Diagnosis codes are used in any practice setting Hospital procedure codes used in hospital settings
Service, Procedure, and Supply Codes			
HCPCS	HCFA[a] Common Procedure Coding System (Three Levels)		
	1. CPT (Current Procedural Terminology) Codes—Physician Medical/Surgical Services, Procedures, and Supplies	99211[b], 99202[b], etc. Evaluation and Management: Office or Other Outpatient Services 99071[b] Educational Supplies	Inpatient and outpatient hospital and other outpatient settings
	2. Alpha-Numeric Medical Products Codes	B4034 Enteral Feeding Supply Kit	Inpatient and outpatient hospital and other outpatient settings
	3. Local Codes assigned by individual Medicare carriers or intermediaries	Check with institutional billing office for which codes apply to you	Inpatient and outpatient hospital and other outpatient settings
AHA Revenue	American Hospital Association Revenue—Supplies, inpatient and outpatient services. Uses UB 92 billing form	510 Clinic 942 Therapeutic Services/Education and Training 949 Therapeutic Services/Other	Inpatient and outpatient hospital settings

[a] HCFA: Health Care Financing Administration.

[b] CPT codes, descriptions, and two-digit numeric modifiers only are copyright 1995, American Medical Association. All rights reserved.

Source: Mathieu-Harris M. Procedure codes for nutrition services. In: Legislation and reimbursement: increasing access to medical nutrition therapy and diabetes self-management training. *On the Cutting Edge.* 1993;14:18–19. Schatz GB. Coding for nutrition services: challenges, opportunities, and guidelines. *J Am Diet Assoc.* 1993;93:471–477.

AMA has not acted on the proposal as of this writing.

Support Needed for Coding Proposals. The CPT Editorial Panel decides on proposed additions to the CPT codes after consultation with appropriate medical specialty societies on the CPT Advisory Committee, such as the American Society for Internal Medicine, the American

Academy of Pediatrics, and the American Academy of Family Physicians. Support for any new codes is needed from physician specialty groups. Physician-clinical experts in the areas of nutrition and diabetes can influence members of their specialty groups who sit on the editorial panels or advisory committees. The process of adopting new codes moves slowly—codes accepted in 1994 would not be published before 1996. The American Dietetic Association and the ADA have supported each other's coding proposals by writing letters and requesting support from appropriate physician groups.

Risks Involved

The availability of uniform and unique codes for medical nutrition therapy and diabetes self-management training will not automatically guarantee reimbursement. More clearly identifying the services may actually make it easier for payers to deny payment. Coverage, or *recognition*, of these services must be attained first to ensure reimbursement.

Keeping Up with Trends in Health Care Benefits Plans

According to a 1992 nationwide health care benefits survey of 2,500 employers, representing 12 million employees and dependents, there are three trends of importance to RD/CDEs.[36] This survey indicates that 61% of all employers offer HMO plans, 39% offer preferred provider organization (PPO) plans, and 67% offer self-funded plans. These trends, two toward managed care (HMOs and PPOs) and one toward employer-financed benefits (self-funded), offer new opportunities for RD/CDEs.

Opportunities in Managed Care

Managed care is an approach to paying for health care in which insurers emphasize cost containment and more efficient use of resources. The economies used may include greater use of primary care physicians or nonphysician providers and discounted purchases of services, supplies, and pharmaceuticals. Although we tend to equate managed care with HMOs and PPOs, almost all third-party payers now incorporate some elements of managed care in their payment decisions. (Exhibit 35-2 provides definitions of terms used in managed care.) RD/CDEs can approach managed care organizations by presenting medical nutrition therapy and diabetes self-management training as a treatment/prevention concept that reduces costs and produces successful outcomes. For example, a person with NIDDM may be able to decrease or discontinue various medications because of nutrition intervention and life-style changes directed at improving blood glucose, blood lipids, and blood pressure. The nutrition intervention produces short-term cost savings on medications and long-term savings on prevention of complications. In the past, insurance companies were not as interested in long-term cost savings as in

Exhibit 35-2 Terms Used in Managed Care

HMO—health maintenance organization. Prepaid plans that finance and provide health care, emphasizing prevention and managed care. Primary care physicians act as gatekeepers for referrals to specialists. Plan subscribers usually can only use providers from within HMO network. Many HMOs employ dietitians on staff or as consultants.

IPA—independent practice association. Health care providers and hospitals who contract with MCOs to use their own offices and facilities to provide services. Can include dietitians and diabetes educators among contracted providers.

MCO—managed care organization. General term used to describe groups offering managed care plans (eg, HMOs, PPOs, IPAs).

POS—point of service. Plans in which members pick primary care physicians from a network list. The primary care physician directs patient care, including referrals to specialists. Patients pay more if they use out-of-network providers.

PPO—preferred provider organization. Plans that negotiate discounted rates with providers. Providers accept lower payments in exchange for a higher volume of patients. Patients pay more if they choose providers outside of the PPO.

short-term savings because the average plan subscriber changed plans frequently. Many HMOs now seek to enroll entire families as long-term members of their plans, therefore increasing interest in looking at long-term outcomes and cost savings of various therapies.

HMOs. Many HMOs employ RD/CDEs on staff and as consultants. The more skills the RD/CDE develops, the greater the opportunities. For example, offering exercise, stress management, and smoking cessation programs in addition to nutrition services increases marketability.[37] Possessing specialty credentials (eg, CDE) will also increase opportunities within managed care organizations.

PPOs. Preferred providers are health care professionals approved by HMOs or PPOs as eligible to receive patient referrals from plan physicians. RD/CDEs in solo private practice or members of groups can obtain preferred provider status.[37]

The Gatekeepers: Physicians and Case Managers. In the managed care scenario, primary care physicians determine the course of treatment, including referrals to other health care providers whether inside or outside the managed care organization. Therefore it is crucial for RD/CDEs to continue to educate physicians on the effectiveness and cost savings of medical nutrition therapy as an integral part of diabetes self-management training. Physicians can learn to appreciate the role of the dietitian on the diabetes management team. Utilization case managers also act as gatekeepers.[38] (*Utilization* case managers are different from *clinical* case managers. Clinical case managers are health care providers and team members responsible for coordinating patient care in a clinical setting.)

Three types of utilization case managers are:

- facility-based case manager. Employed by a health care facility to negotiate reductions in patients' length of stay
- in-house case manager. Full-time employee of the third-party payer. Looks for discounts on services and ways to reduce administrative expenses. Receives annual

profit-sharing bonus, based on negotiated savings
- individual case manager. Independent contractor working as consultant to many different third-party payers. Receives direct compensation based on discounts negotiated with health care providers—a commission.

Identify which type of case manager you are dealing with before releasing pricing information. Be very clear about the details of service provided, and be sure to verify the patient's coverage and reimbursement *before* providing the service.

Provider Networks and Networking. Physicians and other health care professionals have formed alliances or networks in which they join together as a group, pool resources, decrease overhead expenses, and establish a bargaining unit to negotiate discounted fees with third-party payers in exchange for guaranteed referrals. RD/CDEs can join forces to form their own provider networks, or they can contract their services to PPOs or other health care provider networks. The important point for RD/CDEs is to analyze what it costs to provide their services, to establish what profit they would like, and then to negotiate a competitive fee while not underselling themselves.

Opportunities in Self-Funded Plans

Self-funded plans are programs for providing group benefits in which the employer determines and finances health care benefits instead of purchasing coverage from a commercial carrier. The plan may be *administered* (ie, insurance claims processed) by the employer, a commercial carrier, or a third-party administrator. The growth in self-funded plans presents unique opportunities for RD/CDEs to market nutrition services directly to companies and businesses. The RD/CDE can provide preventive services at on-site wellness programs. She or he can also provide medical nutrition therapy at employee clinics or in other practice settings as a covered benefit in the health plan.

Company Benefits Managers. Because they influence employee coverage and reimbursement decisions in self-funded plans, company benefits managers are key contacts for dietitians. The RD/CDE can provide convincing support for coverage and reimbursement by presenting actual cost-saving case studies of client/patient success stories from within the company. Patients/employees, as consumers, can also become advocates for increased coverage. For example, employees having a diagnosis in common, such as diabetes, can form a group to petition the company benefits manager. The group can request coverage and reimbursement for medical nutrition therapy and diabetes self-management training, equipment, and supplies.

MAXIMIZING REIMBURSEMENT IN A TIME OF TRANSITION

As health care reform evolves at national, state, and local levels, RD/CDEs must still operate within the current system's diversity. Dietetics professionals and diabetes educators are seeking ways to maximize reimbursement within current health care financing mechanisms, using all available tips and tools. The following recommendations for maximizing reimbursement are the essential ones generally agreed on by RD/CDEs who are active in reimbursement efforts.[29–31,39–43]

A Step-by-Step Guide for Maximizing Reimbursement for Outpatient Services

1. *Establish charges* based on actual costs of providing services plus desired profit. Be sure to include salary and benefits costs, overhead expenses, and cost of materials and supplies.[44]

2. *Obtain written documentation of physician referral,* including all relevant diagnoses, laboratory data, medications, recommendations, and restrictions. This is the "prescription" authorizing medical nutrition therapy (see sample referral form in Exhibit 35-3). In the private practice setting,

physician referral for nutrition services increased third-party reimbursement by 51%.[12]

3. *Obtain prior authorizations,* if necessary, from HMOs, PPOs and case managers. Be clear about limitations on number of visits. Talk to case managers at insurance companies and benefits managers in self-insured businesses. You may be able to persuade them to change their policy or make exceptions.

4. *Assure payers of quality care.* Indicate use of accepted standards of care, validated practice guidelines, and protocols, which can support reimbursement for a recommended number of visits and plan of care.

5. *Use appropriate codes and terminology. Diagnosis* codes are based on physician referral. Use all codes relevant to the services provided, and place in priority acuity order. *Procedure* codes will vary depending on the insurance plan. Some companies specify which codes to use. When describing services, avoid using terms such as *education* or *counseling*; instead, use *therapy, management, or self-management training.* Refer to Table 35-2 for examples of codes used.

6. *Indicate provider credentials.* If a licensed dietitian, include state dietetic license number on billing statement. If a CDE, include that designation (spelled out) along with signature. Include other credentials such as the Commission on Dietetic Registration specialty board certification in the areas of metabolic nutrition, pediatric nutrition, and renal nutrition.

7. *Include evidence of medical necessity* (service is incidental to physician services or part of treatment plan), usually obvious from diagnoses and physician referral, but a well-written letter may be necessary, especially when refiling an insurance claim (Exhibit 35-4).

8. *Document appropriately.* Documentation should reflect comprehensive outcome-ori-

Exhibit 35-3 Medical Nutrition Therapy and Diabetes Self-Management Training Referral Form

I am referring: _____

                          Name   Daytime Phone

for necessary Medical Nutrition Therapy ❑   Diabetes Self-Management Training ❑

DIAGNOSIS   **ICD-9-CM CODE**

_____
_____
_____
_____

Status of diabetes: Newly diagnosed ❑ or Number of years duration _____
Level of diabetes control: Poor ❑   Fair ❑   Good ❑   Comments: _____
Recurrent hypoglycemia ❑   Recurrent hyperglycemia ❑   Target blood glucose range _____
Other medical conditions:

_____

Relevant lab data (eg, blood glucose, lipids, glycated Hb, urine protein, or microalbumin): _____

_____

Relevant medications: _____

_____
_____

Exercise restrictions/recommendations: _____

_____
_____

Nutrition prescription (check all that apply):
❑   Weight reduction therapy   ❑   Diabetes nutrition therapy
❑   Modified sodium intake   Specifics _____
❑   Modified fat intake   Specifics _____
❑   Modified protein intake   Specifics _____
❑   Hypoglycemia prevention and treatment   ❑   CHO adjustments for exercise
❑   Carbohydrate counting: ❑ CHO consistency   ❑   CHO-to-insulin ratio
❑   Other _____

If medical nutrition therapy is to be determined by registered dietitian, please check ❑

Additional diabetes self-management training:
❑   Self-monitoring of blood glucose   Meter type _____   Other _____

Special instructions: _____

_____
_____

_____
Physician signature

_____
Date   Phone

Source: Courtesy of Sandra J. Gillespie, MMSc, RD/LD, CDE.

Exhibit 35-4 Sample Letter

NIDDM COST BENEFIT STATEMENT
INSURANCE COVERAGE FOR MEDICAL NUTRITION THERAPY
AND DIABETES SELF-MANAGEMENT TRAINING

Date of Service:
Patient's Name:
Insurance ID Number:
Diagnosis/ICD-9-CM Code(s):

This patient was referred for nutrition assessment and therapy to aid in self-management of non–insulin-dependent diabetes mellitus (NIDDM). The referring physician and registered dietitian (RD), as a team, are striving to prevent future medical expenses to your company. From a cost-benefit perspective, nutrition intervention and self-management training by the RD are much less expensive than recurrent office visits or hospitalizations resulting from poor diabetes control. **We all appreciate the fact that if the nutrition service prevents one day of hospitalization, it has paid for itself.**

The American Diabetes Association (ADA) recognizes the importance of goal-directed medical nutrition therapy as a part of the treatment of diabetes. The ADA recommends that every person with diabetes have an individualized meal plan.[1] The RD assesses the patient's nutritional status and tailors nutrition therapy to the individual's eating habits, budget, life style, and goals for management of blood glucose, blood lipids (cholesterol and triglycerides), and blood pressure (if hypertensive). Medical nutrition therapy, directed toward weight reduction and improvement in blood glucose and lipids, and blood pressure of the obese person with NIDDM has great potential for significant positive effects on morbidity and mortality. In addition, medical nutrition therapy leading to improvements in blood glucose, blood lipids, and blood pressure often results in reduction or discontinuation of medications at considerable cost savings.

The RD is qualified by education, experience, examination, and continuing education to meet the professional standards established by the American Dietetic Association (or state, if state-licensed). The RD is a health professional with the background and expertise needed to most effectively provide medical nutrition therapy.

Medical nutrition therapy is perhaps a new aspect of your policy coverage or one that you are considering. This insured patient, (patient name), would appreciate your careful review of this physician-prescribed nutrition services claim. Please contact this office if you have any questions concerning this claim and the services provided.

Thank you for your cooperation in this matter.

Sincerely,

[1] American Diabetes Association. Standards of medical care for patients with diabetes mellitus. *Diabetes Care*. 1994;17:616–623.

ented, goal-directed medical nutrition therapy and diabetes self-management training services based on accepted practice guidelines and standards of care. Include assessment, baseline laboratory values and anthropometric measurements, treatment plan, process, and outcomes. Documentation should reflect time spent and scope of service. Include evidence of hands-on activities (eg, blood glucose monitoring, blood pressure, and anthropometrics). Standardized progress notes can be developed to cue the provider to include information required by third-party payers (see sample initial visit progress note in Exhibit 35-5).

9. *Identify the practice setting.* Practice settings in descending order of reimbursement potential are hospital outpatient departments, county or community health depart-

Exhibit 35-5 Diabetes Nutrition History and Initial Visit Progress Note (To be used as companion to Nutrition and Diabetes Self-Management Flow Sheet. See Exhibit 35-6.)

Name: _____

Usual Intake: _____

Time/Meal   **Location**

B: _____   _____

_____   _____

_____   _____

L: _____   _____

_____   _____

_____   _____

S: _____   _____

_____   _____

_____   _____

Snacks: AM _____

PM _____

HS _____

Food Frequency (average per day*): %RDA (<, >, =)

Milk: _____   Calcium _____

Fruit: _____   Vit. A _____

Veg.: _____   Vit. C _____

Starch: ~ _____ g carbohydrate   Fiber _____

Meat: ~ _____ g protein   Iron _____

Fat: ~ _____ g fat

_____ mg sodium

_____ Approx. calories consumed

* Based on exchanges.

Recommended Meal Plan _____ calories

No. per d.	Exch.	Daily Totals			Meals			Snacks		
		C	P	F	B	L	S	1	2	3
	Milk									
	Fruit									
	Veg.									
	Starch									
	Carb choices									
	Meat									
	Fat									
	Total gm	C	P	F	C	C	C	C	C	C

Referring Physician: _____

Date: _____

Present at Visit: _____ Pt. _____ Other _____

S:

Food allergies: _____

Food intolerances: _____

Food shopping: _____ Food preparation: _____

Living situation: _____

Occupation: _____

Work schedule: _____

Concerns about meal plan: _____

Vitamin/mineral supplements: _____

Water _____ oz/d   Other fluids: _____ oz/d

Sweets: _____

Sugar substitutes: _____

Alcohol: _____

Caffeine: _____

Salt/Na: _____

Dining out: _____

Disabilities/limitations: _____

Feet: _____

Exercise: _____

Dental: _____

Hypoglycemia history and treatment: _____

Smoking history: _____

Weight in past year: _____

Reasonable goal weight: _____

O:

Ht. _____   Wt. _____   DBW _____   B/P _____

BMI _____   Waist _____   Hip _____   Ratio _____

Age: _____

See nutrition flow sheet for meds, labs

Literature provided, educational materials used:

_____

A: See food frequency for summary/adequacy of current intake

Estimated nutritional needs: _____

Comprehension: _____

Anticipated adherence: _____

Goals for medical nutrition therapy: _____

P:

Time spent _____

Additional visits recommended _____

_____

(Signature)

Source: Courtesy of Sandra J. Gillespie, MMSc, RD/LD, CDE.

Exhibit 35-6 Nutrition and Diabetes Self-Management Flow Sheet

(To be used with Diabetes Nutrition History and Initial Visit Progress Note. See Exhibit 35-5.)

Patient Name:_____D.O.B. _____Physician: _____

Phone: H (   ) _____W (   ) _____Diagnosis: _____ Onset of DM __/__/__

Pt. Goal Wt.:_____lb   BG Target Range:_____to_____   Insulin Supplement Formula: _____

Pt. Glucose Meter: _____ Frequency of Monitoring _____

Date	Wt. Lb.	Wt. Δ	B/P	Total Chol.	HDL/ LDL	TG	BG	HbA$_{1c}$	BUN/ CR	Urine Pro/ MA	Other	Meds	Progress Note (Please see initial visit note)

Source: Courtesy of Sandra J. Gillespie, MMSc, RD/LD, CDE.

ment, physicians' offices, and private practice offices.

10. *Use appropriate billing forms.* The HCFA 1500 billing form is considered a universal billing form and is required by Medicare, many state Medicaid programs, and other third-party payers. The HCFA 1500 form is available from most office or computer supply stores or from the HCFA. Individuals may develop their own billing forms.

11. *Use correct procedures* from the time of referral, registration, and the appointment-making process to the time of visit and fee collection. Remind patient in advance of the visit to avoid lost revenues from missed appointments. Be sure patient understands

payment responsibilities. At time of the visit, collect copayments and fees. If patient misses appointment, call to reschedule. Notify referring physician if patient does not keep any appointments.

12. *Submit claims or assist patients with submitting claims*, if necessary. Submit even if the visit was not approved, and the patient decided to self-pay. The claim may still go through and get reimbursed, or if denied, the explanation of benefits can be used for tracking reimbursement or for resubmitting a claim with additional documentation of medical necessity and evidence of patient progress.

13. *Track payments and reimbursement.* Send results for medical nutrition therapy to the American Dietetic Association's computerized reimbursement data base to provide data for your geographic location and practice specialty area. Data collection forms are available from the American Dietetic Association. Assess revenue generated from your services by conducting reimbursement audits. Documentation of revenues generated can be used to justify salary or benefits increases or hiring of additional personnel, purchase of equipment, or expansion of facility. Volunteer to serve as a resource person for the American Dietetic Association's reimbursement department.

14. *Ensure adequate follow-up.* Follow-up visits are essential to provide quality service and to obtain evidence of effectiveness and cost savings. Improvements in glycated hemoglobin, blood lipids, blood pressure, and medications decreased or discontinued must be noted to document outcomes and effectiveness of medical nutrition therapy (see nutrition flow sheet documentation form in Exhibit 35-6). Also indicate if there has been a decrease in number of emergency department visits or annual hospitalizations (eg, fewer diabetic ketoacidosis [DKA] admissions) as a result of medical nutrition therapy and diabetes self-management training services. Be sure to include figures of cost for DKA admissions versus cost of self-management services.

15. *Be persistent.* View every insurance claim denied as an opportunity to educate and negotiate with third-party payers. Help patients refile when the first claim is denied. (More than 50% of claims are denied the first time filed.) Attach a letter of medical necessity, including documentation of any progress, medication discontinued or decreased, and any other cost savings (see sample letter in Exhibit 35-4). In some cases, a letter from the physician, or physician *and* RD/CDE may be more effective. If all else fails, encourage patients to request a *hearing* or a *review board* to reconsider a payment decision by a third-party payer.

16. *Share success stories.* RD/CDEs can improve coverage and reimbursement at the grassroots level by sharing local success stories about which codes and strategies achieve reimbursement, by documenting outcome-oriented services and their cost savings in case studies, and by talking to insurers on behalf of clients and patients seeking reimbursement. Contribute cost-savings case studies to state dietetic associations, dietetic practice groups, and the ADA data collections for health care reform efforts. See section later in this chapter on cost-savings case studies collections.

17. *Establish and develop referral sources.* Local sources include those obtained by networking with other health professionals through organizations such as local chapters, districts, and affiliates of AADE, state dietetic associations, and the ADA. Volunteer work such as speaking to diabetes support groups, conducting grocery store tours and cooking classes, and writing articles for local newspapers can provide publicity and lead to referrals. Visit physician offices. Always carry your business cards

with you and perhaps a brochure describing your credentials and services in case you identify a good prospect. The American Dietetic Association's Nationwide Nutrition Network can direct you to potential clients and patients seeking a dietitian through its Nutrition Hotline (1-800-366-1655). The American Association of Diabetes Educators has developed a program called "Self-Management Matters. Team up with a Diabetes Educator." Potential clients can call 1-800-TEAMUP4 to obtain a referral to a diabetes educator in their area.

Many of these same steps can be used for maximizing reimbursement in the inpatient setting.

ASSURANCE OF EFFECTIVENESS AND QUALITY CARE

Health care providers are being held accountable for achieving desired outcomes at the least cost. This demand for cost-effective, quality care has led to the development of quality assurance processes and outcome measures[44-48] (see Exhibit 35-7 for definitions). Splett and Russo[45] describe a five-phase process for evaluating clinical effectiveness of nutrition care.

1. Define protocols for nutrition care. Clearly define the level, content, and frequency of nutrition care that is appropriate for the disease or condition.
2. Identify outcome indicators. Specify the end result that nutrition care is expected to achieve.
3. Deliver care consistently. Document both the processes and outcomes of care.
4. Assess the rate of success of nutrition services. Collect and summarize data from patients' records and evaluate the results.
5. Act on the findings. Use the results to report effectiveness results to others and to redefine protocols for improved outcomes in the future.

Exhibit 35-7 Terms Used in Quality Assessment and Effectiveness Evaluation

Clinical effectiveness—the degree to which a desired change in outcome indicators related to the patient's disease state is achieved as a result of specific intervention used under ordinary conditions ("real world," rather than laboratory, conditions).

Cost-effectiveness analysis—an approach to evaluation that takes into account both costs and outcomes of intervention for a specific purpose. The analysis is especially useful for comparing alternative methods of intervention.

Cost-benefit analysis—an extension of cost-effectiveness; places a dollar value on the outcomes.

Continuous quality improvement (CQI)—an approach to quality management that follows patient/client care, focusing on processes, customer satisfaction, and continuously improving quality over time.

Critical pathways—diagnosis-specific maps or blueprints of key events in patient's hospital stay or continuum of care, designed to achieve maximum quality of care at minimal cost.

Intervention—a purposefully planned action designed to achieve a defined outcome.

Outcome—an end result of the health care process; a measurable change in the patient's state of health or functioning.

Practice guidelines—systematically developed statements or specifications designed to help practitioners and/or patients/clients choose appropriate health care in "typical" clinical or foodservice systems circumstances.

Protocol—detailed guidelines for care that are specific to the disease or condition and type of patient.

Quality assurance—certification of continuous, optimal, effective, and efficient health and nutrition care.

Quality assessment—measurement of technical and interpersonal aspects of health care and services and the outcomes of the care and service.

Standards of practice—statements of dietetics practitioner's responsibility for providing quality nutrition care.

PRACTICE GUIDELINES FOR DIABETES NUTRITION MANAGEMENT

Practice guidelines are standards of care, such as nutrition care protocols, and are based on the best available research and professional judgment. They must be validated by field testing by a reasonable pool of practitioners.[46]

NIDDM, IDDM, and Gestational Diabetes

The Diabetes Care and Education Practice Group of the American Dietetic Association is currently developing, field testing, and evaluating nutrition practice guidelines for IDDM and gestational diabetes. Mazze et al[49] and Franz et al[50] developed, field tested, and conducted cost-benefit analysis on practice guidelines for nutrition care for persons with NIDDM. The Massachusetts Dietetic Association has developed, field tested, and evaluated practice guidelines for NIDDM, gestational diabetes, hypertension, and hypercholesterolemia.[51]

DOCUMENTING OUTCOMES, EFFECTIVENESS, AND COST SAVINGS

Without documentation we cannot show that medical nutrition therapy and diabetes self-management training are part of quality treatment and are effective, cost-effective, and manageable.[52] Positioning these services as a prevention-treatment concept with documented cost savings is crucial to becoming part of the payment picture. Data documenting effectiveness can be used to justify coverage and reimbursement for these services.

RESEARCH

Third-party payers want the *science* to support any claims for effectiveness and cost-effectiveness.[53] Results of clinical trials demonstrating the cost-effectiveness of diabetes nutrition management can support coverage and reimbursement efforts. A single well-conducted investigation will have greater impact on health care financing decision makers than many less rigorous studies.[54] Examples of such studies are the DCCT[1] and the NIDDM Diabetes Guidelines Cost-Effectiveness Study.[50]

The NIDDM Diabetes Guidelines Cost-Effectiveness Study

The NIDDM Diabetes Guidelines Cost-Effectiveness Study, funded by the American Dietetic Association, was a short-term, prospective clinical trial of adults with NIDDM. Franz et al[50] found significant improvement in glycemic control when patients received medical nutrition therapy from RDs. Two hundred and three study subjects from three geographic locations (Colorado, Florida, and Minnesota) were randomly assigned to basic nutrition care (BC) (one visit with the RD) and practice guidelines care (PGC) (three visits with the RD). The objective of the six-month trial was to conduct cost analysis and to determine cost-effectiveness of BC versus PGC. The outcomes of a sample of 179 subjects from the two groups are summarized in Table 35-3.

A nonrandomized comparison group followed in primary care during the same time period with no RD intervention showed no improvement in HbA[1c]. This cost-effectiveness study demonstrates the achievement of significant improvements in blood glucose control with a relatively small investment of resources when patients receive medical nutrition therapy provided by registered dietitians.

Cost Savings Case Studies Data Collection

Many states and dietetic practice groups have contributed to the American Dietetic Association's collection of more than 1,600 case studies documenting successful outcomes and cost savings of medical nutrition therapy. These case studies are useful in approaching legislators and third-party payers when enlisting their support for coverage and reimbursement of medical nutrition therapy services (see example in Exhibit 35-8).

Table 35-3 NIDDM Diabetes Guidelines Cost-Effectiveness Study Outcomes

Outcome Measures	Basic Care	Practice Guidelines Care
Number of visits with RD	1 (1 hour)	3 (2 1/2 hours)
Mean reduction in fasting plasma glucose (FPG)	7.3 mg/dL	19.2 mg/dL
Mean reduction in HbA$_{1c}$	0.69%	0.93%
Average cost per patient[a]	$41.95	$112.07
Average 1-year cost savings based on changes in therapy (primarily decreases in medications)	$3.13	$31.49
Cost effectiveness ratio (when cost savings factored in)	$5.32 per mg/dL decrease in FPG	$4.20 per mg/dL decrease in FPG

[a] Costs included time spent by RDs and support staff, education materials and supplies, laboratory tests, and overhead expenses.

Source: Franz MS, Splett PL, Monk A, et al. Cost effectiveness of medical nutrition therapy provided by dietitians for persons with non–insulin-dependent diabetes mellitus. *J Am Diet Assoc.* 1995;95:1018–1024.

Exhibit 35-8 Case Study: Cost Savings of Medical Nutrition Therapy and Diabetes Self-Management Training in Gestational Diabetes

Site:	Community Hospital Clinic, Springfield, Massachusetts
Patient:	Pregnant woman with gestational diabetes
Medical Nutrition Therapy:	Individualized treatment, 3 visits
Health Outcome:	Able to control blood glucose levels, control weight gain
Resources Saved:	Avoided need for insulin and potential hospitalization to initiate insulin therapy
Medical Nutrition Therapy Cost:	$135
Cost Savings:	$2,265—cost of use of insulin for 10 weeks and 2-day hospital stay to initiate insulin therapy

Author's Note: Uncontrolled gestational diabetes can result in a large infant requiring a cesarean delivery. According to 1991 data collected by the Health Insurance Association of America, the cost of a cesarean delivery is $3,100 more than the cost of a normal delivery. Therefore, the total cost savings for the above case study could total $5,365 (Health Insurance Association of America. *Source Book of Health Insurance Data* 1993. Washington, DC: Health Insurance Association of America; 1994:92).

Source: Reprinted from Folkman JW, Johnson EQ, Lynch M, Rowan ML, Tiller S. *Nutrition Services Improve Health and Save Money: Evidence from Massachusetts* (p 18) with permission of the Massachusetts Dietetic Association, © 1993.

The American Dietetic Association's Position on Cost-Effectiveness of Medical Nutrition Therapy

The American Dietetic Association recently issued a paper on cost-effectiveness of medical nutrition therapy. The position statement reads:

"It is the position of the American Dietetic Association that medical nutrition therapy is effective in treating disease and preventing disease complications, resulting in health benefits and cost savings for the public. Therefore, medical nutrition therapy provided by dietetics professionals is an essential reimbursable component of com-

Exhibit 35-9 Health Care Policy and Financing Decision Makers and Influencers: Our Customers

Government
- Legislators
- Government Regulatory Agencies: Medicare
- State Departments of Medical Assistance: Medicaid
- State and County Health Departments
- State and County Boards of Health
- State Insurance Commissioners

Insurance Industry
- Managed Care Organizations: HMOs, PPOs
- Blue Cross Blue Shield Associations
- Commercial Insurance Companies
- Medical Directors of Insurance Companies
- Directors of Provider Relations
- Medical Utilization/Case Managers
- Third-Party Administrators

Corporations and Businesses
- Company Chief Executive Officers (CEOs)
- Employer Self-Insured Programs
- Employee Benefits Managers
- Employer Health Care Alliances
- Pension Administrators
- Chamber of Commerce
- Small Business Association

Health Care Providers
- Primary Care Physicians, Nurses, and Other *Gatekeepers* (Referral Sources)
- Hospitals/Administrators
- Professional Associations (eg, American Medical Association, State Medical Societies)
- American Hospital Association, State Hospital Associations

Patient/Consumer Advocacy Groups
- American Diabetes Association, Juvenile Diabetes Association
- Clients/Patients and Their Families (Consumers and Constituents)

prehensive health care services."[55] The position paper includes scientific studies and case studies documenting the effectiveness and cost savings of medical nutrition therapy in a variety of settings for diseases and conditions (including diabetes) in all phases of the life cycle. The paper also lists health care advocacy and government groups that have published recommendations that include medical nutrition therapy.

ACHIEVING COVERAGE THROUGH ADVOCACY—A MARKETING APPROACH

"Marketing is, very simply, identifying a need, assisting potential clients in recognizing that need, and then providing fulfillment for the need."[56] The national focus on health care reform presents unique opportunities for dietitians and diabetes educators to educate and influence health care policy and financing decision makers (see Exhibit 35-9). By viewing these decisions makers as *customers* with a need—a need for cost containment and quality care—we can demonstrate to them how our services can fulfill that need.

Start in Your Own Backyard

RD/CDEs can look at their own health care plans to see if medical nutrition therapy and diabetes self-management training are covered services. If not, they can approach employers with a proposal to include these services as a covered benefit.[57] Collecting cost-savings case studies from one's own practice setting and area of expertise can help persuade employers to provide coverage and reimbursement for these same services in employee health plans.

The Power of Numbers

Enlisting the support of physicians and other referral sources and establishing coalitions of professional and consumer groups can increase leverage with health care financing decision makers. Professional, voluntary, and consumer groups can join forces to lobby for mutual interests. Health care coalitions are alliances formed by groups concerned about health care costs—employers, professional organizations, and health care providers. These alliances develop programs and services of mutual benefit and interest such as wellness councils or benefits managers groups, which provide opportunities for education and sharing. Formally presenting the benefits and cost savings of medical nutrition therapy and diabetes self-management training to alliance group programs provides a unique marketing opportunity for dietitians and diabetes educators.

Coalitions of diabetes voluntary organizations have lobbied successfully with state legislatures in Florida, Minnesota, New York, and Wisconsin. These states have passed laws requiring insurance coverage of diabetes self-management training, equipment, and supplies.[58]

LOOKING AHEAD

Demand Projections for Dietitians and Nutritionists in 2005

The U.S. Bureau of Labor Statistics (BLS) develops and publishes 10- to 15-year projections predicting employment for specific occupations.[59] For employment of dietitians and nutritionists in the year 2005, the BLS 1994 publication estimates 40 to 60% increases in health and fitness facilities and diet workshops, 54% growth in physicians' offices, 63% growth in offices of other health practitioners, and 91% growth in home health care services. Substantial growth (87%) is projected for establishments providing social services and rehabilitation services. These social service agencies include child day care services and residential care. The least growth is predicted for what once were traditional employment settings for dietitians and nutritionists—hospitals 7% and government 0.5%.

The Age of Empowerment

Funnell et al[60] have defined the process of empowerment as

> the discovery and development of one's inherent capacity to be responsible for one's life. People are empowered when they have sufficient knowledge to make rational decisions, sufficient control and resources to

implement their decisions and sufficient experience to evaluate the effectiveness of their decisions. . . . Empowerment is an interactive process of cultivating the power in others through the sharing of knowledge, expertise, and resources.

RD/CDEs can empower themselves and each other, as well as their patients. By sharing strengths and experiences, we can all grow individually and as a profession. RD/CDEs can use employment projections to plan for the future. They can position themselves in the best possible place—*the right niche*—to use their unique skills and qualifications, marketing techniques, and the power of persuasion to achieve the goal of increased access to medical nutrition therapy and diabetes self-management training.

REFERENCES

1. Diabetes Control and Complications Trial Research Group. The effect of intensive treatment of diabetes on the development and progression of long-term complications in insulin-dependent diabetes mellitus. *N Engl J Med*. 1993;329:977–986.

2. Diabetes Control and Complications Trial Research Group. Expanded role of the dietitian in the Diabetes Control and Complications Trial: implications for clinical practice. *J Am Diet Assoc*. 1993;93:758–764,767.

3. Diabetes Control and Complications Trial Research Group. Nutrition interventions for intensive therapy in the Diabetes Control and Complications Trial. *J Am Diet Assoc*. 1993;93:768–772.

4. Delahanty LM, Halford BN. The role of diet behaviors in achieving improved glycemic control in intensively treated patients in the Diabetes Control and Complications Trial. *Diabetes Care*. 1993;16:1453–1458.

5. Delahanty LM, ed. Message from the theme editor. In: Challenges and lessons from the Diabetes Control and Complications Trial. *On the Cutting Edge*. 1994;15:1.

6. Delahanty LM, ed. A new image and a redefined role for dietitians in intensive diabetes therapy. In: Challenges and lessons from the Diabetes Control and Complications Trial. *On the Cutting Edge*. 1994;15:5.

7. American Diabetes Association. Standards of medical care for patients with diabetes mellitus. *Diabetes Care*. 1994;17:616–623.

8. American Diabetes Association. Third-party reimbursement for outpatient diabetes education and counseling. *Diabetes Care*. 1992;15(suppl 2):41.

9. American Diabetes Association. *Diabetes. 1993 Vital Statistics*. Alexandria, Va.: American Diabetes Association, 1993.

10. National Institute of Diabetes, Digestive and Kidney Diseases. *Metabolic Control Matters Nationwide Translation of the Diabetes Control and Complications Trial: Analysis and Recommendations*. Washington, DC: U.S. Department of Health and Human Services, National Institutes of Health; May 1994. NIH Publication No. 94-3773.

11. Wylie-Rosett J. What are the implications of the DCCT for health-care financing? In: Challenges and lessons from the Diabetes Control and Complications Trial. *On the Cutting Edge*. 1994;15:22–23.

12. Crawford GL. *Tracking Third-Party Reimbursement for Nutrition Services Provided by Registered Dietitians in the Private Practice Setting*. Denton, Tex: Department of Nutrition and Food Sciences, College of Health Sciences, Texas Woman's University, 1992. Thesis.

13. American Dietetic Association. *ADA Reimbursement Database Preliminary Data*. Chicago, Ill: American Dietetic Association; 1994.

14. Hood RS, Griffith M. The Ohio NSPS statewide survey of third-party reimbursement policies for nutrition services. *J Am Diet Assoc*. 1993;93:181–182.

15. Tobin CT. Health care policy, finance, and law: report on the AADE survey for third-party reimbursement. *Diabetes Educ*. 1993;19:62–68.

16. Wheeler ML, Warren-Boulton E. Diabetes patient education programs: quality and reimbursement. *Diabetes Care*. 1992;15(suppl 1):36–40.

17. Savage NK. Reimbursement database to serve DCE members. In: Legislation and reimbursement: increasing access to medical nutrition therapy and diabetes self-management training. *On the Cutting Edge*. 1993; 14:19–20.

18. American Dietetic Association. *Reimbursement for Outpatient Nutrition Services under Medical Assistance Programs*. Chicago, Ill: American Dietetic Association; 1994.

19. Bloomgarden ZT. Perspectives on the News. *Diabetes Care*. 1994;17:1084.

20. U.S. Department of Health and Human Services Health Care Financing Administration. *The Medicare 1993 Handbook*. Baltimore, Md: U.S. Department of Health and Human Services; 1993. Publication no. HCFA 10050.

21. AEtna. *Medicare Special Newsletter*. Savannah, Ga: AEtna; October 1992.

22. American Medical Association. *CPT 1995 Physicians' Current Procedural Terminology*. Chicago, Ill: American Medical Association; 1994.

23. U.S. Department of Health and Human Services Health Care Financing Administration, Institution and Home Care Patient Education Programs. *Medicare Coverage Issues Manual* (section 80-1). Baltimore, Md: U.S. Department of Health and Human Services; 1994.

24. Blue Cross Blue Shield of Georgia. *Notes from Medicare Medical Review*. 1994;2:1–2.

25. U.S. Department of Health and Human Services Health Care Financing Administration, Outpatient Diabetic Education Programs. *Medicare Coverage Issues Manual*. Baltimore, Md: U.S. Department of Health and Human Services; 1994. Transmittal No. 71, section 80-2.

26. American Diabetes Association. *Government Relations Update*; April 1995:3.

27. Tootell M. *A Dietitian's Guide to Diagnosis-Related Groups*. 1993 ed. Columbus, Ohio: Ross Laboratories; 1993:4–9.

28. Gallegher-Allred CR. *Reimbursement Success: Coverage and Reimbursement for Nutrition Services*. Columbus, Ohio: Ross Laboratories; 1993.

29. Smith AE, Smith PE. Reimbursement for clinical nutrition services: a 10-year experience. *J Am Diet Assoc*. 1992;92:1385–1388.

30. Smith, KG, Konkle DR, Semen M. Charging for hospital-based nutrition services. In: *Reimbursement and Insurance Coverage for Nutrition Services*. Chicago, Ill: American Dietetic Association; 1991:35–50.

31. Ceresa C, Chafin S, Davidson S, et al. *The Politics of Reimbursement*. Columbus, Ohio: American Dietetic Association and Ross Laboratories; 1993.

32. Mathieu-Harris M. Procedure codes for nutrition services. In: Legislation and reimbursement: increasing access to medical nutrition therapy and diabetes self-management training. *On the Cutting Edge*. 1993;14:18–19.

33. Schatz GB. Coding for nutrition services: challenges, opportunities, and guidelines. *J Am Diet Assoc*. 1993;93:471–477.

34. Gillespie S. Coverage, coding, and reimbursement: turning obstacles into opportunities. *Diabetes Spectrum*. 1993;6:228–232.

35. Warren-Boulton E. CPT codes for diabetes self-management training. In: Legislation and reimbursement: increasing access to medical nutrition therapy and diabetes self-management training. *On the Cutting Edge*. 1993;14:16–18.

36. Foster Higgins. *Foster Higgins Health Care Benefits Survey 1992*. Atlanta, Ga: Foster Higgins; 1993.

37. Mathieu-Harris, Foltz MB, ed. *Finding Your Niche in the Managed Care Market*. Columbus, Ohio: American Dietetic Association and Ross Products Division, Abbott Laboratories; 1993.

38. NHIA National Home Infusion Association. Negotiating with case managers. *Infusion*. 1994;3:1–4.

39. Fox MK, ed. *Reimbursement and Insurance Coverage for Nutrition Services*. Chicago, Ill: American Dietetic Association; 1991.

40. Gillespie S, Thom SL. Maximizing reimbursement: tips from DCE members. In: Legislation and reimbursement: increasing access to medical nutrition therapy and diabetes self-management training. *On the Cutting Edge*. 1993;14:23–27.

41. Carter M, Dodd J. Finn SC, et al. *The Power of Persuasion: Dialogue for Dollars*. Columbus, Ohio: American Dietetic Association/Ross Laboratories; 1992.

42. Bolonda KL, Sacagnina S, Dahl L, Murphy M, Hunt I. Strategies for increasing third-party reimbursement for nutrition counseling. *J Am Diet Assoc*. 1994;94:390–393.

43. Georgia Dietetic Association. *GDA Nutrition Services Payment Systems Bulletin 1994*. Decatur, Ga: Georgia Dietetic Association; 1994.

44. Cross AT. Practical and legal considerations of private nutrition practice. *J Am Diet Assoc*. 1995;95:21–29.

45. Splett P, Russo P. Documenting the quality and effectiveness of nutrition care. In: *Reimbursement and Insurance Coverage for Nutrition Services*. Chicago, Ill: American Dietetic Association; 1991:96–102.

46. Council on Practice Quality Management Task Force, The American Dietetic Association. Learning the language of quality care. *J Am Diet Assoc*. 1993;93:531–532.

47. Disbrow DD, Dowling RA. Cost-effectiveness and cost-benefit analyses: research to support practice. In: Monsen ER, ed. *Research: Successful Approaches*. Chicago, Ill: American Dietetic Association; 1991:272–294.

48. Dwyer WM, Johnson EQ, Nagy-Nero D, Smith KG, Viall C. *Winning the Managed Care Game*. Columbus, Ohio: American Dietetic Association and Ross Products Division, Abbott Laboratories; 1994:42–53.

49. Mazze RS, Franz MJ, Monk A, et al. Methodologies for field-testing and cost-effectiveness analysis. *J Am Diet Assoc*. 1992;92:1139–1142.

50. Franz MS, Splett PL, Monk A, et al. Cost effectiveness of medical nutrition therapy provided by dietitians for persons with non–insulin-dependent diabetes mellitus. *J Am Diet Assoc*. 1995;95:1018–1024.

51. MDA Reimbursement Committee. *Patient Care Protocols*. Plainville, Mass: Massachusetts Dietetic Association; 1992.

52. Maryniuk MD, ed. Measuring outcomes in diabetes and education. *On the Cutting Edge*. 1995;16:1–26.

53. Tobin CT, ed. Economic issues of diabetes care and management. *Diabetes Spectrum*. 1995;8:145–168.

54. Vinicor F. Reimbursement: scientific evidence and the political process. In: Legislation and reimbursement: increasing access to medical nutrition therapy and diabetes self-management training. *On the Cutting Edge*. 1993;14:7–8.

55. American Dietetic Association. Position of the American Dietetic Association: cost effectiveness of medical nutrition therapy. *J Am Diet Assoc*. 1995;95:87–91.

56. American Dietetic Association. *The Competitive Edge, Marketing Strategies for the Registered Dietitian*. Chicago, Ill: American Dietetic Association; 1986:7.

57. Weese N, Jones J, Miller MA. Successful strategies for reimbursement of outpatient nutrition services. *J Am Diet Assoc*. 1993;93:458–459.

58. American Diabetes Association. *Government Relations Update*; June 1995:5.

59. Kornblum TH. Professional demand for dietitians and nutritionists in the year 2005. *J Am Diet Assoc*. 1994;94:21–22.

60. Funnell MM, Anderson RM, Arnold MS, et al. Empowerment: an idea whose time has come in diabetes education. *Diabetes Educ*. 1991;17:37–41.

Chapter 36

View from the Mountain

Kristen McNutt

The world's work is done in the valleys, hemmed in, surrounded by the rush and bustle and routine, but from the mountain top comes the perspective, the meaning of all that you do through the busy day . . .
Do not let your work bury you so that you cannot climb to the mountain top and get a broader, finer vision of what your work means.

The advice above was offered over 40 years ago to young dietitians by Dr. E. Neige Todhunter.[1] Her words are even more relevant today for readers of this book, people who help people who have diabetes.

- The rush to meet deadlines is draining.
- The bustle to balance patients' needs and colleagues' requests is frustrating.
- The routine of paperwork seems meaningless.
- Relationships diminish to associations.
- Days blur together.
- No wonder, at times, life seems overwhelming.

When we hardly have enough energy to put one foot in front of the other, Todhunter's suggestion to climb a mountain sounds ridiculous. But she was busier than anyone I have known.[2] She accomplished so much because the perspective she recommends was for her, as it can be for us, the source of inner strength, purposeful motivation, and a contagious joy for life.

WHY CLIMB?

Everyone has a skillion reasons not to take the time and look for that *broader, finer vision of what our work means*. But the view from the mountain can increase job satisfaction, improve relationships, and enhance our effectiveness.

The work you do is precious. *You have earned the right to enjoy your accomplishments.* When you climb that mental mountain, you will see that your gift to others is far more than healthful years.

- Your caring gives a happier life to your patients and their loved ones.
- Your teaching makes the constraints of diabetes less constraining.
- Your counseling puts people in control, rather than feeling buffeted through life.

The second reason to look for the big picture flows from the first. Your feeling hemmed in and stressed out *has an effect on those you care for, professionally and personally*. Because you feel required to give so much of yourself, often there is simply nothing left inside. Climbing that mental mountain will restore your emotional reserve, thus better enabling you to handle the needs of others.

The third benefit of climbing the mountain is to *improve your job performance*. When you can see beyond your own problems, you gain a sensitivity to those faced by your colleagues. When you stop to contemplate the past, you recall the progress that has been made in treatment options. Appreciating what can be done today for patients offsets, to a degree, your heartache from limitations that remain. Looking into the future, knowing that further advances are just over the horizon, brings hope, which you, in turn, can give to those you counsel and console.

HOW TO CLIMB

The thought of climbing a whole mountain is intimidating. But it is hardly necessary to use an entire vacation day for your first introspective excursion. Start with a few little knolls, moments here and there that help you appreciate the big picture and your role in it. Once you consciously start looking, you may discover that much of what you are searching for has been there all along.

The critical step is the first one, deciding that the view from the mountain will make your life better. Once you believe the trip is worth the effort, you will find the road.

The way you squeeze mental mountain climbing into your calendar is very personal. The time and place must fit your life, in a manner analogous to how you teach your patients to fit their diet and medication into their lives. Your mountain, the place from which you go to view the big picture, may be your exercise bicycle. The only time available for others may be after the kids have finally gone to sleep. Some people may have the luxury of being able, for a short time on some days, to shut a door and take the phone off the hook. You may prefer to think about your role in the big picture in quiet alone but, if you want to, take a friend, one who shares special parts of life, up the mountain with you.

COME BACK DOWN

Just as some people hide from life by filling their hours with busyness, others can bury themselves in introspection. The purpose of climbing the mountain is to make your day-to-day life bet-

ter. The danger is using the experience as an escape.

Todhunter's advice continues:

But do not linger too long on the mountain tops entranced with what you can see. Come down to the valley to work and to be part, just a small part it is true, but nevertheless a vital, functional part among those who work to serve their fellow man.

What you do when you return from the mental mountain depends on why you went up in the first place. Often, the primary life-style difference is simply feeling better about yourself and less stressed by your responsibilities. Your workload remains the same, but your refreshed perspective results in a greater sense of satisfaction.

Your view from the mountain may, however, lead to different behaviors. One potential learning from the mountain is that *some things you thought had to be done, do not*. On the treadmill of life, it is almost impossible to slow down long enough to see which tasks might be nice, but not really necessary, in the big-picture context. Where possible, drop nonessential activities from your to-be-done list and use that time for more vital purposes.

Some time allocation changes may only be possible with your boss's permission, and unilaterally rearranging priorities does not work for team projects. But most people have some discretion about how they spend at least a portion of their days' hours. Look for opportunities to use your time better, even if it requires *investing a little now to save more later*. For example,

- Spending 4 hours now setting up a better system for a routine activity could save 40 hours during the next year.
- A task might be done in half the time if scheduled during the hours when you do that type of work most efficiently.

- Completing a job in one block of time with no interruptions rather than in snatches here and there is obviously more time-efficient and quality-enhancing.
- Rather than wasting time complaining, use those hours to learn a computer skill, take a management course, or do whatever will correct the cause of your energy-costly frustration.

The view from the mountain top might also motivate you to re-assess *the balance of how your life-time is allocated.* Is your current role in the big picture what you want it to be, or have you simply fallen into a pattern by chance or circumstance rather than by choice?

- You might do a better job at work if you spent more time fixing things at home.
- You might be more productive in the office if you invested more of yourself in interpersonal relations than in using your technical skills.
- You might help your patients more by listening rather than teaching.

A related inquiry, which is more comfortable to ask from the mountain than from the valley, is whether the tasks that take most of your time use your best skills. If not, the situation might be corrected by yourself; it may require renegotiating your job, or perhaps it is time to move elsewhere.

SMALL IN PERSPECTIVE

For people who previously had not sufficiently appreciated their contributions, the mountain view can be uplifting. But seeing the smallness of our roles relative to the whole of what life is all about has benefits as well. Realizing that, in the broader context, our roles are quite small can *put into perspective what seem to be major problems.*

From the mountain top, it is safe to ask whether we ourselves create some, although certainly not all, of the pressures of life. The vitalness of our responsibilities can reassure us that our lives have value. But aggrandizing the importance of what we do simply to inflate our sense of self-worth can be destructive:

- Upsets become crises.
- Disappointments become disasters.
- An innocent slight becomes an insulting slander.

However, when we remember how small our challenges are compared with the big picture, what might otherwise have been a draining day becomes a reasonable one with a few little glitches plus some pleasant encounters.

YOU HAVE BRIGHTENED MY VIEW

The mountain is within each of us, not really far away. The invitation to share these thoughts with you led me up my mountain. Thinking about our shared world has given me a broader, finer vision of what is done by you and other nutritionists, dietitians, and health professionals *as we labor together in the valleys to serve our fellow man.*

REFERENCES

1. Todhunter EN. Dietetics from the mountain top. *J Am Diet Assoc.* 1950;26:191.
2. McNutt KW. Biographical article; E. Neige Todhunter (1901–1991). *J Nutr.* 1993;123:603–609.

Index

F

G

I